Revision Anterior Cruciate Ligament Reconstruction

Michael J. Alaia • Kristofer J. Jones
Editors

Revision Anterior Cruciate Ligament Reconstruction

A Case-Based Approach

Springer

Editors
Michael J. Alaia
Department of Orthopedic Surgery
Division of Sports Medicine
New York University Langone Health
New York, NY, USA

Kristofer J. Jones
Department of Orthopaedic Surgery
Division of Sports Medicine
David Geffen School of Medicine
at UCLA
Los Angeles, CA, USA

ISBN 978-3-030-96995-0 ISBN 978-3-030-96996-7 (eBook)
https://doi.org/10.1007/978-3-030-96996-7

This Springer imprint is published by the registered company Springer Nature Switzerland AG
The registered company address is: Gewerbestrasse 11, 6330 Cham, Switzerland

Foreword

Drs. Alaia and Jones have assembled an outstanding group of clinicians and researchers to perform an in-depth review of the management and treatment of failed anterior cruciate ligament (ACL) reconstruction surgeries. The first direct repair of an ACL/PCL injury was performed in 1903, and the importance of the ACL was described in 1911. Jones remarked in 1916 that "stitching of the ligaments was futile," and eventually in the mid-1970s, Feagin and Curl concluded that primary ACL repair without augmentation was of minimal value. Hamstring grafts began to be used in the 1920s, fairly successfully, with patellar tendon grafts soon to follow. In the early 1960s, bone-patellar tendon-bone autografts began to be popularized. Synthetic grafts, beginning with carbon fiber, were attempted in the 1970s and 1980s, but quickly fell out of favor. Interestingly, the usage of various grafts such as fascia lata and meniscus for primary repair were still in vogue during my training years at the Mayo Clinic in the late 1970s. Allografts began to be utilized more frequently during the 1980s beginning with fascia lata and freeze dried bone-ACL-bone allografts. Surgical techniques were becoming more refined and debated in the 1980s regarding the "outside in" method vs. the "inside out" method as well as the usage of "extra-articular procedures" which were the "standard of care" at that time. In 2003, the "double bundle" graft technique became popular despite the technical challenges of performing this procedure.

Utilizing many of these various constructs often resulted in tunnel malposition, residual ligamentous laxity, and osteolysis of the tibial and femoral tunnels. Furthermore, debate over which graft material to utilize at what age and when has unintentionally created significant failure modes requiring creative methods of repair.

In this book, indications for ACL revision as well as graft options will be reviewed. In addition, the majority of this treatise will deal with the management of failed primary and revision ACL reconstructions. Not only are there soft tissue and structural repair issues that are critically important but also bone deficit lesions created by the initial surgery as well as concomitant issues such as meniscal insufficiency or bony malalignment.

Any surgeon who is performing ACL surgery should have this book available to deal with complex problems associated with the various failure modes which can occur regardless of whether the initial procedure was well performed. I commend Drs. Alaia and Jones and their contributors on an outstanding collection of chapters which literally cover the vast majority of issues associated with failed ACL surgery and management of unintended complications.

Jack M. Bert, MD, FAAOS
University of Minnesota School of Medicine
Past President Arthroscopy Association of North America, Cartilage Restoration Center of Minnesota, Woodbury Bone & Joint Specialists, Ltd
Woodbury, MN, USA

Acknowledgment

It has been an honor and a privilege to develop this book with some of the top knee and ACL surgeons in the country and the world. I would like to thank my co-editor, Dr. Kristofer Jones, for his friendship, teamwork, and dedication, a true master of his craft. To my residents, fellows, and colleagues at the NYU Hospital for. Joint Diseases – your devotion, skill, and love of orthopedics and sports medicine is unparalleled. To the mentors I have been fortunate enough to work with at every step of the way – your expertise both in and out of the operating room has developed my ideals as a physician, a father, and a husband. Finally, to my parents, my wife and partner in crime Erin, as well as our budding little physician Scarlett, words will never express my gratitude for your unwavering love and support.

Michael J. Alaia, MD

It is with great pleasure that Dr. Michael Alaia and I present this comprehensive textbook covering all topics related to revision ACL reconstruction. This was quite an endeavor, and I am thankful that I was able to collaborate with a dear friend to provide such a valuable educational resource. As a co-editor, I would like to thank the talented surgeons who contributed to this text because without their expertise and interest it would not be possible to compile such important knowledge into a single book. I would strongly urge the reader to focus on the basic principles highlighted in each chapter, for even as this field continues to evolve, the basics will remain the same. On a personal note, I would like to thank all of my mentors, especially those at the Hospital for Special Surgery, who helped me develop and grow as an orthopedic surgeon. The early lessons that I learned will never be forgotten and they remain a foundation for my approach to patient care. Lastly, and most importantly, I would like to thank my family, wife (Myriam), and sons (Owen and Ethan) for their steadfast support of my career. I would not be able to do any of this without you.

Kristofer J. Jones, MD

Contents

Contributors

Erin F. Alaia Department of Radiology, NYU Langone Health, New York, NY, USA

Michael J. Alaia Department of Orthopedic Surgery, Division of Sports Medicine, New York University Langone Health, New York, NY, USA

Michelle E. Arakgi Fowler Kennedy Sport Medicine Clinic, University of Western Ontario, London, ON, Canada

Justin W. Arner The Steadman Clinic and Steadman Philippon Research Institute, Vail, CO, USA

Lachlan M. Batty Fowler Kennedy Sport Medicine Clinic, University of Western Ontario, London, ON, Canada

St Vincent's Hospital Melbourne, Fitzroy, VIC, Australia

Evan Boyd Department of Orthopaedics and Rehabilitation, The Robert Larner, M.D., College of Medicine at The University of Vermont, Burlington, VT, USA

Colin Burgess Department of Orthopaedic Surgery, Northwell Health System, Donald and Barbara Zucker School of Medicine at Hofstra/Northwell, Huntington Hospital, Huntington, NY, USA

Kirk A. Campbell New York University Langone Health, Department of Orthopedic Surgery, New York, NY, USA

Cordelia W. Carter Department of Orthopedic Surgery, Division of Sports Medicine, NYU Langone Health, New York, NY, USA

Brian M. Cash Division of Sports Medicine and Shoulder Surgery, Department of Orthopaedic Surgery, David Geffen School of Medicine at UCLA, Los Angeles, CA, USA

Jorge Chahla Midwest Orthopaedics at RUSH, Chicago, IL, USA

Kristofer Eastman Chenard Spine and Orthopedic Center, Plantation, FL, USA

Randy M. Cohn Northwell Health, Garden City, NY, USA

Matthew J. Craig Department of Orthopedic Surgery – Hip and Knee Preservation, University of Utah, Salt Lake City, UT, USA

Robert S. Dean Twin Cities Orthopedics, Edina, MN, USA

Nicholas N. DePhillipo Twin Cities Orthopedics, Edina, MN, USA

Oslo Sports Trauma Research Center, Oslo, Norway

Michael G. Doran NYU Langone Department of Orthopedic Surgery, New York, NY, USA

Nathan K. Endres Department of Orthopaedics and Rehabilitation, The Robert Larner, M.D., College of Medicine at The University of Vermont, Burlington, VT, USA

Anthony A. Essilfie New York University Langone Orthopedic Hospital, New York, NY, USA

David G. Fanelli Department of Orthopaedic Surgery and Sports Medicine, Geisinger Medical Center, Danville, PA, USA

Gregory C. Fanelli Department of Medical Education, Geisinger Commonwealth School of Medicine, Scranton, PA, USA

Department of Orthopaedic Surgery and Sports Medicine, Danville, PA, USA

Matthew G. Fanelli Department of Orthopaedic Surgery and Sports Medicine, Geisinger Medical Center, Danville, PA, USA

Rachel M. Frank Department of Orthopaedic Surgery, University of Colorado School of Medicine, Aurora, CO, USA

Ian Gao Department of Orthopaedic Surgery, Stanford University, Stanford, CA, USA

Ignacio Garcia-Mansilla Division of Sports Medicine and Shoulder Surgery, Department of Orthopaedic Surgery, David Geffen School of Medicine at UCLA, Los Angeles, CA, USA

Matthew Geswell Medical University of South Carolina, Lancaster Medical Center, MUSC Lancaster Orthopaedics and Sports Medicine, Lancaster, SC, USA

Alan M. J. Getgood Fowler Kennedy Sport Medicine Clinic, University of Western Ontario, London, ON, Canada

Aaron M. Gipsman Department of Orthopedic Surgery, NYU Langone Health, New York, NY, USA

Alexander Golant Department of Orthopedics and Rehabilitation, New York Presbyterian Queens, Flushing, NY, USA

Guillem Gonzalez-Lomas Orthopaedic Department, Sports Medicine Division, New York University Langone Health, New York City, NY, USA

Trevor Gulbrandsen University of Iowa Hospitals and Clinics, Iowa City, IA, USA

F. Winston Gwathmey, MD Department of Orthopaedic Surgery, University of Virginia, University of Virginia Health System, Charlottesville, VA, USA

Sarah N. Harangody Palos Northwestern Medicine, Department of Orthopaedic Surgery, Palos Heights, IL, USA

S. Mark Heard Orthopaedic Surgery, Banff Sport Medicine, Banff, AB, Canada

Wendell M. R. Heard Department of Orthopaedic Surgery, Tulane University School of Medicine, New Orleans, LA, USA

Jonathan D. Hughes Department of Orthopaedic Surgery, University of Pittsburgh, UPMC Freddie Fu Sports Medicine Center, Pittsburgh, PA, USA

Eoghan T. Hurley New York University Langone Health, Department of Orthopedic Surgery, New York, NY, USA

Paul M. Incan Department of Orthopaedic Surgery, Washington University School of Medicine, St. Louis, MO, USA

Laith M. Jazrawi Orthopaedic Department, Sports Medicine Division, New York University Langone Health, New York City, NY, USA

Kristofer J. Jones Department of Orthopaedic Surgery, Division of Sports Medicine, David Geffen School of Medicine at UCLA, Los Angeles, CA, USA

Patrick W. Joyner Orthocollier, Naples, FL, USA

Ajay C. Kanakamedala Department of Orthopedic Surgery, NYU Langone Health, New York, NY, USA

Daniel J. Kaplan Orthopaedic Department, Sports Medicine Division, New York University Langone Health, New York City, NY, USA

Michaela Kopka Orthopaedic Surgery, Banff Sport Medicine, Banff, AB, Canada

Joseph D. Lamplot Emory University, Department of Orthopedic Surgery, Atlanta, GA, USA

Robert F. LaPrade Twin Cities Orthopedics, Edina, MN, USA

Cort D. Lawton OrthoIllinois, Algonquin, IL, USA

Bryson P. Lesniak Department of Orthopaedic Surgery, University of Pittsburgh, UPMC Freddie Fu Sports Medicine Center, Pittsburgh, PA, USA

Travis G. Maak Department of Orthopedic Surgery – Hip and Knee Preservation, University of Utah, Salt Lake City, UT, USA

Amit K. Manjunath New York University Langone Health, Department of Orthopedic Surgery, New York, NY, USA

Brian J. Mannino Orthopaedic Department, Sports Medicine Division, New York University Langone Health, New York City, NY, USA

Robert G. Marx Hospital for Special Surgery, Sports Medicine Institute, New York, NY, USA

Bogdan A. Matache New York University Langone Health, Department of Orthopedic Surgery, New York, NY, USA

Matthew J. Matava Department of Orthopaedic Surgery, Washington University School of Medicine, St. Louis, MO, USA

Robert J. Meislin New York University Langone Orthopedic Hospital, New York, NY, USA

Mark D. Miller, MD Department of Orthopaedic Surgery, University of Virginia, University of Virginia Health System, Charlottesville, VA, USA

Jill K. Monson Twin Cities Orthopedics, Edina, MN, USA

Kenneth Dale Montgomery New York Jets, Tri-County Orthopedics, Cedar Knolls, NJ, USA

Mary K. Mulcahey Women's Sports Medicine Program, Department of Orthopaedic Surgery, Tulane University School of Medicine, New Orleans, LA, USA

Volker Musahl Department of Orthopaedic Surgery, University of Pittsburgh, UPMC Freddie Fu Sports Medicine Center, Pittsburgh, PA, USA

Darren S. Nabor Department of Orthopaedic Surgery, Wake Forest University, Winston-Salem, NC, USA

Stephen J. Nicholas New York Orthopedics, New York, NY, USA

Olivia O'Reilly University of Iowa Hospitals and Clinics, Iowa City, IA, USA

Franklin Paulino Department of Orthopaedic Surgery, Northwell Health System, Donald and Barbara Zucker School of Medicine at Hofstra/Northwell, Long Island Jewish Medical Center, New Hyde Park, NY, USA

Courtney A. Quinn, MD Department of Orthopaedic Surgery, Inova Health System Fairfax, VA, USA

Anil S. Ranawat Hospital for Special Surgery, Sports Medicine Institute, New York, NY, USA

Joseph J. Ruzbarsky The Steadman Clinic and Steadman Philippon Research Institute, Vail, CO, USA

Michael J. Sayegh Department of Orthopaedic Surgery, Northwell Health System, Donald and Barbara Zucker School of Medicine at Hofstra/Northwell, Long Island Jewish Medical Center, New Hyde Park, NY, USA

Nicholas A. Sgaglione Department of Orthopaedic Surgery, Northwell Health System, Donald and Barbara Zucker School of Medicine at Hofstra/Northwell, Great Neck, NY, USA

Mehul Shah New York University Langone Health, Department of Orthopedic Surgery, New York, NY, USA

Seth L. Sherman Department of Orthopaedic Surgery, Stanford University, Stanford, CA, USA

Eric J. Strauss New York University Langone Health, Department of Orthopedic Surgery, New York, NY, USA

Alec Sundet Department of Orthopaedics and Rehabilitation, The Robert Larner, M.D., College of Medicine at The University of Vermont, Burlington, VT, USA

Christopher J. Tucker Department of Orthopaedic Surgery, Walter Reed National Military Medical Center, Bethesda, MD, USA

Evan E. Vellios Sports Medicine and Shoulder Surgery Service, Sports Medicine Institute, Hospital for Special Surgery, New York, NY, USA

Armando F. Vidal The Steadman Clinic and Steadman Philippon Research Institute, Vail, CO, USA

Brian R. Waterman Department of Orthopaedic Surgery, Wake Forest Baptist Health, Winston-Salem, NC, USA

Philip L. Wilson Department of Orthopedic Surgery, Scottish Rite for Children, University of Texas Southwestern Medical Center, Frisco, TX, USA

Initial Workup of the Failed ACL Reconstruction

1

Justin W. Arner, Joseph J. Ruzbarsky, Rachel M. Frank, and Armando F. Vidal

Causes of ACL Failure

The definition of ACL reconstruction failure remains somewhat controversial. It is perhaps best to view failure through the lens of success. Successful ACL reconstruction is defined as a stable, functional knee that allows the patient to return to all fitness and sporting activities without restriction or limitation. Therefore, failure can be defined as any deviation from that definition. The causes of failure and inability to return to function can be broad and beyond the scope of this chapter. This chapter will narrowly focus on ACL graft rupture, although it is noted that this is not the only defining feature of surgical failure.

ACL reconstruction failures can typically be attributed to technical considerations (most common), failure to recognize or address concomitant ligament injuries, malalignment, biologic failure, rehabilitation failure, or new trauma. These causes are not mutually exclusive and frequently coexist in the same patient. Identification of the contributors to failure is paramount to allow the surgeon to appropriately manage the revision scenario and to optimize the outcome from the revision procedure.

Technical Considerations

Technical considerations leading to failure of a primary ACL reconstruction play a role in approximately 50% of cases [1–3]. Specifically, femoral and/or tibial tunnel malposition, which can lead to rotational instability or graft impingement, is the foremost cause. Additionally, failure of fixation, small graft size, and mal-tensioning of the graft are less frequent but notable technical considerations in evaluating failures.

It is well accepted that femoral tunnel malposition is the most common technical cause of ACL graft failure. Anterior placement of the femoral tunnel is the most typical pattern encountered and is likely secondary to challenges with visualization [1–8]. Despite an expanded understanding of ACL anatomy and increased awareness of the role of tunnel placement in ACL failure, this still remains the primary source of failure [8]. Biomechanically, anterior femoral tunnel placement results in abnormal knee kinematics and increased graft tension in flexion [9, 10].

Tibial tunnel malposition is a less common but notable consideration in failure [2]. Anterior placement results in roof impingement in extension. This results in either a loss of extension, high graft tension, or stretching of the graft [11,

J. W. Arner · J. J. Ruzbarsky · A. F. Vidal (✉)
The Steadman Clinic and Steadman Philippon Research Institute, Vail, CO, USA

R. M. Frank
Department of Orthopaedic Surgery, University of Colorado School of Medicine, Aurora, CO, USA

M. J. Alaia, K. J. Jones (eds.), *Revision Anterior Cruciate Ligament Reconstruction*,
https://doi.org/10.1007/978-3-030-96996-7_1

12]. Posterior tibial tunnel placement can result in abnormal kinematics secondary to increased verticality of the graft or stretching of the graft resulting from PCL impingement.

In summary, a complete understanding of insertional anatomy is paramount to the success of primary ACL reconstruction and evaluation of surgical failures. The importance of well-positioned tunnels is essential for appropriate function of the graft as well as avoidance of impingement [13].

Fixation and tensioning technical failures can also occur. Both over-tensioning and under-tensioning can lead to complications. Over-tensioning the graft may lead to decreased vascularity and graft incorporation, an increase in intraarticular pressure, as well as decreased range of motion and pain [14]. Under-tensioning the graft can result in residual knee instability, which can lead to injury to other knee structures.

Failure to Address Concomitant Ligamentous Injury

Concomitant injuries to the collateral ligaments, posterolateral corner (PLC), and posterior cruciate ligament (PCL) should be evaluated closely with any failed ACL reconstruction, as missed injuries may lead to higher ACL graft stress and thus failure. Upwards of 15% of ACL reconstruction failures may be secondary to a missed associated injury [14].

Missed lateral collateral ligament injuries (LCL) and PLC injuries have been cited to be the most commonly missed concomitant ligament injury leading to ACL graft failure and considerable morbidity. One radiologic study found that 19.7% of patients had at least one injury to the PLC and 75% of those had lateral compartment bone bruising [15]. However, not all PLC injuries require surgical intervention, and this can lead to difficult surgical decision-making. Kinsella et al. reported that 52% of patients had PLC injuries with 14% being complete tears and older individuals more likely to have pathology. This study found that PLC injuries are commonly missed when an ACL tear occurs, and this missed injury leads to poor clinical outcomes. The authors admit that further research is required to determine the true incidence of ACL reconstruction failure associated with PLC injury as it is not known [16]. In a recent study by the MOON cohort, 1.1% of ACLs underwent concurrent PLC surgery, and both groups had good outcomes at 6 year follow-up [17]. Pacheco et al. reported on 68 patients who were referred to a complex knee specialist and found that 72% of PLC injuries were not identified at initial presentation. They cite the importance of a careful physical examination to prevent missed injuries [18].

MCL injuries are cited to occur in 3–31% of ACL injuries [19]. Although less commonly missed than PLC injuries, MCL injuries that initially were believed to be appropriately treated nonoperatively may not heal adequately to provide a stable endpoint and stable knee. Careful physical examination is imperative; however, indications for MCL treatment remain unclear. The authors recommend surgical treatment of acute grade III tibial sided lesions as well as chronic or revision cases with grade III opening in full extension or increased opening on stress radiography.

Stress X-rays are essential for complete evaluation of the MCL and PLC structures. The PLC is particularly complex as it involves different injury patterns which may require different surgical reconstructions [20]. Coronal alignment should also be assessed with consideration regarding which collateral ligament requires reconstruction to minimize the stress on that graft reconstruction. PCL tears occur less commonly with an ACL tear and are less commonly missed, but still should be carefully evaluated and appropriately treated. PCL stress radiographs also are an important adjunct to physical examination when the clinical context warrants.

Other Missed Concomitant Injuries

The role of the menisci in ACL graft failure is controversial but should be considered – especially in patients with multiple failed ACL reconstructions (i.e., failed revision and/or re-revision

ACL reconstruction). The medial meniscus is a secondary stabilizer to anterior tibial translation. In the setting of meniscal deficiency or equivalent states (previous subtotal meniscectomy, posterior medial meniscal root tear), a larger pivot shift has been described [1]. With these injuries, higher ACL graft forces may be seen. Small partial medial meniscectomies are unlikely to impact graft forces in the setting of ACL reconstruction [21]. Additionally, the lateral meniscus is an consequential restraint to anterior tibial translation and pivoting and therefore must be scrutinized closely, particularly in regard to root tears [22]. This is an emerging field of study in which recommendations are continually developing.

There has been a recent focus on the anterolateral knee as well as the posteromedial structures in evaluation of rotatory laxity; however, clinical studies are still needed to best define the injury pattern and role of repair and reconstruction. There is concern regarding overconstraint of the knee if lateral extraarticular tenodesis or anterolateral ligament (ALL) reconstruction is performed. Basic science studies have been conflicted regarding this fact [23–26]. Due to the variability in anatomic reports and surgical techniques, it is difficult to make clear conclusions regarding this adjunctive treatment. Its use in the primary and revision setting is also controversial [27–29]. Currently, many use the pivot shift test to help determine the degree of rotatory instability and the subsequent need for augmentation [30–34]. Studies evaluating the predictability of visualization of these injuries on MRI and ultrasound are also mixed [35, 36].

Malalignment

Proper knee alignment is essential to decrease ACL graft forces and to allow proper knee kinematics. Sagittal malalignment (increased tibial slope) has recently gained much attention particularly in the setting of the multiply failed ACL reconstruction. With sagittal malalignment, typically increased posterior tibial slope, abnormal biomechanics, and higher graft forces can be seen which has been associated with ACL injury and graft failure [37]. Increased posterior tibial slope has historically been an underrecognized risk factor for ACL reconstruction failure. Recent biomechanical studies have demonstrated reduced graft forces/strain as well as reduction of anterior translation of the tibia following slope changing osteotomy in the knees with increased tibial slope [38]. However, numerous recent studies have illustrated its importance in ACL injury and graft failure, particularly in non-contact injuries [39–41]. This is likely less of a contributor to ACL graft failure when compared with increased tibial slope; however, varus malalignment may also lead to higher graft forces and therefore should also be scrutinized closely [42].

Both coronal and sagittal alignment should be assessed clinically and radiographically. The authors recommend bilateral standing radiographs to assess coronal alignment as well as a true lateral for sagittal alignment evaluation. In these cases, osteotomies about the knee may be indicated to decrease the risk of reinjury. MRI and CT scans also can provide information regarding these parameters as well as other bony morphology that may contribute to failure, which include a narrow notch or lateral femoral condyle abnormalities [43]. Although no treatment guidelines exist for these abnormalities, this is a larger issue in the setting of osteoarthritis, osteochondral defects, or meniscal deficiency, which often exist in these patients.

Biologic Considerations

ACL reconstructions need to function both mechanically and biologically. While most studies have focused on the biomechanics and kinematics of reconstructive techniques, there has been increased attention on the role of allograft tissue in ACL failure in recent years. The correlation of allograft tissue use in ACL reconstruction failure in young patients is well-established. Two studies have reported a 4.4 hazard ratio and a 4 times greater risk for graft failure when comparing allograft with autograft in patients under 18 [44, 45]. Additionally, higher serum inflammatory markers and increased anterior knee translation have been documented in patients with allograft reconstructions [46]. Allografts have also been shown to have delayed incorporation and healing when compared with autografts [47].

Although allograft failure rates are higher than that of autograft, overall, allograft failures are still relatively low [48–50]. In young active patients, graft rupture is higher than that of older, less active patients. In those under 25 years of age, reoperation and revision rates have been reported to be 30.8% and 20.5%, respectively [49]. In older and less active patients, allograft failure rates vary, but studies have shown no to little difference when compared with autograft [48–50]. Data has shown that use of allograft in patients younger than 40 years of age results in significantly high rates of re-rupture [44]. When comparing types of allograft, looped tibialis anterior and posterior have been shown to have the highest load to failure, while the highest stiffness is seen in quadriceps allografts [48]. Graft sterilization also plays a role as low-dose gamma irradiated grafts have shown a mixed effect on biomechanical properties with one study reporting a 20% reduction in stiffness and others showing no difference. With higher levels of irradiation, decreased load to failure has been consistent [48]. Non-irradiated allografts have been shown to have a decreased failure rate (5–7% vs. 7–13%) [50].

In addition to correct tunnel placement, autograft tissue selection is critical in athletes to optimize ACL reconstruction outcomes. Autograft type has also been studied extensively with hamstring, patellar tendon, and quadriceps tendon being the most commonly used. Although controversial, large knee registries have suggested that hamstring grafts may have a higher rate of failure when compared to patellar tendon, with one study citing a 2.1 times higher rate of revision with hamstring autograft in young patients with females being at highest risk [51–53]. Quadriceps tendon has gained attention in recent years with initial reports being favorable but with some reporting increased complications including quadriceps weakness [54, 55]. Inadequate graft size also can be a cause of failure. A diameter of 8 mm or less has been shown in active young patients to have a higher risk of re-tear in a retrospective review, while a systematic review found hamstring autograft of 8 mm or more to have a reduced failure rate [56, 57].

Hyperlaxity must also be closely evaluated on physical examination with Beighton score being a useful objective metric. Knee motion including hyperextension should be examined, as should generalized ligamentous laxity which may be associated with higher risk of ACL injury and graft failure [58]. Biologic healing also plays a very important role in graft success or failure. This can be due to failure of fixation, whether it be technical or related to poor bone quality, or lack of graft incorporation for numerous reasons [2]. Failure of graft incorporation can be secondary to excessive tension, aggressive activities during ligamentization, infection, or immune reaction [59].

Lastly, infection, albeit rare, can have a very negative impact on ACL reconstruction biology and outcome. Fortunately, this is rare in ACL surgery with a rate of 0.3–0.8% but is devastating to young athletes undergoing elective surgery [60]. Clinical signs of fever, elevated inflammatory markers, knee effusion, and pain are typical. Aspiration is helpful in diagnosis. If suspected, immediate joint irrigation and debridement is essential. Although early lavage many times can salvage the graft, its change in biology, structure, and mechanical properties is not known. Further, fibrous adhesions can occur which may trigger arthrofibrosis leading to clinical failure. If the graft appears to be incompetent, the infection should first be cleared before revision surgery is considered [61].

Rehabilitation Considerations

A well-planned and executed therapy program is essential to a successful outcome. Inadequate rehabilitation and early return to play before appropriate strength deficits are addressed leads to risk of graft rupture [2]. Graft failure can occur if the graft has not yet incorporated and if loads exceed the ability of the graft to resist this amount of tension, such as in the setting of premature return to unrestricted sporting activity. These injuries typically occur during the ligamentization period where the graft is particularly sensitive [59]. Animal models have shown that patellar tendon integrates more quickly than soft tissue grafts, but this has not been well established clinically [62, 63]. The amount of time for soft tissue or bony graft incorporation is not known in large human studies. One study found that both hamstrings and bone patellar tendon bone grafts still have small amounts of micromotion (1–3 mm) at 1 year postoperatively [63]. The authors recommend comprehensive return to play testing which include dynamic functional evaluation prior to return to play [64, 65].

Trauma

If the previously outlined reasons for failure were completely evaluated and have not revealed any cause of graft re-tear and a new trauma occurred, by process of elimination, it can be assumed that the new traumatic injury is the cause. Studies have reported similar rates of contralateral ACL tears compared with graft ruptures, indicating that certain re-tears may be due to trauma or underlying, uncorrectable patient-specific biomechanical factors [53]. Nevertheless, a complete evaluation of all contributing factors should be done and the specifics discussed with the patient (Table 1.1).

Evaluation of ACL Failure

The first and most important step in evaluating a failed ACL reconstruction is determining all the contributors to failure (see Table 1.1). It is important to note that multiple contributors often coexist in the same patient and are not mutually exclusive (Fig. 1.1). Once a cause(s) has been determined, a well thought out surgical plan must be developed. Important additional considerations include prior surgical approaches/incisions, retained hardware, and other technical aspects often detailed in operative reports and image documentation.

Table 1.1 Considerations of causes of ACL graft failure

Technical considerations	Femoral and/or tibial tunnel malposition
	Small graft size
	Mal-tensioning of graft
	Improper graft fixation
Missed concomitant ligamentous injury	Lateral collateral ligament (LCL)
	Posterolateral corner (PLC)
	Medial collateral ligament (MCL)
	Posterior cruciate ligament (PCL)
Other missed concomitant injury	Previous total medial meniscectomy
	Medial meniscus root tear
	Lateral meniscus root tear
Malalignment	Sagittal plane – increased tibial slope
	Coronal plane – varus
Biologic	Allograft in young and/or active patients
	Hyperlaxity
	Lack of graft incorporation
	Infection
Rehabilitation	Excessively aggressive
	Inadequate therapy before return to activities
	Inappropriate early return to activities
Diagnosis of exclusion	Trauma

Data Collection

The first step when considering revision surgery in any patient who previously had an ACL reconstruction is to obtain the previous surgeon's office records, operative reports, and intraoperative arthroscopy photos if possible. Knowing the prior graft choice(s), adjunctive procedures, and hardware implanted is extremely valuable for both planning and preparation purposes. Small subtleties can have a huge implication on decision-making. For example, there have been cases where the primary surgeon initially harvests the hamstring tendons and then determines that these were inadequate size (less than 8 mm in diameter), before switching to a BTB autograft [66]. Understanding these important details is crucial when planning and discussing with the patient for the upcoming reconstruction.

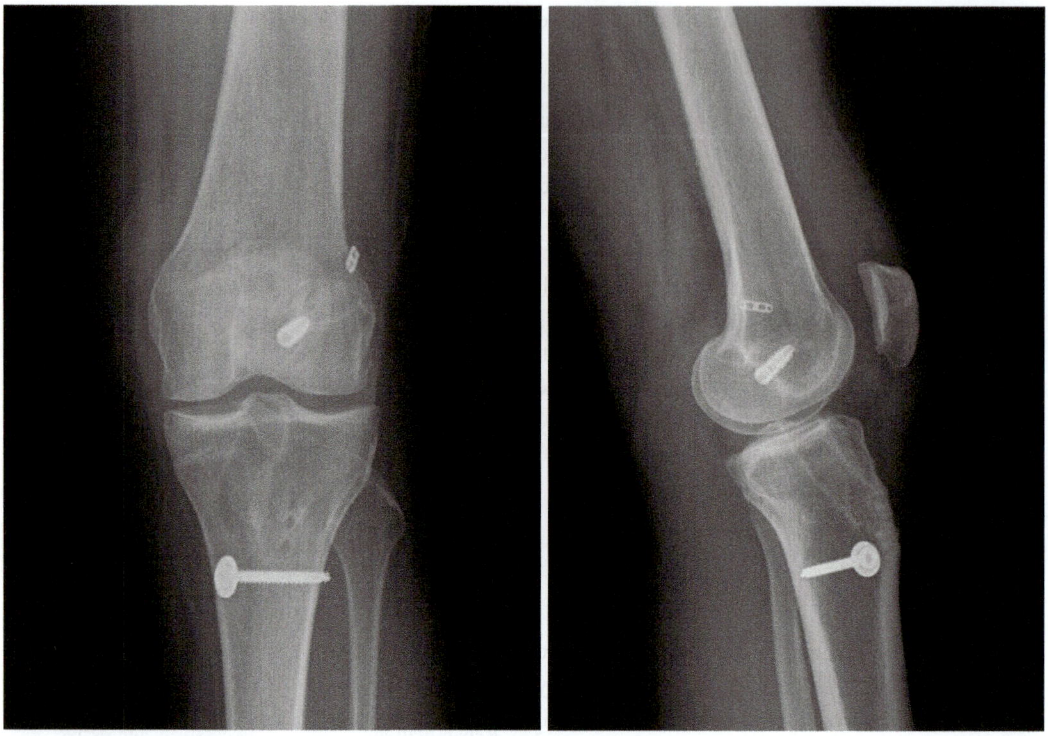

Fig. 1.1 Example of a poorly placed femoral tunnel with tibial tunnel dilation and retained hardware in the femur and tibia

Operative photos can be more valuable than the description in an operative report when visualizing the extent of a meniscectomy or an articular cartilage defect. These types of details prevent surprises and can allow for a surgeon to be better prepared for a cartilage restoration procedure or meniscal transplant at the time of revision reconstruction.

Skin Incisions

In the multiply revised knee, a variety of incisions can be present from prior surgeries including transverse hamstring or BTB harvest incisions, oblique open meniscal repairs or meniscectomies, or longitudinal alternatives to both. Careful attention to prior skin incisions is extremely important given the important considerations regarding skin flaps and vasculature about the knee. Although wound complications are relatively rare in ACL revision surgery, such complications can be devastating (Fig. 1.2) and can compromise an otherwise well-executed surgery [67]. When performing a revision ACL surgery, a primary effort should be made to utilize a prior incision. Given the mobility of the superficial tissues about the knee, an old incision with or without strategic extension can often accomplish multiple goals including both the tibial tunnel preparation in addition to the BTB and hamstring harvest. If more than one incision is required, whether it be for a collateral reconstruction, meniscus repair, or extraarticular tenodesis, these should be accounted for in the surgical plan. Although traditional teaching in knee arthroplasty revision surgery advises against creation of skin bridges of less than 7 cm, this estimate is probably conservative, and an incision bridge of 5 cm, especially if made parallel, is likely safe [68, 69]. When making an incision not parallel, a prior well-healed incision should be crossed perpendicularly, as the skin peninsula at intersections of less than 60° is at high risk for vascular insufficiency [70]. Finally,

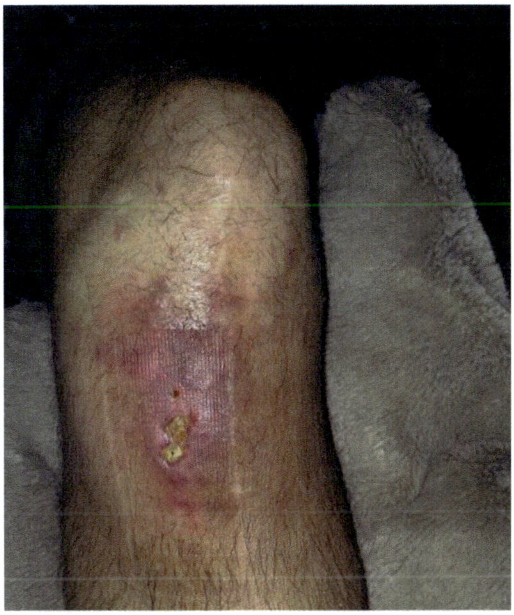

Fig. 1.2 Example of skin necrosis central to two longitudinal incisions at the knee spaces less than 5 cm apart

when choosing among incisions, the most lateral incision that can reasonably accomplish the operative goal should be chosen as the primary incision. Anatomic studies have demonstrated the superficial blood supply to the anterior knee flows mostly from medial to lateral, and furthermore, in cases of a medial skin incision, the lateral flap has shown to have a decreased oxygen tension [71]. The same pattern of vascularity is true for the patella, and therefore, the previous arthrotomy should also be utilized [72].

Graft Choice

Data collection should include all previous graft harvests or attempts at graft harvest. An inventory of available autograft options should be performed before endeavoring on a revision. In cases of revision surgery in patients less than 40 years old or older individuals with a high-impact activity profile, the senior authors' preferred graft is a patellar tendon autograft from the ipsilateral knee if available, followed by the patellar tendon from the contralateral knee in most circumstances. If those grafts are not available, then strong consideration should be given to alternative autograft options. Consideration should be given to the contralateral knee as an autograft choice if the clinical situation warrants.

The Multicenter ACL Revision Study (MARS) group data has demonstrated that revisions with autograft are 2.78× less likely to re-tear when compared to allografts. In addition, higher patient-reported outcome measures (PROMs) are seen with the use of autograft [73]. The bone blocks on each end of the patellar tendon graft allows not only for bone to bone healing, but also for variation of bone block harvesting, if necessary [74]. Quadriceps tendon autograft +/− bone block and hamstring autograft remain important choices as well, depending on the patient's activity profile, i.e., a wrestler who may want to avoid a BTB autograft due to the significant time and activity spent on his knees. Allograft cases are reserved for an older, less active population.

Staging

The guiding principle in revision surgery should always be to achieve an outcome as close to a primary surgery as possible. As such, the treating surgeon should avoid making compromises if possible. In such cases, staging maybe necessary to optimize graft placement. Performing a single versus two stage reconstruction should always be discussed with patients during the preoperative visit when considering ACL revision. Three-dimensional imaging including CT scans and MRIs can give an accurate estimate of the size and position of the prior tibial and femoral tunnels, but the final determination is made at the time of arthroscopic evaluation [75].

Criteria for staging varies by author. It is generally accepted that tunnel dilation of 15 mm on either tunnel should warrant consideration for a staged approach. However, smaller tunnels that are malpositioned but in direct proximity to the surgeon's ideal tunnel can create equally challenging clinical scenarios and can warrant staging. Additionally, an understanding of the vast choices in ACL hardware is critical in making this decision. Removal of the existing hardware can result in bone loss or compromise of traditional fixation methods. It is imperative that as part of the preoperative data gathering, a surgeon familiarizes him/herself with the nuances of previously placed hardware. Attention should also be given to the integrity of the backwall on preoperative imaging in this regard. In many cases, a poorly placed tunnel can allow for creation of a new tunnel in the appropriate location without convergence (Fig. 1.3).

Prior to proceeding with an ACL revision, a surgeon should be prepared for a variety of graft fixation options including interference screws, buttons, posts, and staples in order to allow for versatile fixation and backup fixation options. Furthermore, a surgeon's preferred bone graft and adjuncts should be available if the decision is made to stage the revision.

Other considerations when deciding to stage a revision are alignment and stiffness. If either the coronal or sagittal alignment is sufficiently anomalous and requires an osteotomy for correction, osteotomy and bone grafting with subsequent revision in a second stage should be considered. In some cases, anteroposterior or coronal stability improves, and further ligamentous reconstructions are not required. Finally, in the setting of a failed ACL reconstruction with associated loss of motion, an initial lysis of adhesion, tunnel bone grafting, and manipulation under anesthesia will allow for full motion prior to proceeding with an ACL revision.

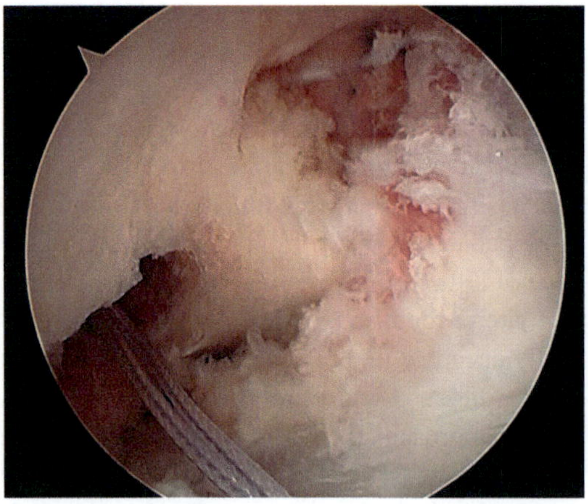

Fig. 1.3 An arthroscopic image using a 30-degree arthroscope viewing from the anterolateral portal demonstrating a nonanatomic high femoral tunnel which allows for placement of an anatomic femoral tunnel without convergence

Prior Hardware

Although addressed in the previous section, the influence of prior hardware in planning a revision cannot be overemphasized. The prior operative report(s) and implant records are critical in determining the exact implants used to help ensure the appropriate tools and sets are available. Understanding if the hardware needs to be removed, how it can be removed, and the impact of removal on the planned revision is critical (Fig. 1.4). General hardware removal and broken

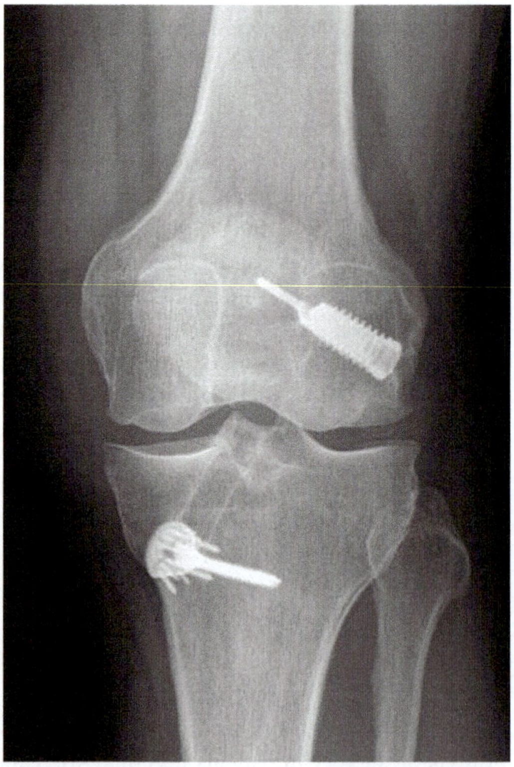

Fig. 1.4 Complex hardware removal that requires special instruments must be considered preoperatively. In this example, a WasherLoc (Zimmer Biomet, Warsaw IN) device in the tibia and Bone Mulch Screw (Zimmer Biomet, Warsaw IN) in the femur require special instrumentation, can be difficult to remove, and lead to significant bone loss

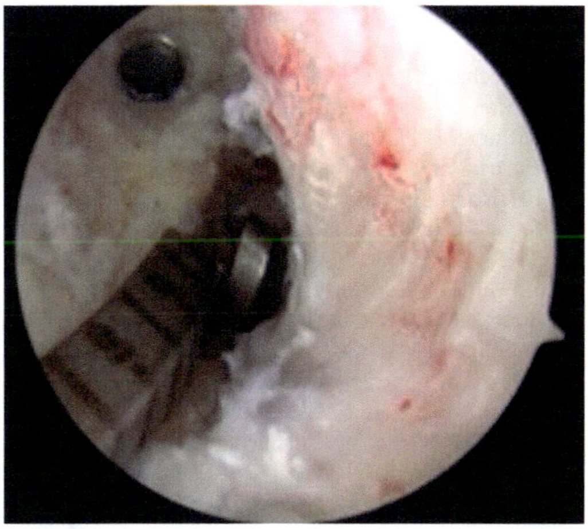

Fig. 1.5 An arthroscopic image using a 30-degree arthroscope viewing from the anterolateral portal demonstrating a femoral interference screw left in place that does not interfere with placement of an anatomic femoral tunnel

screw removal sets should be available in the event of a stripped or broken screwhead. Tibial interference screws and external posts on the tibia are most commonly removed as these have a tendency to disrupt or interrupt new tunnels or ancillary tibial fixation. Under some circumstances, however, the prior hardware is not in the way of the planned new tunnels, and therefore, it can be left in place (Fig. 1.5) [68]. Polyether ether ketone (PEEK) or bioabsorbable implants can often be reamed or drilled through in instances where they cannot be removed. Furthermore, suspensory fixation buttons, especially those on the femoral side, can be ignored as they will not interfere with the femoral tunnel or fixation.

Case Example

A 31-year-old active female previously underwent a hamstring ACL reconstruction 6 years prior in another state. She had no issues until a recent fall while rock climbing in which she felt a pop in her knee. Her other activities included tennis and fitness classes. She attempted physical therapy; however, she had continued episodes of knee shifting with activities of daily living. Her operative report was obtained where she underwent a 7.5-mm hamstring autograft with medial portal flexible reamer drilling utilizing suspensory fixation on the femur and a PEEK compression device in the tibia. She also underwent a prior partial lateral meniscectomy. X-rays showed mild valgus alignment within the tibial spines with a posterior tibial slope of 4°. Stress X-rays showed no injury to the collateral ligaments. An MRI was obtained and showed a prior partial lateral meniscectomy and a complete ACL graft rupture. Measures on CT and X-rays showed a tibial tunnel that was 12 mm in diameter and a femoral tunnel that was 9 mm. Both tunnels appeared to be in anatomic position. It was determined that her ACL graft rupture was likely due to a new trauma, and a one-stage revision was planned.

A diagnostic knee arthroscopic was performed, and the findings were consistent with preoperative imaging. The torn graft was debrided and the tunnels were exposed. The PEEK compression device was easily removed with a rongeur utilizing the proximal portion of the previous incision. A guide pin was placed up the previous tibial tunnel and reamed sequentially up to a size 11 where circumferential healthy bone was encountered. As the previous medial portal drilling technique utilized flexible reamers, the femoral tunnel was then reamed by hand to a depth of 28 mm and a diameter of 10 mm. Both tunnels were dilated, and an 8-mm dilatator was utilized as a guide to pass a pin through the skin to pass a suture through the femoral tunnel. A 10-mm quadriceps tendon autograft was then harvested and prepared, then passed in a retrograde fashion. This was fixed with a larger adjustable loop button on the femur and an 11-mm biocomposite interference screw on the tibia. An X-ray was taken to ensure the femoral button was appropriately flipped and not caught on the previous femoral button before tibial fixation. The Lachman and pivot shift was normalized. Physical therapy was started 3 days postoperatively with home exercises starting immediately. Dynamic exercises, including running, were slightly delayed as was return to sports with the plan to begin cutting and pivoting sports at 9–12 months.

Summary

ACL failures are complex and often multifactorial clinical challenges. A systematic and detailed analysis of the possible contributors of ACL graft failure must be performed for every case. A checklist approach can help the surgeon ensure that all factors are being considered (Table 1.1). Evaluation of patient expectations, operative notes, implant records, notes from the perioperative period, as well as arthroscopic and radiographic images is essential for proper evaluation and operative planning. A preoperative plan with consideration of prior incisions and hardware as well as tunnel location and diameter is imperative. The surgeon should be flexible and prepared during revision surgery with a well-designed plan and specific postoperative strategy. Comfort and flexibility with various techniques is necessary for a successful outcome.

References

1. Trojani C, Sbihi A, Djian P, Potel JF, Hulet C, Jouve F, et al. Causes for failure of ACL reconstruction and influence of meniscectomies after revision. Knee Surg Sports Traumatol Arthrosc. 2011;19(2):196–201.
2. Carson EW, Anisko EM, Restrepo C, Panariello RA, O'Brien SJ, Warren RF. Revision anterior cruciate ligament reconstruction: etiology of failures and clinical results. J Knee Surg. 2004;17(3):127–32.
3. Johnson DL, Coen MJ. Revision ACL surgery. Etiology, indications, techniques, and results. Am J Knee Surg. 1995;8(4):155–67.
4. Colosimo AJ, Heidt RS Jr, Traub JA, Carlonas RL. Revision anterior cruciate ligament reconstruction with a reharvested ipsilateral patellar tendon. Am J Sports Med. 2001;29(6):746–50.
5. Redler A, Iorio R, Monaco E, Puglia F, Wolf MR, Mazza D, et al. Revision anterior cruciate ligament reconstruction with hamstrings and extra-articular tenodesis: a mid- to long-term clinical and radiological study. Arthroscopy. 2018;34(12):3204–13.
6. Safran MR, Harner CD. Technical considerations of revision anterior cruciate ligament surgery. Clin Orthop Relat Res. 1996;325:50–64.
7. Greis PE, Johnson DL, Fu FH. Revision anterior cruciate ligament surgery: causes of graft failure and technical considerations of revision surgery. Clin Sports Med. 1993;12(4):839–52.
8. Burnham JM, Herbst E, Pauyo T, Pfeiffer T, Johnson DL, Fu FH, et al. Technical considerations in revision anterior cruciate ligament (ACL) reconstruction for operative techniques in orthopaedics. Oper Tech Orthop. 2017;27(1):63–9.
9. Bylski-Austrow DI, Grood ES, Hefzy MS, Holden JP, Butler DL. Anterior cruciate ligament replacements: a mechanical study of femoral attachment location, flexion angle at tensioning, and initial tension. J Orthop Res J Orthop Res. 1990;8(4):522–31.
10. Harner CD, Irrgang JJ, Paul J, Dearwater S, Fu FH. Loss of motion after anterior cruciate ligament reconstruction. Am J Sports Med. 1992; 20(5):499–506.
11. Howell SM, Clark JA, Farley TE. A rationale for predicting anterior cruciate graft impingement by the intercondylar roof. A magnetic resonance imaging study. Am J Sports Med. 1991;19(3):276–82.
12. Howell SM, Taylor MA. Failure of reconstruction of the anterior cruciate ligament due to impingement by the intercondylar roof. J Bone Joint Surg Am. 1993;75(7):1044–55.
13. Forsythe B, Kopf S, Wong AK, Martins CA, Anderst W, Tashman S, et al. The location of femoral and tibial tunnels in anatomic double-bundle anterior cruciate ligament reconstruction analyzed by three-dimensional computed tomography models. J Bone Joint Surg Am. 2010;92(6):1418–26.
14. Getelman M, Schepsis A, Zimmer J. Revision ACL reconstruction: autograft versus allograft. Arthroscopy. 1995;11(1):378.
15. Temponi EF, de Carvalho Junior LH, Saithna A, Thaunat M, Sonnery-Cottet B. Incidence and MRI characterization of the spectrum of posterolateral corner injuries occurring in association with ACL rupture. Skelet Radiol. 2017;46(8):1063–70.
16. Kinsella SD, Rider SM, Fury MS, Tepolt FA, Ecklund K, Kocher MS. Concomitant posterolateral corner injuries in skeletally immature patients with acute anterior cruciate ligament injuries. J Pediatr Orthop. 2020;40(6):271–6.
17. Westermann RW, Marx RG, Spindler KP, Huston LJ, Amendola A, Andrish JT, et al. No difference between posterolateral corner repair and reconstruction with concurrent ACL surgery: results from a prospective multicenter cohort. Orthop J Sports Med. 2019;7(7):2325967119861062.
18. Pacheco RJ, Ayre CA, Bollen SR. Posterolateral corner injuries of the knee: a serious injury commonly missed. J Bone Joint Surg. 2011;93(2):194–7.
19. Wright RW, Huston LJ, Spindler KP, Dunn WR, Haas AK, Allen CR, et al. Descriptive epidemiology of the Multicenter ACL Revision Study (MARS) cohort. Am J Sports Med. 2010;38(10):1979–86.
20. LaPrade RF, Heikes C, Bakker AJ, Jakobsen RB. The reproducibility and repeatability of varus stress radiographs in the assessment of isolated fibular collateral ligament and grade-III posterolateral knee injuries. An in vitro biomechanical study. J Bone Joint Surg Am. 2008;90(10):2069–76.
21. Gupta R, Kapoor A, Mittal N, Soni A, Khatri S, Masih GD. The role of meniscal tears and meniscectomy in the mechanical stability of the anterior cruciate ligament deficient knee. Knee. 2018;25(6):1051–6.
22. Musahl V, Citak M, O'Loughlin PF, Choi D, Bedi A, Pearle AD. The effect of medial versus lateral meniscectomy on the stability of the anterior cru-

ciate ligament-deficient knee. Am J Sports Med. 2010;38(8):1591–7.
23. Marcacci M, Zaffagnini S, Giordano G, Iacono F, Presti ML. Anterior cruciate ligament reconstruction associated with extra-articular tenodesis: a prospective clinical and radiographic evaluation with 10- to 13-year follow-up. Am J Sports Med. 2009;37(4):707–14.
24. Monaco E, Maestri B, Conteduca F, Mazza D, Iorio C, Ferretti A. Extra-articular ACL reconstruction and pivot shift: in vivo dynamic evaluation with navigation. Am J Sports Med. 2014;42(7):1669–74.
25. Saragaglia D, Pison A, Refaie R. Lateral tenodesis combined with anterior cruciate ligament reconstruction using a unique semitendinosus and gracilis transplant. Int Orthop. 2013;37(8):1575–81.
26. Novaretti JV, Arner JW, Chan CK, Polamalu S, Harner CD, Debski RE, et al. Does lateral extra-articular tenodesis of the knee affect ACL graft in situ forces and tibiofemoral contact pressures? Arthroscopy. 2020;36(5):1365–73.
27. Claes S, Vereecke E, Maes M, Victor J, Verdonk P, Bellemans J. Anatomy of the anterolateral ligament of the knee. J Anat. 2013;223(4):321–8.
28. Dodds AL, Halewood C, Gupte CM, Williams A, Amis AA. The anterolateral ligament: anatomy, length changes and association with the Segond fracture. Bone Joint J. 2014;96-b(3):325–31.
29. Vincent JP, Magnussen RA, Gezmez F, Uguen A, Jacobi M, Weppe F, et al. The anterolateral ligament of the human knee: an anatomic and histologic study. Knee Surg Sports Traumatol Arthrosc. 2012;20(1):147–52.
30. Getgood A, Bryant D, Firth A. The Stability study: a protocol for a multicenter randomized clinical trial comparing anterior cruciate ligament reconstruction with and without Lateral Extra-articular Tenodesis in individuals who are at high risk of graft failure. BMC Musculoskelet Disord. 2019;20(1):216.
31. Getgood A, Brown C, Lording T, Amis A, Claes S, Geeslin A, et al. The anterolateral complex of the knee: results from the International ALC Consensus Group Meeting. Knee Surg Sports Traumatol Arthrosc. 2019;27(1):166–76.
32. Offerhaus C, Balke M, Arner JW, Musahl V, Hoher J. Reefing of the posteromedial capsule in anteromedial rotatory instability. Arthrosc Tech. 2018;7(5):e547–e51.
33. Musahl V, Rahnemai-Azar AA, Costello J, Arner JW, Fu FH, Hoshino Y, et al. The influence of meniscal and anterolateral capsular injury on knee laxity in patients with anterior cruciate ligament injuries. Am J Sports Med. 2016;44(12):3126–31.
34. Magnussen RA, Reinke EK, Huston LJ, Hewett TE, Spindler KP, Amendola A, et al. Effect of high-grade preoperative knee laxity on 6-year anterior cruciate ligament reconstruction outcomes. Am J Sports Med. 2018;46(12):2865–72.
35. Devitt BM, O'Sullivan R, Feller JA, Lash N, Porter TJ, Webster KE, et al. MRI is not reliable in diagnosing of concomitant anterolateral ligament and anterior cruciate ligament injuries of the knee. Knee Surg Sports Traumatol Arthrosc. 2017;25(4):1345–51.
36. Faruch Bilfeld M, Cavaignac E, Wytrykowski K, Constans O, Lapegue F, Chiavassa Gandois H, et al. Anterolateral ligament injuries in knees with an anterior cruciate ligament tear: contribution of ultrasonography and MRI. Eur Radiol. 2018;28(1):58–65.
37. Rahnemai-Azar AA, Yaseen Z, van Eck CF, Irrgang JJ, Fu FH, Musahl V. Increased lateral tibial plateau slope predisposes male college football players to anterior cruciate ligament injury. J Bone Joint Surg Am. 2016;98(12):1001–6.
38. Imhoff FB, Mehl J, Comer BJ, Obopilwe E, Cote MP, Feucht MJ, et al. Slope-reducing tibial osteotomy decreases ACL-graft forces and anterior tibial translation under axial load. Knee Surg Sports Traumatol Arthrosc. 2019;27(10):3381–9.
39. Lee CC, Youm YS, Cho SD, Jung SH, Bae MH, Park SJ, et al. Does posterior tibial slope affect graft rupture following anterior cruciate ligament reconstruction? Arthroscopy. 2018;34(7):2152–5.
40. Bernhardson AS, Aman ZS, Dornan GJ, Kemler BR, Storaci HW, Brady AW, et al. Tibial slope and its effect on force in anterior cruciate ligament grafts: anterior cruciate ligament force increases linearly as posterior tibial slope increases. Am J Sports Med. 2019;47(2):296–302.
41. Dejour D, Pungitore M, Valluy J, Nover L, Saffarini M, Demey G. Tibial slope and medial meniscectomy significantly influence short-term knee laxity following ACL reconstruction. Knee Surg Sports Traumatol Arthrosc. 2019;27(11):3481–9.
42. Hinckel BB, Demange MK, Gobbi RG, Pecora JR, Camanho GL. The effect of mechanical varus on anterior cruciate ligament and lateral collateral ligament stress: finite element analyses. Orthopedics. 2016;39(4):e729–36.
43. Pfeiffer TR, Burnham JM, Hughes JD, Kanakamedala AC, Herbst E, Popchak A, et al. An increased lateral femoral condyle ratio is a risk factor for anterior cruciate ligament injury. J Bone Joint Surg Am. 2018;100(10):857–64.
44. Kaeding CC, Aros B, Pedroza A, Pifel E, Amendola A, Andrish JT, et al. Allograft versus autograft anterior cruciate ligament reconstruction: predictors of failure from a MOON prospective longitudinal cohort. Sports Health. 2011;3(1):73–81.
45. Engelman GH, Carry PM, Hitt KG, Polousky JD, Vidal AF. Comparison of allograft versus autograft anterior cruciate ligament reconstruction graft survival in an active adolescent cohort. Am J Sports Med. 2014;42(10):2311–8.
46. Li J, Wang J, Li Y, Shao D, You X, Shen Y. A prospective randomized study of anterior cruciate ligament reconstruction with autograft, gamma-irradiated allograft, and hybrid graft. Arthroscopy. 2015;31(7):1296–302.
47. Gulotta LV, Rodeo SA. Biology of autograft and allograft healing in anterior cruciate ligament reconstruction. Clin Sports Med. 2007;26(4):509–24.

48. Lansdown DA, Riff AJ, Meadows M, Yanke AB, Bach BR Jr. What factors influence the biomechanical properties of allograft tissue for ACL reconstruction? A systematic review. Clin Orthop Relat Res. 2017;475(10):2412–26.
49. Lenehan EA, Payne WB, Askam BM, Grana WA, Farrow LD. Long-term outcomes of allograft reconstruction of the anterior cruciate ligament. Am J Orthop (Belle Mead NJ). 2015;44(5):217–22.
50. Brown MJ, Carter T. ACL allograft: advantages and when to use. Sports Med Arthrosc Rev. 2018;26(2):75–8.
51. Persson A, Fjeldsgaard K, Gjertsen JE, Kjellsen AB, Engebretsen L, Hole RM, et al. Increased risk of revision with hamstring tendon grafts compared with patellar tendon grafts after anterior cruciate ligament reconstruction: a study of 12,643 patients from the Norwegian Cruciate Ligament Registry, 2004-2012. Am J Sports Med. 2014;42(2):285–91.
52. Rahr-Wagner L, Thillemann TM, Pedersen AB, Lind M. Comparison of hamstring tendon and patellar tendon grafts in anterior cruciate ligament reconstruction in a nationwide population-based cohort study: results from the danish registry of knee ligament reconstruction. Am J Sports Med. 2014;42(2):278–84.
53. Spindler KP, Huston LJ, Zajichek A, Reinke EK, Amendola A, Andrish JT, et al. Anterior cruciate ligament reconstruction in high school and college-aged athletes: does autograft choice influence anterior cruciate ligament revision rates? Am J Sports Med. 2020;48(2):298–309.
54. Perez JR, Emerson CP, Barrera CM, Greif DN, Cade WH 2nd, Kaplan LD, et al. Patient-reported knee outcome scores with soft tissue quadriceps tendon autograft are similar to bone-patellar tendon-bone autograft at minimum 2-year follow-up: a retrospective single-center cohort study in primary anterior cruciate ligament reconstruction surgery. Orthop J Sports Med. 2019;7(12):2325967119890063.
55. Fukunaga T, Johnson CD, Nicholas SJ, McHugh MP. Muscle hypotrophy, not inhibition, is responsible for quadriceps weakness during rehabilitation after anterior cruciate ligament reconstruction. Knee Surg Sports Traumatol Arthrosc. 2019;27(2):573–9.
56. Magnussen RA, Lawrence JT, West RL, Toth AP, Taylor DC, Garrett WE. Graft size and patient age are predictors of early revision after anterior cruciate ligament reconstruction with hamstring autograft. Arthroscopy. 2012;28(4):526–31.
57. Conte EJ, Hyatt AE, Gatt CJ Jr, Dhawan A. Hamstring autograft size can be predicted and is a potential risk factor for anterior cruciate ligament reconstruction failure. Arthroscopy. 2014;30(7):882–90.
58. Akhtar MA, Bhattacharya R, Keating JF. Generalised ligamentous laxity and revision ACL surgery: is there a relation? Knee. 2016;23(6):1148–53.
59. Arnoczky SP. Biology of ACL reconstructions: what happens to the graft? Instr Course Lect. 1996;45:229–33.
60. Brophy RH, Wright RW, Huston LJ, Nwosu SK, Spindler KP. Factors associated with infection following anterior cruciate ligament reconstruction. J Bone Joint Surg Am. 2015;97(6):450–4.
61. Burks RT, Friederichs MG, Fink B, Luker MG, West HS, Greis PE. Treatment of postoperative anterior cruciate ligament infections with graft removal and early reimplantation. Am J Sports Med. 2003;31(3):414–8.
62. Lui P, Zhang P, Chan K, Qin L. Biology and augmentation of tendon-bone insertion repair. J Orthop Surg Res. 2010;5:59.
63. Irvine JN, Arner JW, Thorhauer E, Abebe ES, D'Auria J, Schreiber VM, et al. Is there a difference in graft motion for bone-tendon-bone and hamstring autograft ACL reconstruction at 6 weeks and 1 year? Am J Sports Med. 2016;44(10):2599–607.
64. DeFrancesco CJ, Lebrun DG, Molony JT Jr, Heath MR, Fabricant PD. Safer and cheaper: an enhanced milestone-based return to play program after anterior cruciate ligament reconstruction in young athletes is cost-effective compared with standard time-based return to play criteria. Am J Sports Med. 2020;363546520907914
65. Kaplan Y, Witvrouw E. When is it safe to return to sport after ACL reconstruction? Reviewing the criteria. Sports Health. 2019;11(4):301–5.
66. Magnussen RA, Kaeding CC, Taylor DC. Solutions to small hamstring autograft harvest. Curr Orthop Pract. 2015;26(1):42–4.
67. Grassi A, Kim C, Marcheggiani Muccioli GM, Zaffagnini S, Amendola A. What is the mid-term failure rate of revision ACL reconstruction? A systematic review. Clin Orthop Relat Res. 2017;475(10):2484–99.
68. Carlisle J, Parker R, Matava M. Technical considerations in revision anterior cruciate ligament surgery. J Knee Surg. 2010;20(04):312–22.
69. Rao S, Vijayan S. Surgical approaches to total knee arthroplasty. Knee surgery. Jaypee Brothers Medical Publishers (P) Ltd; 2014. p. 26.
70. Della Valle CJ, Berger RA, Rosenberg AG. Surgical exposures in revision total knee arthroplasty. Clin Orthop Relat Res. 2006;446:59–68.
71. Vince KG, Abdeen A. Wound problems in total knee arthroplasty. Clin Orthop Relat Res. 2006;452:88–90.
72. Lazaro LE, Cross MB, Lorich DG. Vascular anatomy of the patella: implications for total knee arthroplasty surgical approaches. Knee. 2014;21(3):655–60.
73. Group M, Wright RW. Effect of graft choice on the 6 year outcome of revision anterior cruciate ligament reconstruction in the multicenter ACL revision study (MARS) cohort. Orthop J Sports Med. 2019;7(7_suppl5):2325967119S0028.
74. Horvath A, Senorski EH, Westin O, Karlsson J, Samuelsson K, Svantesson E. Outcome after anterior cruciate ligament revision. Curr Rev Musculoskelet Med. 2019;12(3):397–405.
75. Wilde J, Bedi A, Altchek DW. Revision anterior cruciate ligament reconstruction. Sports Health. 2014;6(6):504–18.

Radiographic Workup of the Failed ACLR

2

Ajay C. Kanakamedala, Aaron M. Gipsman, Michael J. Alaia, and Erin F. Alaia

Introduction

A greater understanding of the role of imaging in the diagnosis and treatment of the failed ACLR is critical for all surgeons performing revision ACLR. Plain radiographs, computed tomography (CT), and magnetic resonance (MR) imaging all have various roles and can be helpful for identifying the etiology of a prior ACLR failure, as well as assist in preoperative planning. The focus of this chapter is on the use of imaging in the workup and treatment of the failed ACLR.

Radiographic Landmarks for Anatomic ACL Reconstruction

Multiple studies have shown that non-anatomic tunnel placement, specifically femoral tunnel placement, is associated with higher rates of ACLR failure [1, 2]. While anteromedial portal femoral tunnel drilling was introduced to facilitate a more anatomic and horizontal femoral tunnel position and has been shown to accomplish this goal [3], recent studies have found high rates of non-anatomic tunnel placement with both methods, which highlights the importance of careful tunnel position identification regardless of surgical technique [4].

There are several radiographic landmarks that can be used to evaluate femoral tunnel position. In the coronal plane, whether on an anteroposterior (AP) radiograph or the coronal cut of MRI or CT imaging, the clock-face method is often used to evaluate the femoral tunnel position. Using this method, the femoral tunnel is either placed at the 10 o'clock or 2 o'clock position for a right or left knee, respectively (Fig. 2.1). Of note, this method has been shown to have poor inter-rater reliability, and many, including the authors of this chapter, have moved away from this method as it is not reliable and does not accurately correspond to bony morphology [5, 6]. In the sagittal plane, the quadrant method has been described to evaluate the femoral tunnel position (Fig. 2.2). Using this method, a grid is superimposed on the femoral condyles. The ideal tunnel position is just inferior to the most superoposterior quadrant [7]. This corresponds to a point in center of the ACL footprint which leaves about 1–2 mm of the posterior cortical wall of the femur intact.

With regard to the tibial tunnel, in the coronal plane, the tibial ACL footprint corresponds to a point between the intercondylar eminences about

A. C. Kanakamedala (✉) · A. M. Gipsman
Department of Orthopedic Surgery, NYU Langone Health, New York, NY, USA

M. J. Alaia
Department of Orthopedic Surgery, Division of Sports Medicine, New York University Langone Health, New York, NY, USA

E. F. Alaia
Department of Radiology, NYU Langone Health, New York, NY, USA

M. J. Alaia, K. J. Jones (eds.), *Revision Anterior Cruciate Ligament Reconstruction*,
https://doi.org/10.1007/978-3-030-96996-7_2

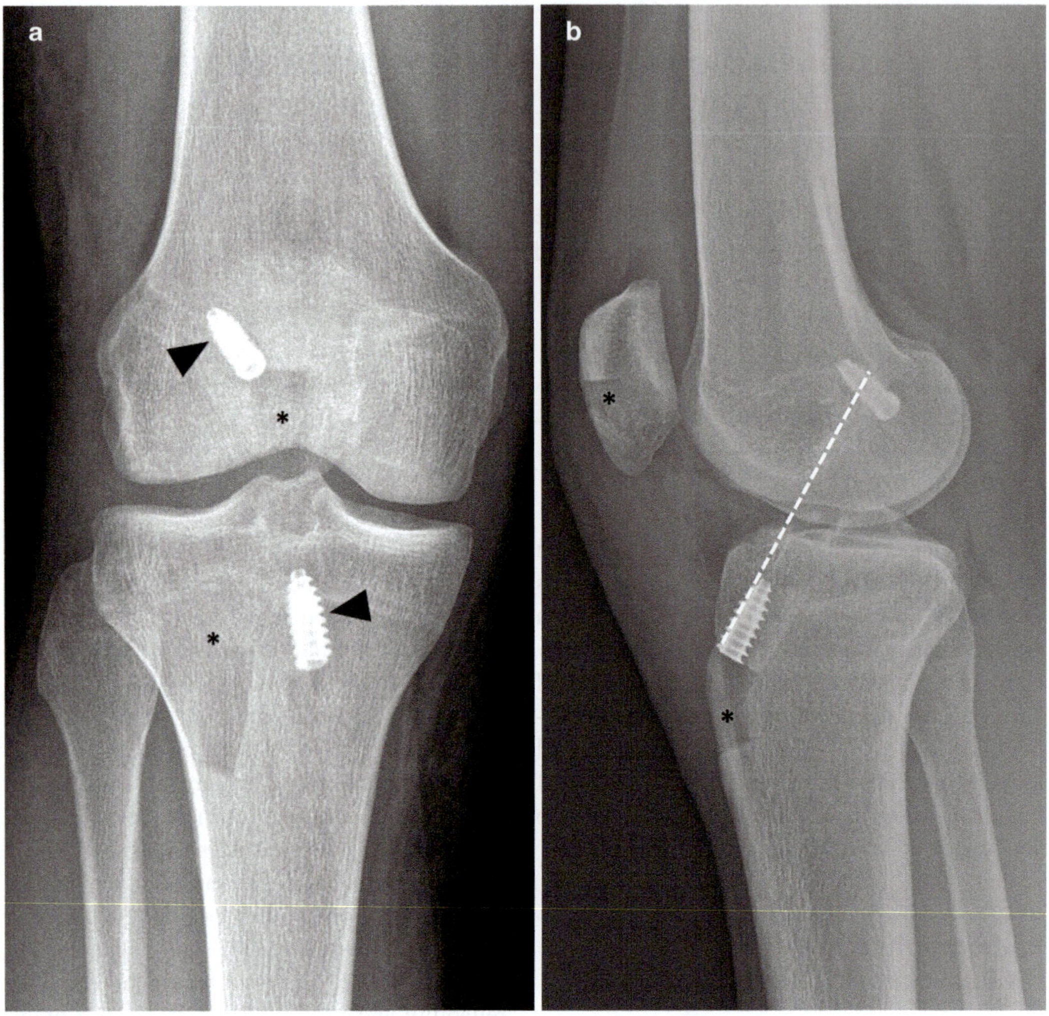

Fig. 2.1 Normal radiographic appearance after anterior cruciate ligament reconstruction. Frontal and lateral radiographs of the knee demonstrate typical postoperative changes after bone-patellar tendon-bone autograft harvesting, with geographic defects along the central patella and the tibial tuberosity at the bone plug harvest site (asterisks). The femoral tunnel interference screw is in standard position, at the 10 o'clock position (femoral arrowhead, **a**). The tibial tunnel should lie posterior to where Blumensaat's line intersects the tibia (dotted line, **b**)

2/5 of the way from the medial to lateral eminence [8]. In the sagittal plane, traditionally the tibial tunnel was recommended to be placed parallel to the slope of the intercondylar roof, i.e., Blumensaat's line [9]. Using this model, the ideal tibial ACL footprint lies just posterior to where Blumensaat's line intersects the surface of the tibia (Fig. 2.1). Recent studies have suggested that use of the intercondylar roof may not always be a reliable landmark, however, and have identified that the center of the tibial ACL footprint can more consistently be located at a point between 43% and 45% of the anteroposterior length of the tibia (Fig. 2.3) [10]. This is based on anatomic studies showing consistency in the location of the tibial ACL footprint relative to the length of the tibial plateau despite variation in intercondylar roof angles. Moreover the tibial tunnel angle will occasionally need to be altered depending on the length of the harvested graft to avoid graft tunnel mismatch [11]. To avoid graft impingement in the intercondylar notch during extension, the tibial tunnel angle is typically recommended to be parallel to the intercondylar roof inclination

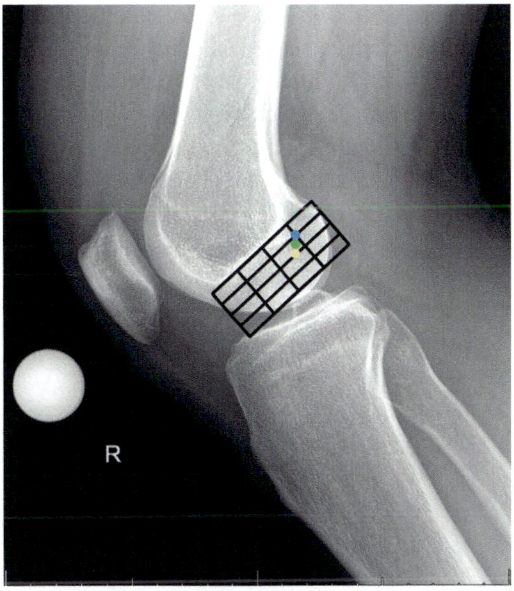

Fig. 2.2 Quadrant method for identifying anatomic ACL origin and correct femoral tunnel position. A grid is superimposed on the femoral condyles parallel to Blumensaat's line. Each dimension is split into quartiles. The anatomic origin of the anteromedial bundle is about 25% anterior and deep to the posterosuperior most aspect of the femoral condyle (blue dot). The anatomic origin of the posterolateral bundle is about 33% anterior and 50% deep to the posterosuperior most aspect of the femoral condyle (yellow dot). The center of the ACL between these two points is shown by the green dot

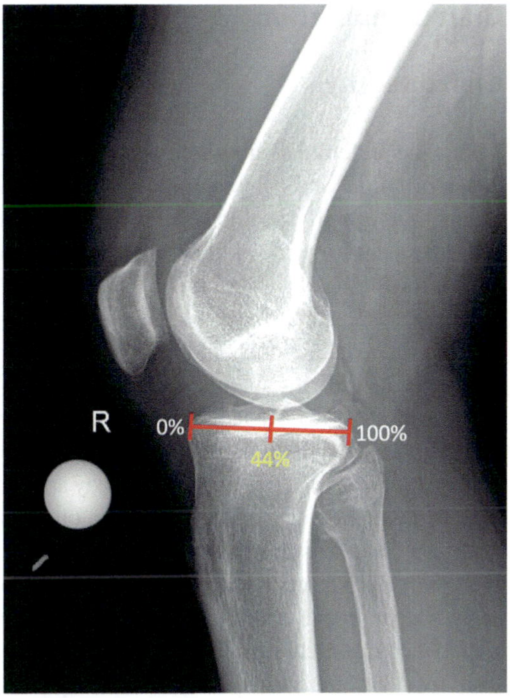

Fig. 2.3 Tibial tunnel location based on the anteroposterior length of the tibial plateau. The method of Stäubli et al. is shown for identifying the ideal tibial tunnel location. A point 44% from the anterior to the posterior edge of the tibia is noted which corresponds to the average location of the ACL insertion

angle, which has been reported to be, on average, 36.8° in men and 35.2° in women [12].

It is worth noting that, while plain radiographs can provide valuable information, multiple studies have shown poor inter-rater reliability and validity with the use of plain radiographs for the evaluation of tunnel placement when compared to MR and CT imaging. Moreover, it is often difficult to even identify bony tunnels on plain radiograph. Some authors recommend routinely obtaining CT imaging for the most accurate identification of prior tunnel position whenever precise measurements are needed [13]. Three-dimensional CT reconstructions can also be extremely helpful, as they can directly examine the aperture on both the femur and the tibia, especially when the medial femoral condyle is subtracted, as this allows a direct en face view of the lateral femoral condyle wall and the tibial plafond (Fig. 2.4).

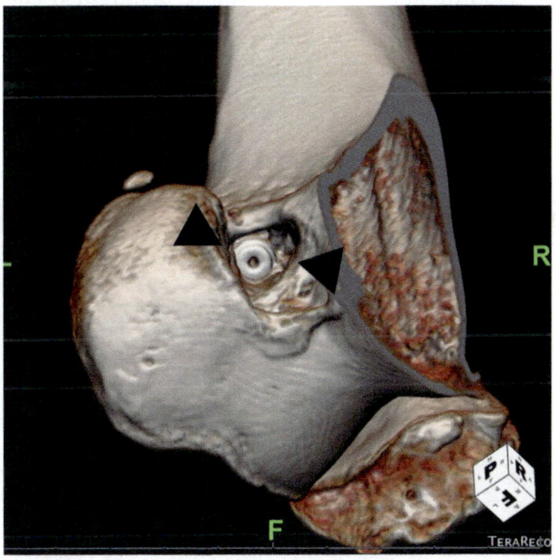

Fig. 2.4 Utility of 3D CT in the evaluation of the ACL graft tunnel. A 3D reconstructed CT image with medial femoral condyle subtraction demonstrates the aperture of the femoral tunnel (arrowheads), which appears widened, with gapping between the tunnel wall and the femoral interference screw

Graft Complications

Graft Integrity

MRI is the preferred diagnostic modality for evaluation of partial and complete graft tear, demonstrating an overall specificity of 86.7% and a positive predictive value of 93.5% [14]. Similar to evaluating the native anterior cruciate ligament, the anterior cruciate ligament graft should be evaluated in the axial, coronal, and sagittal planes on every knee MRI. In the authors' experience, tear of the graft is most readily identified in the axial or coronal plane, typically in close proximity to the femoral tunnel entrance site. Graft tear may appear as frank disruption of graft fibers with an obvious defect on fluid-sensitive images (Fig. 2.5); however, graft fiber discontinuity may be difficult to appreciate in more chronic tears with scarring around the graft. Occasionally in chronic tears, the graft may become largely resorbed and poorly visualized. On sagittal images, orientation of graft fibers should be closely scrutinized. Normally the graft should remain taut and parallel to Blumensaat's line (Fig. 2.6), with a more horizontal orientation and any fiber redundancy being important clues in subtle tears.

Additionally, it is important to distinguish partial graft tear or low-grade sprain injury from the normal process of ligamentization seen in the immature graft. This process is often described as consisting of three phases: an initial healing phase during the first 6 months after surgery, a second remodeling stage which typically continues for another 6 months, and a final maturation phase which starts around 1 year after surgery and has been shown to continue at 2 years after surgery [15]. Ligamentization during the early healing

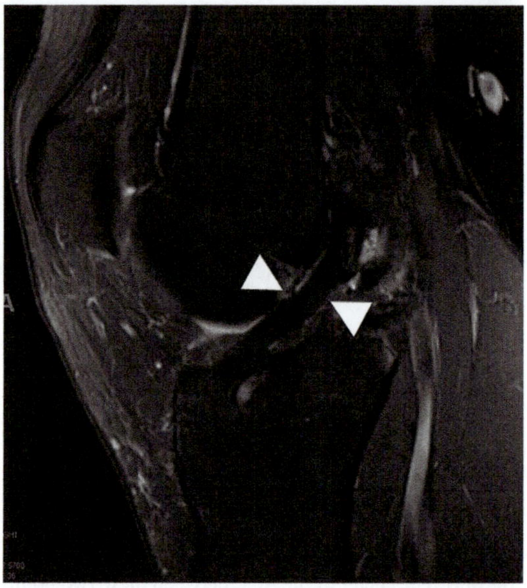

Fig. 2.6 Normal ACL graft. The normal ACL graft is homogeneously low in signal on fluid-sensitive images, with graft fibers intact and taut, and parallel to Blumensaat's line

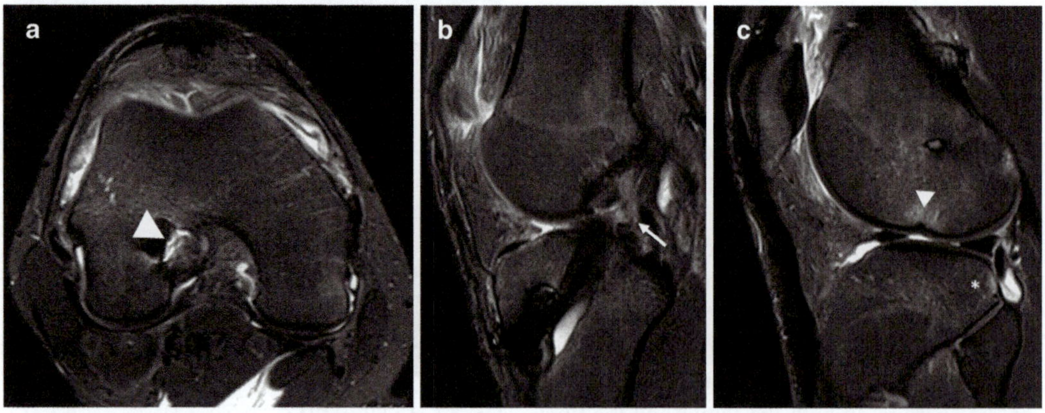

Fig. 2.5 Complete ACL graft tear on MRI. Axial image (**a**) demonstrates a fluid filled full-thickness defect (arrowhead) of graft fibers adjacent to the femoral tunnel. Sagittal image (**b**) demonstrates redundancy of graft fibers, which are normally taut, and important secondary findings, including an impaction fracture of the lateral femoral condyle (arrowhead), contusion of the posterolateral tibial plateau (asterisk), and anterior tibial translation (**c**)

phase will manifest on MRI as focal areas of intermediate signal within the graft that should not be misinterpreted as pathologic (Fig. 2.7). This signal intensity tends to slowly decrease as the graft matures [16]. While numerous studies have found varying timelines for ligamentization, some have reported that ligamentization may persist for up to 4 years following graft reconstruction [9].

Aside from discrete graft tear, secondary findings may be useful in diagnosing a graft tear, including the presence of a large joint effusion, contusion of the lateral femoral condyle and posterior lateral tibial plateau, and anterior tibial translation, imaging findings which are commonly seen in primary ACL tears (Fig. 2.5) [9].

It is important to note, though, that MR imaging is not completely sensitive to graft rupture. One retrospective review of 50 revision ACL cases found that in 24% of cases, the graft was read on MR imaging as intact despite no intact graft on arthroscopic or clinical examination [17]. The sensitivity of MR imaging for detecting ACL graft rupture has been reported to range from 59% to 72% [14, 17, 18]. It is important that any findings on MR imaging are combined with clinical and arthroscopic findings when evaluating for graft rupture after ACLR.

Graft Impingement

Graft impingement is a significant complication of ACLR and can lead to graft rupture, anterior knee pain, knee effusions, and loss of range of motion, particularly extension [19]. Graft impingement occurs when the graft makes contact with the walls of the femoral intercondylar notch, typically during extension. This can occur due to anterior positioning of the tibial tunnel or anterior positioning of the femoral tunnel [19]. Findings of graft impingement on MR imaging include evidence of graft contact with the intercondylar roof, posterior bowing of the graft, and altered signal intensity in the graft, typically in the anterior two thirds (Fig. 2.8) [9, 20]. It is important to distinguish graft impingement from a partial graft tear with anterior tibial translation, as they can have similar findings including

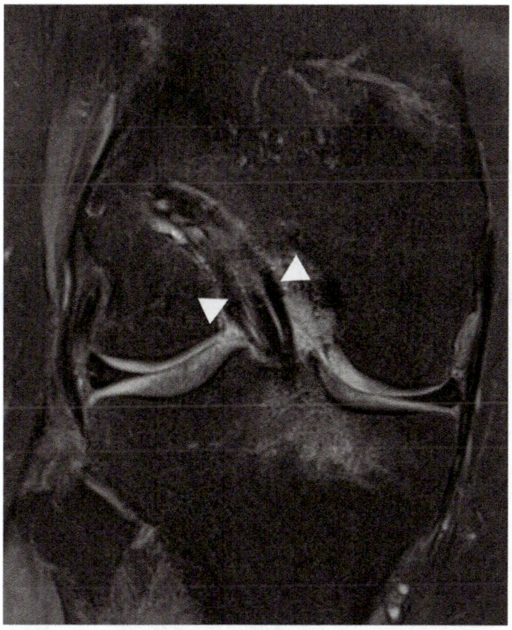

Fig. 2.7 Normal ligamentization of an ACL graft. Coronal MRI image shows thin longitudinal fluid signal along intact fibers of the ACL graft (arrowheads), representing the normal process of ligamentization in this patient 3 months following ACL reconstruction

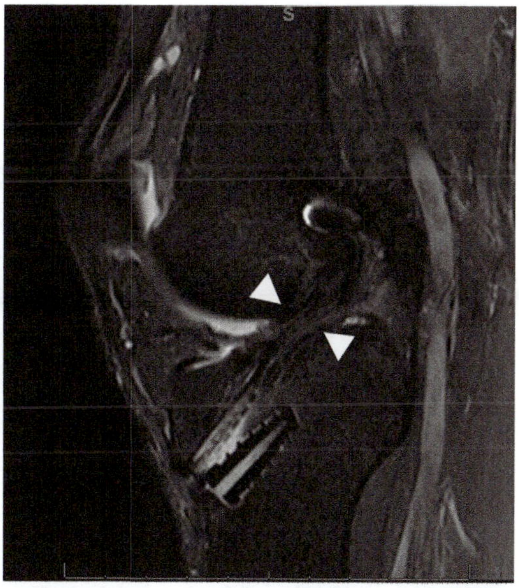

Fig. 2.8 Roof impingement following ACL reconstruction. Sagittal MRI image shows evidence of roof impingement, with anterior graft fibers (arrowheads) mildly frayed and kinked along the undersurface of the intercondylar notch. The tibial tunnel has an anterior position relative to where Blumensaat's line intersects the tibia, predisposing to roof impingement

anterior position of the tibia relative to the femur, buckling of graft fibers, and altered graft signal intensity. Anterior positioning of the tibial tunnel and the presence of a true cyclops lesion [21] are findings that might suggest graft impingement rather than a partial graft tear. It is important to distinguish a true cyclops lesion from a "pseudo-cyclops" lesion which can occur in partial graft tears when the torn fibers flip into the intercondylar notch and create a mass-like appearance – these can be distinguished from true cyclops lesions as these fibers can be traced back to the femoral or tibial tunnels [22].

A less common form of graft wall impingement is sidewall impingement, which may occur between the graft and the medial wall of the lateral femoral condyle if the tibial tunnel is placed too laterally, which appears as a medial indentation in the graft [23]. It can also occur as a result of osteophyte formation at the site of notchplasty or an interference screw protruding into the intercondylar notch [24, 25].

Hardware Complications

ACLR failure can occur as a result of failure of graft fixation. Fixation devices such as metal or bioabsorbable interference screws can rarely loosen and migrate intra-articularly (Fig. 2.9) [26, 27]. As mentioned above, if the screw is not placed entirely within the tunnel and is slightly protruding intra-articularly, it can lead to graft impingement [24]. Occasionally, the tibial interference screw will have a proud position and may irritate the overlying soft tissues, with potential for formation of an adventitial bursa.

Other Complications

Arthrofibrosis

Arthrofibrosis after ACLR is defined as the presence of scar tissue within the knee joint and is reported to occur in 1–10% of patients after ACLR. There are two main forms: focal arthrofibrosis (otherwise known as the cyclops lesion) and diffuse arthrofibrosis.

A cyclops lesion is a nodular mass of fibroproliferative tissue and can sometimes contain osseous or cartilaginous tissue and, in such cases, are sometimes referred to as "true cyclops" lesions as opposed to cyclopoid scars, which only contain fibrous tissue [28]. True cyclops

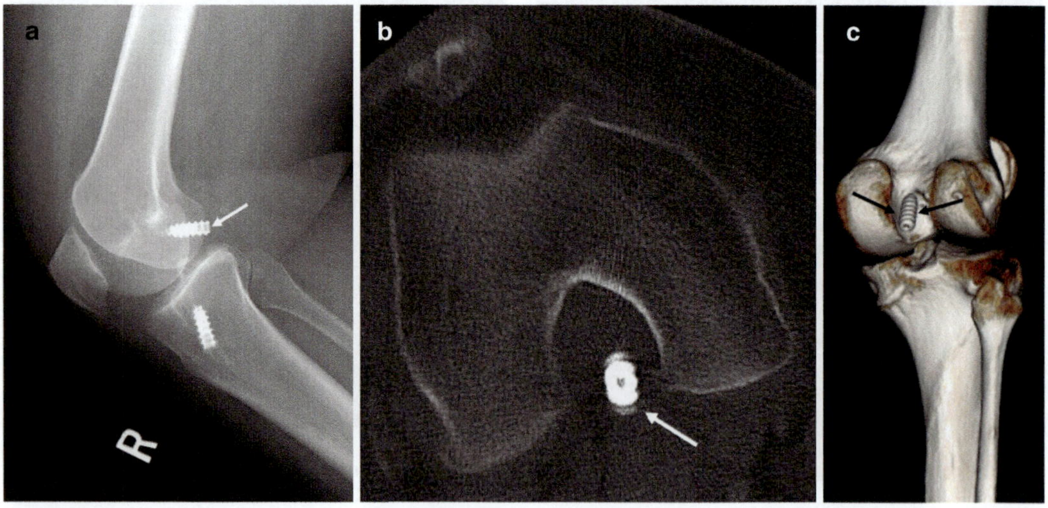

Fig. 2.9 Displaced femoral interference screw following ACL reconstruction. Lateral radiograph (**a**), axial CT (**b**), and 3D CT reconstructed images (**c**) demonstrate displacement of the femoral interference screw into the posterior intercondylar notch (arrows)

lesions are more likely to cause loss of extension since, unlike cyclopoid scars, they cannot be easily compressed. They appear on MR imaging as a well-circumscribed nodule with an average size of 10–15 mm [29] (Fig. 2.10). They are typically located in the anterior intercondylar notch and subsequently can cause impingement in extension and loss of extension. They most commonly occur at 6–12 months postoperatively after ACLR [30]. It is important to distinguish pseudocyclops lesions from cyclops lesions, as stated above [22].

Arthrofibrosis can also occur in a diffuse form and is more common in patients with poor preoperative range of motion [31]. It appears on MR imaging as hypointense fibrous tissue surrounding the graft and extending to the posterior joint capsule and possibly in the infrapatellar fat pad. This is in contrast to a distinct mass-like lesion as in the case of cyclops lesions. The differential for arthrofibrosis includes nodular synovitis (focal pigmented villonodular synovitis) and synovial chondromatosis.

Tunnel Cysts/Osteolysis

Role of CT in Cases of Suspected Tunnel Widening

It is common for small amounts of fluid to be present in the tibial and femoral graft tunnels up to 18 months after ACLR [32]. This fluid is typically reabsorbed within 18 months and does not constitute a true cyst or lead to tunnel expansion, ganglion formation, or graft failure. When tunnel cysts do form, they can occur in the pretibial space, in the tibial tunnel, and in the femoral tunnel. They can also be classified as communicating or non-communicating depending on whether they communicate with the joint space.

While their etiology is not completely understood, tunnel cysts and widening have been attributed to several causes, including excess graft motion in the tunnel, accumulation of osteolytic cytokines from synovial fluid in the tunnel secondary to incomplete graft incorporation, early accelerated rehabilitation prior to complete

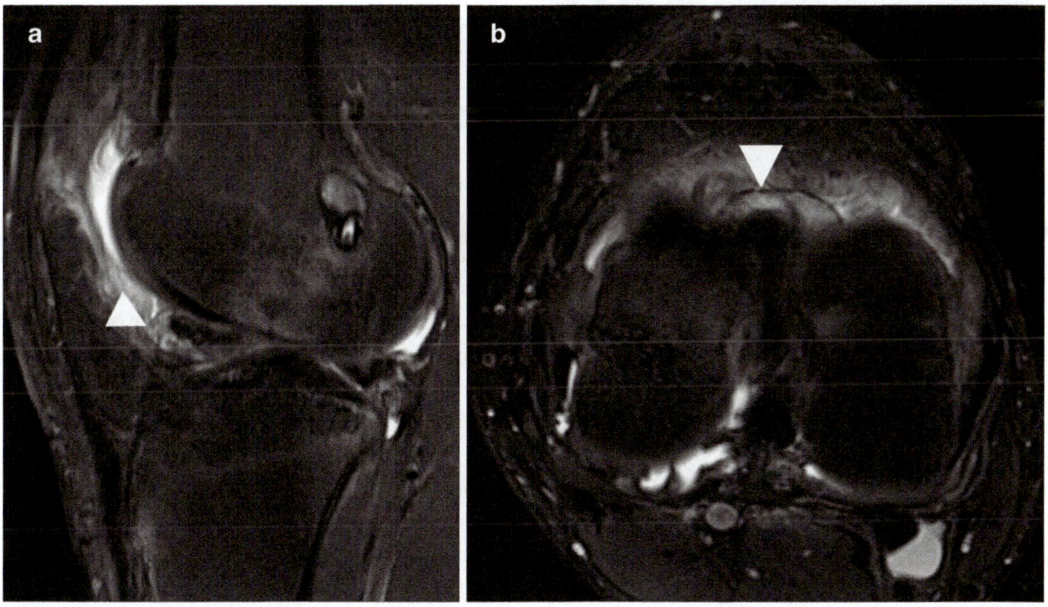

Fig. 2.10 Focal arthrofibrosis following ACL reconstruction. Sagittal (**a**) and axial (**b**) images of the knee demonstrate a heterogeneously T2 hyperintense nodule along the anterior intercondylar notch (arrowheads), compatible with focal arthrofibrosis (cyclops lesion)

graft incorporation, and host response to hardware such as bioabsorbable interference screws [33, 34].

With regard to findings on imaging, plain radiographs may show tunnel widening around the fixation device [35, 36], as well as sclerotic borders identifying the geographic limits of the tunnel. MR imaging can show fluid in the tunnel, tunnel widening, or simple or loculated cysts (Fig. 2.11). These findings are most adequately visualized on STIR or fat-suppressed T2 sequences, especially since STIR images are less affected by metal artifact from certain fixation devices. These cysts extend into the pretibial space, intercondylar notch, or popliteal fossa.

CT imaging is also often used to evaluate tunnel widening and cyst formation (Fig. 2.12). One comparative study found that neither plain radiographs nor MRI was reliable in evaluating tunnel widening and found greatest intra-rater and inter-rater reliability for the evaluation of tunnel widening with CT imaging [37].

The differential for tunnel widening/osteolysis includes foreign body granulomas, which appear as a heterogenous mass that enhance with intravenous gadolinium contrast, and screw extrusion in which there will be a cyst in the tunnel but the screw will be visibly extruded from the tunnel. While there is no evidence that the development of a tunnel cyst is associated with increased rates of graft failure, it is important to note the formation of a tunnel cyst or tunnel widening on imaging for the purposes of preoperative planning for revision ACLR. In some cases, a two-stage procedure may be required with an initial bone grafting procedure followed by a second definitive ACLR once there is adequate bone stock for tunnel drilling.

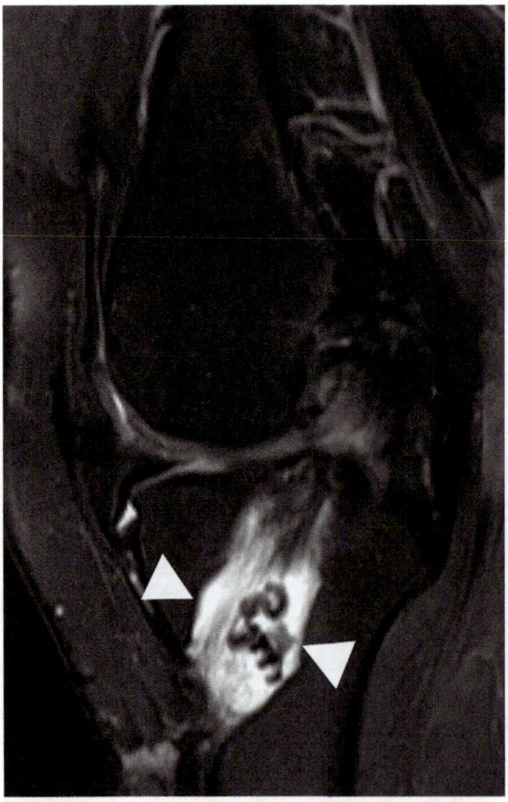

Fig. 2.11 Tunnel osteolysis on MRI after anterior cruciate ligament reconstruction. Sagittal MRI image demonstrates osteolysis of the tibial tunnel, with marked tunnel cystic widening (arrowheads)

Additional Factors That May Contribute to Risk of Graft Re-rupture or Recurrent Instability

Alignment

Coronal Plane

Assessment of tibiofemoral alignment in the coronal plane is a critical component of the evaluation of any patient with an ACL injury. There are several ways of assessing varus or valgus alignment. Methods include drawing the mechanical axis, which can be depicted as a line from the center of the femoral head to the center of the tibiotalar joint, and assessing whether this line passes medial or lateral to the center of the tibiofemoral joint, indicating varus or valgus alignment, respectively.

Varus alignment has been shown to increase the forces placed across both the native and reconstructed ACL, thus putting patients at risk for increased risk of ACL injury as well as ACLR failure [38]. Varus alignment combined with ACL deficiency can also lead to increased development of arthritis [39]. As a result, multiple authors have advocated for performing high tibial osteotomies (HTO), either combined or in staged

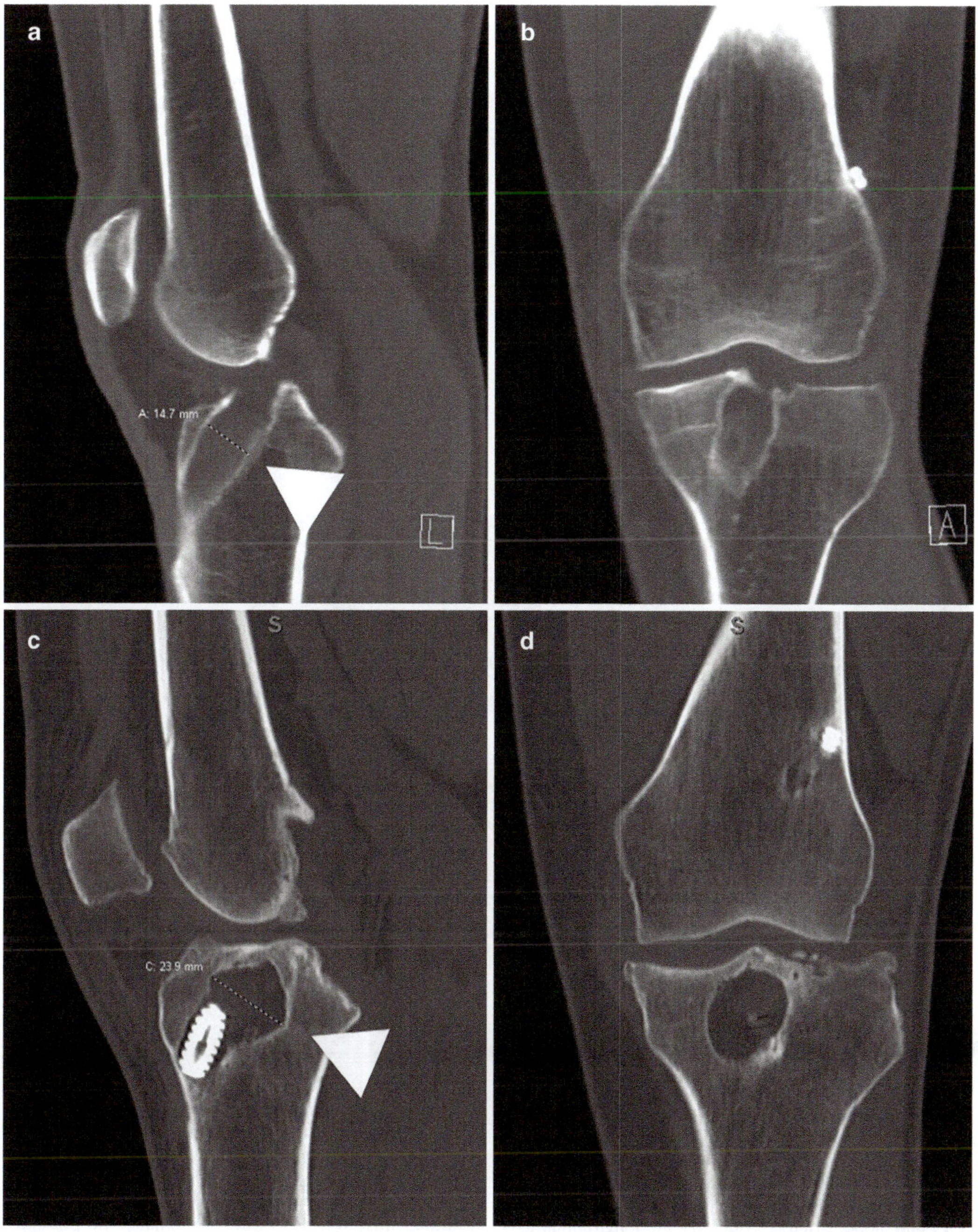

Fig. 2.12 Tunnel osteolysis on CT after anterior cruciate ligament reconstruction. Sagittal (**a** and **c**) and coronal (**b** and **d**) images demonstrate examples of osteolysis of the tibial tunnel in two separate knees. Measurement of tunnels at their widest point are shown on the sagittal images (arrowheads). The first patient (**a** and **b**) was noted to have maintained cylindricity of their tunnel, whereas the second patient (**c** and **d**) was found to have a more cavitary area of bone loss

fashion with revision ACLR, to address ACL deficiency, prevent or delay the progression of medial compartment osteoarthritis, and reduce the risk of revision ACLR failure. Several studies have found favorable functional and clinical outcomes with this approach [40, 41].

Tibial Sagittal Slope

Assessment of sagittal alignment is an important part of the preoperative planning process. The most commonly used parameter of sagittal alignment is posterior tibial slope (PTS), which can be measured as the angle formed by the intersection of a line parallel to the tibial shaft and another line tangential to the articular surface of the tibial plateau (Fig. 2.13).

Multiple studies have found increased rates of ACLR failure as well as primary ACL injuries with increased posterior tibial slope (PTS), with some studies identifying a particularly large increase in risk with a posterior tibial slope of 12 degrees or greater [42, 43]. Biomechanical studies have confirmed that increased forces are seen across the ACL with increased PTS [44]. As a result, several authors have suggested performing proximal tibial slope-reducing osteotomies to decrease the posterior slope in patients with excessive PTS and reduce the rate of ACLR failure [42, 45]. It remains unclear whether there is more value to measuring the PTS on the medial or lateral tibial plateau. While some authors recommended using the medial tibial plateau as it is more recognizable [46], the lateral tibial plateau PTS has also been shown to be associated with increased risk of ACL injury and ACLR failure [43, 47].

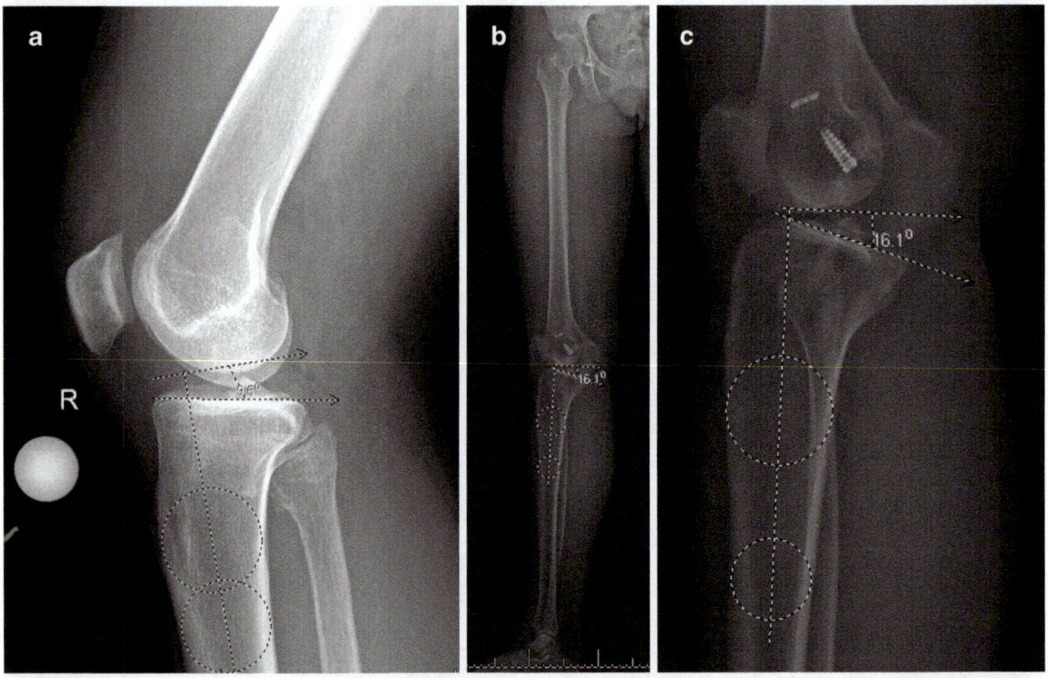

Fig. 2.13 Measurement of posterior tibial slope. A lateral radiograph (**a**) is shown with a measurement of the posterior tibial slope. Briefly, to identify the longitudinal axis of the tibia, a line is drawn connecting the center of the tibia at 2 points about 5 cm apart and with the distal point as distal in the tibia as possible. A second line is drawn connecting the anterior and posterior most points on the tibial plateau. The angle between a line perpendicular to the longitudinal axis of the tibia and the line tangential to the tibial plateaus is the posterior tibial slope angle, which is 9.5 degrees in this radiograph. (**b**) is the full-length standing film from a 24-year-old female who presented with recurrent ACL reconstruction failure after three prior ACL reconstructions. Her posterior tibial slope, which is measured in (**b**, **c**), is 16.1 degrees, and she was indicated for a closing wedge high tibial osteotomy, along with revision ACL reconstruction, to decrease her posterior tibial slope and decrease her chance of recurrent graft failure

Other Sources of Persistent Instability

Meniscus Pathology

The menisci are important secondary stabilizers of the ACL-deficient knee, and meniscal injuries can increase the forces on the reconstructed ACL graft. The medial meniscus has been shown to contribute primarily to anteroposterior stability, whereas the lateral meniscus contributes more to rotatory stability by preventing anterior tibial translation during pivot-shift maneuvers involving a valgus and internal rotation load [48]. Concomitant meniscectomy with ACLR has been shown to be associated with worse clinical outcomes and increased radiographic development of osteoarthritic changes compared to ACLR alone [49]. The combination of chronic anterior tibial translation with posterior meniscus deficiency can specifically lead to increased chondral wear posteriorly. One radiographic marker of this is the "cupola" sign, or an osteophyte on the posteromedial corner of the tibia that develops in response to chronic anterior tibial translation [50]. One study of 103 patients undergoing total knee arthroplasty found that all 43 patients who had a cupola sign on preoperative radiographs were confirmed intraoperatively to have a ruptured ACL [51]. Thus, it is important to recognize meniscal pathology and perform meniscal repair when possible (Fig. 2.14), and studies have shown that lateral meniscus root repair can improve stability in the ACL-deficient knee [52].

There is also now increasing awareness of the importance of identifying lesions involving the peripheral attachment of the posterior medial meniscus, termed "ramp" lesions, which have been reported to be present in 9.3–17% of ACL injuries [53, 54]. These lesions can manifest as a meniscocapsular avulsion, a meniscotibial ligament avulsion, or a combination of these two. Cadaveric studies have found that ramp lesions lead to increased anterior tibial translation and external rotation in the ACL-deficient knee and that ACLR alone did not restore these parameters but ACLR with ramp repair did [55, 56]. On the other hand, one prospective randomized study of ACLR with repair of concomitant stable ramp lesions has found no difference in clinical outcomes or anterior tibial translation [57].

Although only unstable ramp lesions may require surgical intervention, it is important to identify them using MR imaging. These tend to occur in a posteromedial "blind spot," which is difficult to view with the traditional arthroscopic portals. They can, however, easily be visualized through the Gillquist position, which will be discussed in other chapters [58]. Studies of the sensitivity of MR imaging for identifying ramp lesions report widely varying values from 0% to 84.6% [53, 59, 60], which reflects a variety of factors including that some studies only looked at the official reports in the medical record, in which ramp lesions might not have been specifically examined for. One author hypothesized that the low sensitivity of MR imaging might be related to MR imaging being performed when the knee is in extension, which can lead to the meniscocapsular separation being reduced.

Ramp lesion findings on MR imaging include the presence of a thin fluid signal between the posterior horn of the medial meniscus and adjacent posteromedial capsule, representing meniscocapsular separation [61], or may appear as a vertical longitudinal tear in the red-red zone of the medial meniscus posterior horn [62]. This can be accompanied by a high signal irregularity involving the capsular margin of the posterior horn of the medial meniscus on the fluid-sensitive images (Fig. 2.15) [63].

Anterolateral Capsular/Structural Insufficiency

There has been a large amount of interest recently in the anterolateral complex of the knee. There is increasing awareness now that traditional single-bundle ACLR may not reliably restore rotatory stability, which has been shown to have a significant effect on clinical outcomes [64, 65], and that the anterolateral complex significantly contributes to the rotatory stability of

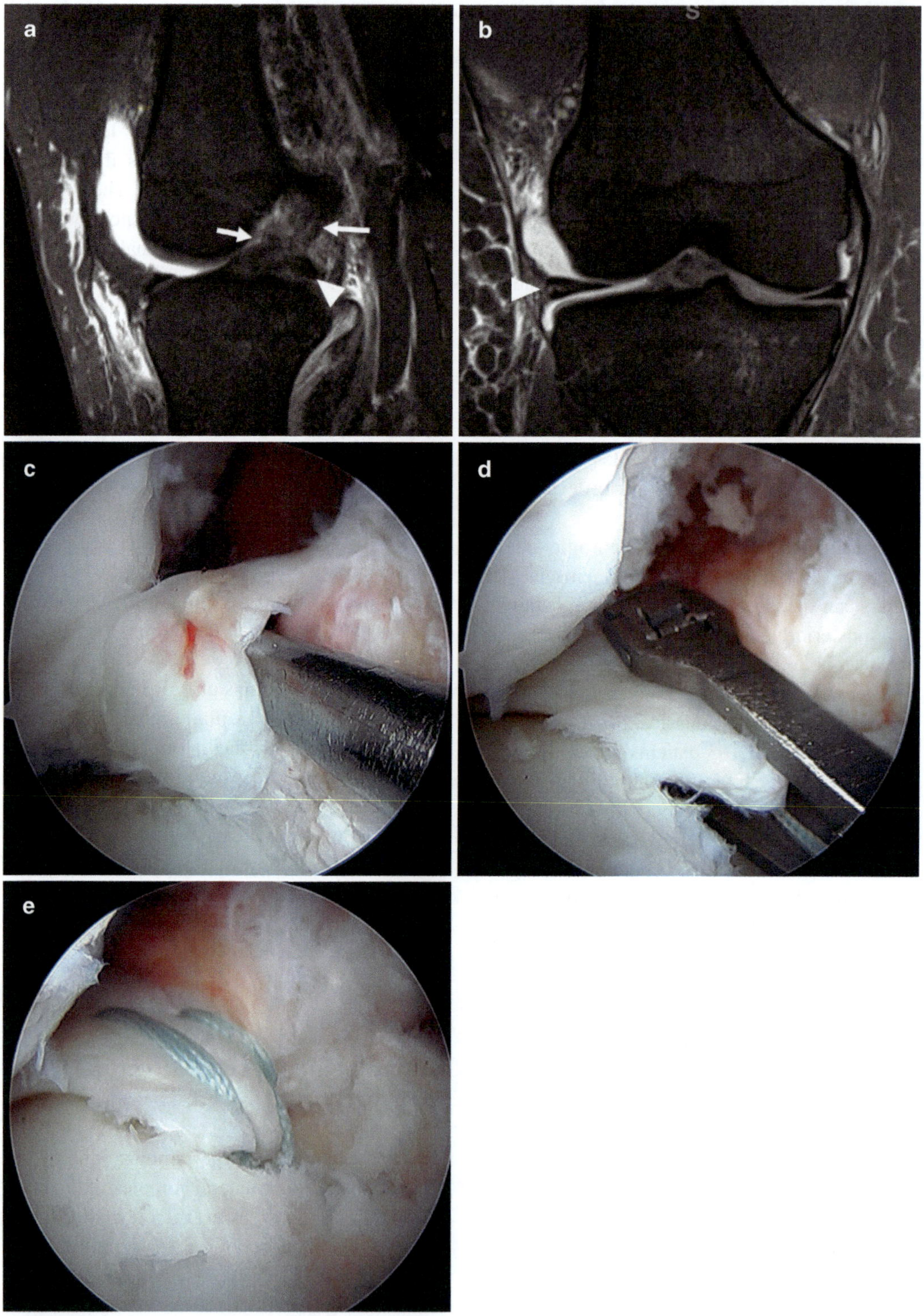

Fig. 2.14 Meniscal root injury with anterior cruciate ligament (ACL) rupture. Sagittal and coronal MRI images demonstrate an ACL tear (arrows, **a**) with meniscal root injury (arrowhead, **a**) with meniscal extrusion (arrowhead, **b**). Intraoperative arthroscopy confirms meniscal root injury (**c**, **d**). Meniscal root repair was performed concomitantly with ACL reconstruction (**e**)

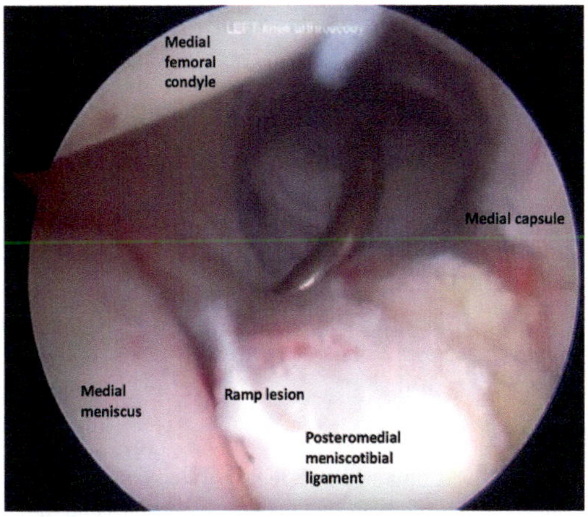

Fig. 2.15 Arthroscopic image of ramp lesion. This image depicts a ramp lesion as seen through the Gillquist view during an arthroscopic anterior cruciate ligament reconstruction. The peripheral attachment of the posterior horn of the medial meniscus, specifically the posteromedial meniscotibial ligament, has been disrupted. MRI has varying sensitivity for detecting these lesions, and it is important to evaluate for them intraoperatively, as unstable ramp lesions may require additional surgical intervention

the knee [66, 67]. The anterolateral complex contains the lateral collateral ligament (LCL), the anterolateral capsule, the iliotibial band, as well as a thickening of the anterolateral capsule that has been termed the "anterolateral ligament" (ALL). While there is controversy on whether this structure constitutes a discrete ligament versus a thickening of the capsule, part of the iliotibial band, or both, evaluation of the anterolateral complex is nevertheless an important component of the preoperative planning process given its critical role in rotatory stability [68]. While there is variation in its reported appearance, the ALL has been described on MR imaging as a sheetlike structure connecting the distal femur to the proximal tibia. There is still some controversy surrounding the ALL's origin, but most people think its origin is proximal and posterior to the LCL attachment and that it courses anteriorly and inferiorly until it inserts on the lateral meniscus and lateral tibial plateau, 6.5 mm below the articular surface [69, 70].

The reported sensitivity of MR imaging for identification of the intact ALL ranges from 11% to 100% [71, 72], and the reported incidence of concomitant ALL abnormalities with ACL injuries ranges from 33% to 90% [73–75]. While ultrasonography has been investigated for its utility in evaluating ALL injuries, prior studies have found contrasting results, with one study reporting 100% sensitivity for identifying ALL injuries on ultrasound [76], while others have found that ultrasound cannot even accurately identify or visualize the ALL [77].

Identification of these injuries is important because it may influence the decision to perform additional procedures during ACLR, such as extra-articular tenodesis or ALL reconstruction [78, 79]. Further work is being done to characterize the anatomy and role of the anterolateral ligament and the entire anterolateral complex, and this is an aspect of ACLR that is continuing to rapidly evolve.

Collateral Ligament Insufficiency

Evaluation of concomitant injuries to the medial collateral ligament (MCL), lateral collateral ligament (LCL), posteromedial corner, and posterolateral corner is an important component of the evaluation of the failed ACLR. Various studies have found that untreated concomitant ligamentous laxity tends to account for 3–5% of revision ACL cases [1, 80]. While these injuries can occur at the time of the initial ACL rupture, it is also important to note that concomitant ligamentous laxity can also develop over time in the ACL-deficient knee in the absence of the stabilizing effect of the ACL. The ACL has been shown to provide both valgus and varus stability, particularly in the absence of a competent medial- or lateral-sided ligamentous structures. In these chronic situations where there is ligamentous laxity without a discrete tear, especially in the setting of a history of subjective instability, stress radiography can be particularly helpful (Fig. 2.16). Prior studies have found that side-to-side differences on stress radiographs of 2.7 mm for isolated LCL, 3.2 mm for MCL, and 4 mm for PLC are suggestive of grade III ligamentous injuries [81].

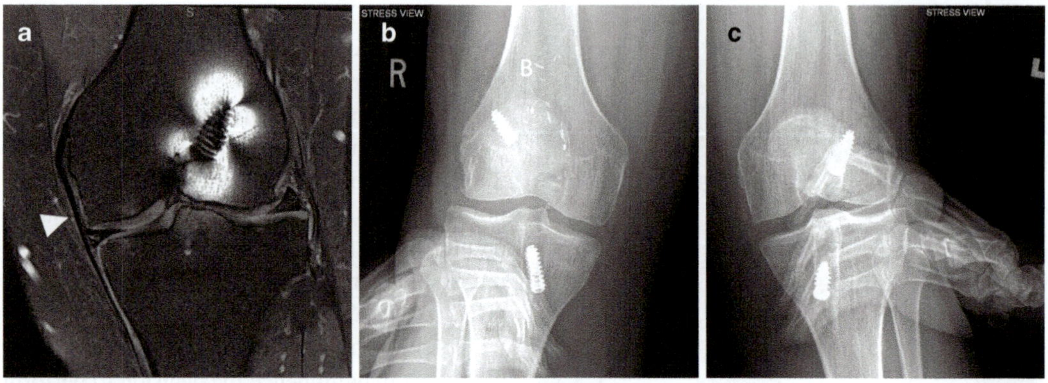

Fig. 2.16 Stress radiographs indicating left knee medial collateral ligament laxity. This patient was a 38-year-old male who had undergone bilateral prior anterior cruciate ligament reconstructions and presented with recurrent left knee instability and laxity to valgus stress on exam. A left knee MRI was obtained and demonstrated complete ACL graft rupture, with nonvisualization of the graft, and intact MCL (arrowhead, **a**). Stress radiographs were obtained and were notable for 8 mm and 12 mm of opening to valgus stress in the right (**b**) and left (**c**) knees, respectively

Conclusion

Surgeons should obtain advanced imaging as a critical component of the preoperative planning process. MR imaging is often the preferred modality for identifying various postoperative complications including graft rupture, impingement, and arthrofibrosis. CT imaging, however, is a useful adjunct and the most reliable method for assessing tunnel location and size. MR imaging can be used to both identify various causes of the failed ACLR and to diagnose additional injuries, such as ALC disruption or ramp lesions, which may require additional procedures.

References

1. Trojani C, Sbihi A, Djian P, Potel J-F, Hulet C, Jouve F, et al. Causes for failure of ACL reconstruction and influence of meniscectomies after revision. Knee Surg Sports Traumatol Arthrosc. 2011;19(2):196–201.
2. Parkinson B, Robb C, Thomas M, Thompson P, Spalding T. Factors that predict failure in anatomic single-bundle anterior cruciate ligament reconstruction. Am J Sports Med. 2017;45(7):1529–36.
3. Venosa M, Delcogliano M, Padua R, Alviti F, Delcogliano A. Femoral tunnel positioning in anterior cruciate ligament reconstruction: anteromedial portal versus transtibial technique—a randomized clinical trial. Joints. 2017;5(01):034–8.
4. Jaecker V, Zapf T, Naendrup J-H, Pfeiffer T, Kanakamedala AC, Wafaisade A, et al. High non-anatomic tunnel position rates in ACL reconstruction failure using both transtibial and anteromedial tunnel drilling techniques. Arch Orthop Trauma Surg. 2017;137(9):1293–9.
5. Mehta V, Petsche T, Rawal AM. Inter-and intrarater reliability of the femoral tunnel clock-face grading system during anterior cruciate ligament reconstruction. Arthroscopy. 2017;33(2):394–7.
6. Rayan F, Nanjayan SK, Quah C, Ramoutar D, Konan S, Haddad FS. Review of evolution of tunnel position in anterior cruciate ligament reconstruction. World J Orthop. 2015;6(2):252.
7. Bernard M, Hertel P, Hornung H, Cierpinski T. Femoral insertion of the ACL. Radiographic quadrant method. Am J Knee Surg. 1997;10(1):14–21; discussion −2.
8. Hwang MD, Piefer JW, Lubowitz JH. Anterior cruciate ligament tibial footprint anatomy: systematic review of the 21st century literature. Arthroscopy. 2012;28(5):728–34.
9. Bencardino JT, Beltran J, Feldman MI, Rose DJ. MR imaging of complications of anterior cruciate ligament graft reconstruction. Radiographics. 2009;29(7):2115–26.
10. Scheffel PT, Henninger HB, Burks RT. Relationship of the intercondylar roof and the tibial footprint of the ACL: implications for ACL reconstruction. Am J Sports Med. 2013;41(2):396–401.
11. Shaffer B, Gow W, Tibone JE. Graft-tunnel mismatch in endoscopic anterior cruciate ligament reconstruction: a new technique of intraarticular measurement and modified graft harvesting. Arthroscopy. 1993;9(6):633–46.

12. Stäubli H-U, Rauschning W. Tibial attachment area of the anterior cruciate ligament in the extended knee position. Knee Surg Sports Traumatol Arthrosc. 1994;2(3):138–46.
13. Hoser C, Tecklenburg K, Kuenzel KH, Fink C. Postoperative evaluation of femoral tunnel position in ACL reconstruction: plain radiography versus computed tomography. Knee Surg Sports Traumatol Arthrosc. 2005;13(4):256–62.
14. Collins MS, Unruh KP, Bond JR, Mandrekar JN. Magnetic resonance imaging of surgically confirmed anterior cruciate ligament graft disruption. Skelet Radiol. 2008;37(3):233–43.
15. Pauzenberger L, Syré S, Schurz M. "Ligamentization" in hamstring tendon grafts after anterior cruciate ligament reconstruction: a systematic review of the literature and a glimpse into the future. Arthroscopy. 2013;29(10):1712–21.
16. Weiler A, Peters G, Mäurer J, Unterhauser FN, Südkamp NP. Biomechanical properties and vascularity of an anterior cruciate ligament graft can be predicted by contrast-enhanced magnetic resonance imaging: a two-year study in sheep. Am J Sports Med. 2001;29(6):751–61.
17. Waltz RA, Solomon DJ, Provencher MT. A radiographic assessment of failed anterior cruciate ligament reconstruction: can magnetic resonance imaging predict graft integrity? Am J Sports Med. 2014;42(7):1652–60.
18. Van Dyck P, Gielen JL, Vanhoenacker FM, Wouters K, Dossche L, Parizel PM. Stable or unstable tear of the anterior cruciate ligament of the knee: an MR diagnosis? Skelet Radiol. 2012;41(3):273–80.
19. Iriuchishima T, Shirakura K, Fu FH. Graft impingement in anterior cruciate ligament reconstruction. Knee Surg Sports Traumatol Arthrosc. 2013;21(3):664–70.
20. Iriuchishima T, Shirakura K, Horaguchi T, Morimoto Y, Fu FH. Full knee extension magnetic resonance imaging for the evaluation of intercondylar roof impingement after anatomical double-bundle anterior cruciate ligament reconstruction. Knee Surg Sports Traumatol Arthrosc. 2011;19(1):22–8.
21. Watanabe BM, Howell SM. Arthroscopic findings associated with roof impingement of an anterior cruciate ligament graft. Am J Sports Med. 1995;23(5):616–25.
22. Simpfendorfer C, Miniaci A, Subhas N, Winalski CS, Ilaslan H. Pseudocyclops: two cases of ACL graft partial tears mimicking cyclops lesions on MRI. Skelet Radiol. 2015;44(8):1169–73.
23. Papakonstantinou O, Chung CB, Chanchairujira K, Resnick DL. Complications of anterior cruciate ligament reconstruction: MR imaging. Eur Radiol. 2003;13(5):1106–17.
24. Bents RT, Jones RC, May DA, Snearly WS. Intercondylar notch encroachment following anterior cruciate ligament reconstruction: a prospective study. Am J Knee Surg. 1998;11(2):81–8.
25. May D, Snearly W, Bents R, Jones R. MR imaging findings in anterior cruciate ligament reconstruction: evaluation of notchplasty. AJR Am J Roentgenol. 1997;169(1):217–22.
26. Bush-Joseph CA, Bach B Jr. Migration of femoral interference screw after anterior cruciate ligament reconstruction. Am J Knee Surg. 1998;11(1):32.
27. Appelt A, Baier M. Recurrent locking of knee joint caused by intraarticular migration of bioabsorbable tibial interference screw after arthroscopic ACL reconstruction. Knee Surg Sports Traumatol Arthrosc. 2007;15(4):378–80.
28. Minne C, Velleman MD, Suleman FE. MRI findings of cyclops lesions of the knee. SA Orthop J. 2012;11(2):56–60.
29. Zappia M, Capasso R, Berritto D, Maggialetti N, Varelli C, D'Agosto G, et al. Anterior cruciate ligament reconstruction: MR imaging findings. Musculoskelet Surg. 2017;101(1):23–35.
30. Gohil S, Falconer TM, Breidahl W, Annear PO. Serial MRI and clinical assessment of cyclops lesions. Knee Surg Sports Traumatol Arthrosc. 2014;22(5):1090–6.
31. Mayr HO, Weig TG, Plitz W. Arthrofibrosis following ACL reconstruction—reasons and outcome. Arch Orthop Trauma Surg. 2004;124(8):518–22.
32. Sanders TG, Tall MA, Mulloy JP, Leis HT. Fluid collections in the osseous tunnel during the first year after anterior cruciate ligament repair using an autologous hamstring graft: natural history and clinical correlation. J Comput Assist Tomogr. 2002;26(4):617–21.
33. Ghazikhanian V, Beltran J, Nikac V, Feldman M, Bencardino JT. Tibial tunnel and pretibial cysts following ACL graft reconstruction: MR imaging diagnosis. Skelet Radiol. 2012;41(11):1375–9.
34. Sprowson AP, Aldridge SE, Noakes J, Read J, Wood DG. Bio-interference screw cyst formation in anterior cruciate ligament reconstruction—10-year follow up. Knee. 2012;19(5):644–7.
35. Lamprakis AA, Fortis AP, Dimas A. Rejection reaction to stabilizing bolts after ACL reconstruction: a case report. Knee Surg Sports Traumatol Arthrosc. 2008;16(1):19–23.
36. Tsuda E, Ishibashi Y, Tazawa K, Sato H, Kusumi T, Toh S. Pretibial cyst formation after anterior cruciate ligament reconstruction with a hamstring tendon autograft. Arthroscopy. 2006;22(6):691.e1–6.
37. Marchant MH, Willimon SC, Vinson E, Pietrobon R, Garrett WE, Higgins LD. Comparison of plain radiography, computed tomography, and magnetic resonance imaging in the evaluation of bone tunnel widening after anterior cruciate ligament reconstruction. Knee Surg Sports Traumatol Arthrosc. 2010;18(8):1059–64.
38. Jan van de Pol G, Arnold MP, Verdonschot N, van Kampen A. Varus alignment leads to increased forces in the anterior cruciate ligament. Am J Sports Med. 2009;37(3):481–7.
39. Noyes FR, Schipplein OD, Andriacchi TP, Saddemi SR, Weise M. The anterior cruciate ligament-deficient

knee with varus alignment: an analysis of gait adaptations and dynamic joint loadings. Am J Sports Med. 1992;20(6):707–16.
40. Zaffagnini S, Bonanzinga T, Grassi A, Muccioli GMM, Musiani C, Raggi F, et al. Combined ACL reconstruction and closing-wedge HTO for varus angulated ACL-deficient knees. Knee Surg Sports Traumatol Arthrosc. 2013;21(4):934–41.
41. Noyes FR, Barber-Westin SD, Hewett TE. High tibial osteotomy and ligament reconstruction for varus angulated anterior cruciate ligament-deficient knees. Am J Sports Med. 2000;28(3):282–96.
42. Webb JM, Salmon LJ, Leclerc E, Pinczewski LA, Roe JP. Posterior tibial slope and further anterior cruciate ligament injuries in the anterior cruciate ligament–reconstructed patient. Am J Sports Med. 2013;41(12):2800–4.
43. Christensen JJ, Krych AJ, Engasser WM, Vanhees MK, Collins MS, Dahm DL. Lateral tibial posterior slope is increased in patients with early graft failure after anterior cruciate ligament reconstruction. Am J Sports Med. 2015;43(10):2510–4.
44. McLean SG, Oh YK, Palmer ML, Lucey SM, Lucarelli DG, Ashton-Miller JA, et al. The relationship between anterior tibial acceleration, tibial slope, and ACL strain during a simulated jump landing task. J Bone Joint Surg. 2011;93(14):1310–7.
45. Dejour D, Saffarini M, Demey G, Baverel L. Tibial slope correction combined with second revision ACL produces good knee stability and prevents graft rupture. Knee Surg Sports Traumatol Arthrosc. 2015;23(10):2846–52.
46. Dejour H, Bonnin M. Tibial translation after anterior cruciate ligament rupture. Two radiological tests compared. J Bone Joint Surg Br. 1994;76(5):745–9.
47. Rahnemai-Azar AA, Yaseen Z, van Eck CF, Irrgang JJ, Fu FH, Musahl V. Increased lateral tibial plateau slope predisposes male college football players to anterior cruciate ligament injury. J Bone Joint Surg Am. 2016;98(12):1001–6.
48. Musahl V, Citak M, O'Loughlin PF, Choi D, Bedi A, Pearle AD. The effect of medial versus lateral meniscectomy on the stability of the anterior cruciate ligament-deficient knee. Am J Sports Med. 2010;38(8):1591–7.
49. Wu WH, Hackett T, Richmond JC. Effects of meniscal and articular surface status on knee stability, function, and symptoms after anterior cruciate ligament reconstruction: a long-term prospective study. Am J Sports Med. 2002;30(6):845–50.
50. Brunkhorst J, Johnson DL. Radiographic evidence of anterior cruciate ligament insufficiency. Orthopedics. 2014;37(11):759–62.
51. Mullis BH, Karas SG, Kelley SS. Characterization of a consistent radiographic finding in chronic anterior cruciate ligament deficiency: the posteromedial osteophyte. Am J Orthop (Belle Mead NJ). 2007;36(9):494.
52. Forkel P, von Deimling C, Lacheta L, Imhoff FB, Foehr P, Willinger L, et al. Repair of the lateral posterior meniscal root improves stability in an ACL-deficient knee. Knee Surg Sports Traumatol Arthrosc. 2018;26(8):2302–9.
53. Bollen S. Posteromedial meniscocapsular injury associated with rupture of the anterior cruciate ligament: a previously unrecognised association. J Bone Joint Surg. 2010;92(2):222–3.
54. Liu X, Feng H, Zhang H, Hong L, Wang XS, Zhang J. Arthroscopic prevalence of ramp lesion in 868 patients with anterior cruciate ligament injury. Am J Sports Med. 2011;39(4):832–7.
55. Stephen JM, Halewood C, Kittl C, Bollen SR, Williams A, Amis AA. Posteromedial meniscocapsular lesions increase tibiofemoral joint laxity with anterior cruciate ligament deficiency, and their repair reduces laxity. Am J Sports Med. 2016;44(2):400–8.
56. Peltier A, Lording T, Maubisson L, Ballis R, Neyret P, Lustig S. The role of the meniscotibial ligament in posteromedial rotational knee stability. Knee Surg Sports Traumatol Arthrosc. 2015;23(10):2967–73.
57. Liu X, Zhang H, Feng H, Hong L, Wang X-s, Song G-Y. Is it necessary to repair stable ramp lesions of the medial meniscus during anterior cruciate ligament reconstruction? A prospective randomized controlled trial. Am J Sports Med. 2017;45(5):1004–11.
58. Strobel MJ. Manual of arthroscopic surgery. Berlin: Springer Science & Business Media; 2013.
59. Arner JW, Herbst E, Burnham JM, Soni A, Naendrup J-H, Popchak A, et al. MRI can accurately detect meniscal ramp lesions of the knee. Knee Surg Sports Traumatol Arthrosc. 2017;25(12):3955–60.
60. Edgar C, Ware J, Obopilwe E, Ziegler C, Reed D, Arciero R, editors. Posteromedial meniscocapsular tear: prevalence, detection sensitivity, biomechanics, and repair technique. AAOS Annual Meeting; 2016.
61. Hash TW. Magnetic resonance imaging of the knee. Sports Health. 2013;5(1):78–107.
62. Greif DN, Baraga MG, Rizzo MG, Mohile NV, Silva FD, Fox T, et al. MRI appearance of the different meniscal ramp lesion types, with clinical and arthroscopic correlation. Skelet Radiol. 2020;49:677.
63. Hatayama K, Kimura M, Ogoshi A, Takagishi K, editors. Ramp lesion associated with anterior cruciate ligament rupture. International society of arthroscopy, knee surgery and orthopaedic sports medicine biennial congress, Toronto, Canada; 2013.
64. Kocher MS, Steadman JR, Briggs KK, Sterett WI, Hawkins RJ. Relationships between objective assessment of ligament stability and subjective assessment of symptoms and function after anterior cruciate ligament reconstruction. Am J Sports Med. 2004;32(3):629–34.
65. Ayeni OR, Chahal M, Tran MN, Sprague S. Pivot shift as an outcome measure for ACL reconstruction: a systematic review. Knee Surg Sports Traumatol Arthrosc. 2012;20(4):767–77.
66. Nitri M, Rasmussen MT, Williams BT, Moulton SG, Cruz RS, Dornan GJ, et al. An in vitro robotic assessment of the anterolateral ligament, part 2: anterolateral ligament reconstruction combined with anterior

cruciate ligament reconstruction. Am J Sports Med. 2016;44(3):593–601.
67. Musahl V, Rahnemai-Azar AA, Costello J, Arner JW, Fu FH, Hoshino Y, et al. The influence of meniscal and anterolateral capsular injury on knee laxity in patients with anterior cruciate ligament injuries. Am J Sports Med. 2016;44:3126.
68. Musahl V, Herbst E, Burnham JM, Fu FH. The anterolateral complex and anterolateral ligament of the knee. J Am Acad Orthop Sur. 2018;26(8):261–7.
69. Helito CP, Demange MK, Bonadio MB, Tírico LEP, Gobbi RG, Pécora JR, et al. Anatomy and histology of the knee anterolateral ligament. Orthop J Sports Med. 2013;1(7):2325967113513546.
70. Helito CP, Helito PVP, Costa HP, Bordalo-Rodrigues M, Pecora JR, Camanho GL, et al. MRI evaluation of the anterolateral ligament of the knee: assessment in routine 1.5-T scans. Skelet Radiol. 2014;43(10):1421–7.
71. Taneja AK, Miranda FC, Braga CA, Gill CM, Hartmann LG, Santos DC, et al. MRI features of the anterolateral ligament of the knee. Skelet Radiol. 2015;44(3):403–10.
72. Kosy JD, Mandalia VI, Anaspure R. Characterization of the anatomy of the anterolateral ligament of the knee using magnetic resonance imaging. Skelet Radiol. 2015;44(11):1647–53.
73. Van Dyck P, Clockaerts S, Vanhoenacker FM, Lambrecht V, Wouters K, De Smet E, et al. Anterolateral ligament abnormalities in patients with acute anterior cruciate ligament rupture are associated with lateral meniscal and osseous injuries. Eur Radiol. 2016;26(10):3383–91.
74. Claes S, Bartholomeeusen S, Bellemans J. High prevalence of anterolateral ligament abnormalities in magnetic resonance images of anterior cruciate ligament-injured knees. Acta Orthop Belg. 2014;80(1):45–9.
75. Helito CP, Helito PVP, Costa HP, Demange MK, Bordalo-Rodrigues M. Assessment of the anterolateral ligament of the knee by magnetic resonance imaging in acute injuries of the anterior cruciate ligament. Arthroscopy. 2017;33(1):140–6.
76. Cavaignac E, Wytrykowski K, Reina N, Pailhé R, Murgier J, Faruch M, et al. Ultrasonographic identification of the anterolateral ligament of the knee. Arthroscopy. 2016;32(1):120–6.
77. Capo J, Kaplan DJ, Fralinger DJ, Adler RS, Campbell KA, Jazrawi LM, et al. Ultrasonographic visualization and assessment of the anterolateral ligament. Knee Surg Sports Traumatol Arthrosc. 2017;25(10):3134–9.
78. Dodds A, Gupte C, Neyret P, Williams A, Amis A. Extra-articular techniques in anterior cruciate ligament reconstruction: a literature review. J Bone Joint Surg. 2011;93(11):1440–8.
79. Sonnery-Cottet B, Thaunat M, Freychet B, Pupim BH, Murphy CG, Claes S. Outcome of a combined anterior cruciate ligament and anterolateral ligament reconstruction technique with a minimum 2-year follow-up. Am J Sports Med. 2015;43(7):1598–605.
80. Lind M, Menhert F, Pedersen AB. Incidence and outcome after revision anterior cruciate ligament reconstruction: results from the Danish registry for knee ligament reconstructions. Am J Sports Med. 2012;40(7):1551–7.
81. James EW, Williams BT, LaPrade RF. Stress radiography for the diagnosis of knee ligament injuries: a systematic review. Clin Orthop Relat Res. 2014;472(9):2644–57.

Indications for Revision Anterior Cruciate Ligament Reconstruction

3

Alec Sundet, Evan Boyd, Patrick W. Joyner, and Nathan K. Endres

Introduction

Rupture of the anterior cruciate ligament (ACL) occurs in up to 250,000 patients each year in the United States [1]. Annually, 175,000 to 200,000 primary reconstructive procedures (ACL-R) are performed [2]. Failure of ACL-R, as defined by pathologic knee laxity or graft rupture, occurs in 2–6% of patients undergoing primary ACL-R [3, 4]. Risk factors for ACL-R failure include male gender, return to sport, use of allograft during the primary reconstruction, and age younger than 25 years [5–11]. When ACL-R fails, revision reconstruction is considered [12]. Satisfactory outcomes have been seen in 75–97% of patients undergoing ACL revision [13–15]. This chapter discusses the indications and contraindications for ACL revision reconstruction.

Indications

The indications for revision ACL reconstruction are listed in Table 3.1. It is important to note that not all patients experiencing a failed ACL reconstruction require ACL revision. The primary goal of a revision reconstruction is similar to a primary ACL reconstruction, that is, to restore functional stability to the knee. In addition to improving function, restoring knee stability protects the menisci and articular cartilage from injury.

Table 3.1 Indications for revision of failed ACL reconstruction

Early failure (<1 year)
Young patient (<25 years old)
Failed ACL-R in a high-level athlete in a high-risk cutting sport
Failed ACL-R with functional instability
Failed ACL-R in patient undergoing concomitant ligament reconstruction
Failed ACL-R in patient undergoing meniscal repair or transplant
Failed ACL-R in patient undergoing cartilage repair or restoration procedure

Failed ACL-R can be categorized as early (<1 year) or late (>1 year). Early failures frequently occur due to technical errors, failure of graft incorporation, premature return to activity, overly aggressive rehabilitation, or unrecognized concomitant injuries [8, 16–19]. Late (>1 year) failure is frequently associated with repeat trauma [7]. Knee instability resulting from ACL-R failure can lead to chondral injuries in both the tibiofemoral and patellofemoral compartments [7]. The Multicenter ACL Revision Study (MARS) group reported that 90% of knees undergoing

A. Sundet · E. Boyd · N. K. Endres (✉)
Department of Orthopaedics and Rehabilitation, The Robert Larner, M.D., College of Medicine at The University of Vermont, Burlington, VT, USA

P. W. Joyner
Orthocollier, Naples, FL, USA

M. J. Alaia, K. J. Jones (eds.), *Revision Anterior Cruciate Ligament Reconstruction*,
https://doi.org/10.1007/978-3-030-96996-7_3

revision ACL reconstruction had meniscal or chondral injury, with previous partial meniscectomy associated with a higher incidence of articular cartilage lesions [20]. ACL injury is associated with early-onset osteoarthritis [21–24]. Restoring knee stability, especially in the young, active patient with failed ACL-R, should be considered to potentially prevent further meniscal and chondral damage. Timing of revision reconstruction is a consideration. When compared to patients undergoing early revision (< 6 months), patients undergoing delayed revision (> 6 months) have a higher degree of articular cartilage damage [31].

In the athlete with a failed ACL-R, a discussion should be held regarding the chances of returning to sport and the difference between returning to sport and returning to preinjury level of activity. Although unpredictable, 49–75% of patients undergoing revision will return to some level of sport, but only 43% will return to their preinjury level of activity [32–34]. Return-to-sport rates are significantly lower when compared to return to sport following primary ACL-R [32]. However, revision ACL-R may yield the best chance of restoring knee stability [8] and provide athletes the best chance of return to competitive play.

Any patient with failed ACL-R undergoing meniscal repair or transplantation, articular cartilage repair or restorative procedures, or ligamentous reconstruction (PCL, PLC, PMC) should undergo concomitant or staged ACL revision reconstruction. Failing to address pathologic laxity related to ACL insufficiency significantly increases the likelihood of any of these procedures failing. [7, 25–30]

Contraindications

Several technical- and patient-related factors are associated with poorer outcomes and higher rates of failure after revision ACL reconstruction. Thus, it is important to identify these and consider them in surgical planning. A well-executed revision ACL that restores biomechanical stability may meet objective measures of success and yet still fail clinically. Firm contraindications to revision ACL surgery include active infection and significant knee stiffness/arthrofibrosis. The latter of the two is particularly relevant given that over 50% of patients undergoing revision ACL reconstruction report a history of trauma as the cause of their recurrent instability [2]. A summary of contraindications to revision ACL reconstruction are listed in Table 3.2.

Table 3.2 Contraindications for revision of failed ACL reconstruction

Active infection
Arthrofibrosis
Lower demand, older individual without functional instability
Patient unwilling/unable to comply with postoperative rehabilitation and precautions.
Morbid obesity
Advanced arthritis
Uncorrected malalignment
Unaddressed meniscal root tears/meniscal deficiency
Unaddressed pathologic laxity due to posterolateral corner, posteromedial corner, or PCL injuries
Unrealistic patient expectations
Regional pain syndromes

The goal of revision ACL surgery is restoration of functional knee stability, and the patient's goals should be clearly defined prior to the procedure. Older individuals with lower functional demands may not benefit from the procedure, especially if they are not having functional instability. Patients pursuing the procedure for pain-related purposes should be counseled accordingly, and this should be clearly addressed in any patient with symptomatic arthritis, obesity, or regional pain syndromes. Articular cartilage damage (grade 2 or greater) is independently associated with inferior clinical outcomes [10, 35]. Thus, regardless of the surgeon's technical skill and expertise, the presence of symptomatic chondrosis may negatively impact the final outcome.

At baseline, revision ACL surgery has 3–4 times the failure rate of primary ACL reconstruction and is associated with inferior clinical outcomes, including lower Cincinnati, Lysholm, Tegner, IKDC, and KOOS scores [36]. Therefore, patients with unrealistic functional expectations may be unhappy with the final result. In a similar fashion, surgeons should consider carefully any patient that might be unwilling or unable to comply with postoperative rehabilitation or surgical precautions.

Malalignment and concomitant ligamentous injury is a contraindication to revision ACL-R if not corrected prior to, or at the time of surgery. Varus malalignment causes graft strain [37] and potentially graft failure. In addition to coronal malalignment, sagittal malalignment (increased tibial slope) should be taken into account when planning a revision surgery. Unaddressed posterolateral and posteromedial corner injuries also places strain on the ACL graft which can lead to failure [37, 38] as does untreated meniscal injury or meniscal deficiency. Careful attention should be paid to the presence of meniscal root tears when considering a revision ACL-R. Meniscal deficiency in the setting of a failed primary ACL-R may be an indication for meniscal transplantation.

Illustrative Cases

Case 1 The patient is a 26-year-old male who underwent primary left ACL-R with patella tendon autograft. He returned to all activities, including competitive soccer at 9 months after surgery. Fourteen months after surgery, he re-injured his knee in a traumatic fashion playing soccer. Physical examination was consistent with ACL graft tear, which was confirmed by MRI. No meniscal tear or concomitant ligament injury was identified. He had symmetric, passive knee hyperextension. The etiology of graft failure was felt to be recurrent trauma, ligamentous laxity and increased tibial slope. Because of his desire to return to competitive soccer, he elected to proceed with revision ACL surgery. He underwent a single-stage revision ACL-R with contralateral patella tendon autograft and lateral extra-articular tenodesis (modified Lemaire procedure) (see Figs. 3.1 and 3.2).

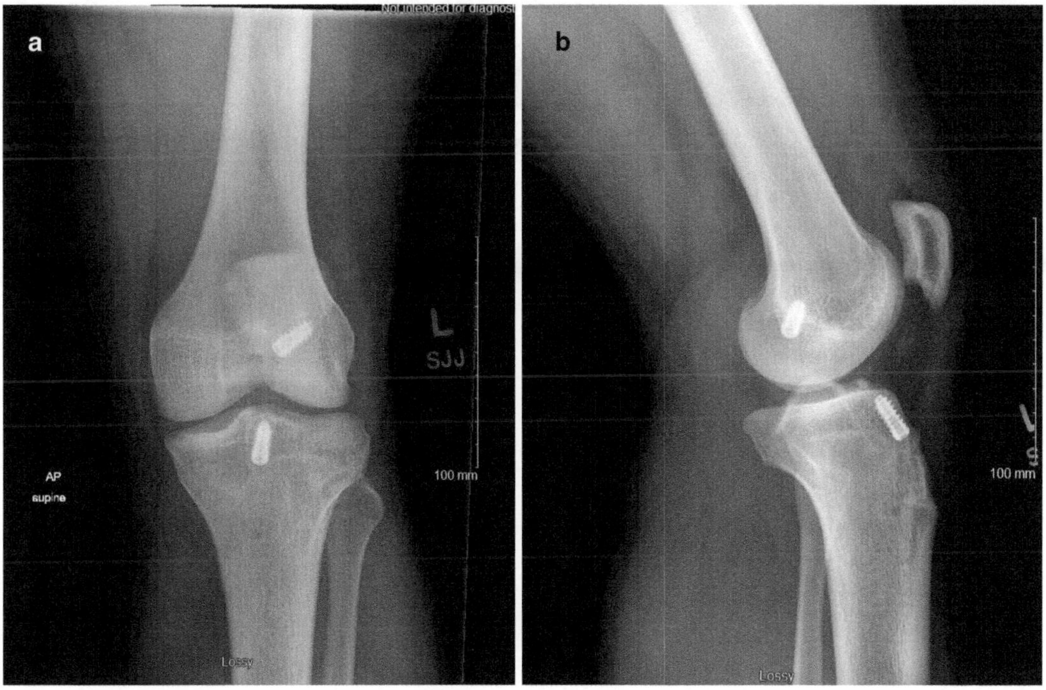

Fig. 3.1 AP (**a**) and lateral (**b**) preoperative radiographs of the left knee prior to ACL revision procedure

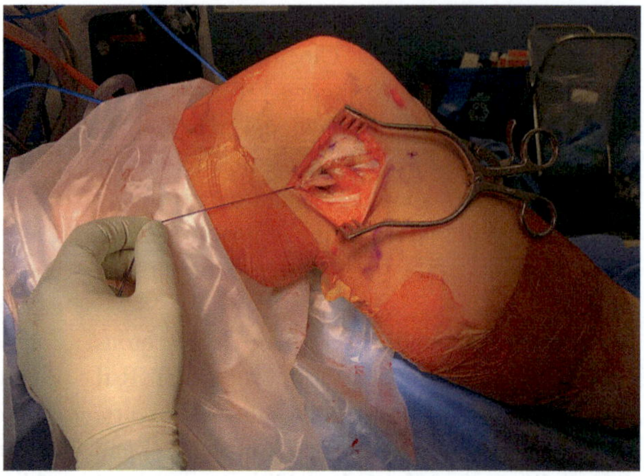

Fig. 3.2 Intraoperative image demonstrating the lateral extra-articular tenodesis with iliotibial band graft tunneled deep to the fibular collateral ligament

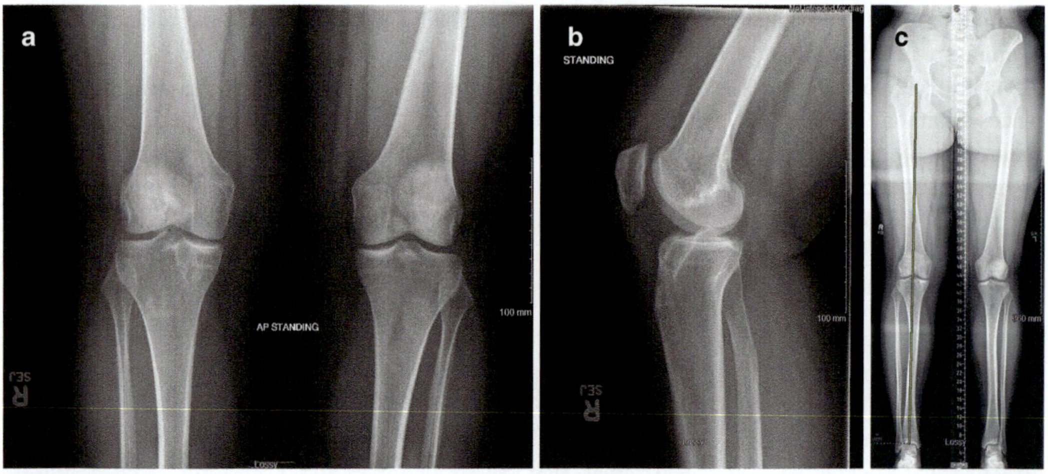

Fig. 3.3 Preoperative radiographs of AP view of bilateral knees (**a**), lateral of the right knee (**b**), and mechanical axis view demonstrating a neutral mechanical axis (**c**)

Case 2 The patient is a 25-year-old female with anterior knee pain and knee instability. She underwent an ACL-R with hamstring graft and partial lateral meniscectomy 8 years prior to presentation. She has had functional instability, including ADLs, since a minor ski injury 1 year ago. Physical examination was consistent with ACL insufficiency, including a high-grade pivot shift. Plain radiographs revealed no arthrosis or malalignment. MRI confirmed a chronic appearing ACL graft tear, lateral meniscus root tear, and vertical and longitudinal tear of the medial meniscus. The etiology of the graft failure was felt to be multifactorial and not related to recurrent trauma. Because of her functional instability, young age, and reparable meniscal tears, revision ACL-R was indicated and she elected to proceed. She underwent revision ACL-R with patella tendon autograft, lateral meniscus root repair, medial meniscus repair, and lateral extra-articular tenodesis (modified Lemaire procedure) (see Fig. 3.3).

References

1. Gianotti SM, Marshall SW, Hume PA, Bunt L. Incidence of anterior cruciate ligament injury and other knee ligament injuries: a national population-based study. J Sci Med Sport. 2009;12(6):622–7.
2. Wright RW, Huston LJ, Spindler KP, et al. Descriptive epidemiology of the Multicenter ACL Revision Study (MARS) cohort. Am J Sports Med. 2010;38(10):1979–86.
3. Freedman KB, D'Amato MJ, Nedeff DD, Kaz A, Bach BR Jr. Arthroscopic anterior cruciate ligament reconstruction: a metaanalysis comparing patellar tendon and hamstring tendon autografts. Am J Sports Med. 2003;31(1):2–11.
4. Yunes M, Richmond JC, Engels EA, Pinczewski LA. Patellar versus hamstring tendons in anterior cruciate ligament reconstruction: a meta-analysis. Arthroscopy. 2001;17(3):248–57.
5. Allen MM, Pareek A, Krych AJ, et al. Are female soccer players at an increased risk of second anterior cruciate ligament injury compared with their athletic peers? Am J Sports Med. 2016;44(10):2492–8.
6. Wright RW, Dunn WR, Amendola A, et al. Risk of tearing the intact anterior cruciate ligament in the contralateral knee and rupturing the anterior cruciate ligament graft during the first 2 years after anterior cruciate ligament reconstruction: a prospective MOON cohort study. Am J Sports Med. 2007;35(7):1131–4.
7. Chen JL, Allen CR, Stephens TE, et al. Differences in mechanisms of failure, intraoperative findings, and surgical characteristics between single- and multiple-revision ACL reconstructions: a MARS cohort study. Am J Sports Med. 2013;41(7):1571–8.
8. George MS, Dunn WR, Spindler KP. Current concepts review: revision anterior cruciate ligament reconstruction. Am J Sports Med. 2006;34(12): 2026–37.
9. Shelbourne KD, Gray T, Haro M. Incidence of subsequent injury to either knee within 5 years after anterior cruciate ligament reconstruction with patellar tendon autograft. Am J Sports Med. 2009;37(2):246–51.
10. Salmon LJ, Pinczewski LA, Russell VJ, Refshauge K. Revision anterior cruciate ligament reconstruction with hamstring tendon autograft: 5- to 9-year follow-up. Am J Sports Med. 2006;34(10):1604–14.
11. Kaeding CC, Aros B, Pedroza A, et al. Allograft versus autograft anterior cruciate ligament reconstruction: predictors of failure from a MOON prospective longitudinal cohort. Sports Health. 2011;3(1):73–81.
12. Osti L, Buda M, Osti R, Massari L, Maffulli N. Preoperative planning for ACL revision surgery. Sports Med Arthrosc Rev. 2017;25(1):19–29.
13. Chalmers PN, Mall NA, Moric M, et al. Does ACL reconstruction alter natural history?: a systematic literature review of long-term outcomes. J Bone Joint Surg Am. 2014;96(4):292–300.
14. Baer GS, Harner CD. Clinical outcomes of allograft versus autograft in anterior cruciate ligament reconstruction. Clin Sports Med. 2007;26(4):661–81.
15. Bach BR Jr. Revision anterior cruciate ligament surgery. Arthroscopy. 2003;19(Suppl 1):14–29.
16. Borchers JR, Kaeding CC, Pedroza AD, Huston LJ, Spindler KP, Wright RW. Intra-articular findings in primary and revision anterior cruciate ligament reconstruction surgery: a comparison of the MOON and MARS study groups. Am J Sports Med. 2011;39(9):1889–93.
17. Johnson DL, Swenson TM, Irrgang JJ, Fu FH, Harner CD. Revision anterior cruciate ligament surgery: experience from Pittsburgh. Clin Orthop Relat Res. 1996;325:100–9.
18. Uribe JW, Hechtman KS, Zvijac JE, Tjin ATEW. Revision anterior cruciate ligament surgery: experience from Miami. Clin Orthop Relat Res. 1996;325:91–9.
19. Harner CD, Giffin JR, Dunteman RC, Annunziata CC, Friedman MJ. Evaluation and treatment of recurrent instability after anterior cruciate ligament reconstruction. Instr Course Lect. 2001;50:463–74.
20. Brophy RH, Wright RW, David TS, et al. Association between previous meniscal surgery and the incidence of chondral lesions at revision anterior cruciate ligament reconstruction. Am J Sports Med. 2012;40(4):808–14.
21. Argentieri EC, Sturnick DR, DeSarno MJ, et al. Changes to the articular cartilage thickness profile of the tibia following anterior cruciate ligament injury. Osteoarthr Cartil. 2014;22(10):1453–60.
22. Chaudhari AM, Briant PL, Bevill SL, Koo S, Andriacchi TP. Knee kinematics, cartilage morphology, and osteoarthritis after ACL injury. Med Sci Sports Exerc. 2008;40(2):215–22.
23. von Porat A, Roos EM, Roos H. High prevalence of osteoarthritis 14 years after an anterior cruciate ligament tear in male soccer players: a study of radiographic and patient relevant outcomes. Ann Rheum Dis. 2004;63(3):269–73.
24. Gillquist J, Messner K. Anterior cruciate ligament reconstruction and the long-term incidence of gonarthrosis. Sports Med. 1999;27(3):143–56.
25. Indelicato PA, Bittar ES. A perspective of lesions associated with ACL insufficiency of the knee. A review of 100 cases. Clin Orthop Relat Res. 1985;198:77–80.
26. Allen CR, Wong EK, Livesay GA, Sakane M, Fu FH, Woo SL. Importance of the medial meniscus in the anterior cruciate ligament-deficient knee. J Orthop Res. 2000;18(1):109–15.
27. Osti L, Del Buono A, Maffulli N. Anterior medial meniscal root tears: a novel arthroscopic all inside repair. Transl Med UniSa. 2015;12:41–6.
28. Meniscal and articular cartilage predictors of clinical outcome after revision anterior cruciate ligament reconstruction. Am J Sports Med. 2016;44(7):1671–9.
29. Kamath GV, Redfern JC, Greis PE, Burks RT. Revision anterior cruciate ligament reconstruction. Am J Sports Med. 2011;39(1):199–217.
30. Zantop T, Schumacher T, Diermann N, Schanz S, Raschke MJ, Petersen W. Anterolateral rotational knee

instability: role of posterolateral structures. Winner of the AGA-DonJoy Award 2006. Arch Orthop Trauma Surg. 2007;127(9):743–52.
31. Ohly NE, Murray IR, Keating JF. Revision anterior cruciate ligament reconstruction: timing of surgery and the incidence of meniscal tears and degenerative change. J Bone Joint Surg Br. 2007;89(8):1051–4.
32. Lefevre N, Klouche S, Mirouse G, Herman S, Gerometta A, Bohu Y. Return to sport after primary and revision anterior cruciate ligament reconstruction: a prospective comparative study of 552 patients from the FAST cohort. Am J Sports Med. 2017;45(1):34–41.
33. Battaglia MJ 2nd, Cordasco FA, Hannafin JA, et al. Results of revision anterior cruciate ligament surgery. Am J Sports Med. 2007;35(12):2057–66.
34. Andriolo L, Filardo G, Kon E, et al. Revision anterior cruciate ligament reconstruction: clinical outcome and evidence for return to sport. Knee Surg Sports Traumatol Arthrosc. 2015;23(10):2825–45.
35. Group M. Predictors of clinical outcome following revision anterior cruciate ligament reconstruction. J Orthop Res. 2020;38(6):1191–203.
36. Wright RW, Gill CS, Chen L, et al. Outcome of revision anterior cruciate ligament reconstruction: a systematic review. J Bone Joint Surg Am. 2012;94(6):531–6.
37. Noyes FR, Barber-Westin SD, Hewett TE. High tibial osteotomy and ligament reconstruction for varus angulated anterior cruciate ligament-deficient knees. Am J Sports Med. 2000;28(3):282–96.
38. Getelman MH, Friedman MJ. Revision anterior cruciate ligament reconstruction surgery. J Am Acad Orthop Surg. 1999;7(3):189–98.

4 Graft Options in the Revision ACL Setting

Darren S. Nabor, Christopher J. Tucker, and Brian R. Waterman

Introduction

Revision anterior cruciate ligament (ACL) reconstruction is indicated for management of failed primary reconstruction in an active patient population, as this can restore stability and facilitate reliable rates of return to sport between 56% and 100% in a recent systematic review [1–3]. Graft selection in revision ACL reconstruction can be complex, as previous surgery and concomitant pathology can have significant repercussions on surgical decision-making and subsequent outcomes [4]. Graft availability may be limited in the revision setting and frequently depends on previous graft use, retained implants or hardware, and relative tunnel placement. It is important to consider each patient's functional goals as well as their demographics (i.e., age, sex, and activity level) and anatomic variables (i.e., patella height, sagittal and coronal alignment, muscle strength and coordination). An awareness of the merits and disadvantages of each respective graft option is important for ultimate revision graft selection.

D. S. Nabor
Department of Orthopaedic Surgery, Wake Forest University, Winston-Salem, NC, USA

C. J. Tucker
Department of Orthopaedic Surgery, Walter Reed National Military Medical Center, Bethesda, MD, USA

B. R. Waterman (✉)
Department of Orthopaedic Surgery, Wake Forest Baptist Health, Winston-Salem, NC, USA

Patellar Bone-Tendon-Bone Graft

Patellar bone-tendon-bone (BTB) autograft has long been considered the traditional gold standard in ACL reconstruction surgery, and the advantages have been well documented including a strong graft, direct osseous healing, and faster incorporation times. Accordingly, young competitive athletes remain the ideal candidates for BTB in the revision scenario. In patients with a previous hamstring tendon (HT) or free quadriceps tendon (QT) autograft harvest, utilization of an ipsilateral BTB may serve as a reasonable option, especially among the younger athletic population. During revision ACL reconstruction, the tibial bone harvest can also be customized to a larger size in order to address osteolysis or widened tunnels while also obtaining rigid aperture screw fixation. The disadvantages to using BTB in ACL revision are similar to that seen with its use during primary reconstruction, primarily rates of anterior knee pain or crepitation, osteoarthritis of the knee, and patella fracture [5, 6]. In patients with previous QT autograft harvest and persistent extensor weakness, consideration of an ipsilateral BTB may cause a "second hit" phenomenon to the extensor mechanism.

M. J. Alaia, K. J. Jones (eds.), *Revision Anterior Cruciate Ligament Reconstruction*,
https://doi.org/10.1007/978-3-030-96996-7_4

Initially popularized by Shelbourne for primary ACL reconstruction, contralateral BTB grafts have been used to facilitate greater parity in side-to-side strength without significant complications [7]. One must consider the potential harvest site morbidity to the contralateral extremity and take this into consideration during rehabilitation and recovery times for high-level athletes. Given the comparatively decreased rates of re-rupture in the young athletic population, the benefits of harvesting a contralateral BTB graft, including early bone-to-bone healing, customizable graft size, and low rates of soft tissue creep, may outweigh the disadvantages with bilateral lower extremity rehabilitation.

While repeated ipsilateral BTB harvesting after primary autologous BTB reconstruction has been reported, the data supporting its use is scarce. Prior advanced imaging studies have shown reconstitution of the central third of the BTB donor site, but the histologic composition at the tendon-bone interface largely reflects scar tissue rather than a traditional enthesis with four distinct zones of transition. There are limited reports from Europe detailing successful re-harvesting of BTB 4 years after primary reconstruction [8], but ipsilateral re-harvest of the BTB for ACL revision has been associated with inferior short- and long-term patient-reported outcomes [9, 10]. Based on these findings, this graft often is not recommended for ACL revision reconstruction.

Case 1

A 14-year-old male sustained a non-contact injury while playing football. He noted immediate pain and inability to bear weight and presented with a large effusion and positive 2B Lachman and grade I pivot shift exam. Radiographs revealed skeletal immaturity with open physes and ill-defined tibial tubercle apophysis. MRI was consistent with a right ACL intra-substance tear. He underwent a five-strand, HT autograft ACL reconstruction using a hybrid "physeal kind" technique with physeal-sparing, outside-in drilling of the femur, and central transphyseal tibial drilling. Suspensory fixation was utilized on the femoral side, and bio-composite screw fixation was employed on the tibial side with backup staple fixation (Fig. 4.1). Rehabilitation was successful, and the patient was

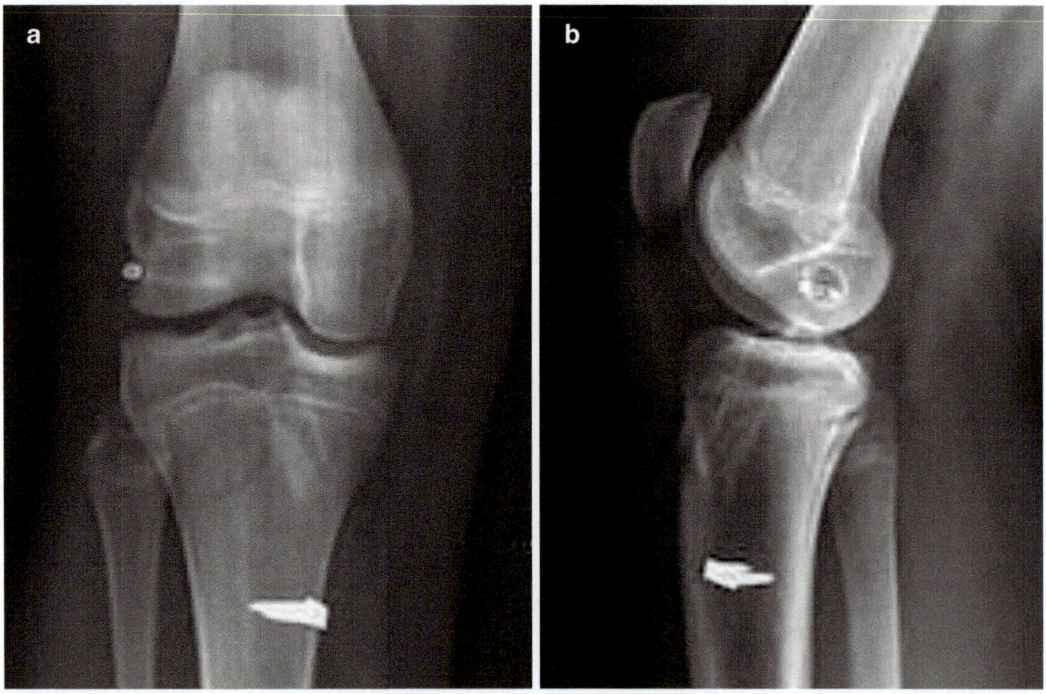

Fig. 4.1 (**a**) AP view (**b**) Lateral view status post primary HT ACL reconstruction

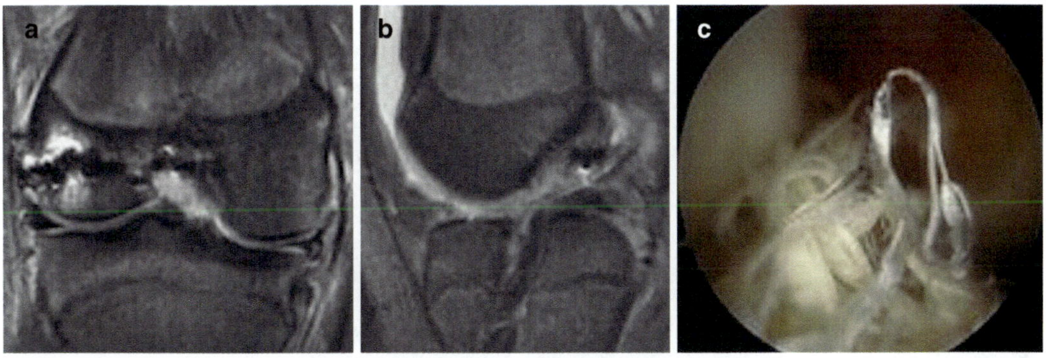

Fig. 4.2 (**a**) Coronal MRI (**b**) Sagittal MRI (**c**) Arthroscopic imaging of ACL graft failure

able to return to sport after comprehensive functional testing by physical therapy.

At approximately 10 months postoperatively, he sustained a twisting injury playing basketball and sustained a complete mid-substance graft tear (Fig. 4.2). Given his young age and multisport involvement, revision ACL reconstruction was recommended.

When considering graft selection for this patient, several factors were considered including his young age, involvement in competitive level 1 cutting and pivoting sports, and recent physeal closure. Given these risk factors, autograft was selected given the higher failure rates with allograft, with discussion between ipsilateral BTB or QT. Previous tunnel location and assessment for minimal widening were also considered.

Given the previous physeal-sparing-femoral tunnel, we elected for use of ipsilateral BTB graft with new divergent femoral tunnel across the physeal scar (so-called funnel technique), while the primary tibial tunnel was drilled until encountering healthy metaphyseal bone with punctate bleeding, with the use of a larger diameter bone block for optimal fill. The tunnel walls were found to be competent, and the BTB autograft was deployed and subsequently fixated with metallic interference screws on both sides (Fig. 4.3). Given his high-grade pivot shift and prior autograft failure, an extra-articular iliotibial band (ITB) tenodesis was also performed using the modified Lemaire technique. He successfully completed rehabilitation with objective return to sport testing and was able to return to football at 10 months after his revision BTB ACL reconstruction. He has remained stable without re-injury at approximately 3 years follow-up.

Hamstring Tendon Graft

HT autograft is commonly used in primary ACL reconstruction with favorable results [11], although there can be wide variability in preparation techniques and fixation constructs. In patients with previous BTB or QT autograft, harvesting an ipsilateral or contralateral HT remains a potential option. The advantages are similar to primary reconstruction including smaller incisions and less perioperative donor site morbidity, specifically less kneeling pain as compared to BTB. Fixation strength may be less than BTB, and caution is advised in females due to concerns about compromise of the posterior kinetic chain, residual hamstring weakness with loss of secondary stabilizers, and slightly higher risk of re-rupture. Traditionally, surgeons have also exercised caution to avoid HT autografts in athletes who compete in high-flexion (e.g., wrestling, hurdling) or hamstring-dominant sports such as skiing or soccer, although there is little evidence to support this theory. In contradistinction to primary ACL reconstruction, similar out-

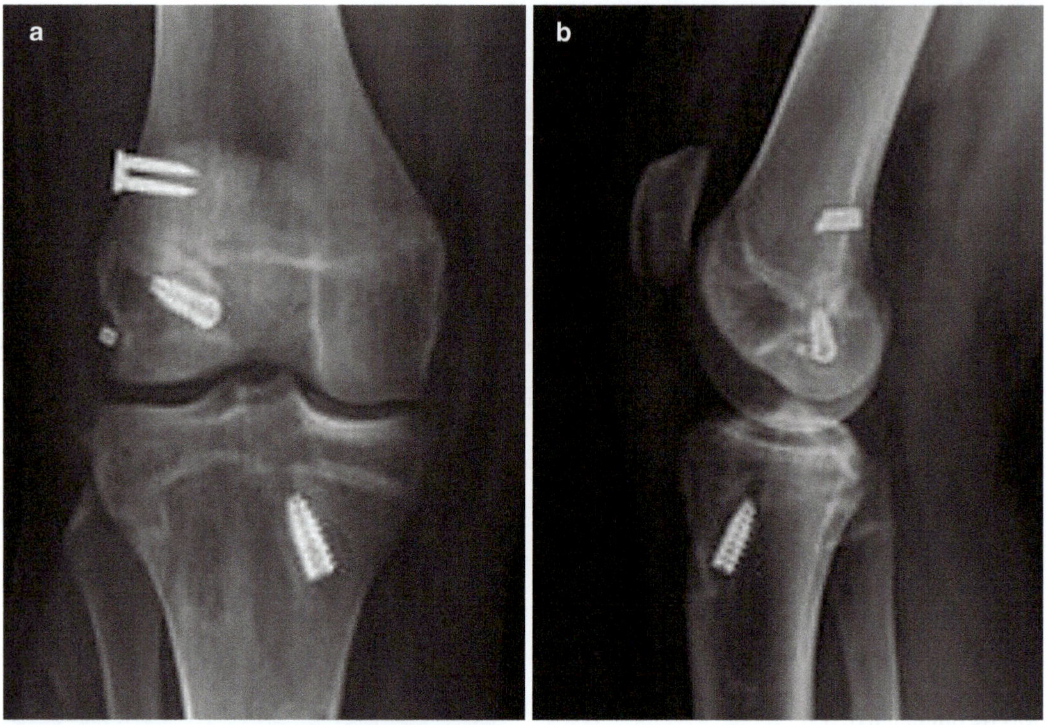

Fig. 4.3 (**a**) AP view (**b**) Lateral view status post ACL revision reconstruction with BTB autograft

comes and graft rupture rates between HT and BTB autograft in the revision setting have been shown across numerous large-scale database studies [2]. A recent meta-analysis showed patients treated with BTB autograft had inferior objective IKDC grades compared with HT autograft and non-irradiated allografts presumably from increased donor site morbidity in the BTB group [12].

Studies on contralateral HT harvest for ACL revision report this as a feasible option with similar clinical and patient-reported outcomes compared with ipsilateral HT harvest and allograft [13, 14]. While a valid option, caution should be taken in young females due to elevated risk of a contralateral ACL rupture secondary to hamstring weakness at index ACL surgery [15]. The ideal candidates for HT autograft are active patients without evidence of hyperlaxity, those seeking to avoid donor site morbidity associated with other graft options, and those objecting to allograft use.

Case 2

An 18-year-old male NCAA Division 1 offensive lineman sustained a non-contact twisting injury to his right knee. He presented with a large effusion and positive 2B Lachman and grade 1 pivot shift exam. Plain film radiographs of his right knee were unremarkable, and MRI was consistent with complete mid-substance ACL tear. He underwent a right ACL reconstruction with BTB autograft using suspensory fixation on the femur and a metal interference screw on the tibia (Fig. 4.4).

He was able to return to Division 1 football activity; however, 2 years after his primary reconstruction, he sustained a second non-contact twisting injury during a game. His exam was consistent with re-rupture of the BTB graft, which was confirmed with MRI (Fig. 4.5). Given his young age and goals to return to Division 1 football, revision ACL reconstruction was recommended.

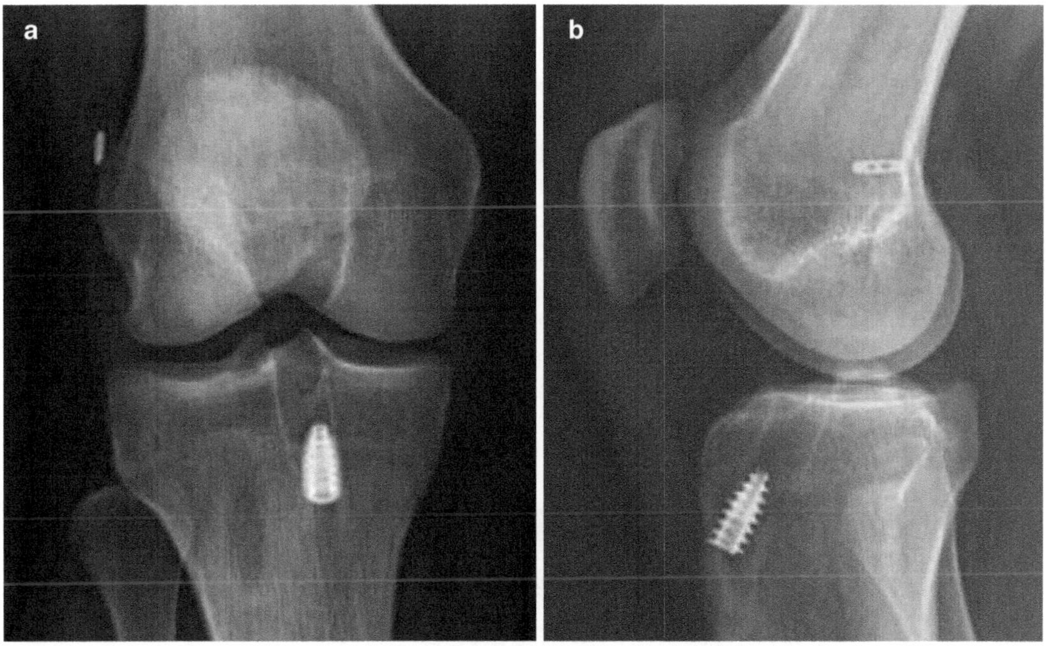

Fig. 4.4 (**a**) AP view (**b**) Lateral view status post primary BTB ACL reconstruction

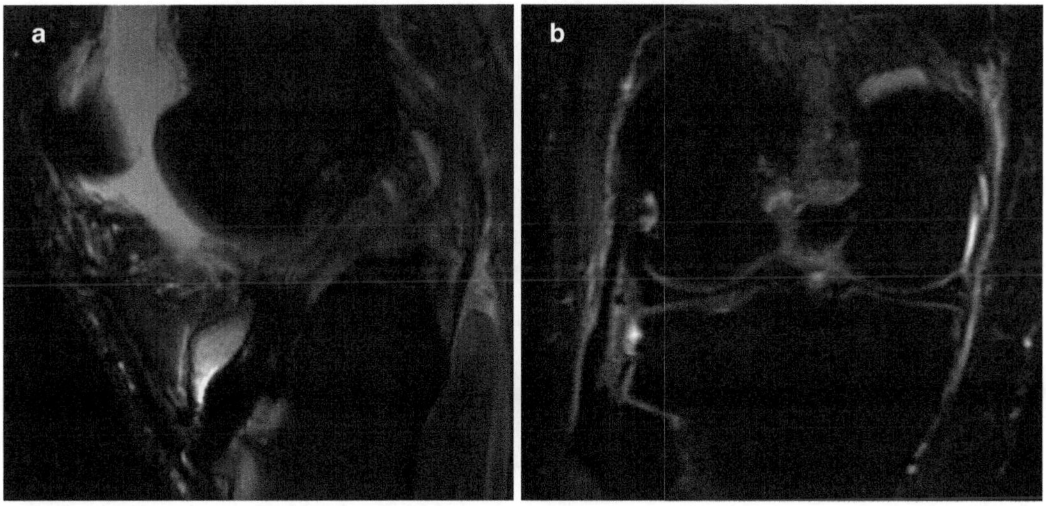

Fig. 4.5 (**a**) Sagittal MRI (**b**) Coronal MRI cuts of ACL graft failure

When considering graft selection for this patient, several factors were considered including his young age and involvement in high-level intercollegiate cutting and pivoting athletics. In view of these variables, autograft was selected, with deliberation between ipsilateral HT or QT. Contralateral BTB was also discussed with the athlete; however, he wished to avoid donor site morbidity to his healthy, unaffected extremity. Given the previous non-anatomic femoral tunnel location and minimal widening, HT autograft was selected for the revision reconstruction.

At the time of revision, an all-inside technique was utilized. The semitendinosus and gracilis grafts were harvested from the ipsilateral knee and fashioned to a four-strand 10-mm diameter. The femoral and tibial tunnels were reamed with an outside-in technique. The previous bone plugs from the primary reconstruction were completely consolidated with no tunnel widening. The tibial metal interference screw was removed to ream the tibial tunnel to healthy metaphyseal bone. The tunnel walls were found to be competent, and the HT autograft was deployed and subsequently secured with suspensory fixation on both sides (Fig. 4.6). He successfully completed rehabilitation with objective return to sport testing and was able to return to football 10 months after his revision HT ACL reconstruction.

Quadriceps Tendon Graft

The quadriceps tendon (QT) has gained increasing attention as an option for both primary and revision ACL reconstruction. Given its larger average graft thickness, the QT can be harvested with or without a bone block and either using two or three layers of the QT. The thickness of the QT has been measured to be an average of 18 mm in males and 16 mm in females [16, 17]. This thickness is compared with a thickness of less than 6 mm for normal BTB grafts [16–18]. The intra-articular volume of harvested QT has also been found to be 87.5% greater than harvested BTB,

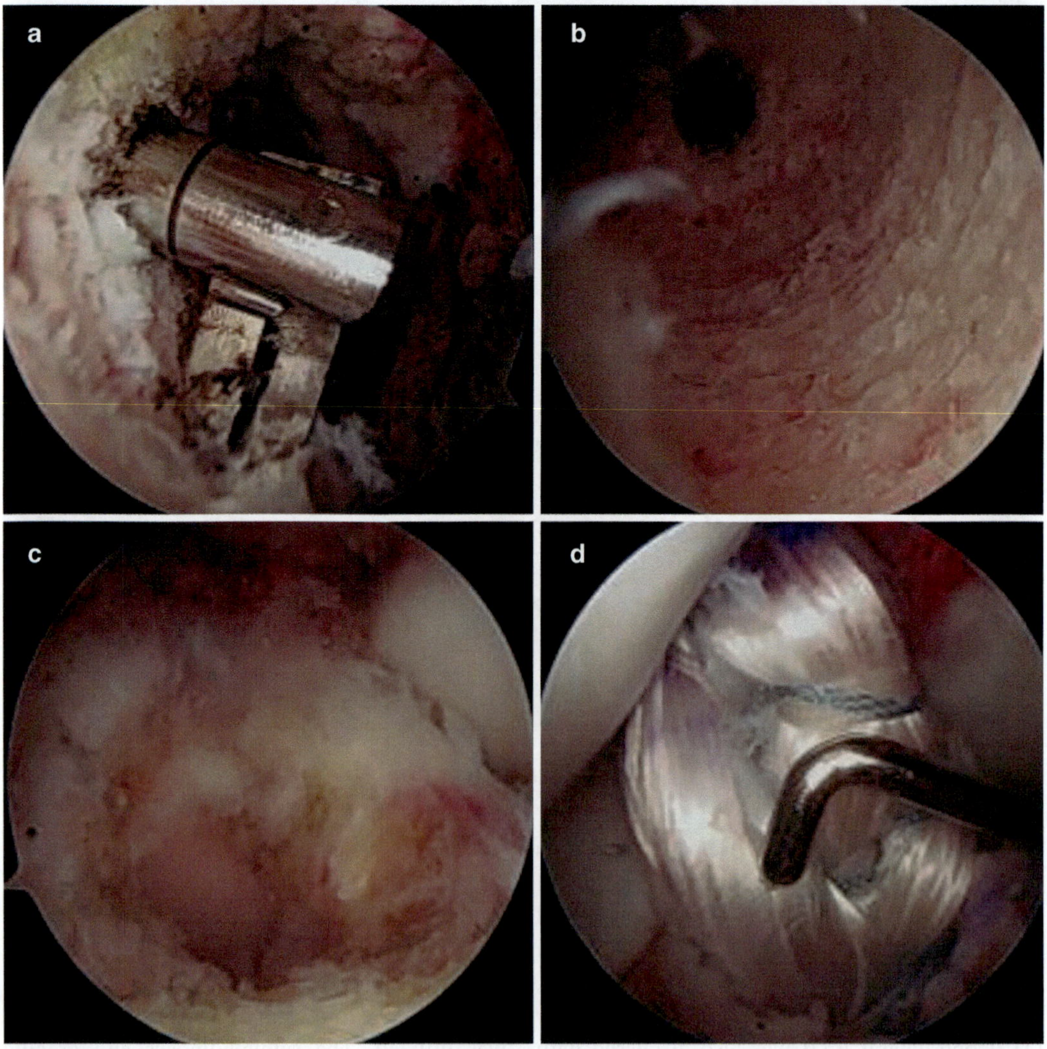

Fig. 4.6 (**a**) Arthroscopic imaging of retrograde reamer (femur) (**b**) Femoral tunnel (**c**) Tibial tunnel (**d**) HT autograft

and after the harvest, there was significantly more QT remaining than BTB [18]. Similar to the BTB bone plug, a quadriceps bone block can also be used to augment bone loss from widened tunnels with the possibility of less donor site morbidity. In addition to robust tissue volume, the QT has lower donor site morbidity and equivalent outcomes to other autograft types [19–21].

A recent study compared ipsilateral QT with contralateral HT autograft for ACL revision and found no differences in revision rates, postoperative knee joint stability, or patient-reported outcomes [22]. Utilizing a contralateral QT autograft is also an option; however, there is little literature regarding this option. As with any contralateral autograft, the primary reservations often center around the potential donor site morbidity to the uninvolved extremity. Younger athletic patients, particularly those with open physes, patella alta, or pre-existing anterior knee pain or patellar tendinopathy, are among the ideal candidates for QT autografts.

Case 3

A 17-year-old male with previous history of left HT autograft ACL reconstruction sustained a non-contact twisting injury during a high school football game. He felt immediate pain and swelling. Pivot shit and Lachman examination were positive, and MRI confirmed re-rupture of the HT autograft with prior anatomic tunnel position. Given his young age and wish to continue competitive high-demand sports, revision ACL reconstruction was recommended.

Interestingly the patient also had evidence of patella alta with a large patellar tendon enthesophyte at the inferior pole of the patella (Fig. 4.7). Given his age and commitment to play collegiate football, QT autograft was recommended in order to prevent concerns related to graft tunnel mismatch or pre-existing tendinopathy. His previous surgery was performed with suspensory fixation on both the femur and tibia. A QT autograft with patellar bone block was considered for modest tunnel widening due to the previous soft tissue graft. Alternatively, QT could also be harvested without the bone block if one was more comfortable with soft tissue fixation and tunnel lysis was not a concern. Relative contraindications to BTB in this case included pre-existing enthesopathy with large accessory ossicle and patella alta (Insall-Salvati index 1.5).

At the time of surgery, the central third 10 × 70 mm of the QT was harvested taking a 10 × 20 mm bone block (Fig. 4.8). An over-the-top femoral footprint guide and tibial guide were used to create a 10-mm and 10.5-mm tunnel, respectively, after sequential tunnel dilation.

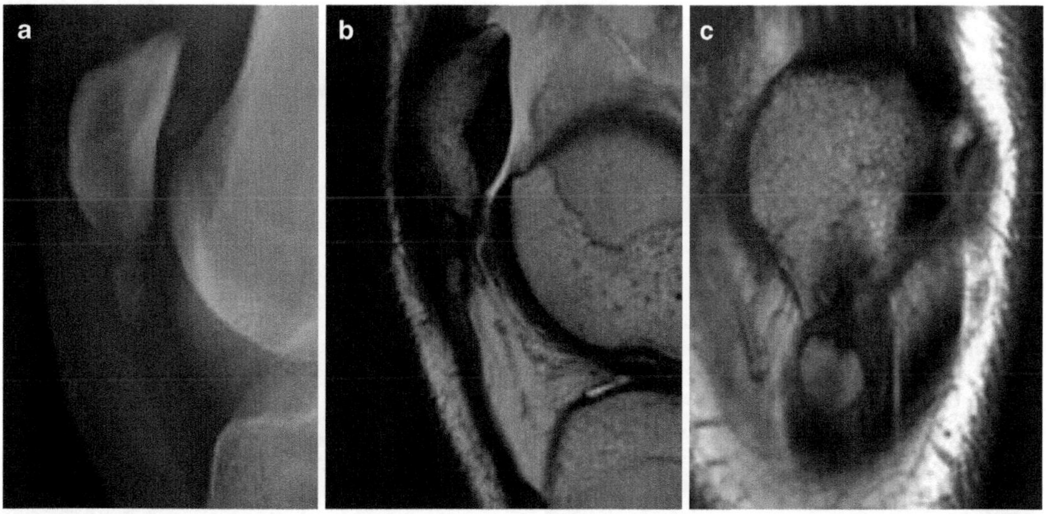

Fig. 4.7 (**a**) Lateral X-ray (**b**) Sagittal MRI (**c**) Coronal MRI showing enthesophyte at inferior pole of patella

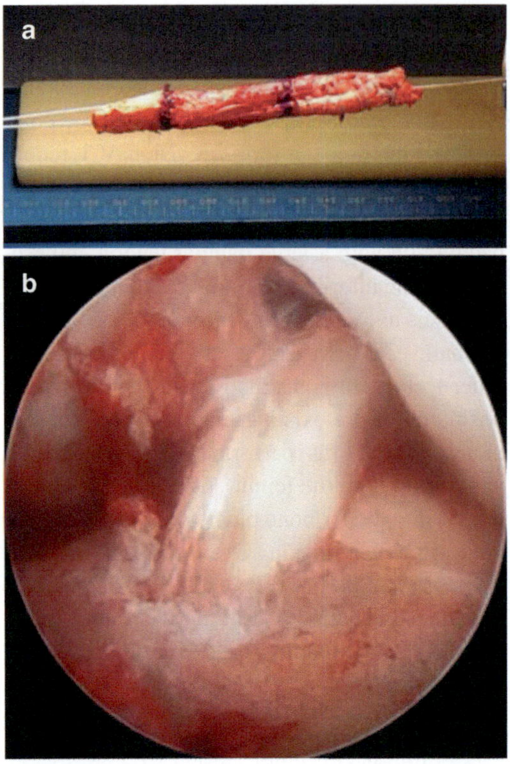

Fig. 4.8 (**a**) QT autograft after harvest (**b**) QT autograft after fixation

Careful scrutiny and direct "tunneloscopy" revealed a competent back wall with surrounding healthy reamed bone devoid of prior graft tissue. The QT graft was then deployed with the bone plug on the femoral side and soft tissue end towards the tibia (Fig. 4.9). After tapping, two PEEK interference screws were then placed in the femur and tibia, with sizes 7 mm and 10 mm utilized, respectively (Fig. 4.9).

By nearly 10 months postoperatively, the patient had a successful rehabilitation with no donor site morbidity, residual strength deficits, or limitations in terminal range of motion, and he has been able to return to competitive sport.

Allograft

Unlike primary ACL reconstruction, graft choice during revision cases can be limited by prior autograft use. Among these, numerous allograft options exist for revision ACL reconstruction and may offer the advantages of shorter operative times, smaller incisions, single- or two-staged reconstruction, and ability to obviate

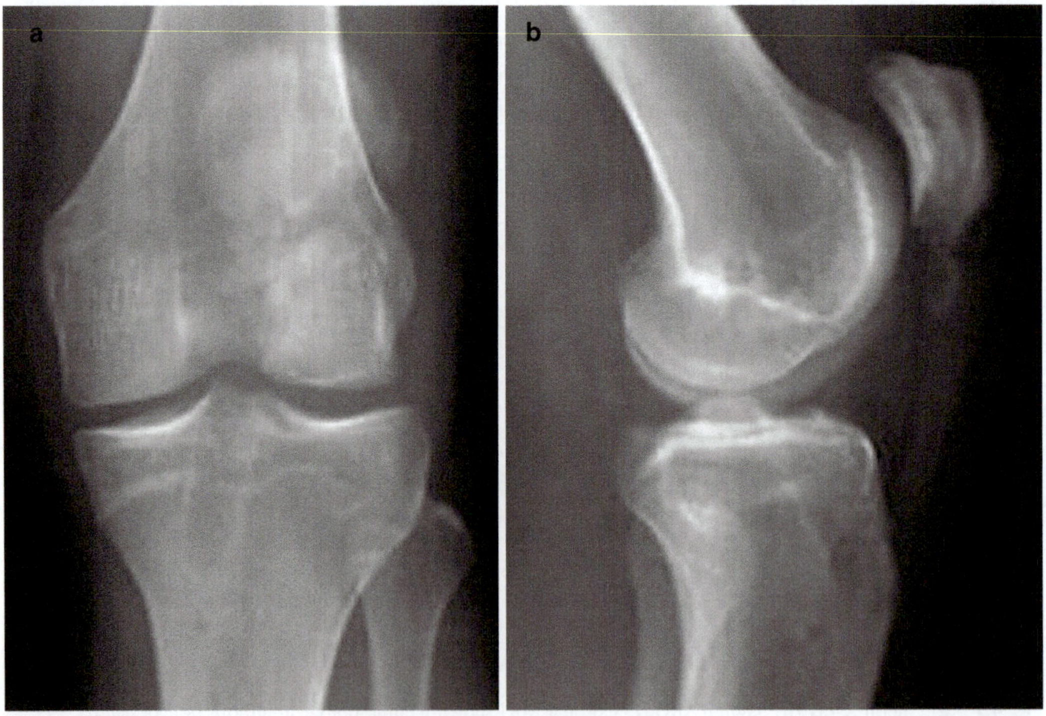

Fig. 4.9 (**a**) AP view (**b**) Lateral view status post revision QT ACL reconstruction

donor site morbidity. BTB, HT, posterior tibialis (PT), and Achilles allografts are commonly used in the revision setting. Use of a larger allograft, such as an Achilles allograft and hemi-patellar (or whole tendon) allograft, can allow for customization of bone block sizing to accommodate larger tunnel diameters seen with prior interference screw fixation, tunnel osteolysis, or subtle tunnel malposition. However, the disadvantages need to be dually considered, including longer incorporation times, potential disease transmission, and higher cost. It has been well documented that younger patients experience disproportionally higher re-rupture rates during revision surgery with allograft use [4, 12]. Several large-scale studies have also reported up to four times higher failure rates for primary [23] and two times higher in the revision setting [24]. Conversely, patients of increased age (i.e., >40 years) and/or lower physical demands are more appropriate candidates for allograft, and their use should be used with caution in young competitive athletes.

Furthermore, tissue processing and sterilization of allografts also must be taken into consideration. Several studies have demonstrated that non-irradiated and fresh allografts have similar failure rates to autograft. Conversely, there is a corresponding higher rate of failure in irradiated allografts, even at lower doses [4, 12, 25]. A systematic review compared autograft to non-chemically treated and non-irradiated allograft tissue during primary ACL reconstruction. The authors noted no differences between the two groups in terms of Lysholm scores, IKDC scores, Lachman examinations, pivot shift testing, KT-1000 measurements, or failure rates [25]. In addition, another group evaluated 5986 primary ACL reconstruction cases and found the use of BioCleanse and graft irradiation of >1.8 Mrad were associated with a higher risk of revision when compared with all other methods of processing [26]. A recent meta-analysis including 32 studies looked at outcomes of revision ACL reconstruction, comparing the use of autograft and irradiated (2.5 mRad; 2 studies) and non-irradiated allograft (7 studies) [12]. Autografts exhibited better outcomes than allografts, with lower postoperative laxity and rates of complication and reoperations. However, outcomes were similar between autografts and allografts after exclusion of irradiated allografts.

One of the goals of the Multicenter ACL Revision Study (MARS) cohort was to determine if revision ACL graft choice predicts outcomes related to sports function, activity level, OA symptoms, graft re-rupture, and reoperation at 2 years following revision [4]. In this study, 1205 patients underwent revision ACL reconstruction at a mean age of 26 years old, and the distribution of graft selection was 48% autograft, 49% allograft, and 3% hybrid autograft/allograft. The use of autograft predicted improved score on the IKDC, KOOS subscale Sports and Recreation, and KOOS subscale Quality of Life. Importantly, the use of an autograft resulted in patients 2.8 times less likely to sustain a subsequent graft rupture than if an allograft was utilized. No differences were noted in re-rupture or patient-reported outcomes between soft tissue and BTB autografts.

Case 4

A 42-year-old male sustained a twisting injury at work and felt immediate pain and swelling. His exam was consistent with a left ACL tear which was confirmed with MRI. He underwent soft tissue allograft ACL reconstruction via a trans-tibial technique by an outside surgeon with suspensory fixation on the femur and bioabsorbable screw on the tibia (Fig. 4.10). He was able to rehabilitate his knee and return to recreational sports; however, while playing basketball he sustained a twisting injury and was diagnosed with a re-tear of his allograft ACL reconstruction.

Given his age and activity goals, it was recommended he undergo revision ACL reconstruction. His goals were to return to recreational sports including basketball and running. Preoperative imaging was obtained including MRI and CT scan to evaluate for tunnel widening (Fig. 4.11). The MRI revealed complete rupture of the allograft, and CT scan revealed tunnel widening of approximately 14 mm on the tibial side and 12 mm on the femoral side. Given this information it was determined the revision would be

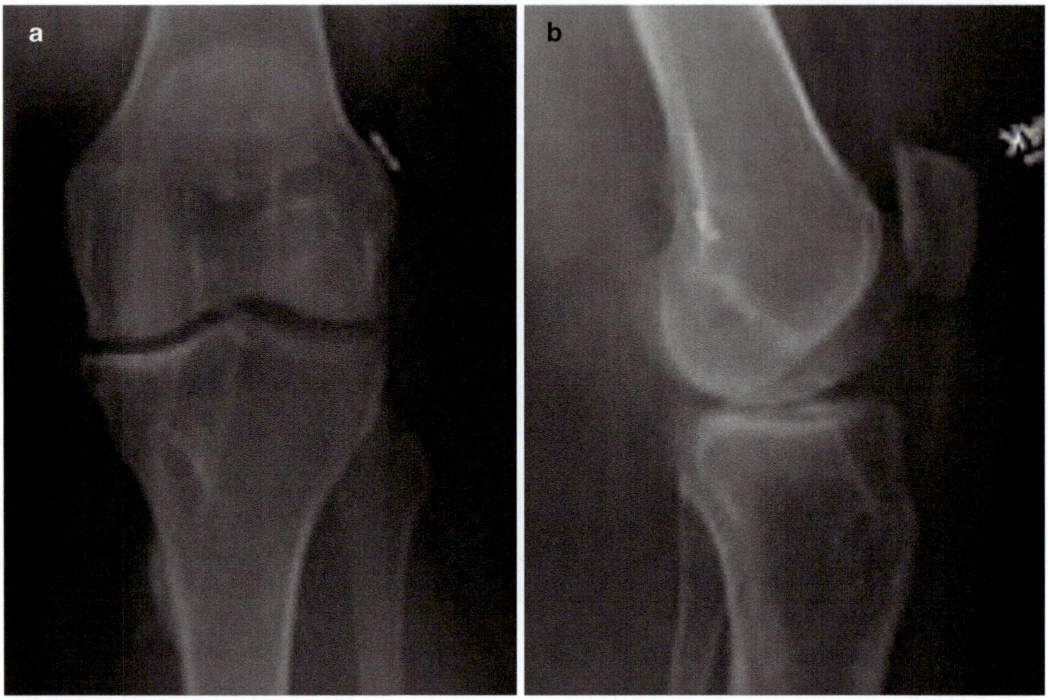

Fig. 4.10 (**a**) AP view (**b**) Lateral view status post primary allograft HT ACL reconstruction

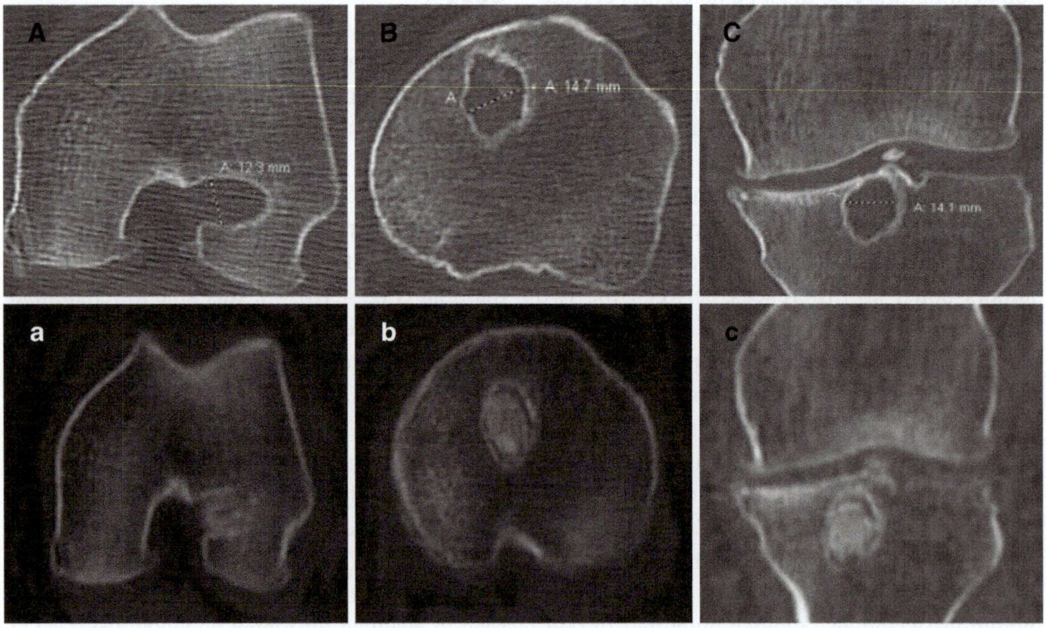

Fig. 4.11 (**A**) Axial CT (femur) (**B**) Axial CT (tibia) (**C**) Coronal CT pre-bone grafting. (**a**) Axial CT (femur) (**b**) Axial CT (tibia) (**c**) Coronal CT post-bone grafting

staged with bone grafting of the defects followed by revision ACL reconstruction.

Taking into consideration the patient's age, activity goals, and previous surgical confounders including tunnel widening, allograft was selected for the revision reconstruction. In choosing between the multiple allograft options, BTB was selected to allow for the possibility of utilizing the bone block to fill any residual tunnel widening and obtain secure fixation with screws.

At the time of surgery, both the femoral and tibial bone grafts had consolidated. With an anteromedial portal technique, an over-the-top footprint guide was utilized for the femur, and a 10 mm socket was reamed. The tibial guide was then used to ream a tunnel in anatomic position. A BTB allograft was then deployed into the tunnels with good fit, and metal screws were then placed with excellent purchase (Figs. 4.12 and 4.13). His postoperative course including reha-

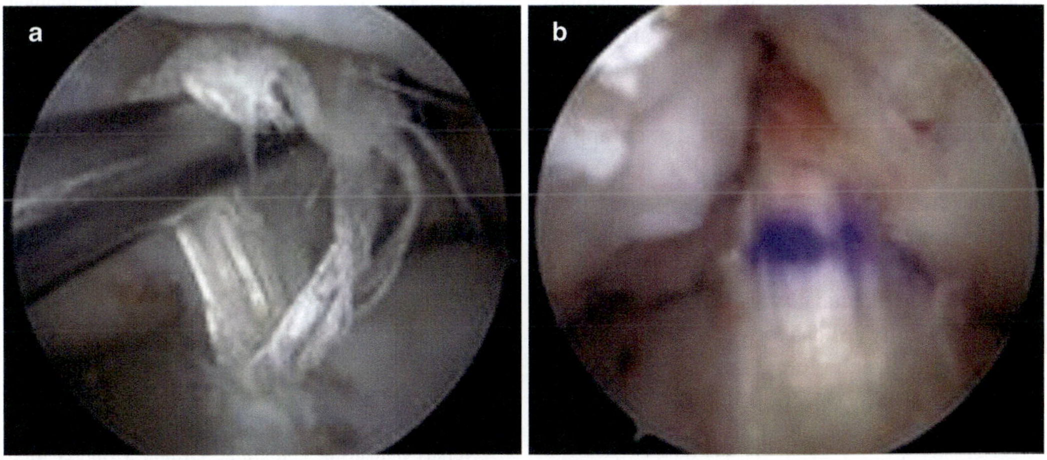

Fig. 4.12 (**a**) Arthroscopic image of failed primary ACL reconstruction (**b**) Revision BTB allograft reconstruction

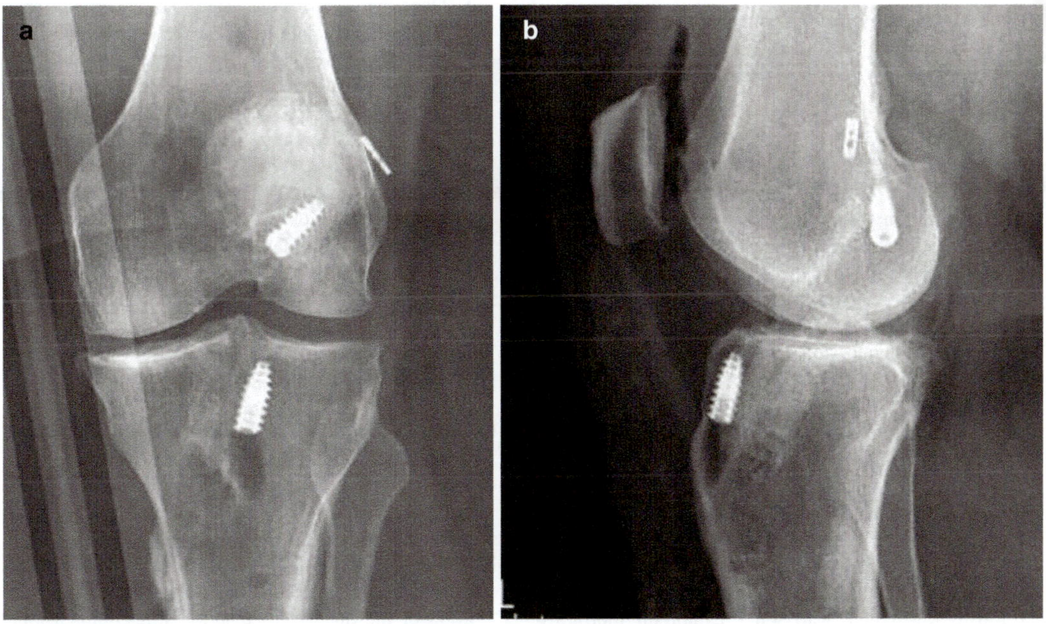

Fig. 4.13 (**a**) AP view (**b**) Lateral view status post BTB allograft revision reconstruction

bilitation was successful, and he has been able to return to activities of daily living and recreational athletics without further instability.

Conclusion

In summary, there are multiple options for graft selection during revision ACL reconstruction, with numerous relative advantages and limitations. In planning for revision ACL surgery, consideration of technical aspects of primary reconstruction, risk factors for failure, and unique patient-specific variables is critical during this decision-making process to ensure an optimal outcome. In addition to patient demographics, one must also evaluate factors such as prior surgical procedures, prior graft use, presence of tunnel widening, previous fixation methods, and patient goals with anticipated future level of activity. Ultimately, a technically well-performed ACL reconstruction is critical for early graft remodeling, function, and longer-term survivorship, regardless of graft selection. However, in many cases, graft selection can impact patient-reported outcomes and surgical success rates, and preoperative planning is essential for appropriate graft selection.

References

1. Ahn JH, Lee YS, Ha HC. Comparison of revision surgery with primary anterior cruciate ligament reconstruction and outcome of revision surgery between different graft materials. Am J Sports Med. 2008;36:1889–95.
2. Denti M, Lo Vetere D, Bait C, et al. Revision anterior cruciate ligament reconstruction: causes of failure, surgical technique, and clinical results. Am J Sports Med. 2008;36:1896–902.
3. Glogovac G, Schumaier A, Grawe B. Return to sport following revision anterior cruciate ligament reconstruction in athletes: a systematic review. Arthroscopy. 2019;35:2222–30.
4. MARS Group. Effect of graft choice on the outcome of revision anterior cruciate ligament reconstruction in the Multicenter ACL Revision Study (MARS) Cohort. Am J Sports Med. 2014;42(10):2301–10.
5. Kartus J, Movin T, Karlsson J. Donor-site morbidity and anterior knee problems after anterior cruciate ligament reconstruction using autografts. Arthroscopy. 2001;17:971–80.
6. Xie X, Xiao Z, Li Q, et al. Increased incidence of osteoarthritis of knee joint after ACL reconstruction with bone-patellar tendon-bone autografts than hamstring autografts; a meta-analysis of 1,443 patients at a minimum of 5 years. Eur J Orthop Surg Traumatol. 2015;25:149–59.
7. Shelbourne KD, Beck MB, Gray T. Anterior cruciate ligament reconstruction with contralateral autogenous patellar tendon graft: evaluation of donor site strength and subjective results. Am J Sports Med. 2015;43(3):648–53.
8. Karns DJ, Heidt RS Jr, Holladay BR, Colosimo AJ. Case report: revision anterior cruciate ligament reconstruction. Arthroscopy. 1994;10:148–51.
9. Liden M, Ejerhed L, Sernert N, Bovaller A, Karlsson J, Kartus J. The course of the patellar tendon after reharvesting its central third for ACL revision surgery: a long-term clinical and radiographic study. Knee Surg Sports Traumatol Arthrosc. 2006;14(11):1130–8.
10. Stener S, Ejerhed L, Movin T, Sernert N, Papadogiannakis N, Kartus J. The reharvested patellar tendon has the potential for ligamentization when used for anterior cruciate ligament revision surgery. Knee Surg Sports Traumatol Arthrosc. 2012;20(6):1168–74.
11. Poehling-Monaghan K, Salem H, Ross K, Secrist E, Ciccotti M, Tjoumakaris F, Ciccotti M, Freedman K. Long-term outcomes in anterior cruciate ligament reconstruction: a systematic review of patellar tendon versus hamstring autografts. Orthop J Sports Med. 2017;5(6):2325967117709735.
12. Grassi A, Nitri M, Moulton GM, Marcheggiani Muccioli GM, Bondi A, Romagnoli M, Zaffagnini S. Does the type of graft affect the outcome of revision anterior cruciate ligament reconstruction? Bone Joint J. 2017;99-B:714–23.
13. Ferretti A, Monaco E, Capema L, Palma T, Conteduca F. Revision ACL reconstruction using contralateral hamstrings. Knee Surg Sports Traumatol Arthrosc. 2013;21(3):690–5.
14. Legnani C, Peretti G, Borgo E, Zini S, Ventrua A. Revision anterior cruciate ligament reconstruction with ipsi- or contralateral hamstring tendon grafts. Eur J Orthop Surg Traumatol. 2017;27(4):533–7.
15. Andernord D, Desai N, Bjornsson H, Gillen S, Karlsson J, Samuelsson K. Predictors of contralateral anterior cruciate ligament reconstruction: a cohort study of 9061 patients with 5-year follow-up. Am J Sports Med. 2015;43(2):295–302.
16. Harris NL, Smith DA, Lamoreaux L, Pernell M. Central quadriceps tendon for anterior cruciate ligament reconstruction. Part 1: morphometric and biomechanical evaluation. Am J Sports Med. 1997;25:23–8.
17. Xerogeanes JW, Mitchel PM, Karasev PA, Kolesov IA, Romine SE. Anatomic and morphological evaluation of the quadriceps tendon using 3-dimensional magnetic resonance imaging reconstruction: applica-

tions for anterior cruciate ligament choice and procurement. Am J Sports Med. 2013;41:2392–9.
18. Staubli HU, Schatzmann L, Brunner P, Ricon L, Nolte LP. Mechanical tensile properties of the quadriceps tendon and patellar ligament in young adults. Am J Sports Med. 1999;27:27–34.
19. Belk JW, Kraeutler MJ, Marshall HA, Goodrich JA, McCarty EC. Quadriceps tendon autograft for primary anterior cruciate ligament reconstruction: a systematic review of comparative studies with minimum 2-year follow-up. Arthroscopy. 2018;34(5):1699–707.
20. Hurley ET, Calvo-Gurry M, Withers D, Farrington SK, Moran R, Moran CJ. Quadriceps tendon autograft in anterior cruciate ligament reconstruction: a systemic review. Arthroscopy. 2018;34(5):1690–8.
21. Sheean AJ, Musahl V, Slone HS, Xerogeanes JW, Milinkovic D, Fink C, et al. Quadriceps tendon autograft for arthroscopic knee ligament reconstruction: use it now, use it often. Br J Sports Med. 2018;52(11):698–701.
22. Haner M, Bierke S, Petersen W. Anterior cruciate ligament revision surgery: ipsilateral quadriceps versus contralateral semitendinosus-gracilis autografts. Arthroscopy. 2016;32(11):2308–17.
23. Kaeding C, Aros B, Pedroza A, Pifel E, Amendola A, Andrish J, Dunn W, Marx R, McCarty E, Parker R, Wright R, Spindler K. Allograft versus autograft anterior cruciate ligament reconstruction. Sports Health. 2011;3(1):73–81.
24. Nissen K, Eysturoy N, Nielsen T, Lind M. Allograft use results in higher re-revision rate for revision anterior cruciate ligament reconstruction. Orthop J Sports Med. 2018;6(6):2325967118775381.
25. Lamblin C, Waterman B, Lubowitz J. Anterior cruciate ligament reconstruction with autografts compared with non-irradiated, non-chemically treated allografts. Arthroscopy. 2013;29(6):1113–22.
26. Tejwani SG, Chen J, Funahashi TT, Love R, Maletis GB. Revision risk after allograft anterior cruciate ligament reconstruction; association with graft processing techniques, patient characteristics, and graft type. Am J Sports Med. 2015;43(11):2696–705.

Game-Day Preparation for Revision ACL Surgery

5

Anthony A. Essilfie, Randy M. Cohn, Robert J. Meislin, and Michael J. Alaia

Background

Anterior cruciate ligament (ACL) reconstructions are one of the most common procedures performed in orthopedic surgery. It is estimated that over 200,000 ACL reconstructions are performed annually in the United States [1–3]. Many of these patients are highly motivated to return to their sport of choice. The return to play from primary ACL reconstruction ranges from 63% to 98% depending on the sport [4].

Even though most athletes return to sport after primary ACL reconstruction, there are several possible complications that could necessitate revision ACL reconstruction surgery. The Multicenter Orthopaedic Outcomes Network (MOON) group reported that there was an 8% rate for revision ACL reconstruction in the ipsilateral knee, with the median time to revision ACL reconstruction being 17 months from the primary procedure [5]. Revision ACL reconstructions have inferior outcomes compared to primary ACL reconstruction [6]. Moreover, these patients have increased postoperative osteoarthritis when compared to primary ACL reconstruction [7]. These suboptimal outcomes have also been highlighted in the pediatric and adolescent patient population who are particularly at risk for revision ACL reconstruction [8, 9].

Given the inferior results of revision ACL reconstruction, it is imperative that every effort is made to make the revision ACL surgery as efficacious as possible and understand the many relevant factors when planning for the procedure, many of which are highlighted elsewhere in this textbook. With that in mind, this chapter will provide practical game-day preparation for the revision ACL reconstruction and impart tips and tricks that have been effective for us in a complex knee surgery practice.

Preoperative Evaluation

History

One must ascertain why the primary ACL reconstruction may have failed, and as is highlighted in the other chapters in this book, the list of reasons can be quite robust. It is possible that the patient fully healed the primary ACL reconstruction and sustained another traumatic event leading to a graft tear [10]. Nevertheless, the most common technical reason for ACL reconstruction failure is poor tunnel placement. Particularly, femoral tunnel malposition has been cited as the reason for failure for almost 50% of cases [11]. Many patients

A. A. Essilfie (✉) · R. J. Meislin
New York University Langone Orthopedic Hospital, New York, NY, USA

R. M. Cohn
Northwell Health, Garden City, NY, USA

M. J. Alaia
Department of Orthopedic Surgery, Division of Sports Medicine, New York University Langone Health, New York, NY, USA

M. J. Alaia, K. J. Jones (eds.), *Revision Anterior Cruciate Ligament Reconstruction*, https://doi.org/10.1007/978-3-030-96996-7_5

that have a failed primary ACL reconstruction change their surgeon [12]. As such, it is important to obtain the history regarding the initial mechanism of injury, the operative report, and the arthroscopic images from the initial procedure. Additionally, it is critical to determine if there were any complications during the postoperative course. It is also paramount that the surgeon determines where along the rehabilitation process the patient was when he or she started having recurrent instability symptoms. Furthermore, the patient should be asked about general ligamentous laxity or connective tissue disorders at baseline.

Physical Exam

A thorough physical examination is vital in planning for revision ACL surgery. The patient's previous skin incisions should be carefully assessed. A decision should be made whether the incisions can be re-used for revision surgery or if it is best to avoid the initial incisions. Moreover, the knee should be examined for signs of infection. A general assessment of varus or valgus alignment should be made. Range of motion of the injured knee should be compared to the contralateral side. Prone heel heights can help detect slight differences in extension. Examination should assess for the presence of an effusion. A comprehensive evaluation of stability is essential. Commonly performed physical examination maneuvers pertinent to detect ACL tears include the Lachman, anterior drawer, and pivot shift examination. Gait should be assessed for any valgus or varus thrust as this may indicate concomitant laxity to the posteromedial or posterolateral corner, respectively. Menisci are commonly injured in the setting of an ACL injury and should be assessed on physical exam. Additionally, knees should be assessed for the presence of knee hyperextension. (For a more detailed workup for revision ACL tears, refer to Chap. 2.)

Radiographs

Weight-bearing AP, PA with 45 degrees of knee flexion, lateral, and merchant views should be obtained. Tunnel placement and possible tunnel expansion should be carefully scrutinized. It is also important to note if there is any hardware that may require removal. Careful attention should be focused on the posterior slope of the tibia as it has been found that increased posterior slope greater than 12 degrees may result in greater pivot shifts and higher ACL reconstruction failures [13, 14]. In our practice, hip to ankle standing alignment films are obtained in all patients with a failed reconstruction. Stress radiographs can help determine the degree of instability which can aid treatment decision-making. It is critical to obtain an MRI to assess for integrity of the ACL graft as well as any concomitant knee injury. Lastly, if tunnel widening is concerning on XR, a CT scan should be ordered [15]. There is great variability in the threshold of tunnel enlargement that would prompt a two-stage revision ACL reconstruction. Generally, tunnel enlargement greater than 15–16 mm necessitates a two-stage revision ACL reconstruction with initial bone grafting of the tunnels and subsequent ACL reconstruction [16–19].

Shared Decision-Making Discussion

A failed primary ACL reconstruction is a devastating event for the patient. From the patient's perspective, the patient has undergone a surgical procedure and then invested time and resources into a prolonged rehabilitation program of 6 months or longer in an attempt to return to an active lifestyle. This reality must not be lost on the surgeon when discussing the decision to undergo a revision ACL reconstruction. It is important that patients have appropriate expectations after revision ACL reconstruction. It has been shown that patients have lower outcome scores and return to sport after a revision ACL reconstruction when compared to primary ACL reconstruction [7, 20, 21]. It is also important to discuss potential graft options and harvest sites. The advantages and disadvantages of each autograft should be tailored to the patient's physiologic age, lifestyle, and physical demands. Additionally, consideration of allograft as a possible graft source should be discussed, based on patient age, activity level, and expectations. (For further detail on graft options, refer to Chap. 5.) If concomitant injuries are identified, a through discussion regarding additional procedures and their impact on outcomes is essential. A discussion over supplemental anterolateral procedures such as lateral extra-articular tenodesis (LET) and anterolateral ligament reconstruction is presented in Chaps. 17 and 18, respectively. Furthermore, the medial sided structures may be injured and require repair versus reconstruction as discussed in Chap. 13.

Game-Day Preparation and Pearls for Revision ACL Reconstruction

Game-day success begins with preparation. A thorough physical examination, appropriate radiographic studies, and intensive patient counseling will all contribute to your success. However, as there are many potential intraoperative pitfalls that you may encounter (e.g., hardware complications, tunnel issues), you should have a game plan that not only includes your preferred surgical approach but also a plan to resolve potential pitfalls with bailouts or alternative options. The best way to handle intraoperative difficulties is to anticipate them; this sort of preparation will keep you composed in the heat of the moment should an issue arise. A checklist of special equipment and availability should be created ahead of the scheduled surgery date to ensure availability.

Prior to the day of surgery, attempt to figure out who will be part of your surgical team. Who will be your anesthesiologist, circulator, and surgical technician? Who will be your assistant? Will it be a physician assistant, or, for those with trainees, will it be a resident or fellow? It is important that all members of the team are familiar with the procedure in order to optimize the quality of care provided to the patient. The anesthesiologist should be familiar with a regional nerve block that will allow appropriate pain control for the perioperative period. The circulator should ensure that all items on the picklist are in the room or readily available to minimize the amount of time spent out of the room looking for supplies. The surgical technician and assistants need to be familiar with the steps of the procedure and instrumentation in order to optimize efficiency.

The preoperative consent process should be detailed and hopefully involve a family member as well in the room if possible. The surgeon should go over the plan with the patient in detail, as revision surgeries may change on the fly. We routinely consent for ACL revision surgery with the preferred autograft, as well as the possibility of allograft. Additionally, we typically include meniscal repair or debridement on the consent, as well as removal of hardware, anterolateral or collateral ligament augmentation, and two-staged procedures with bone graft. It is certainly ideal to inform patients of the distinct possibilities prior to making incision; this will not only improve the physician-patient relationship but also set appropriate patient expectations.

Before scrubbing for the case, it is helpful to write down the steps of the procedure on the whiteboard. This serves as a reference for all members of the surgical team and allows everyone to anticipate the next step. If you have planned for an allograft revision, then confirm your choice of allograft is readily available and that there are backups in case the procedure needs to be altered or if the graft has a complication. Once the decision to use an allograft has been determined, it should be opened and thawed to prevent wasted time later on in the procedure. Graft preparation can even be done concurrently with induction of anesthesia to optimize efficiency during the surgical procedure. Additionally, bone grafting options including bone dowels, cancellous chips, or structural allografts should be readily available in case there is excessive osteolysis or significant convergence is encountered and the procedure requires staging.

Our preferred setup is with the patient lying supine with a leg holder proximal on the thigh. We routinely use a tourniquet, placed very proximal on the leg in order to have as much space exposed for any proximally based work or guide pin passage. The leg holder should never be excessively tight; otherwise a venous tourniquet may be created. We ensure that the knee can easily be hyperflexed in the case that hardware needs to be removed or anteromedial (AM) portal femoral drilling is preferred. Depending on surgeon preference, the contralateral leg is supported with either blankets under the distal thigh or a well leg holder with the extremity well abducted and flexed, to allow sufficient space for a posteromedial portal; this is important for combined ACL/PCL reconstruction cases as well as posterior medial ramp lesion fixation. A 70-degree arthroscope in addition to the 30-degree scope should be available for improved viewing posteriorly in the knee.

Although a significant amount of information regarding tunnels can be gathered preoperatively, we recommend diagnostic arthroscopy prior to any autograft harvest in revision cases. This allows the surgeon to obtain critical information regarding the exact positions of prior tunnels and can also help determine if the preferred surgical plan should be altered in terms of drilling method, fixation method, or graft choice (e.g., switch between autograft to allograft or whether or not the procedure should be staged and bone grafting needed). We never want to subject a patient to the morbidity of an autograft harvest to have it jeopardized by a suboptimal environment for fixation.

Although our preference is to maintain preexisting hardware in the tibia or femur, sometimes hardware removal is required, particularly in the tibia. If this is the case, fluoroscopy can be extremely helpful to have in the operating room, not only for incision localization but also to localize the hardware in cases where bone has overgrown the fixation. We prefer to use a mini C-arm and prop the leg up on a ring stand or small table with a stack of towels to pad the heel in order to get appropriate orthogonal images. Make sure that the appropriate screwdriver or hardware removal set is in the room as well as osteotomes to remove bone overgrowth. If a formal osteotomy is planned in addition to the revision ACL reconstruction, a regular C-arm will be helpful. It is incumbent on the surgeon to be familiar with the osteotomy instrumentation. Typically, the femoral ACL tunnel is addressed prior to the tibial osteotomy for varus correction, and the tibial tunnel will be drilled following correction of the varus deformity.

Having the appropriate instrumentation is of critical importance. Ensure that you have different options for graft fixation such as large screws, staples, suture anchors, cortical fixation devices, and large frag screw and washer. Also, large barrel reamers may be needed for cylindrical tunnel reaming. If previous fixation was made with biodegradable or biocomposite hardware, it should be noted that reaming through these materials will not feel like normal bone and the reamer may not pass easily. The surgeon may choose to begin with a smaller reamer and gradually increase the diameter of the tunnel until the desired width is obtained. Additionally, ACL dilators are extremely helpful in revision ACL cases, not only for tunnel creation but also to center a guide pin in a previously made tunnel.

Clinical Cases

Case 1

The patient is a 39-year-old female who underwent a bone-patella tendon-bone (BTB) autograft ACL reconstruction of her right knee 15 years earlier in Europe. Two years prior to presentation at our institution, she had a repeat pivoting injury while surfing. She attempted to treat her knee with rest and activity modification; however, symptoms of instability persisted, and she ultimately had difficulty performing basic activities of daily living.

On physical examination, she had a grade 2B Lachman and a positive pivot glide. Her knee was stable to varus and valgus stress at 0 and 30 degrees of flexion. She had a negative examination of her posterolateral and posteromedial corners with normal alignment which was confirmed with a hip to ankle standing alignment film. Radiographs demonstrated a previous screw and washer fixation with metal wire for cortical fixation on the femoral side, while a metal interference screw was used for tibial fixation (Fig. 5.1). MRI showed an ACL graft tear, anterior tibial

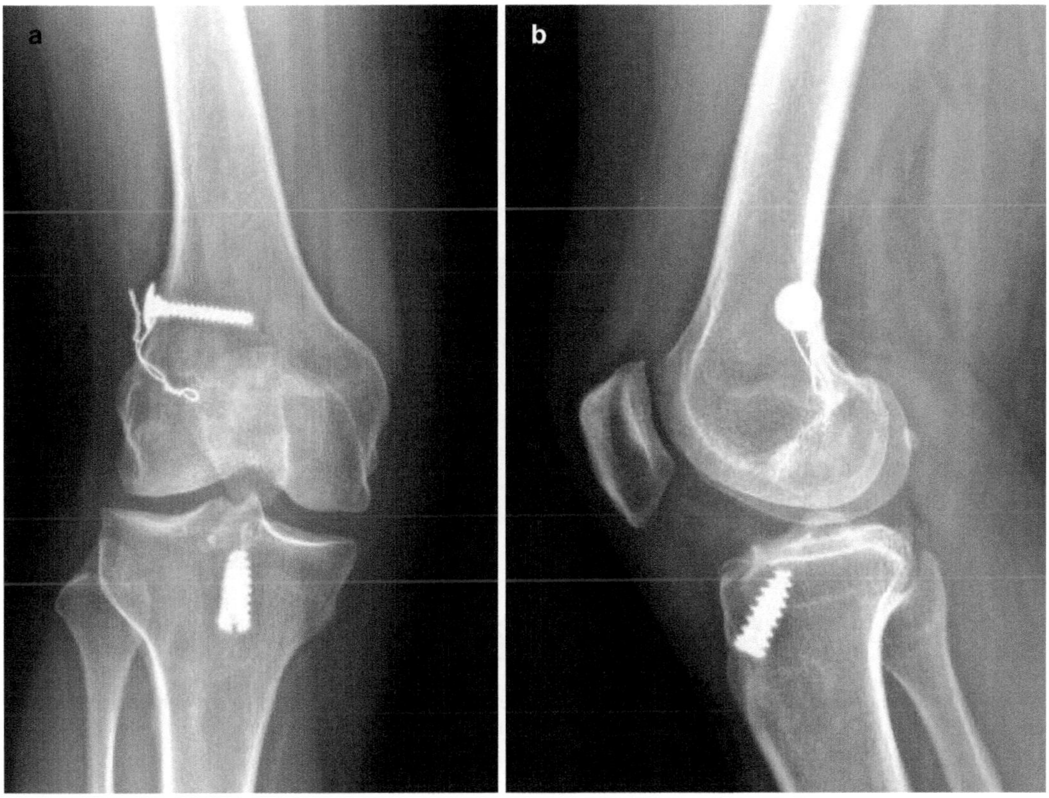

Fig. 5.1 AP (**a**) and lateral (**b**) radiographs of the right knee with previous screw and washer with metal wire used for femoral fixation. A metal interference screw was used for tibial fixation in the index procedure

translation, as well as a complex medial meniscus tear. Given the patient's symptoms and activity level, she elected to undergo a revision ACL reconstruction using bone-patellar tendon-bone allograft.

Prior to the procedure, there were concerns about the location of the femoral and tibial hardware. It was possible that using an AM drilling technique could potentially cause either hardware convergence or inability to pass the graft. Additionally, the tibial screw may have to be removed if it could not be bypassed by the tibial reamer.

In planning for this procedure, we considered possible pitfalls related to the previously placed hardware. We had instrumentation on backup that would allow us to perform outside-in drilling as well as potential bone graft options or larger screw options for the tibia. Intraoperatively, an irreparable medial meniscus tear was found, and a partial meniscectomy was performed. When drilling the femoral tunnel with the knee in hyperflexion through a low AM portal, the guide pin was unable to be passed around the prior hardware. Rather than making an incision to remove the hardware, we elected to drill the femoral tunnel utilizing a separate, outside-in retrograde reaming technique which allowed us to bypass the femoral hardware. Fluoroscopic imaging was available for the procedure to confirm that the tunnels were divergent. Additionally, the tibial screw was removed to allow for a new tunnel to be drilled. Intraoperative fluoroscopy showed appropriate positioning with metal interference screws in the femoral and tibial tunnels (Fig. 5.2). Ultimately, the patient did well from her procedure and had no recurrent episodes of instability.

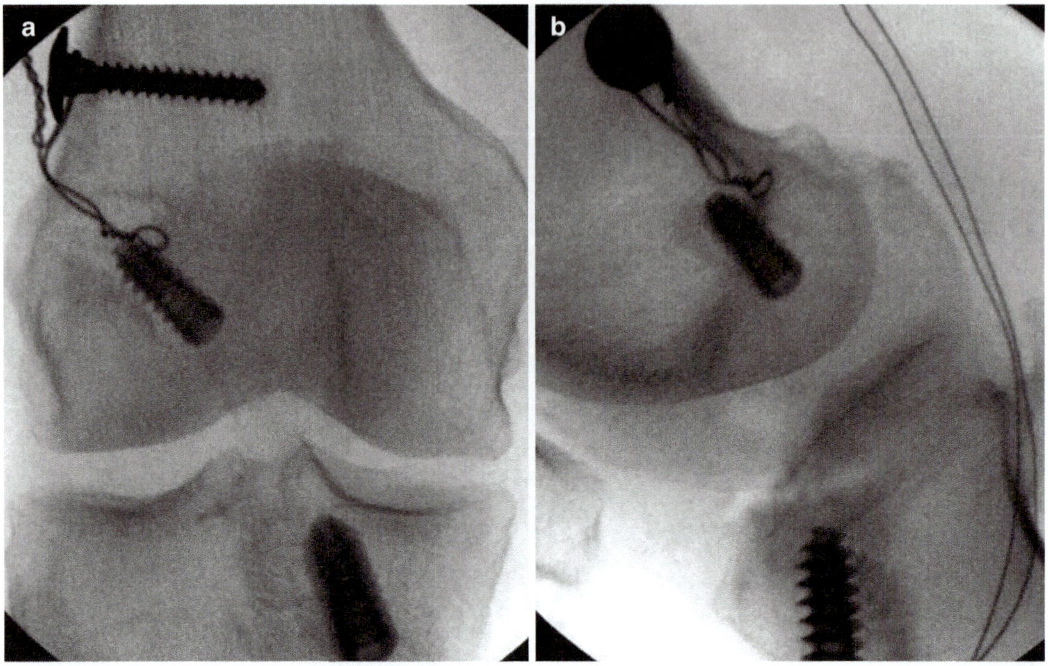

Fig. 5.2 Intraoperative fluoroscopic AP (**a**) and lateral (**b**) views or the right knee showing new interference fixation at the femoral and tibial tunnels with maintained femoral fixation hardware from the index procedure

Case 2

An 18-year-old male recreational athlete underwent an isolated ACL reconstruction with BTB autograft. The primary surgery was performed with a 10-mm retrograde drill for the femoral socket and a 10-mm barrel reamer for the tibial tunnel. Femoral and tibial fixation was achieved with metal interference screws.

Five months postoperatively, the patient sustained a re-rupture when he slipped on a wet floor. On examination, the patient had normal gait and alignment without varus or valgus thrust. He had a mild effusion and full range of motion. There was a 2+ anterior drawer, 2B Lachman examination, and a positive pivot glide in the office. Examination of his collaterals and corners was normal. Radiographs demonstrated appropriate positioning of femoral and tibial tunnels using metal interference screws, and MRI showed a complete rupture of the graft without concomitant meniscal or cartilage injury (Figs. 5.3 and 5.4).

Given his age and activity level, the decision was made to use an ipsilateral hamstring autograft for the revision ACL reconstruction. Additionally, given the prior 10-mm tunnels, the surgeon must consider techniques to ensure sufficient graft diameter to fill the prior tunnels. The possibility of a hybrid autograft-allograft was discussed with patient, in case his hamstring autograft was of insufficient size to fill the prior tunnels. To prepare for this possibility, the surgeon ensured that there was a semitendinosus allograft of sufficient length available. For this patient, a quadrupled semitendinosus autograft had a 10 mm diameter and was thus appropriate for the revision reconstruction, without need to harvest the gracilis tendon.

The next issue to tackle was hardware removal. The prior operative report was reviewed to identify the particular interference screws used in the index procedure and have the appropriate screwdriver available for removal. Additionally, the surgeon planned to have osteotomes and other instruments available in case there was bony

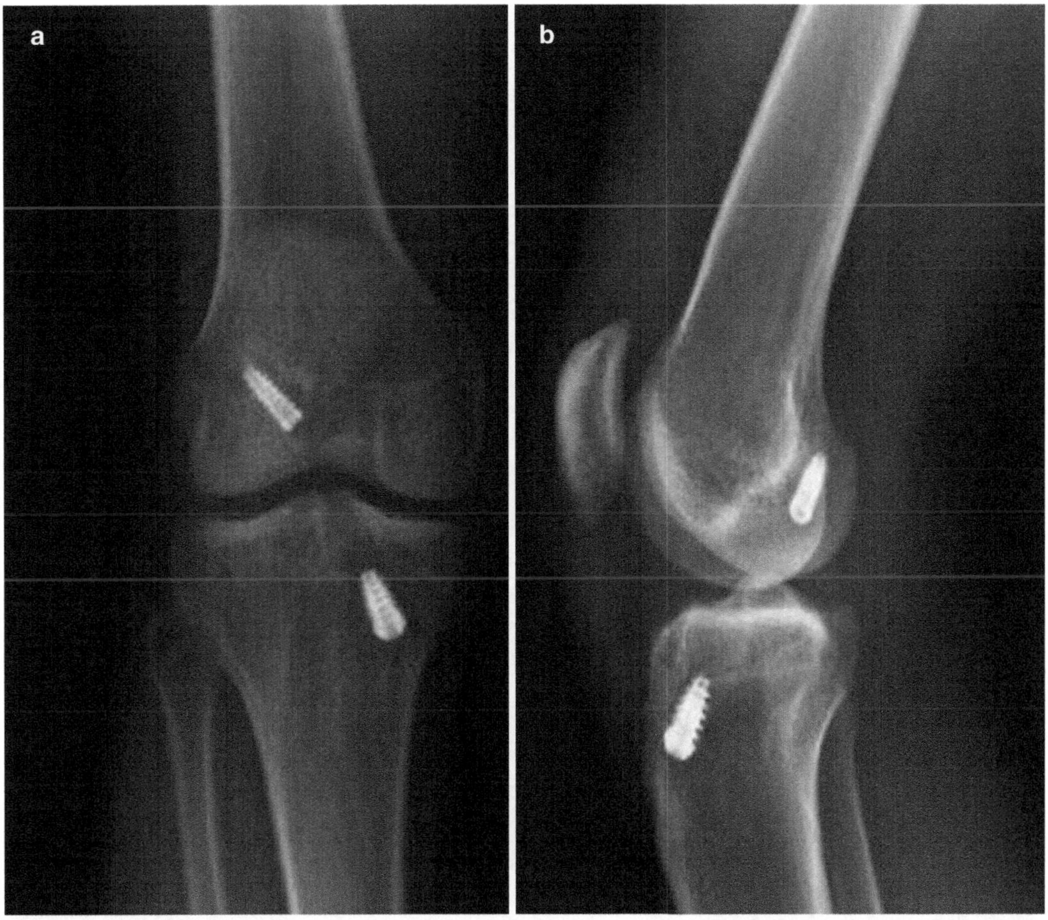

Fig. 5.3 AP (**a**) and lateral (**b**) radiographs of a right knee, status post index ACL reconstruction with metal interference screws

overgrowth encountered during hardware removal. Fluoroscopy should be available if the hardware is not apparent. The surgeon may also plan to leave in the prior metal screws and place new tunnels around them.

After hardware removal and debridement of the prior graft, the next crucial step was creation of femoral and tibial tunnels. The index ACL was performed using an independent outside-in retrograde drill for the femur. The surgeon's preference was to recreate the femoral socket in similar fashion. However, during the revision operation, difficulty was encountered in re-drilling the femoral socket due to the presence of soft tissue within the socket. In planning for this potential issue, the surgeon had requested that low-profile reamers be available. The soft tissue within the planned socket was removed using a 10-mm low-profile reamer, through an accessory low AM portal with the knee in hyperflexion. The thin shaft of the low-profile reamer allows for fine adjustment of the femoral tunnel placement when working around the medial condyle during AM portal drilling. The outside-in retrograde drill was then used to complete femoral socket preparation.

Tibial tunnel preparation and graft fixation also presented challenges in this case. For the index procedure, a 10-mm barrel reamer was used to create the tibial tunnel. As a result, there was no longer cortical bone at the distal aspect of the tibial tunnel, preventing the use of a standard button for cortical fixation. For this patient, the tibial tunnel was recreated using a 10-mm barrel

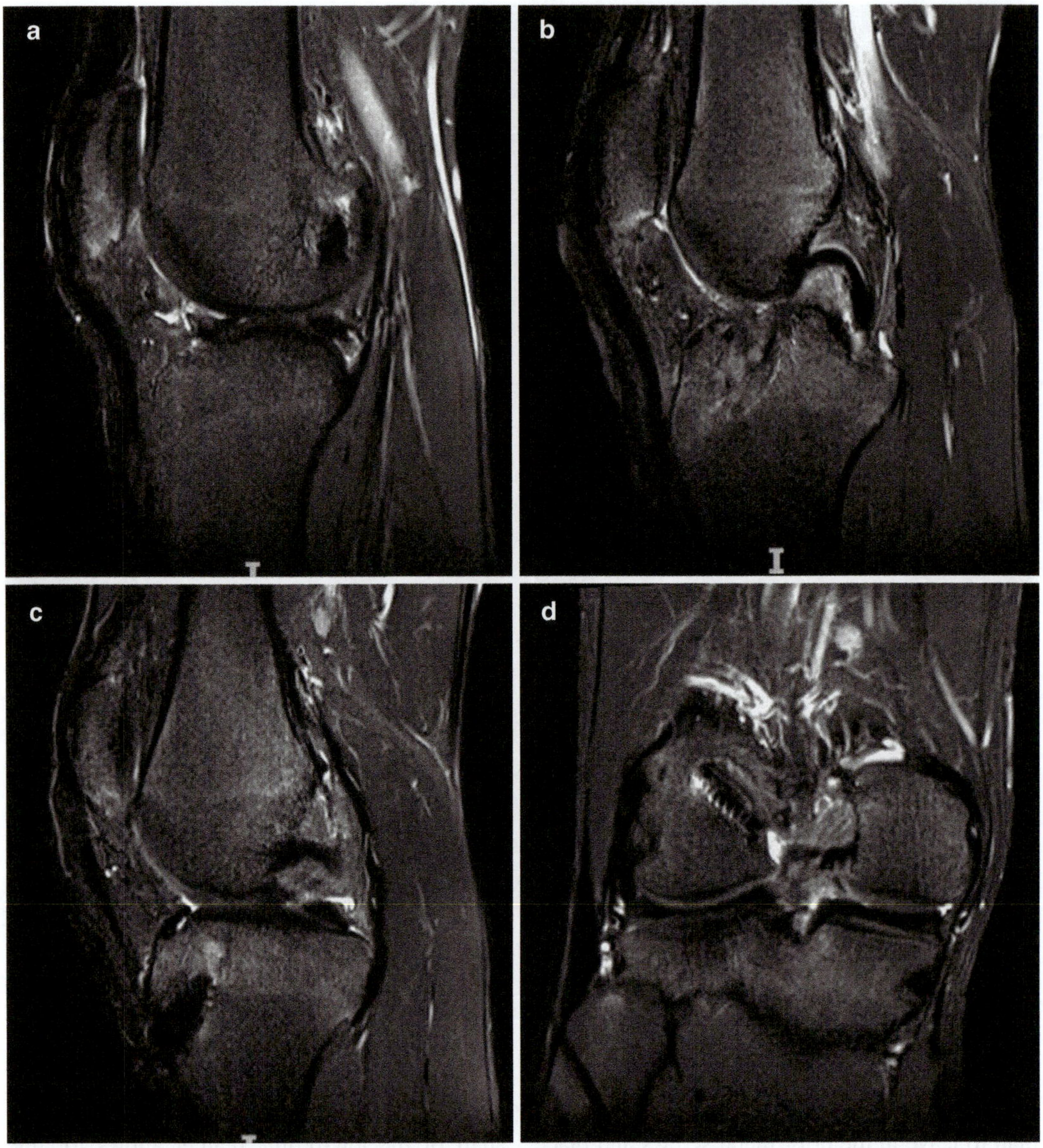

Fig. 5.4 Sagittal (**a**, **b**, **c**) and coronal (**d**) T2 STIR weighted MRI images demonstrating full thickness re-tear of the ACL graft

reamer. In this case, the surgeon preferred to use an "all-inside" technique, given the adequate size of the quadrupled semitendinosus. A cortical button larger than the 10-mm tibial aperture must be available to use this technique. For this patient, a standard femoral button was used along with a 14-mm button for tibial fixation (Fig. 5.5). In this case, the surgeon had to plan ahead in determining graft choice and availability, hardware removal, tunnel preparation, and graft fixation.

Case 3

A 24-year-old male was seen in clinic with a history of left knee ACL reconstruction with autologous hamstring tendons performed at an outside institution 3 years prior. One year following this index surgery, the ACL graft failed, and the surgeon performed a revision ACL allograft procedure. This procedure was complicated by a

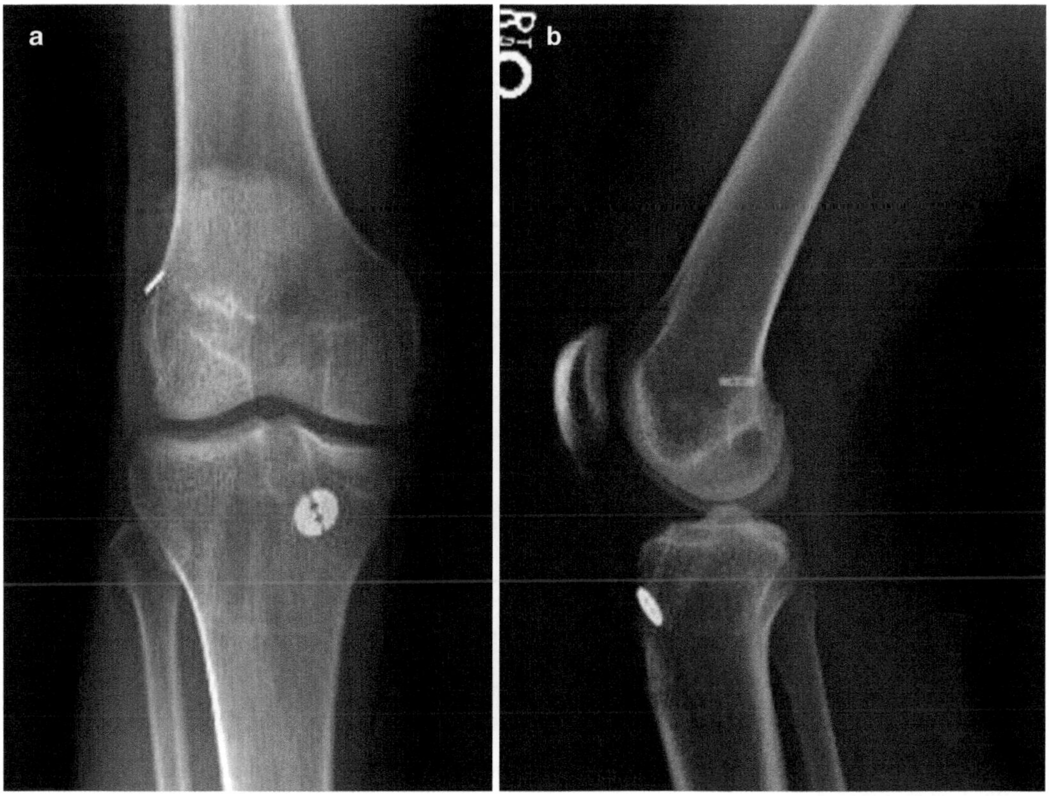

Fig. 5.5 AP (**a**) and lateral (**b**) radiographs of a right knee, status post revision ACL reconstruction with cortical button fixation at the femur and tibia. A 14-mm revision button was used for tibial fixation given the prior failed ACL reconstruction with 10-mm tibial tunnel

postoperative infection necessitating multiple irrigation and debridements as well as intravenous antibiotics. The patient presented 2 years following this second failed ACL surgery.

The patient complained of continued left knee instability including buckling and giving way episodes. His physical examination showed a 3B Lachman with soft endpoint and positive pivot shift. Range of motion with extension of 0 degrees and flexion to 130 degrees, trace effusion, and valgus/varus stress testing was stable at 0 and 30 degrees of flexion. No evidence of posterolateral or posteromedial instability. The overall alignment was normal. Radiographs showed no increase sagittal slope and no metallic hardware present (Fig. 5.6). MRI showed a failed ACL graft with intact menisci.

The patient wished to pursue a third left knee ACL reconstruction. Preoperative workup included a thorough evaluation for any active infection with blood labs drawn including complete blood count with differential, erythrocyte sedimentation rate, and C-reactive protein. All labs were negative. Attempts at tracking down his previous surgical records including pathogen source and antibiotic sensitivities were unsuccessful.

We chose ipsilateral bone-patellar tendon-bone autograft for the revision. Additionally, the patient was indicated for a possible modified Lemaire extra-articular tenodesis (LET) procedure using a central slip of his iliotibial band (ITB) to add an additional checkrein to internal rotation while in flexion to protect the ACL graft. This was ultimately decided with the examination under anesthesia, with a large pivot shift leading us to perform a LET augmentation.

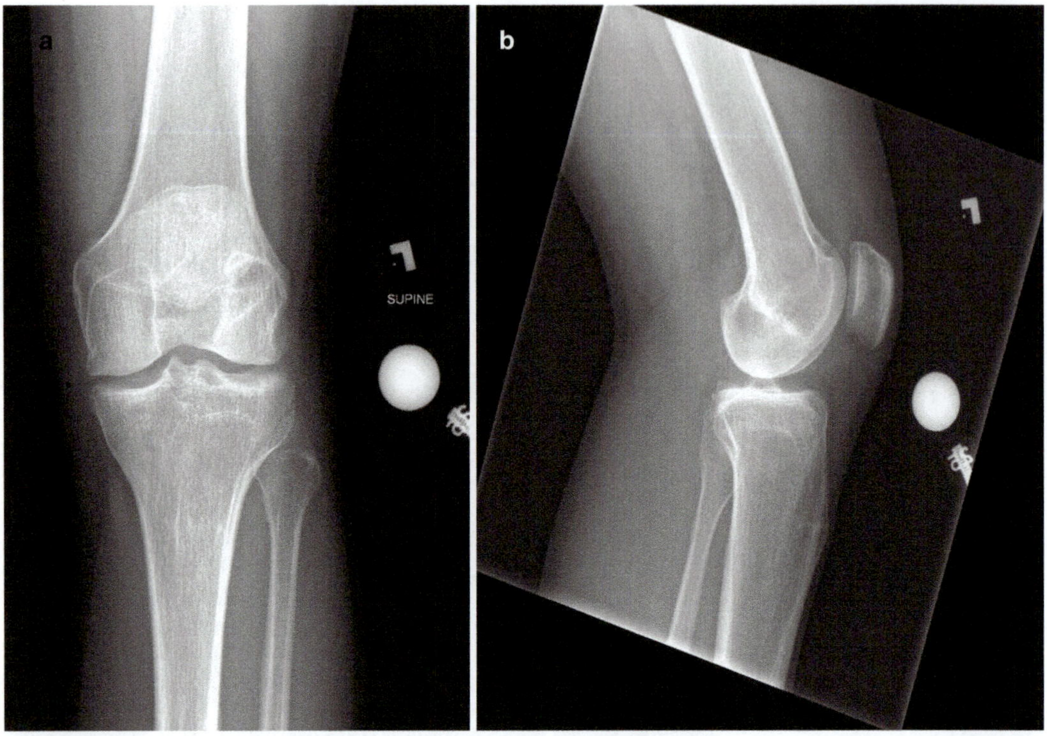

Fig. 5.6 AP (**a**) and lateral (**b**) radiographs of the left knee show mild degenerative changes and minimal osteolysis. No metallic fixation was used

When performing a revision ACL procedure, time is important. If you feel that you may need more than 2 hours of tourniquet use for visualization, the initial diagnostic knee scope can be performed with the tourniquet down. A radiofrequency probe coupled with epinephrine in the saline bag can be helpful for visualization with the tourniquet down.

In this case, the graft was completely torn with little residual remnant and an overgrown intercondylar notch. The notch was prepared, and there was no evidence of a bony femoral socket from previous surgeries. The BTB was harvested with 10-mm bone plugs. The femoral tunnel was created with the use of a flexible Beath pin and flexible reamer. The BTB graft was fixed with biocomposite interference screws in both the femoral and tibial tunnels.

Attention was paid to the LET reconstruction with a distal lateral thigh incision. The central 9 mm of ITB was harvested maintaining its insertion at Gerdy's tubercle. Care is taken not to harvest the posterior ITB since this could disrupt Kaplan's fibers which are located 31.4 mm proximal to the lateral epicondyle [22]. The ITB slip was then tunneled underneath the lateral collateral ligament (LCL) and fixed within a 6-mm tunnel that is slightly proximal at the location of Kaplan's fibers and posterior to the lateral femoral epicondyle. The femoral tunnel for the modified LET tenodesis is drilled in a proximal and anterior direction. The exiting sutures from the ACL passed graft should be maintained to hold the ACL bone block location and to ensure that the femoral tunnel for the modified LET tenodesis is placed away and divergent from the ACL femoral tunnel. The graft was secured with a 6-mm biocomposite screw with the knee flexed 40 degrees and slight internal rotation. Additionally, if there is any concern of convergence, fluoroscopy can confirm relative divergence from prior tunnels. If previously placed hardware from prior surgeries blocks passage of a pin or prevents a blind ending tunnel, the ITB tenodesis can certainly be fixed with a staple as well. Whatever the case, the ACL graft should always be visualized following placement of the modified LET graft to ensure integrity and proper tension.

Summary

Revision ACL reconstruction is fraught with potential variables that can make the case daunting. However, with appropriate planning, revision ACL reconstruction can be straightforward. Making sure that you and the surgical team are prepared for the procedure and potential variables will optimize the quality of care for the patient. Hopefully, with proper planning, your next revision ACL reconstruction will be effective and simplified.

References

1. Fetzer GB, Spindler KP, Amendola A, Andrish JT, Bergfeld JA, Dunn WR, et al. Potential market for new meniscus repair strategies: evaluation of the MOON cohort. J Knee Surg. 2009;22(3):180–6.
2. Mall NA, Chalmers PN, Moric M, Tanaka MJ, Cole BJ, Bach BR, et al. Incidence and trends of anterior cruciate ligament reconstruction in the United States. Am J Sports Med. 2014;42(10):2363–70.
3. Buller LT, Best MJ, Baraga MG, Kaplan LD. Trends in anterior cruciate ligament reconstruction in the United States. Orthop J Sport Med. 2015;3(1):1–8.
4. Mohtadi NG, Chan DS. Return to sport-specific performance after primary anterior cruciate ligament reconstruction: a systematic review. Am J Sports Med. 2018;46(13):3307–16.
5. Hettrich CM, Dunn WR, Reinke EK, Spindler KP. The rate of subsequent surgery and predictors after anterior cruciate ligament reconstruction: two- and 6-year follow-up results from a multicenter cohort. Am J Sports Med. 2013;41(7):1534–40.
6. Grassi A, Ardern CL, Muccioli GMM, Neri MP, Marcacci M, Zaffagnini S. Does revision ACL reconstruction measure up to primary surgery? A meta-analysis comparing patient-reported and clinician-reported outcomes, and radiographic results. Br J Sports Med. 2016;50(12):716–24.
7. Wright RW, Gill CS, Chen L, Brophy RH, Matava MJ, Smith MV, et al. Outcome of revision anterior cruciate ligament. J Bone Joint Surg Am. 2012;94:531–6.
8. Christino MA, Tepolt FA, Sugimoto D, Micheli LJ, Kocher MS. Revision ACL reconstruction in children and adolescents. J Pediatr Orthop. 2020;40(3):129–34.
9. Defrancesco CJ, Storey EP, Flynn JM, Ganley TJ. Pediatric ACL reconstruction and return to the operating room: revision is less than half of the story. J Pediatr Orthop. 2019;39(10):516–20.
10. Chen JL, Allen CR, Stephens TE, Haas AK, Huston LJ, Wright RW, et al. Differences in mechanisms of failure, intraoperative findings, and surgical characteristics between single- and multiple-revision ACL reconstructions: a MARS cohort study. Am J Sports Med. 2013;41(7):1571–8.
11. Morgan JA, Dahm D, Levy B, Stuart MJ, MARS Study Group. Femoral tunnel malposition in ACL revision reconstruction. J Knee Surg. 2012;25(5):361–8.
12. Sutherland K, Clatworthy M, Chang K, Rahardja R, Young SW. Risk factors for revision anterior cruciate ligament reconstruction and frequency with which patients change surgeons. Orthop J Sport Med. 2019;7(11):1–8.
13. Brandon ML, Haynes PT, Bonamo JR, Flynn MII, Barrett GR, Sherman MF. The association between posterior-inferior Tibial slope and anterior cruciate ligament insufficiency. Arthrosc J Arthrosc Relat Surg. 2006;22(8):894–9.
14. Christensen JJ, Krych AJ, Engasser WM, Vanhees MK, Collins MS, Dahm DL. Lateral Tibial posterior slope is increased in patients with early graft failure after anterior cruciate ligament reconstruction. Am J Sports Med. 2015;43(10):2510–4.
15. van Eck CF, Schreiber VM, Liu TT, Fu FH. The anatomic approach to primary, revision and augmentation anterior cruciate ligament reconstruction. Knee Surg Sport Traumatol Arthrosc. 2010;18(9):1154–63.
16. Groves C, Chandramohan M, Chew C, Subedi N. Use of CT in the management of anterior cruciate ligament revision surgery. Clin Radiol [Internet] 2013;68(10):e552–9. Available from: https://doi.org/10.1016/j.crad.2013.06.001.
17. Mayr R, Rosenberger R, Agraharam D, Smekal V, El Attal R. Revision anterior cruciate ligament reconstruction: an update. Arch Orthop Trauma Surg. 2012;132(9):1299–313.
18. Rizer M, Foremny GB, Rush A, Singer AD, Baraga M, Kaplan LD, et al. Anterior cruciate ligament reconstruction tunnel size: causes of tunnel enlargement and implications for single versus two-stage revision reconstruction. Skeletal Radiol [Internet] 2017;46(2):161–9. Available from: https://doi.org/10.1007/s00256-016-2535-z
19. Voos JE, Wickiewicz TL, Warren RF. Tunnel widening in revision anterior cruciate ligament. J Am Acad Orthop Surg. 2010;18(11):695–706.
20. Andriolo L, Filardo G, Kon E, Ricci M, Della Villa F, Della Villa S, et al. Revision anterior cruciate ligament reconstruction: clinical outcome and evidence for return to sport. Knee Surg Sport Traumatol Arthrosc. 2015;23(10):2825–45.
21. Reinhardt KR, Hammoud S, Bowers AL, Umunna BP, Cordasco FA. Revision ACL reconstruction in skeletally mature athletes younger than 18 years. Clin Orthop Relat Res. 2012;470(3):835–42.
22. Godin JA, Chahla J, Moatshe G, Kruckeberg BM, Muckenhirn KJ, Vap AR, et al. A comprehensive reanalysis of the distal iliotibial band: quantitative anatomy, radiographic markers, and biomechanical properties. Am J Sports Med. 2017;45(11):2595–603.

Management of the Structurally Intact ACL with Residual Instability

6

Alexander Golant, Matthew Geswell, and Stephen J. Nicholas

Diagnosis of Structurally Intact but Abnormally Lax ACL Graft

Firstly, it's important to differentiate between laxity on exam and true symptomatic instability. Inadequate rehabilitation and lack of lower extremity neuromuscular control can result in symptoms of instability, even without any objective evidence of laxity after ACL reconstruction [1]. In contrast, some asymptomatic and fully functional patients may demonstrate positive exam findings of laxity on such tests as the Lachman, anterior drawer, pivot shift tests, and arthrometer measurements.

For patients who have exhausted rehabilitative measures and continue to exhibit symptomatic instability, a follow-up MRI must be obtained to assess integrity of the ACL graft and evaluate for other pathologies. In the setting of an intact graft, the following most common scenarios that can lead to residual instability must be considered:

A. Golant (✉)
Department of Orthopedics and Rehabilitation, New York Presbyterian Queens, Flushing, NY, USA

M. Geswell
Medical University of South Carolina, Lancaster Medical Center, MUSC Lancaster Orthopaedics and Sports Medicine, Lancaster, SC, USA

S. J. Nicholas
New York Orthopedics, New York, NY, USA

1. Proper graft position, but insufficient graft tension
2. Improper graft position/orientation
3. Unrecognized or unaddressed additional injuries/conditions

Below, we discuss a step-by-step approach to recognizing and surgically addressing each of the above factors.

Scenario 1: Properly Positioned Graft with Insufficient Tension

One potential cause of an unstable knee with a structurally intact ACL graft is laxity of the graft itself. Detailed physical examination and dedicated imaging are important to rule out additional contributing factors (discussed below), such as erroneous tunnel placement, other ligamentous injuries, and malalignment. Arthroscopic evaluation of the graft will reveal an intact graft in correct position/orientation, with abnormal laxity to probing (case 1, Fig. 6.2). In this case, the graft may be lax for the following reasons: (a) inadequate initial tension, (b) failure of rigid fixation, and (c) graft stretching over time.

Inappropriate Intraoperative Tension

Inadequate initial intraoperative tension on an ACL graft may result from: (a) failure to pretension the graft prior to implantation, (b) failure

M. J. Alaia, K. J. Jones (eds.), *Revision Anterior Cruciate Ligament Reconstruction*,
https://doi.org/10.1007/978-3-030-96996-7_6

to place the knee into correct position during graft fixation, and (c) failure to apply adequate tension during graft fixation.

Pre-tensioning the graft is important in order to remove the creep (i.e., plastic deformation) prior to implantation. Biomechanical studies show that higher loads and longer application times leave the graft with higher residual tension and lower potential for stretching [2, 3]. In the clinical setting, application of 80–90 N load to the graft for a minimum of 15 minutes is recommended. *Surgical tip:* be sure to re-check and adjust the tension on the graft a few minutes after the initial load is applied – as plastic deformation occurs, the graft stretches slightly, and the tension experienced decreases.

For a single-bundle ACL reconstruction, the graft should be fixed with the knee in full extension, while a reverse Lachman force is applied [4]. Failure to apply this force may result in graft fixation with the tibia in the excessively anterior position (case 1, Fig. 6.1b).

Applying adequate force to the ACL graft during fixation represents a balance between preventing laxity and avoiding over-tightening, with

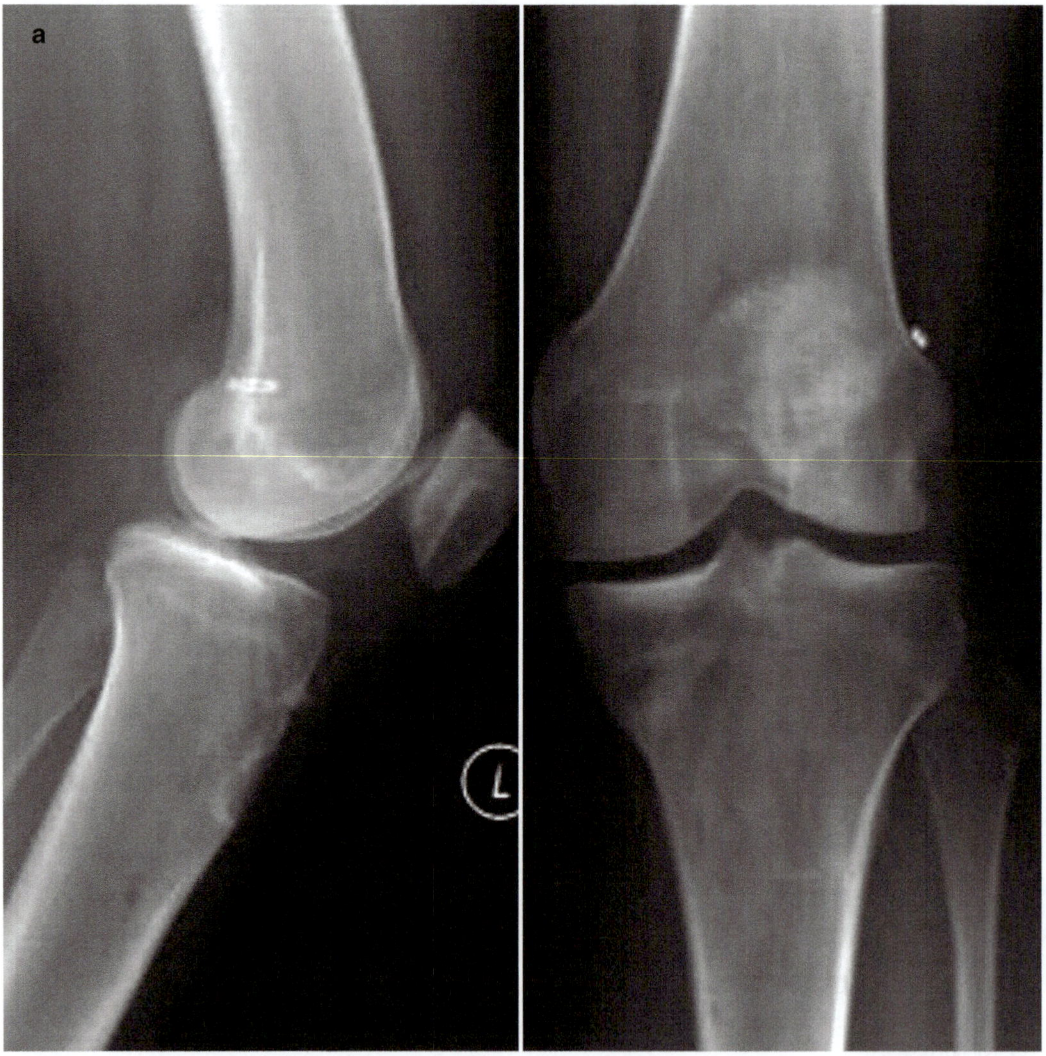

Fig. 6.1 (**a**) Plain radiographs show neutral alignment and appropriate tunnel position. (**b**) MRI confirmed appropriate tunnel position/orientation and an intact graft, but also showed significant (8 mm) anterior tibial translation

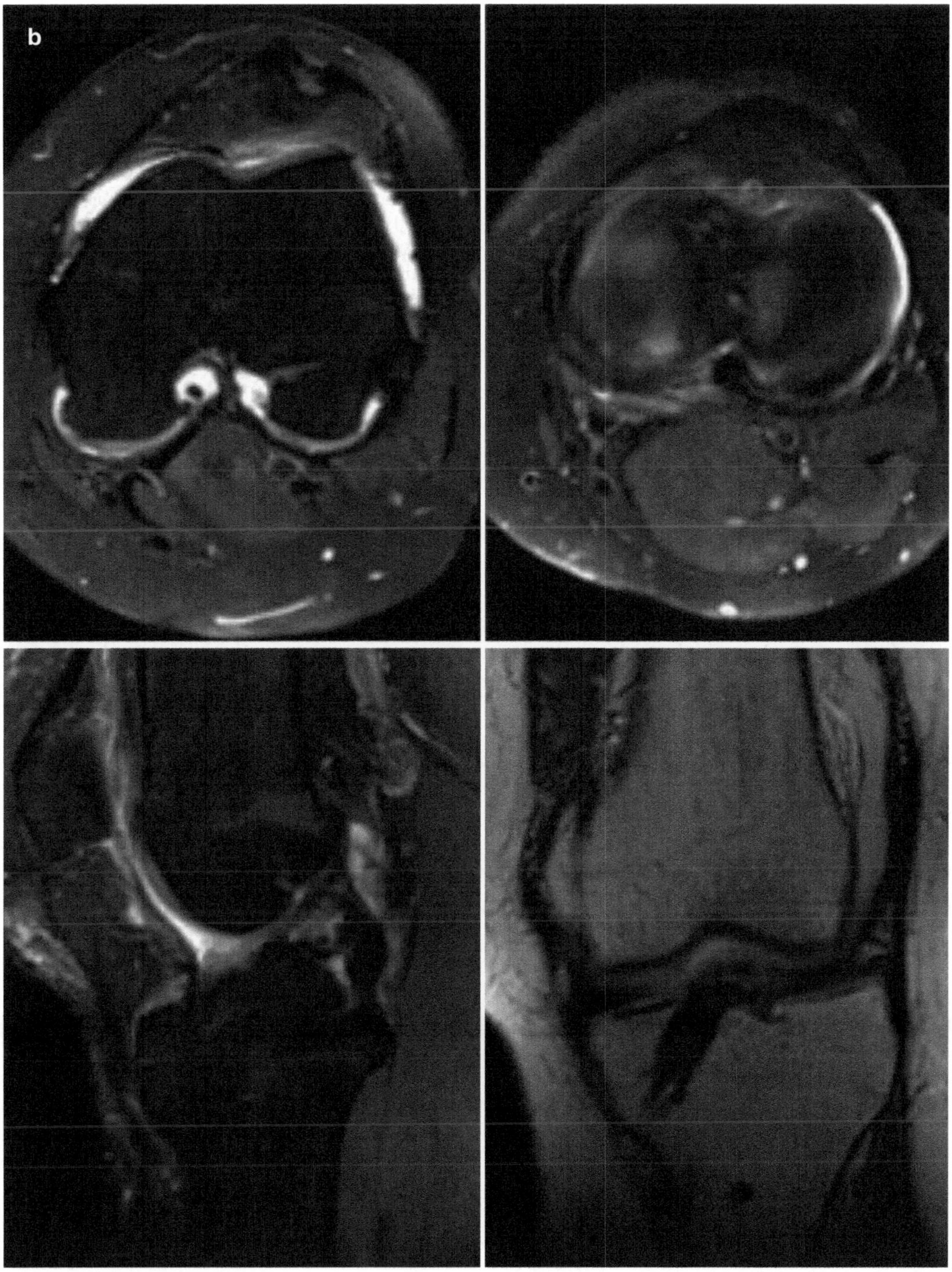

Fig. 6.1 (continued)

a minimum of 20 N of force recommended [5]. It is essential to verify appropriate graft tension at the conclusion of the case by checking knee stability manually via Lachman, anterior drawer, and pivot shift tests and by probing the graft under direct arthroscopic visualization.

Loss of Rigid Graft Fixation (i.e. Graft Slippage)

A wide variety of options for securing the ACL graft exist, broadly divided into the main types of aperture fixation and suspensory fixation. Aperture fixation at the intra-articular opening of the tunnel results in the shortest possible distance of the unfixed graft. Suspensory fixation leaves more of the graft unsecured, allowing a "windshield-wiper effect" and possible tunnel widening, which can theoretically allow the graft to shift into a suboptimal position, potentially producing graft laxity [6, 7]. Additionally, laxity can result when fixation mode itself fails, such as button pull through, adjustable loop lengthening, suture failure, and graft slippage past the interference screw [8, 9].

Graft Stretch

Due to intrinsic properties, some grafts are predisposed to greater likelihood of stretching over time. Studies have shown higher risk of re-rupture with allografts than with autografts [9–11]; additionally, hamstring grafts are more likely to experience stretch than bone-patellar tendon-bone (BPTB) grafts are [8, 9]. Although differences in overall clinical outcomes are debatable, a number of studies have demonstrated greater anterior knee laxity with hamstring grafts, compared to that of BPTB grafts [12–14]. Chapter 5 focuses specifically on graft options for ACL revision reconstruction.

Table 6.1 Surgical tips and tricks

How to manage instability after ACLR with an intact graft		
Why is the knee unstable?	What to do	How to do it
Graft is in good position but too lax Poorly tensioned Failed fixation Graft stretched	Revise the graft	Use same tunnels/sockets (if anatomically placed) Use stiffer graft Ensure maximal pre-tensioning of the graft Ensure reverse Lachman during fixation Use more rigid fixation (consider dual fixation on each side)
Poorly positioned graft Femoral tunnel too anterior Tibial tunnel too posterior Vertical graft	Option 1: Revise completely Option 2: Add PL bundle (for rotational-only instability) Option 3: Add ALL reconstruction	Identify anatomic locations for femoral and tibial tunnels Ensure adequate bone stock for new tunnels or graft old tunnels to rebuild stock Use outside-in or AM portal drilling and fluoroscopic imaging to avoid tunnel collisions
Additional pathology Varus deformity High posterior tibial slope PLC insufficiency Meniscal lesions	HTO De-flexion osteotomy PLC reconstruction Meniscal repair or reconstruction	See respective chapters for details

Surgical Approach to a Properly Positioned Graft with Insufficient Tension

For a symptomatic patient with an ACL graft that is properly positioned but lax on clinical and arthroscopic examination, revision ACL reconstruction is required, as there is currently no clinically proven way to "tighten" such a graft in situ. In this situation, the surgeon must consider and address all possible contributing issues, discussed above, as follows (Table 6.1).

1. If possible, choose a stiffer graft, with lower intrinsic likelihood of stretching. If an allograft was used at index surgery, an autograft should be considered for revision. With a previously used hamstring, consider BPTB or quadriceps tendon (QT).
2. Ensure appropriate graft tension during preparation and implantation. Maintain the graft

under at least 80–90N of tension for at least 15 minutes prior to implantation, re-checking the tension every 4–5 minutes. While the graft is being secured, ensure full knee extension and a reverse Lachman force. Consider using a tensiometer to ensure adequate force application at the time of graft fixation, and verify elimination of the Lachman, anterior drawer, and pivot shift tests afterwards.

3. For securing the graft, choose implants that will ensure optimal tension and rigid fixation and have the least likelihood of any postoperative slippage. Aperture fixation produces the shortest and stiffest grafts, while many currently used suspensory devices allow adding graft tension even after fixation is set. In a revision setting, consider employing two modes of fixation on either the femoral or tibial side or even on both sides. For example, you can secure the graft with a button-loop device on the femur and interference screw on the tibia, add tension as needed from the femoral side, finalize femoral fixation by adding an interference screw, and back up tibial fixation by securing the graft sutures distally (to a post or an anchor).

Scenario 2: Improperly Positioned Graft

If the graft has been malpositioned, residual knee laxity and instability may occur, even with a graft that's properly tensioned, well fixed, and intrinsically stiff. Proper graft function depends on anatomic tunnel position [15–17], and thus, erroneous tunnel placement, which is the most common technical error during ACL reconstruction [18], can result in a graft that is structurally intact but functionally insufficient (i.e., lax).

Femoral Tunnel Too Anterior

A femoral tunnel placed too anteriorly has been found to be an important factor leading to graft failure, occurring in ~30% of revision ACL reconstructions [18]. A too anterior tunnel produces a graft that becomes excessively tight in flexion and loose in extension [19].

Tibial Tunnel Too Posterior

The most common mistake of tibial tunnel placement is a too posterior location, which has been shown to result in higher rates of rotational instability and worse subjective outcomes [20]. In contrast, a too-anteriorly placed tibial tunnel may cause graft impingement on the roof of the intercondylar notch in extension and may lead to loss of terminal extension [17].

Vertical Graft

The classically described vertical graft can be stable in the anterior to posterior plane, but has a rotationally unstable component, as seen with a positive pivot shift phenomenon (case 2, Fig. 6.3). Vertical grafts can result from the femoral tunnel placed too anteriorly, the tibial tunnel placed too posteriorly, or a combination of the two [16, 18].

Surgical Approach to an ACL Graft with Non-anatomic Tunnel Placement

Preoperative confirmation of suspected graft/tunnel malposition as cause for residual laxity should be done with imaging, including plain radiographs (which can show too-anterior femoral and/or too-posterior tibial tunnels), MRI (which can show an intact but vertically oriented graft), and CT scan with 3D reconstructions (which can identify locations and orientation of the tunnels, measure tunnel widening, and assess availability of bone stock for revision reconstruction).

Option 1: Graft Revision

If the structurally intact yet lax ACL graft is believed to be due to tunnel malposition, the most obvious solution is a revision ACL reconstruction with proper tunnel placement. For tunnels that are grossly malpositioned but not significantly widened, there may be enough "real estate" to place entirely new tunnels or sockets in proper anatomic locations. In other cases, convergence between new and old tunnels may be unavoidable – techniques to address this problem are discussed in detail in subsequent chapters.

Option 2: Graft Augmentation

Some vertically oriented grafts provide adequate anterior-posterior stability, but lack rotational stability, resulting in patient complaints of the knee giving out – particularly with pivoting and cutting movements. A careful examination demonstrates negative or grade 1A Lachman and anterior drawer tests, with a positive pivot shift. Imaging and arthroscopic exam confirm a graft that is well-positioned in the sagittal plane, but is too vertical in the coronal plane, thereby adequately replicating the anteromedial (AM) bundle of the ACL, but not the posterolateral (PL) bundle. In this scenario, especially if the graft appears well-vascularized and incorporated, it is reasonable to consider augmentation with a small-size graft to replicate the PL bundle, serving to add rotational stability to an already anteriorly stable knee [21].

To add a PL bundle to an existing vertical graft, a similar technique as used to perform selective bundle reconstruction for partial ACL tears with an intact AM bundle should be used. A 5–7-mm diameter graft is sufficient, as larger grafts may cause impingement; a doubled semitendinosus graft readily serves this purpose.

To ensure adequate rotational stability is restored, it is essential to respect anatomic footprints of the PL bundle on the femur and tibia. On the femoral side, the PL bundle inserts distal to the AM bundle, typically just inferior to the bifurcate ridge [22]. Outside-in or AM portal drilling can both be used to place a femoral socket in this location, avoiding convergence with the existing femoral tunnel; fluoroscopy can be used intraoperatively to verify guide-wire position prior to reaming.

On the tibial side, the insertion of the PL bundle is located about 10 mm posterolateral to the center of the AM bundle [22], just medial to the lateral tibial spine. Compared to the typical angle of the tibial tunnel seen in cases with vertical grafts (which is usually about 20–30 degrees in the coronal plate), the angle of the guide-wire when adding the PL bundle reconstruction should be about 20–30 degrees more oblique (i.e., about 40–60 degrees in the coronal plane). The graft should be secured with the knee in 60–70 degrees of flexion and slight external rotation, with a posterior drawer force applied.

An additional consideration for intact grafts with lack of rotational stability (with adequate anterior stability) is the integrity of the anterolateral ligament (ALL) [23]. For patients with this complaint, if the graft appears to be appropriately oriented, secured, and taught to arthroscopic palpation, consideration can be given to adding ALL reconstruction, which will be discussed separately in Chap. 18.

Scenario 3: Unrecognized or Unaddressed Additional Injuries/ Conditions

ACL tears occur frequently in conjunction with other pathologies, including meniscal tears, injuries to other ligaments, lower extremity coronal malalignment, and/or abnormal tibial slope. Failure to recognize and address these issues can result in excessive stress on the ACL graft, leading to graft stretching and laxity, clinical instability, and even graft failure. When encountering a knee with an intact ACL graft and persistent laxity, it is important for the surgeon to perform a thorough workup to identify the aforementioned potential contributing factors and plan accordingly when considering surgical intervention.

Coronal Plane Malalignment

Significant deviations from a normal mechanical axis impart abnormal forces to the knee joint and can contribute to failure of an ACL reconstruction. Varus malalignment, in particular, has been noted in greater proportion of ACL revision cases compared to successful index reconstructions [24–26] and is typically managed with a valgus-producing high tibial osteotomy (HTO), which can be done with a medial opening or lateral closing wedge technique [27, 28]. By correcting alignment, HTO can help normalize knee kinematics, allowing the ACL to function appropriately without excessive stress [29]. Both single-stage and two-stage approaches have been proposed for treating a knee with a failed ACL reconstruction and deformity. In the setting of an intact graft with clinical instability, we feel it best to choose a two-stage approach, as correction of varus deformity (especially if combined with tibial slope decrease) may provide enough stability improvement to obviate the need for graft revision. Details of managing coronal plane deformity are discussed in Chap. 15.

Sagittal Plane Malalignment

Excessively high posterior tibial slope (PTS) increases anterior translation of the tibia in weight-bearing and has been established as an independent predictor of ACL reconstruction failure [30, 31]. It's been reported that a PTS of greater than 12 degrees significantly increases the risk of ACL graft failure [32, 33], whereas biomechanical studies have confirmed that slope-reducing osteotomies decrease ACL graft forces and anterior tibial translation under axial load [34]. A number of clinical studies have shown successful outcomes with ACL revision reconstruction combined with tibial osteotomies that corrected excessive PTS [35, 36]. Sagittal plane deformity is further discussed in Chap. 16.

Additional Ligamentous Injury and Meniscal Deficiency

The most common additional ligamentous insufficiency that contributes to failure of ACL reconstruction is that of the posterolateral corner (PLC) [37]. Careful clinical examination is paramount in identifying this when preparing for ACL revision, as PLC structures may appear intact on imaging, but nevertheless exhibit laxity, especially when the original trauma is chronologically remote. Both isolated PLC reconstruction and those combined with ACL graft revision may be used to address persistent instability in cases of an intact ACL graft with residual instability. Management of the posterolateral corner as part of ACL revision reconstruction is discussed in detail in Chap. 14.

Finally, meniscal deficiency and certain meniscocapsular lesions have been shown to contribute to increased laxity both in ACL-deficient and ACL-reconstructed knees, leading to increased anterior translation and rotation [38–41]. Management of these lesions is discussed in Chaps. 19 and 20.

Summary

Not uncommonly, a patient may present with a clinically failed (i.e., unstable) ACL reconstruction, despite imaging findings of an intact graft. It is the surgeon's job to perform a meticulous evaluation, using detailed history, thorough physical examination, advanced imaging, and sometimes examination under anesthesia, including arthroscopy, to determine the cause for this instability. Dividing the potential causes into three main groups, as described in this chapter, can be helpful to determine the best surgical approach. Grafts that are well positioned may be lax due to failure of fixation, insufficient initial tension, or graft stretching; this scenario requires a revision with a stiffer graft, more rigid fixation, and appropriate intraoperative graft tensioning. Malpositioned grafts usually need to be revised with creation of tunnels in anatomic locations, although in some cases, an isolated posterolateral bundle reconstruction can add rotational stability to an existing graft that demonstrates adequate anterior stability. Finally, other issues that contribute to knee laxity must be sought out and addressed, including varus malalignment, high posterior tibial slope, additional ligamentous injuries, and meniscal deficiency.

Additionally, a surgeon must remember that, from a psychological standpoint, when imaging shows an intact graft, it can be difficult to convince a patient that revision surgery is necessary and that they will need to go through an extensive period of convalescence and rehabilitation all over again. It is, therefore, crucial to engage the patient as an active participant in decision-making, to recognize and acknowledge their goals and expectations, to explain in detail the issues that are contributing to their instability, and to ensure appropriate rehabilitation prior to any repeat surgical intervention.

Case 1

Patient is an 18-year-old collegiate volleyball player who presented 1 year after BTB autograft ACL reconstruction with a medial meniscus repair, complaining of knee pain, mechanical symptoms, and intermittent buckling. She completed a full course of rehabilitation, including a return-to-play protocol with her athletic trainer, and resumed training, but was unable to wean from the brace for athletic participation and did not feel ready to return to competition. Clinical examination demonstrated a normal gait, neutral lower extremity alignment, full range of motion with pain and clicking, tenderness over the medial joint line, and normal strength. Stability examination showed 1B Lachman and anterior drawer tests, while a pivot shift could not be properly assessed due to guarding. The PCL, collateral ligaments, and corners were stable. Imaging showed neutral alignment, good tunnel positions on X-rays (Fig. 6.1), and intact graft in a proper orientation, but with significant anterior tibial translation on MRI (Fig. 6.1b), indicating laxity. Considering these findings, ACL laxity and symptoms of instability were thought to be due to either insufficient initial graft tension (at the time of index surgery) or subsequent graft stretching.

Due to failure of conservative management and significant limitations on her athletic participation, patient was indicated for and elected to proceed with a revision ACL reconstruction. Exam under anesthesia confirmed isolated ACL laxity, with positive Lachman, anterior drawer, and pivot shift tests. Arthroscopy examination showed an intact graft that exhibited significant laxity to probing and anterior tibial translation (Fig. 6.2). Graft orientation and tunnel positions were confirmed to be acceptable. Revision to a quadrupled hamstring autograft was then performed. After the semitendinosus and gracilis tendons were harvested and whipstitched, they were pretensioned at 80–90N for 20–30 minutes. For graft placement, we were able to utilize the same tunnel positions, as the tunnels were well healed from previous BTB graft plugs (Fig. 6.2). The graft was secured to the femur with an adjustable button-loop device. The knee was cycled 20 times and placed into full extension, reverse Lachman force was applied to ensure reduction of the tibia posteriorly, and, while applying maximal manual force to the graft, an interference screw was placed into the tibial tunnel. The knee was cycled again, and the graft was re-tensioned from the femoral side. Excellent graft tension was observed on direct probing (Fig. 6.2) and on stability testing. To decrease the risk slippage, we also secured the distal graft sutures over a post and tied the tensioning sutures on the femoral side.

Patient recovered well, returning to full competition 1 year postoperatively. Her last clinical examination showed no more than 1A Lachman and anterior drawer and a negative pivot shift. She did not complain of any instability sensation or buckling.

Case 2

Patient is a 55-year-old active male who initially injured his knee playing softball and underwent an ACL reconstruction with allograft at an outside institution. He began having recurrent symptoms of instability shortly after weaning from the postoperative brace, and despite extensive rehabilitation, this did not improve. On exam, his gait was normal, and range of motion and strength were full; however, stability examination demonstrated a 2A Lachman, 1A anterior drawer, and a positive pivot shift with a glide. Imaging with plain radiographs (Fig. 6.3) and an MRI (Fig. 6.3b) demonstrated an intact graft in a vertical orientation, largely due to an excessively posterior tibial tunnel position. Due to the patient's persistent symptoms, evidence of instability on exam, and imaging findings of a vertically oriented graft, a decision was made to proceed with revision surgery. Given the patient's

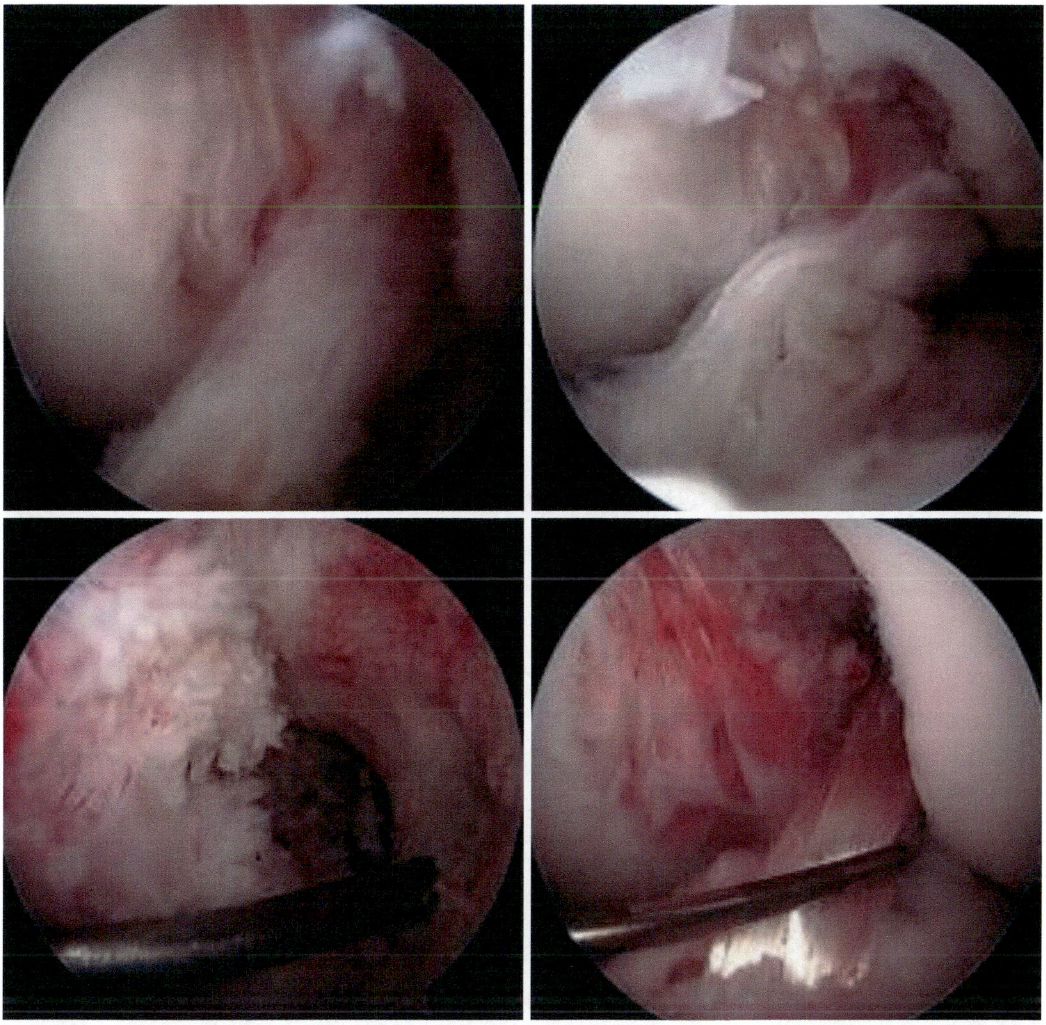

Fig. 6.2 Arthroscopic pictures show an intact graft with significant laxity. The femoral tunnel can be drilled "fresh," as the previous bone plug healed fully. The final graft demonstrated appropriate position and tension

age and activity level, an allograft was selected. Intraoperatively, the previous graft was resected, and completely separate tunnels were drilled (Fig. 6.4), allowing appropriate orientation of the new graft. Secure fixation was obtained on the femoral side with an adjustable button-loop construct, and on the tibial side with an interference screw in the tunnel, backed up by a staple over the distal tail of the graft. At his 1-year follow-up, the patient reported no instability and had a negative Lachman, anterior drawer, and pivot shift tests on exam, and imaging showed appropriate graft orientation and tunnel position (Fig. 6.5).

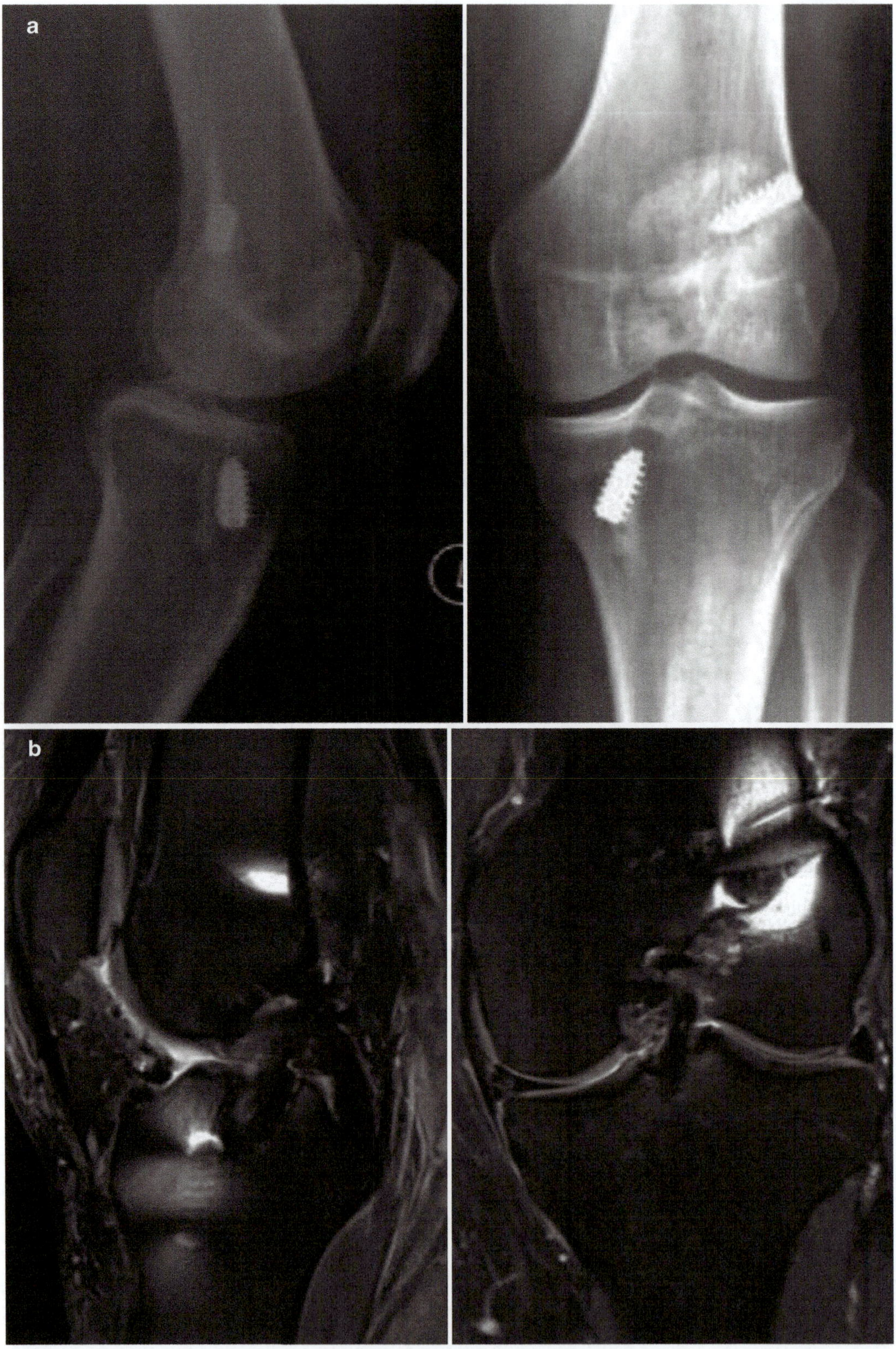

Fig. 6.3 (**a**) Plain radiographs suggest a vertical orientation of the graft, primarily due to a very posterior position of the tibial tunnel. (**b**) MRI confirms vertical orientation of the graft and shows that it is structurally intact

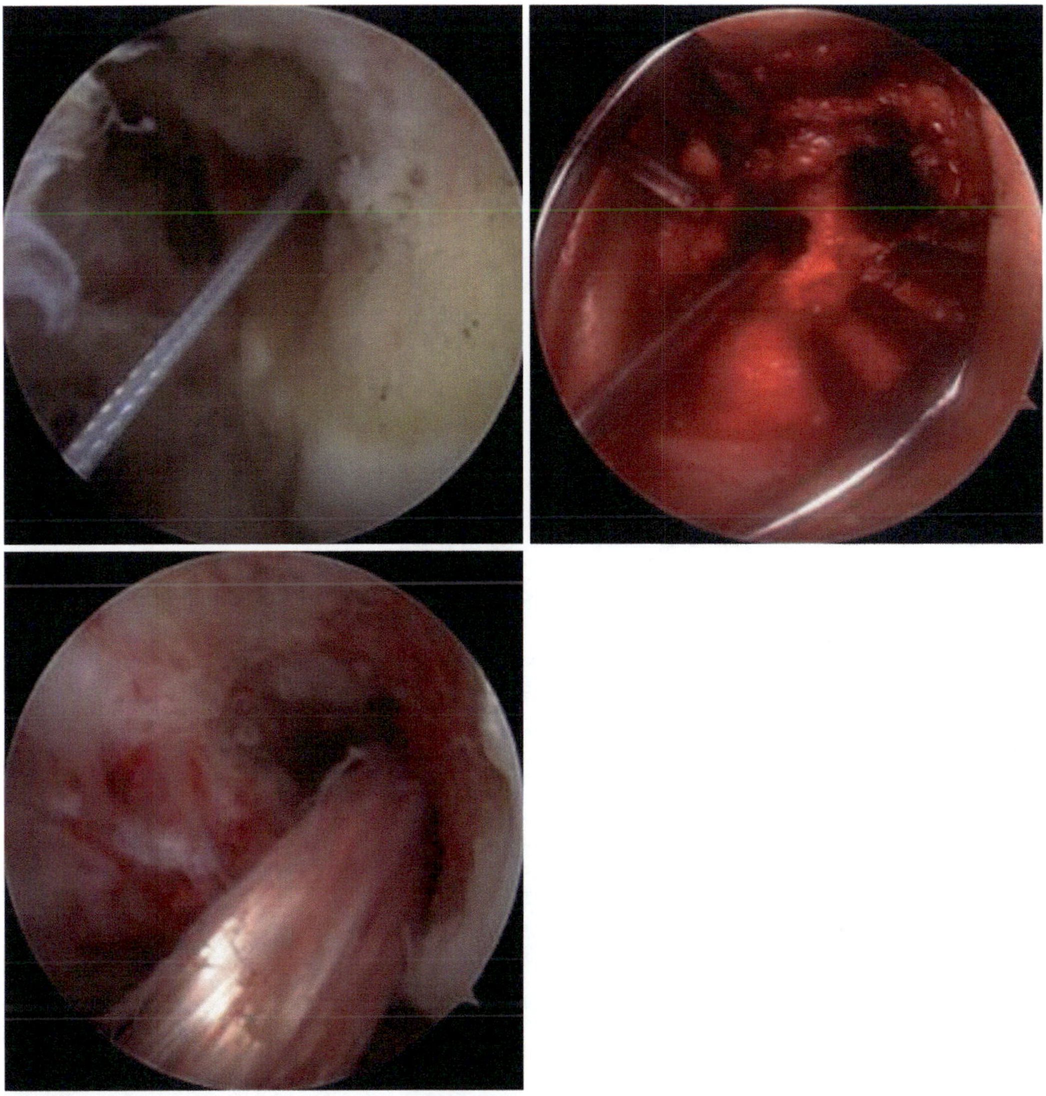

Fig. 6.4 Intraoperative arthroscopy pictures and photographs (left knee). Note the more posterior location of the new femoral tunnel, the more anterior location of the tibial tunnel (metallic suction tip is in the old tunnel), and the proper oblique orientation of the final graft

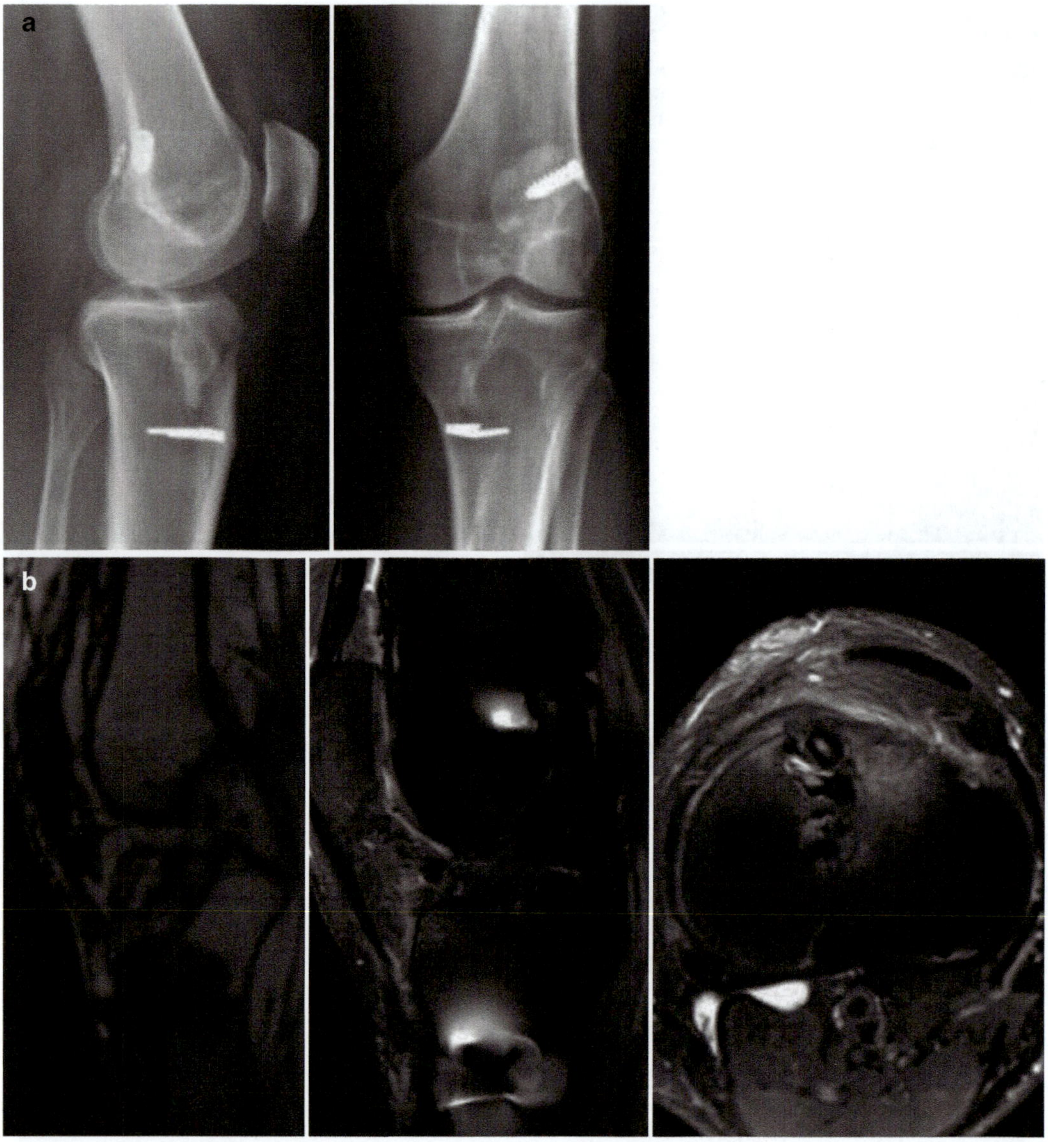

Fig. 6.5 (**a**) One-year postoperative X-rays show proper tunnel position. Note the anterior location of the new tibial tunnel, relative to the old one. (**b**) One-year postoperative MRI shows appropriate orientation of the graft and confirms absence of tunnel convergence

References

1. Risberg MA, Holm I, Myklebust G, Engebretsen L. Neuromuscular training versus strength training during first 6 months after anterior cruciate ligament reconstruction: a randomized clinical trial. Phys Ther. 2007;87(6):737–50.
2. Pilia M, Murray M, Guda T, Heckman M, Appleford M. Pretensioning of soft tissue grafts in anterior cruciate ligament reconstruction. Orthopedics. 2015;38(7):e582–7.
3. Lockwood WC, Marchetti DC, Dahl KD, Mikula JD, Williams BT, Kheir MM, Turnbull TL, LaPrade RF. High-load preconditioning of human soft tissue hamstring grafts: an in vitro biomechanical analysis. Knee Surg Sports Traumatol Arthrosc. 2017;25(1):138–43.
4. Gertel TH, Lew WD, Lewis JL, Stewart NJ, Hunter RE. Effect of anterior cruciate ligament graft tension-

ing direction, magnitude, and flexion angle on knee biomechanics. Am J Sports Med. 1993;21(4):572–81.
5. Van Kampen A. The effect of different graft tensioning in anterior cruciate ligament reconstruction: a prospective randomized study. Arthroscopy. 1998;14(8):845–50.
6. Brown CH Jr, Wilson DR, Hecker AT, Ferragamo M. Graft-bone motion and tensile properties of hamstring and patellar tendon anterior cruciate ligament femoral graft fixation under cyclic loading. Arthroscopy. 2004;20(9):922–35.
7. Kamelger FS, Onder U, Schmoelz W, Tecklenburg K, Arora R, Fink C. Suspensory fixation of grafts in anterior cruciate ligament reconstruction: a biomechanical comparison of 3 implants. Arthroscopy. 2009;25(7):767–76.
8. Steiner ME, Hecker AT, Brown CH Jr, Hayes WC. Anterior cruciate ligament graft fixation: comparison of hamstring and patellar tendon grafts. Am J Sports Med. 1994;22(2):240–7.
9. Maletis GB, Inacio MC, Desmond JL, Funahashi TT. Reconstruction of the anterior cruciate ligament: association of graft choice with increased risk of early revision. Bone Joint J. 2013;95(5):623–8.
10. Mars Group. Effect of graft choice on the outcome of revision anterior cruciate ligament reconstruction in the Multicenter ACL Revision Study (MARS) Cohort. Am J Sports Med. 2014;42(10):2301–10.
11. Magnussen RA, Taylor DC, Toth AP, Garrett WE. ACL graft failure location differs between allografts and autografts. Sports Med Arthrosc Rehabil Ther Technol. 2012;4(1):1–6.
12. Cristiani R, Sarakatsianos V, Engström B, Samuelsson K, Forssblad M, Stålman A. Increased knee laxity with hamstring tendon autograft compared to patellar tendon autograft: a cohort study of 5462 patients with primary anterior cruciate ligament reconstruction. Knee Surg Sports Traumatol Arthrosc. 2019;27(2):381–8.
13. Beynnon BD, Johnson RJ, Fleming BC, Kannus P, Kaplan M, Samani J, Renström P. Anterior cruciate ligament replacement: comparison of bone-patellar tendon-bone grafts with two-strand hamstring grafts: a prospective, randomized study. JBJS. 2002;84(9):1503–13.
14. Freedman KB, D'Amato MJ, Nedeff DD, Kaz A, Bach BR. Arthroscopic anterior cruciate ligament reconstruction: a metaanalysis comparing patellar tendon and hamstring tendon autografts. Am J Sports Med. 2003;31(1):2–11.
15. Burnham JM, Malempati CS, Carpiaux A, Ireland ML, Johnson DL. Anatomic femoral and tibial tunnel placement during anterior cruciate ligament reconstruction: anteromedial portal all-inside and outside-in techniques. Arthrosc Tech. 2017;6(2):e275–82.
16. Rupp S, Müller B, Seil R. Knee laxity after ACL reconstruction with a BPTB graft. Knee Surg Sports Traumatol Arthrosc. 2001;9(2):72–6.
17. Chhabra A, Diduch DR, Blessey PB, Miller MD. Recreating an acceptable angle of the tibial tunnel in the coronal plane in anterior cruciate ligament reconstruction using external landmarks. Arthroscopy. 2004;20(3):328–30.
18. Morgan JA, Dahm D, Levy B, Stuart MJ, MARS Study Group. Femoral tunnel malposition in ACL revision reconstruction. J Knee Surg. 2012;25(5):361.
19. Zavras TD, Race A, Bull AM, Amis AA. A comparative study of 'isometric' points for anterior cruciate ligament graft attachment. Knee Surg Sports Traumatol Arthrosc. 2001;9(1):28–33.
20. Inderhaug E, Strand T, Fischer-Bredenbeck C, Solheim E. Effect of a too posterior placement of the tibial tunnel on the outcome 10–12 years after anterior cruciate ligament reconstruction using the 70-degree tibial guide. Knee Surg Sports Traumatol Arthrosc. 2014;22(5):1182–9.
21. Chhabra A, Starman JS, Ferretti M, Vidal AF, Zantop T, Fu FH. Anatomic, radiographic, biomechanical, and kinematic evaluation of the anterior cruciate ligament and its two functional bundles. JBJS. 2006;88(suppl_4):2–10.
22. Ziegler CG, Pietrini SD, Westerhaus BD, Anderson CJ, Wijdicks CA, Johansen S, Engebretsen L, LaPrade RF. Arthroscopically pertinent landmarks for tunnel positioning in single-bundle and double-bundle anterior cruciate ligament reconstructions. Am J Sports Med. 2011;39(4):743–52.
23. Helito CP, Camargo DB, Sobrado MF, Bonadio MB, Giglio PN, Pécora JR, Camanho GL, Demange MK. Combined reconstruction of the anterolateral ligament in chronic ACL injuries leads to better clinical outcomes than isolated ACL reconstruction. Knee Surg Sports Traumatol Arthrosc. 2018;26(12):3652–9.
24. Won HH, Chang CB, Je MS, Chang MJ, Kim TK. Coronal limb alignment and indications for high tibial osteotomy in patients undergoing revision ACL reconstruction. Clinical Orthopaedics and Related Research®. 2013;471(11):3504–11.
25. Jan van de Pol G, Arnold MP, Verdonschot N, van Kampen A. Varus alignment leads to increased forces in the anterior cruciate ligament. Am J Sports Med. 2009;37(3):481–7.
26. Hinckel BB, Demange MK, Gobbi RG, Ricardo J, Camanho GL. The effect of mechanical varus on anterior cruciate ligament and lateral collateral ligament stress: finite element analyses. Orthopedics. 2016;39(4):e729–36.
27. Zaffagnini S, Bonanzinga T, Grassi A, Muccioli GM, Musiani C, Raggi F, Iacono F, Vaccari V, Marcacci M. Combined ACL reconstruction and closing-wedge HTO for varus angulated ACL-deficient knees. Knee Surg Sports Traumatol Arthrosc. 2013;21(4):934–41.
28. Klek M, Dhawan A. The role of high Tibial osteotomy in ACL reconstruction in knees with coronal and sagittal plane deformity. Curr Rev Musculoskelet Med. 2019;12(4):466–71.
29. Noyes FR, Barber SD, Simon R. High tibial osteotomy and ligament reconstruction in varus angulated, anterior cruciate ligament-deficient knees: a two-to seven-year follow-up study. Am J Sports Med. 1993;21(1):2–12.

30. Bernhardson AS, Aman ZS, Dornan GJ, Kemler BR, Storaci HW, Brady AW, Nakama GY, LaPrade RF. Tibial slope and its effect on force in anterior cruciate ligament grafts: anterior cruciate ligament force increases linearly as posterior tibial slope increases. Am J Sports Med. 2019;47(2):296–302.
31. Arun GR, Kumaraswamy V, Rajan D, Vinodh K, Singh AK, Kumar P, Chandrasekaran K, Santosh S, Kishore C. Long-term follow up of single-stage anterior cruciate ligament reconstruction and high tibial osteotomy and its relation with posterior tibial slope. Arch Orthop Trauma Surg. 2016;136(4):505–11.
32. Webb JM, Salmon LJ, Leclerc E, Pinczewski LA, Roe JP. Posterior tibial slope and further anterior cruciate ligament injuries in the anterior cruciate ligament–reconstructed patient. Am J Sports Med. 2013;41(12):2800–4.
33. Lee CC, Youm YS, Do Cho S, Jung SH, Bae MH, Park SJ, Kim HW. Does posterior tibial slope affect graft rupture following anterior cruciate ligament reconstruction? Arthroscopy. 2018;34(7):2152–5.
34. Imhoff FB, Mehl J, Comer BJ, Obopilwe E, Cote MP, Feucht MJ, Wylie JD, Imhoff AB, Arciero RA, Beitzel K. Slope-reducing tibial osteotomy decreases ACL-graft forces and anterior tibial translation under axial load. Knee Surg Sports Traumatol Arthrosc. 2019;27(10):3381–9.
35. Schuster P, Geßlein M, Schlumberger M, Mayer P, Richter J. The influence of tibial slope on the graft in combined high tibial osteotomy and anterior cruciate ligament reconstruction. Knee. 2018;25(4):682–91.
36. Dejour D, Saffarini M, Demey G, Baverel L. Tibial slope correction combined with second revision ACL produces good knee stability and prevents graft rupture. Knee Surg Sports Traumatol Arthrosc. 2015;23(10):2846–52.
37. Kim SJ, Choi DH, Hwang BY. The influence of posterolateral rotatory instability on ACL reconstruction: comparison between isolated ACL reconstruction and ACL reconstruction combined with posterolateral corner reconstruction. JBJS. 2012;94(3):253–9.
38. Stephen JM, Halewood C, Kittl C, Bollen SR, Williams A, Amis AA. Posteromedial meniscocapsular lesions increase tibiofemoral joint laxity with anterior cruciate ligament deficiency, and their repair reduces laxity. Am J Sports Med. 2016;44(2):400–8.
39. DePhillipo NN, Moatshe G, Brady A, Chahla J, Aman ZS, Dornan GJ, Nakama GY, Engebretsen L, LaPrade RF. Effect of meniscocapsular and meniscotibial lesions in ACL-deficient and ACL-reconstructed knees: a biomechanical study. Am J Sports Med. 2018;46(10):2422–31.
40. Cristiani R, Rönnblad E, Engström B, Forssblad M, Stålman A. Medial meniscus resection increases and medial meniscus repair preserves anterior knee laxity: a cohort study of 4497 patients with primary anterior cruciate ligament reconstruction. Am J Sports Med. 2018;46(2):357–62.
41. Grassi A, Macchiarola L, Urrizola Barrientos F, Zicaro JP, Costa Paz M, Adravanti P, Dini F, Zaffagnini S. Steep posterior tibial slope, anterior tibial subluxation, deep posterior lateral femoral condyle, and meniscal deficiency are common findings in multiple anterior cruciate ligament failures: an MRI case-control study. Am J Sports Med. 2019;47(2):285–95.

Management of Osteolysis in Revision ACL: The Role of Single-Stage Reconstruction

7

Courtney A. Quinn, F. Winston Gwathmey, and Mark D. Miller

Introduction

Planning for revision anterior cruciate ligament (ACL) reconstruction involves consideration of numerous factors to determine the best method and timing for surgery, as certain variables can dictate whether a one- or a two-stage revision is optimal. Performing an ACL revision in a single-stage operation is preferable for many reasons. With a single procedure, the patient is subjected to only one surgery, which has decreased patient morbidity, healthcare costs, and missed work or school. Single-stage revisions allow for faster overall rehabilitation and return to sport. Additionally, delaying definitive ACL reconstruction increases the risk of chondral and meniscal damage to the knee that may be sustained in the ACL-deficient waiting period between the first and second stages [1, 2].

A major factor that dictates the timeline for ACL revision surgery is the degree of widening and the position of the femoral and tibial tunnels made during the index procedure. Tunnel widening, also known as tunnel osteolysis, is a common radiographic and anatomic entity. The clinical implications of tunnel widening on ACL outcomes are largely unknown; there is no clear indication that osteolysis of tunnels is associated with increased graft failure rates or worse patient-reported outcomes [3, 4]. Nevertheless, tunnel osteolysis can present a challenging problem in revision ACL surgery.

The etiology of tunnel widening is not well understood, but it is postulated to be due to mechanical and/or biologic causes. Mechanical concerns are micromotion of the graft within the tunnel ("windshield wipering"), stress shielding on the graft, and possibly accelerated rehabilitation protocols [5]. Suspensory fixation is associated with increased rates of tunnel widening [6]. Graft choice is also a factor, as allograft tissue causes higher rates of osteolysis than autograft [7]. Additionally, hamstring grafts have been shown to be more associated with tunnel osteolysis than bone-patellar tendon-bone grafts [8–10].

Graft micromotion may draw synovial fluid into the tunnel resulting in a high-pressure gradient against the walls, in a so-called bungee cord effect [8]. From a biologic standpoint, synovial fluid entrapment and increased inflammatory response within the tunnel may also increase tunnel diameter [7]. Recently, investigators have suggested that subclinical bacterial colonization is common in patients undergoing revision ACL surgery and is associated with tunnel osteolysis [11], although more studies are needed to further elucidate this.

C. A. Quinn
Department of Orthopaedic Surgery, Inova Health System Fairfax, VA, USA

F. W. Gwathmey (✉) · M. D. Miller
Department of Orthopaedic Surgery, University of Virginia, University of Virginia Health System, Charlottesville, VA, USA

M. J. Alaia, K. J. Jones (eds.), *Revision Anterior Cruciate Ligament Reconstruction*,
https://doi.org/10.1007/978-3-030-96996-7_7

The process of osteolysis is believed to be first appreciated radiographically around 6 months from the index surgery and typically does not progress beyond 2 years postoperatively [5, 12]. The morphology of tunnel expansion can be categorized as linear, cavitary, mushroom, and cone [3] (Fig. 7.1).

Assessment of Tunnel Osteolysis

Typically, plain radiography is used to gauge the degree of osteolysis and can produce accurate measurements [13], although computed tomography (CT) provides more reproducible and reliable measurements of tunnel width and shape

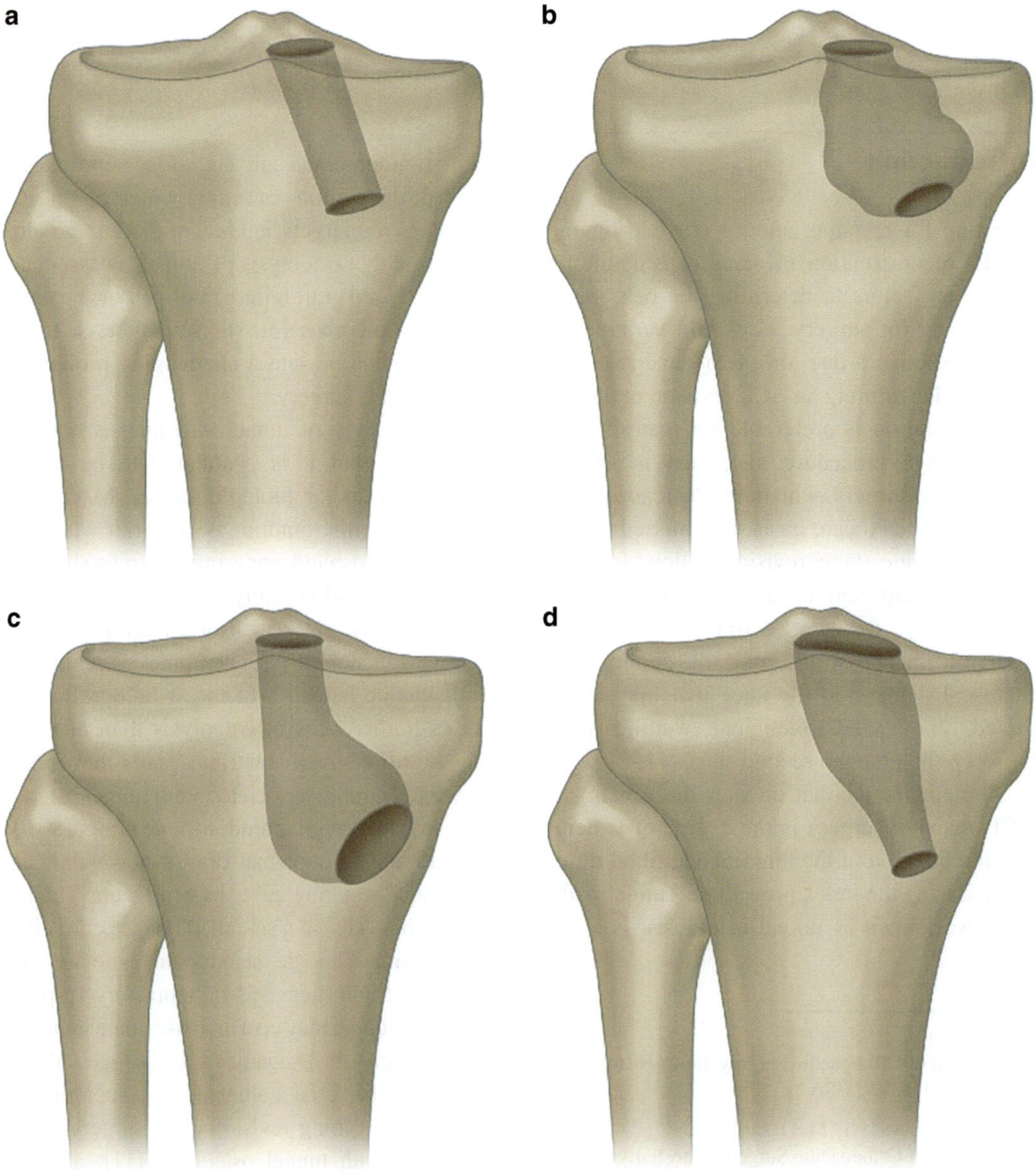

Fig. 7.1 Types of tunnel osteolysis morphology, as described by Klein et al. [3]. (**a**) Linear, (**b**) cavitary, (**c**) mushroom, (**d**) cone

and can also better illustrate tunnel position [14, 15]. Magnetic resonance imaging (MRI) is inferior to plain radiography and CT in determining tunnel anatomy and should not be used in isolation when planning for revision surgery if tunnel widening is suspected.

A CT scan is recommended for preoperative planning in revision ACL surgeries when there is concern for tunnel osteolysis or atypical tunnel morphology. Femoral and tibial tunnel diameter should be measured at the widest visualized diameter on the axial, coronal, and sagittal planes, as seen in Fig. 7.2. There is no concrete consensus in the literature on what degree of osteolysis constitutes a two-stage surgery, but it is generally agreed upon that if tunnel widening is less than 14 mm, a single-stage revision can be accomplished [2, 16, 17]. Measurements ≥15 mm are consistent with significant tunnel osteolysis. With such a degree of widening, it is recommended that a two-stage revision approach be pursued [18–20]. In these circumstances, the tunnels can be prepared and filled with bone graft or other bone substitutes during the first procedure, with the revision ACL reconstruction performed in a delayed fashion. Please refer to Chap. 9 on indications and techniques for two-stage revision reconstruction.

Tunnel Positioning and Osteolysis

Proper tunnel positioning is vital to ACL reconstruction. The principles of tunnel positioning and evaluation of prior tunnel placement are described in detail in Chaps. 3, 10, and 11. Tunnel osteolysis complicates revision ACL surgery by adding a degree of difficulty to achieving anatomic tunnel placement. Prior tunnel positioning can be generally classified into three subtypes [21]:

1. Anatomic: current tunnel is in the anatomic position.
2. Completely nonanatomic: the tunnel is entirely out of the way of where the new anatomic tunnel would be placed, so that the new tunnel could be drilled without any overlap with the prior tunnel.
3. Incompletely nonanatomic: the current tunnel overlaps with where the new tunnel would ideally be placed.

Anatomic tunnels or completely nonanatomic tunnels can be relatively straightforward to address. The management of incompletely anatomic tunnels often provides the greatest challenge in revision ACL surgery if performed in a single-stage, as there are multiple goals of surgery that can be conflicting: filling the bony defect, achieving anatomic new tunnel placement, obtaining adequate graft fixation, and ensuring a proper structural and biologic environment for graft incorporation. We will discuss specific techniques for how to address osteolysis in the setting of these different tunnel positions during a single-stage revision procedure.

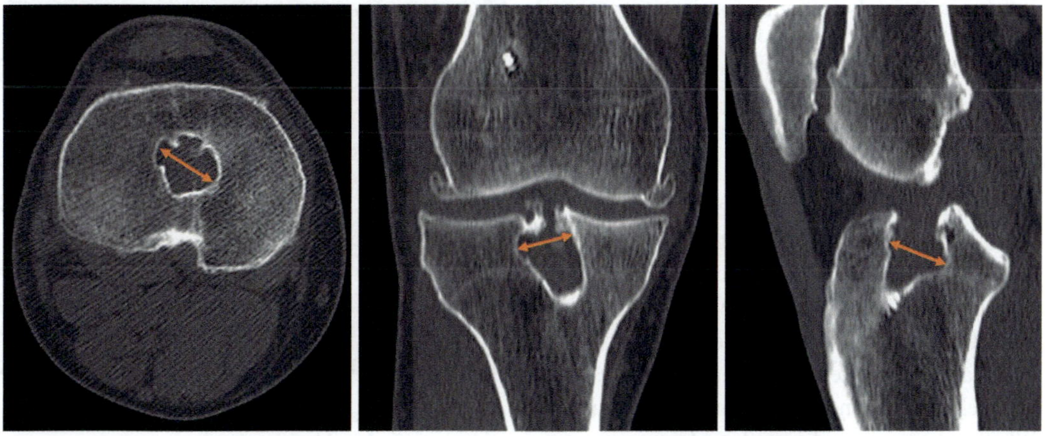

Fig. 7.2 Computed tomography scan with tibial tunnel width measurements made at the tunnel's widest diameter in all three axes (axial, coronal, and sagittal)

Techniques

Prior to surgery, a thorough evaluation of the previous operative reports is imperative to understand which implants were used and how they were applied, as well as to ensure that the implant extraction devices are readily available. Either supine or hemilithotomy positioning can be used, though supine positioning has the advantage of access to the iliac crest for autograft, if desired. A radiolucent table and intraoperative fluoroscopy can be useful for hardware removal and confirmation of tunnel positioning. As is always done, a complete physical examination of both knees is conducted prior to draping.

If the previously made portals are in suboptimal positions, new portals should be made while avoiding narrow skin bridges. Diagnostic arthroscopy is performed to evaluate for other intra-articular pathology, including chondral damage, meniscal tears, and loose bodies, which should be addressed concurrently. Typically, addressing concomitant chondral or meniscal injuries is technically easier while the ACL is absent, so performing these portions of the procedure prior to ACL fixation is recommended. After debridement of the prior ACL stump, and exposure of the anatomic footprints, a limited notchplasty can be performed in patients with notch overgrowth, though the contribution of this step is debated [22].

Anatomic Tunnels

If the prior tunnels are in anatomic positions and there is less than 14 mm of tunnel widening, then a single-stage procedure can be considered. Hardware within the tunnels is removed. If there is asymptomatic backup fixation that was placed outside the tunnel trajectory during the primary reconstruction, this hardware can be left in place. Only hardware that interferes with new graft passage and fixation need be removed.

With hardware removed, the tunnels can be re-cannulated. On the femoral side, a guidewire can be advanced into the tunnel using an offset guide or freehand, depending on surgeon preference. Whether using a rigid or a flexible reaming system, drilling the femoral tunnel in >90 degrees of flexion can improve the surgeon's ability to create an appropriately posterior and oblique tunnel. In the cases of prior soft tissue graft and osteolysis, this guide pin generally advances with ease. Use of intraoperative fluoroscopy will confirm placement of the guide pin centrally within the tunnel on both the AP and lateral views.

For the tibial tunnel, a standard ACL tibial tunnel guide can be used to target the intra-articular footprint. Depending on the prior graft type and hardware used and on the time since the index surgery, it can sometimes be difficult to locate the tunnel opening on the anteromedial tibial cortex. Fluoroscopy can be useful here to aid in localizing the tunnel opening, as well as to confirm central placement of the pin within the tunnel once cannulated.

The tunnels are then reamed sequentially to remove residual graft material and sclerotic bone, which is necessary for incorporation of the new graft. In cases of unexplained or severe osteolysis, the tunnel material should be cultured to rule out indolent infection. The goal of reaming is to achieve circumferential bony margins in the tunnel, as confirmed with direct arthroscopic visualization up the tunnel in Fig. 7.3. If the standard ACL reamers are not wide enough to achieve this goal, the intramedullary reamer set can be used.

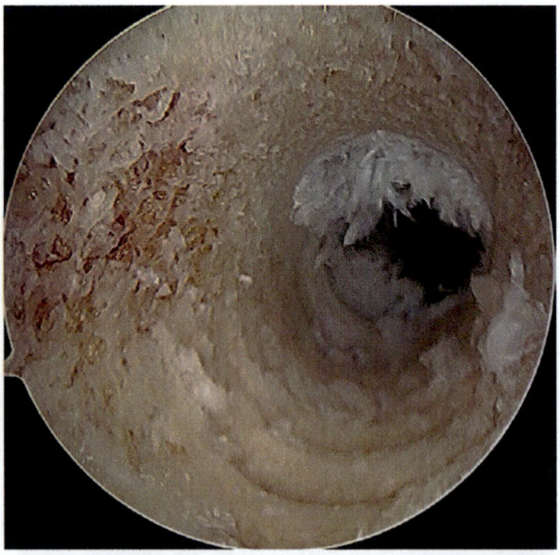

Fig. 7.3 Arthroscopic view up a reamed tibial tunnel with circumferential bony margins

Once reaming is complete, the new graft can be passed in the standard fashion. Graft options are discussed in Chap. 5. In situations in which the resulting tunnel diameter is several millimeters larger than the graft diameter, the difference can be accounted for with one of the several techniques. If planning to use a bone-patellar tendon-bone or quadriceps tendon autograft, a slightly larger than normal graft can be harvested, such as 11-mm or 12-mm diameter. This is a straightforward way to account for tunnel widening and provides the best biologic fixation, but comes at the cost of increased donor site morbidity and possible fracture risk. A larger than typical interference screw can be utilized to obtain adequate graft compression. Stacking interference screws has been used historically [23], but may increase the risk of graft compromise and is biomechanically less stable [24, 25] (Fig. 7.4). Bone graft can also be impacted around the graft in the tunnel prior to fixation. Bone graft can be autograft (usually iliac crest or proximal tibia) or allograft. Allograft can be in the form loose cancellous chips, thin "matchsticks", or as cylindrical bullets [26], as depicted in Fig. 7.5. Once the tunnel

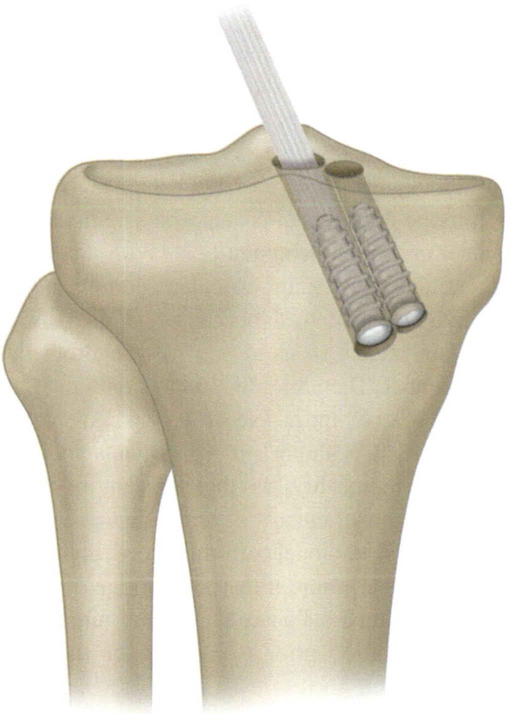

Fig. 7.4 Schematic demonstrating stacking interference screws. Converging or adjacent tunnels can be effectively narrowed by keeping prior or placing new interference screws in nonanatomic tunnels

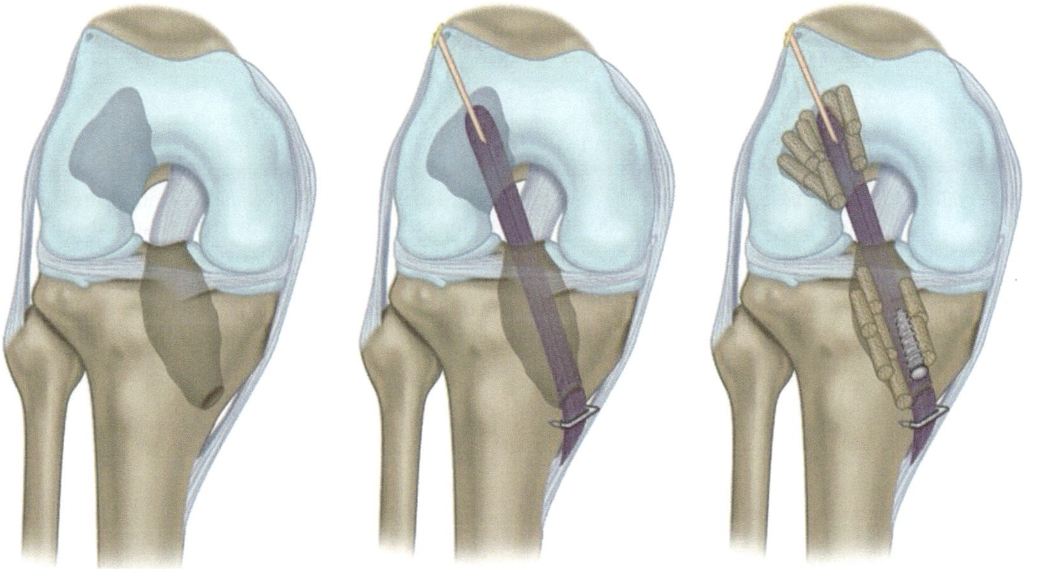

Fig. 7.5 Schematic demonstrating bone graft impaction into widened tunnels after graft passage. (Redrawn from: Ra et al. [37])

is filled around the ACL graft, the graft can be fixed. Interference fixation is generally preferred when possible due to lower rates of osteolysis, but suspensory or cortical fixation is also an appropriate option.

Another technique for single-stage revision in which the prior tunnel is anatomic is a divergent tunnel or funnel technique [27]. With this technique, the tunnel intra-articular aperture at the footprint is maintained, but the new tunnel direction is changed, so as to be divergent from the prior tunnel. Therefore, the tunnels only overlap at the ACL footprint (See Fig. 7.6). With this technique, it is important for patients to have robust bone quality, as the segment of bone between the two tunnels is generally narrow and there is a risk of tunnel perforation and, therefore, loss of graft fixation, if the bone bridge is weak. To avoid tunnel collapse, the former tunnel can be bone grafted prior to drilling of the new tunnel.

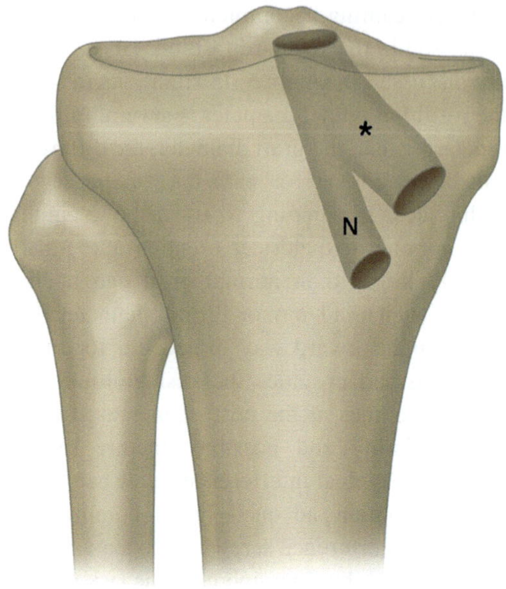

Fig. 7.6 A new tunnel is drilled in a divergent trajectory from the prior tunnel (*) while maintaining the same footprint intra-articularly

Summary of Techniques for Single-Stage Revision with Widened Anatomic Tunnels

Technique	Description	Pro	Con
Use larger ACL graft	Harvesting 11–12-mm BTB or quadriceps tendon graft; tripling semitendinosus for 5-strand total HS graft	No additional steps, better biologic fixation	Donor site morbidity (patella fracture risk, patellar tendon rupture); HS: graft length limitation
Large interference screw	Upsize the interference screw diameter to fill the void	No additional steps	Limited in sizes
Stacking interference screws	Using multiple interference screws around different sides of the graft	Technically easy	Inferior fixation in biomechanical studies; may cut/damage graft
Bone graft tunnel	Using bone graft to narrow the tunnel for a tighter fit around the graft	Avoids need to drill new tunnel; promotes biologic healing/graft incorporation	Technically more challenging; autograft harvest morbidity, if selected
Divergent tunnel/funnel	Using the same anatomic tunnel opening, but using different trajectory	Drilling through native bone to the ideal diameter for the new graft	Thin wall in between tunnels that may collapse

HS hamstrings

Even with effective execution of the above techniques, graft fixation can often be questionable. In any case of concern over fixation integrity, backup fixation of the graft using a suture anchor, a post, or a staple should be employed.

Completely Nonanatomic Tunnels

Prior tunnels that are completely nonanatomic – that is, there will be no overlap between the desired location of the new tunnel and the prior tunnel – are arguably the simplest to treat, even in cases of osteolysis. Nonanatomic tunnels and associated hardware can generally be ignored entirely; the surgeon can proceed with drilling new tunnels in the same fashion as one would with primary ACL reconstruction. If there is an anticipated narrow bone bridge between the former and new tunnel and concern for tunnel collapse, the old tunnel can be bone grafted with auto- or allograft first, to provide a rigid wall against which the new tunnel can be drilled and graft fixation secured.

Incompletely Nonanatomic Tunnels

The most challenging tunnel orientation to treat with a single-stage revision ACL reconstruction is that in which the prior tunnel is nonanatomic, but overlaps with the intended position of the new, anatomic tunnel. Tunnel osteolysis increases the chances of this problem, as the expanded tunnel encroaches upon the anatomic footprint. If tunnel widening is 15 mm or greater, a two-stage reconstruction should be considered, as adequate long-term graft fixation is difficult to achieve in this setting. If widening is 14 mm or less, however, there are several techniques that can be employed to accomplish a successful single-stage outcome.

Dilation Technique

The concept of a dilation method is that as the new tunnel is created adjacent to the original tunnel, bone is impacted outward into the old tunnel, thereby filling the old tunnel as the new one is gradually dilated open. This is in contrast to a standard tunnel technique in which bone is reamed away, which causes tunnel convergence given proximity. With this technique, hardware within the prior tunnel can be kept in place if it will not interfere with the new tunnel, as it acts as a space filler. To create the new tunnel, a guide pin is placed in intact bone – while minimizing contact with the old tunnel whenever possible – in the ideal position for the new tunnel. Often times a divergent tunnel trajectory is needed. Over this pin, a small entry drill (typically around 5-mm diameter) is used to create a narrow tunnel. Through this narrow tunnel, sequentially larger dilators are introduced that slowly expand the tunnel by displacing or impacting cancellous bone in an outwards direction, as opposed to removing the bone as a reamer does. This bone is impacted into the adjacent nonanatomic tunnel. If successful, a wall of bone is maintained between the two tunnels, so that there is minimal convergence. In good quality bone, this technique can be challenging, as the cancellous bone is not easily displaced with a dilator. Depending on the size of the prior tunnel and amount of bone between the new tunnels, there may not be sufficient bone to collapse the prior tunnel entirely. The bridge between the two tunnels can become thin and not uncommonly results in subpar bony fixation for the graft. Biomechanically, this technique is associated with higher rates of graft fixation failure than other techniques [25]. For these reasons, this technique is not commonly used.

Maintaining Prior Hardware

Removing interference screws is not always necessary, as it can be surprisingly difficult to extract, but also can leave the tunnel gap even wider. Because most metallic interference screws are titanium, the stainless steel reamer can be used to drill through part of the screw. This can be accomplished with relative ease and little damage to the reamer if there is minimal overlap between the reamer and the screw – i.e., if used to "smooth" out the peripheral threads of the screw (Fig. 7.7). Metallic debris can be expected but easily irrigated away. If there is significant over-

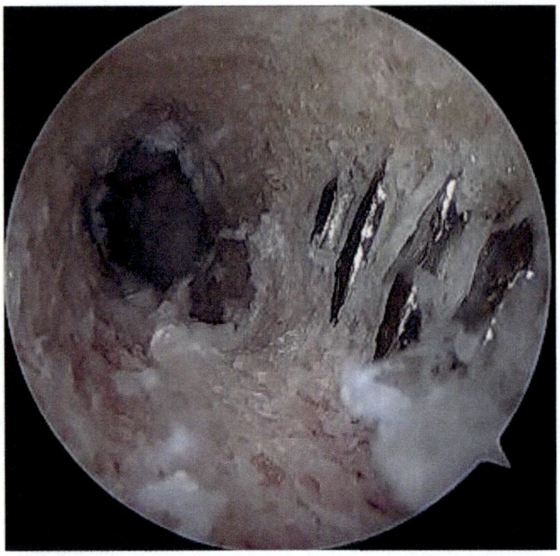

Fig. 7.7 View within a tibial tunnel demonstrating a retained metallic interference screw that has been partially drilled through. This can be performed to avoid the need to remove the screw

lap between the reamer and the screw, this method is not recommended.

Interference screws can also be stacked, as mentioned in the previous section on anatomic tunnels.

Tunnel Filling (With Bone Graft or Bone Substitute) and Immediate Drilling

Bone grafting of prior tunnels has been used extensively to treat malpositioned tunnels or widened tunnels in the two-stage revision setting. Its use in the single-stage setting has gained further popularity in recent years as its efficacy has been proven in the literature [26, 28]. With this technique, the previous tunnel is prepared and then filled with bone graft (autograft or allograft) or bone substitute, then the new tunnel is immediately drilled adjacent to or overlapping with the previous tunnel. Hardware that is in the prior tunnel or is in the way of the new tunnel should be removed so that the prior tunnel can be thoroughly debrided of graft material and sclerotic bone. Reamers, curettes, and the arthroscopic shaver, among other tools, can be utilized to debride the tunnels.

Autologous bone grafting of widened tunnels is described almost exclusively in two-stage revision settings [29]. While autograft is the gold standard for the management of bone defects, there is morbidity with procurement, particularly if the volume of graft needed is substantial. Iliac crest bone graft has the advantage of providing a corticocancellous graft that can be shaped cylindrically. It is recommended to place the cortical portion of the graft posteriorly in the tibial tunnel, as it is the posterior portion of the tunnel that endures the highest compressive force by the tendon grafts after ACL reconstruction [20, 30]. Corticocancellous bone from the proximal tibia can also be used, extracted with the coring tube set used during osteochondral autograft harvesting [31, 32]. While there are other sources of autograft bone described for use in ACL revision surgery (including femoral marrow cavity bone harvested with a reamer-irrigator-aspirator (RIA) system [33]), autograft used in a single-stage setting must have a robust structural property in order to support immediate tendon graft fixation.

The use of allograft bone to fill widened tunnels is more commonly used in single-stage revision ACL reconstruction because it provides ample supply with no donor site morbidity and is commercially available in different shapes and sizes to fit patient-specific needs. Cylindrical allograft dowels allow for a structural, bulk void-filler that can obtain excellent press fit fixation in a tunnel [28, 34, 35]. Postoperative CT imaging studies confirm that there is excellent incorporation of these dowels with the patient's native bone [28]. Cancellous allograft chips can also be used to fill defects, either prior to or after drilling the revision tunnel [26, 36]. Strips (or "matchsticks") of allograft bone can be used in a similar fashion, to act as a "shim" to narrow the tunnel and compress the graft [37, 38], as was depicted similarly in Fig. 7.5.

However, not all tunnels undergo uniform osteolysis in a cylindrical fashion – some are cone-shaped or cystic – meaning that gross widening only occurs at certain portions of the tunnel. Reaming a cavitary tunnel into a cylindrical one (to accept a large bulk bone graft) requires widening the entire tunnel to its widest diameter, resulting in a potentially significant amount of native bone removal. This is one drawback to structural bone grafts.

Bone substitutes have the advantage of being amorphous in their pre-hardened states. Because of this versatility, these substances can fill cavities of any shape without the need to remove excess bone. Investigations have demonstrated the use of fast-setting calcium phosphate bone substitutes in single-stage revision ACL reconstructions to be biomechanically sound in cadaveric studies [39, 40], even when applied arthroscopically in an aqueous environment. This technique has been used in vivo for single-stage reconstruction with good results [41], but demonstration of long-term efficacy is lacking. An ideal bone substitute for single-stage revision ACL reconstruction is one that is easily deliverable into a small space, initially a viscous liquid so that it can take on the shape of the cavity, fast-setting without dissolution arthroscopically, durable over time, and allows for (or at least does not inhibit) tendon graft incorporation. Clinical studies are in the early stages of research with this technique, but may prove to be of high utility in the future, particularly for irregularly shaped bone tunnels.

Authors' Preferred Technique: Allograft Dowels

For cases in which prior tunnels are incompletely nonanatomic but tunnel diameter is less than 14 mm, the authors prefer a single-stage revision ACL reconstruction using freeze-dried allograft dowels to fill the widened tunnels. These grafts provide sufficient structural support to allow immediate redrilling of new tunnels partially through or next to the dowel.

Intraoperatively, a final assessment of tunnel position and osteolysis is made. Hardware is removed, unless it is out of range of the prior tunnels and the intended revision tunnels. The previous tunnels are then thoroughly debrided of graft material. A cannulated dilator is introduced into the tunnel, and then a guide pin is placed through the hole of the dilator to ensure central positioning of the pin prior to reaming. The dilator is then removed, and the tunnel is reamed over the pin. Sequentially larger reamers are used to achieve

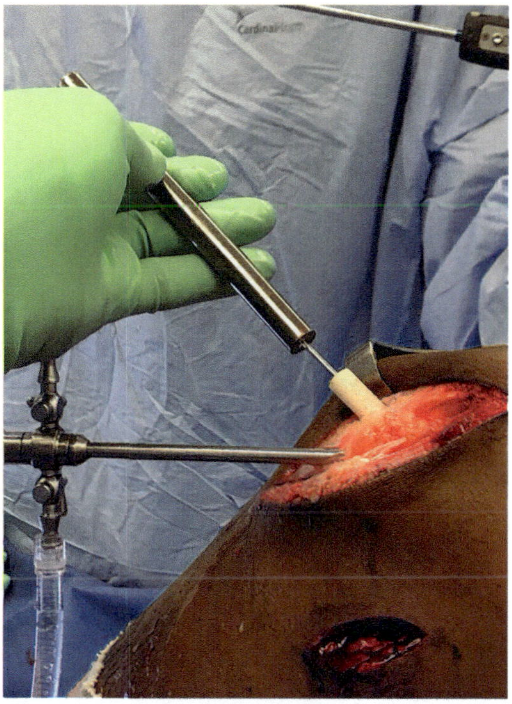

Fig. 7.8 Delivery of a cannulated allograft bone dowel into a femoral tunnel using a cannulated tamp system

circumferential bony margins. Allograft dowels are available in a variety of diameters (typically in increments of 1 mm, ranging 10–18 mm), as well as various lengths. The authors use a cannulated allograft dowel system, with a bulleted end for ease of insertion. It is recommended to use a dowel of the same diameter of the largest reamer used on the tunnel, as this obtains the best press fit while decreasing risk of dowel fracture. The dowel is rehydrated with sterile saline before being impacted into the tunnel using a cannulated tamp (Fig. 7.8). Insertion of the dowel is to be done carefully, as dowel fracture is possible and can lead to insufficient fixation and bony incorporation.

Due to the press fit fixation, the revision tunnel can be drilled immediately adjacent to or overlapping with a portion of the dowel, as long as the overlap is <50% of the dowel (Fig. 7.9). Overlap of the new tunnel with the dowel of >50% increases the risk of dowel fracture and loss of dowel fixation. Efforts should be made to have the tunnels be divergent whenever possible

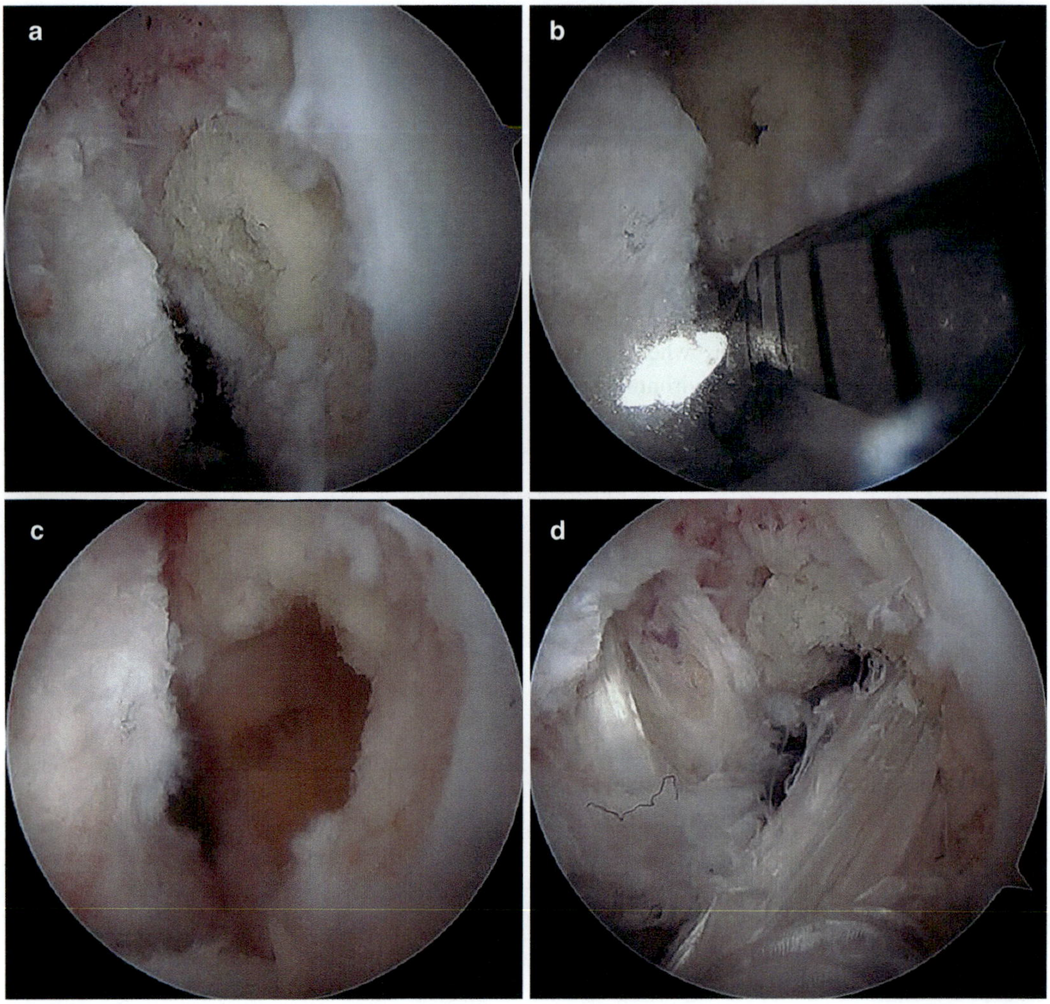

Fig. 7.9 With incompletely nonanatomic tunnels, the prior tunnel can be filled with bone graft and then the new tunnel drilled through part of the tunnel, especially if there is a press fit. These pictures are views of the medial wall of the lateral femoral condyle and the ACL femoral footprint. (**a**) The prior incompletely nonanatomic tunnel was reamed and then filled with a cylindrical cannulated allograft bone dowel. (**b**) The aperture and trajectory for the new femoral tunnel is established via an outside-in technique to ensure a divergent course. (**c**) The new tunnel is drilled with some overlap with the allograft bone, without fracturing the dowel. This is possible due to the press fit of the dowel. (**d**) The new ACL graft is fixed with interference fixation

while keeping the entry point of the revision tunnel anatomic. Using a two-incision outside-in femoral tunnel can be useful in this setting to ensure tunnel divergence. The new ACL graft can be fixed as one would in a primary ACL reconstruction setting, although there is a preference for aperture fixation with interference screws, given a lower risk for tunnel osteolysis compared to suspensory fixation [6]. As with all revision ACL procedures, the surgeon must always have a backup plan for each step of the procedure in the event that technical issues arise or there is inadequate fixation. When in doubt at any step, defaulting to a two-stage procedure is preferable to suboptimal single-stage execution.

Outcomes

Yoon et al. [36] performed a study comparing outcomes of single-stage revision reconstruction in patients with tunnel diameter <12 mm to those with tunnel diameters >12 mm. Patients with tunnels >9 mm in diameter had the tunnels impacted with allograft bone chips to effectively narrow the tunnel prior to fixation. Results demonstrated that there was no difference in subjective outcomes or failure rates between the two groups at a minimum of 5-year follow-up (average follow-up was 7.9 years) but that the group with preoperative tunnel diameter <12 mm had better objective knee stability (Lachman and pivot shift exams and telos measurements).

A study by Mitchell et al. compared single-stage vs two-stage ACL reconstructions in 88 patients with a minimum 2-year follow-up and found that there were no objective or subjective differences between the groups at final follow-up [42]. Single-stage bone grafting with bulk allograft dowels and immediate adjacent drilling has also been shown to be effective in several level IV clinical studies [28, 35]. Werner et al. published favorable results with their series of 12 patients treated in a single-stage revision with use of allograft dowels and average of 2.6-year follow-up. In their series, there were no objective ACL graft failures, and there was excellent incorporation of the bone graft on postoperative CT scan.

Tips and Pearls

- Obtain prior operative notes to ensure the appropriate tools are available for hardware removal.
- Liberal use of intraoperative fluoroscopy is encouraged to assist with localizing prior hardware and identifying tunnel location and trajectory.
- Consider backup fixation of the graft if there is any concern for graft stability,
- Always have a plan B (and C) available for each step of the procedure, as revision reconstruction is commonly unpredictable
- If intraoperative evaluation reveals that a single-stage procedure would result in suboptimal graft fixation, defaulting to a two-stage procedure is encouraged.

Case Examples

Case 1: Completely Nonanatomic and Widened Tibial Tunnel

The patient is a 19-year-old female who presented with right knee pain and instability after a pivot injury sustained 2 weeks prior. She noted immediate swelling and a pop at the time of the injury. She previously had a right ACL reconstruction using hamstring tendon autograft 4 years prior by a different surgeon. Her exam was concerning for a re-tear of her ACL, which was confirmed on MRI. Her plain radiographs at the time are shown in Fig. 7.10, demonstrating an excessively posterior tibial tunnel that was widened to 12 mm. The femoral tunnel appeared to be in an appropriate position with a diameter of 11 mm. There was no coronal or sagittal malalignment.

After discussion with the patient, we elected to proceed with a single-stage ACL reconstruction using bone-patellar tendon-bone (BTB) autograft, assuming our arthroscopic evaluation was consistent with preoperative imaging. The procedure began first with removal of hardware from the femoral tunnel (Fig. 7.11). The AperFix device (Fig. 7.12) (formerly Cayenne Medical, now Zimmer Biomet) was removed, and a 6-mm cannulated dilator was inserted into the femoral tunnel and was used to establish the tunnel's trajectory bluntly. A guide pin was then passed through the cannula, centrally in the tunnel. After the dilator is removed, the tunnel was reamed of soft tissue sequentially to a diameter of 12 mm.

The anteromedial tibia was exposed through the previous incision, and the opening of the tibial tunnel was identified. The PEEK interference screw and sheath were removed (Fig. 7.13). An ACL elbow guide was used to insert a guide pin through the tibial tunnel, exiting at the tunnel's aperture intra-articularly. Starting with a 6-mm reamer and progressing sequentially, the tunnel was reamed over this guide wire until all soft tis-

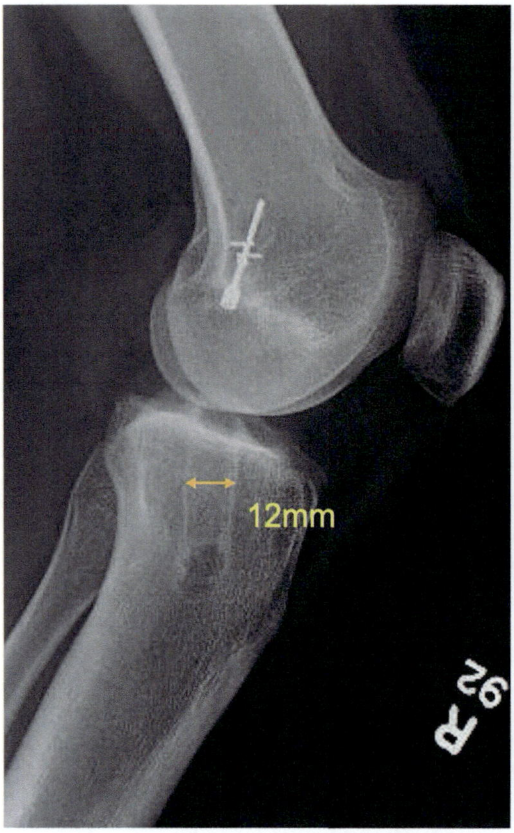

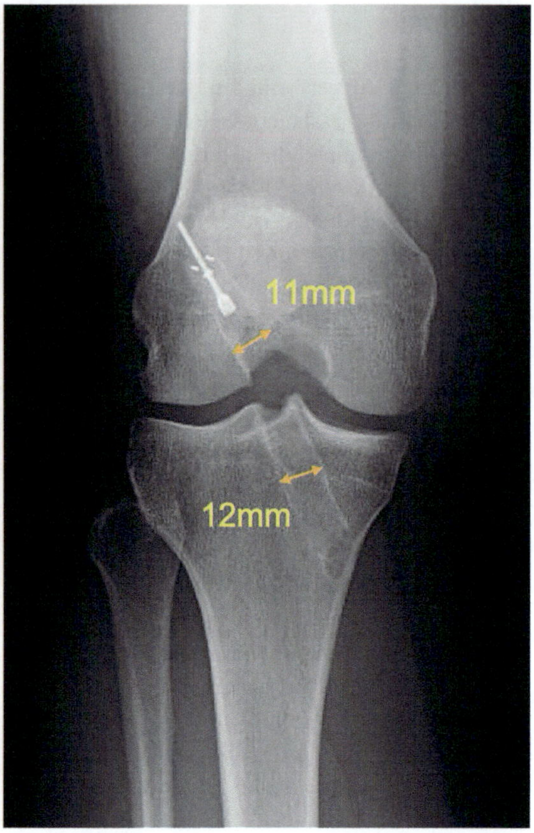

Fig. 7.10 AP and lateral radiographs demonstrating a posteriorly malpositioned tibial tunnel that is 12-mm wide. The femoral tunnel is 11-mm wide, but appears to be in appropriate position. There is an aperture fixation device employed for femoral fixation

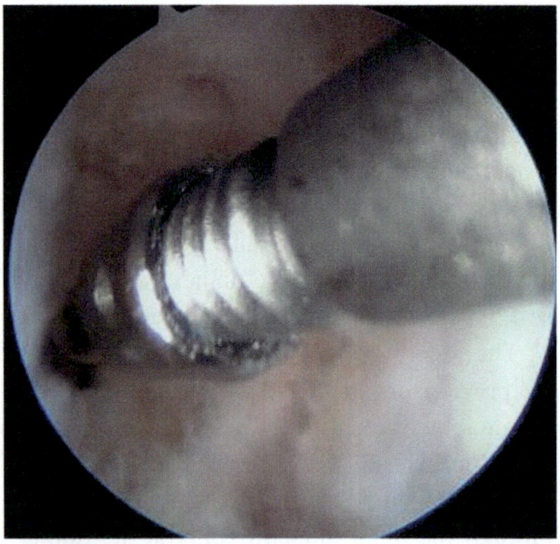

Fig. 7.11 Prior hardware being removed from the femoral tunnel

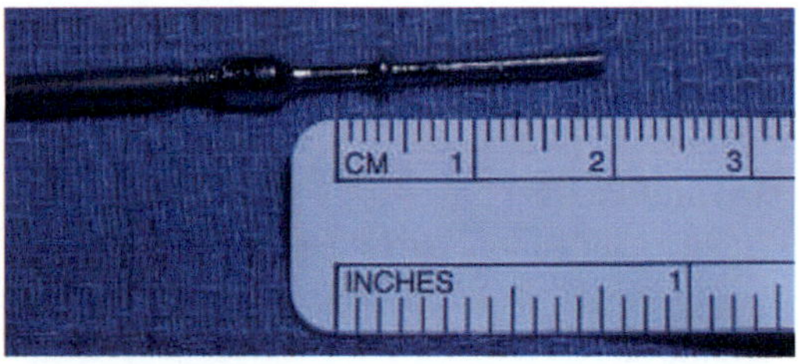

Fig. 7.12 AperFix device (formerly Cayenne Medical, now Zimmer Biomet) from the patient's original hamstrings ACL fixation that was removed from the femoral tunnel during revision surgery

sue was removed from the tunnel, which was accomplished with a 12-mm reamer. The arthroscope was inserted into the tunnel to confirm this clearance of soft tissue (Fig. 7.14). A 12-mm metallic dilator was placed into the tibial tunnel,

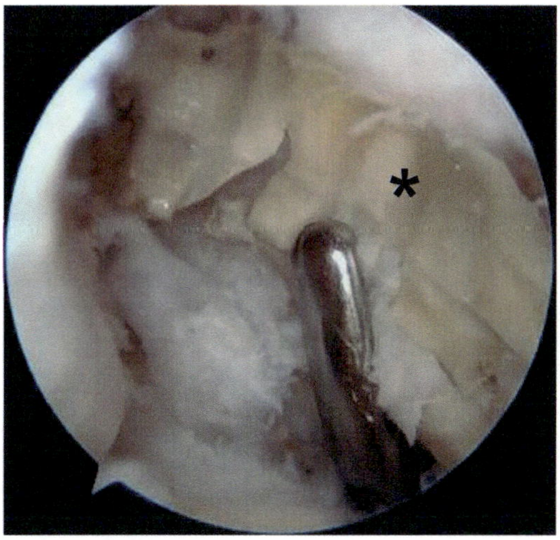

Fig. 7.13 PEEK sheath (*) removed from the tibial tunnel using a grasper

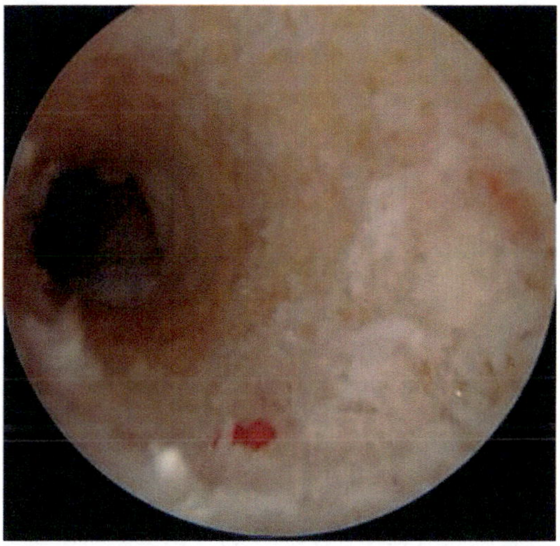

Fig. 7.14 View up the prior malpositioned tibial tunnel that was reamed to 12 mm to clear debris before bone grafting

and fluoroscopy was used to verify that this tunnel was excessively posterior. Given the diameters of both tunnels were <14 mm, a final decision was made to proceed with single-stage reconstruction. With this confirmation, the BTB autograft with 11-mm diameter bone plugs was then harvested.

Returning to the tibial tunnel, a cannulated 12 mm × 30 mm allograft bone dowel (LifeNet

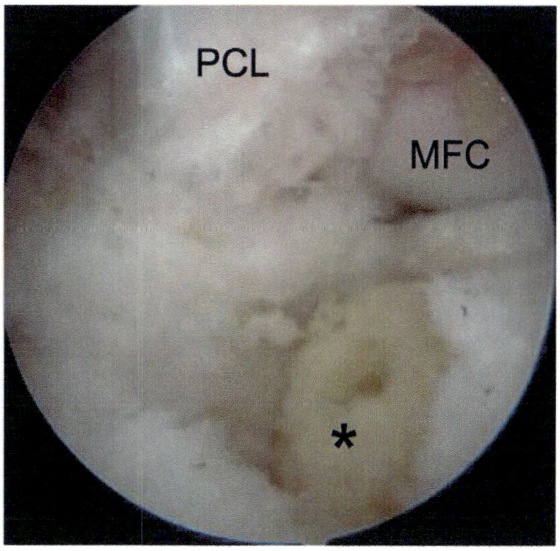

Fig. 7.15 Allograft dowel (*; LifeNet Tissue Service; 12 mm x 30 mm into a 12 mm tunnel) placed in the prior tibial tunnel before drilling new tunnel. The dowel is advanced to the level of the joint surface. View from anterolateral portal. (* allograft bone dowel, MFC medial femoral condyle, PCL posterior cruciate ligament)

Tissue Service) was inserted with gentle impaction using a cannulated tamp, until it was flush with the tibial plateau (Fig. 7.15). With the previous tunnel filled, a guide pin for the new tibial tunnel was passed using an elbow guide into the anatomic footprint location. The position of the pin was confirmed with fluoroscopy. An 11-mm reamer was used to drill the tunnel, placing the entry point on the anterior tibia in between our previous tunnel opening and the tibial tubercle harvest site (Fig. 7.16). There was minimal to no overlap between the two tunnels at the joint surface (Fig. 7.17), but the allograft dowel was necessary to prevent tunnel collapse. The BTB autograft was then able to be passed and fixed with metal interference screws on both the tibial and femoral sides after appropriate tensioning (Fig. 7.18).

The patient was made immediate weight-bearing without a brace, with range of motion encouraged. She progressed through the standard ACL rehabilitation protocol postoperatively and did well returning to recreational exercise without residual instability at 7 months postoperatively.

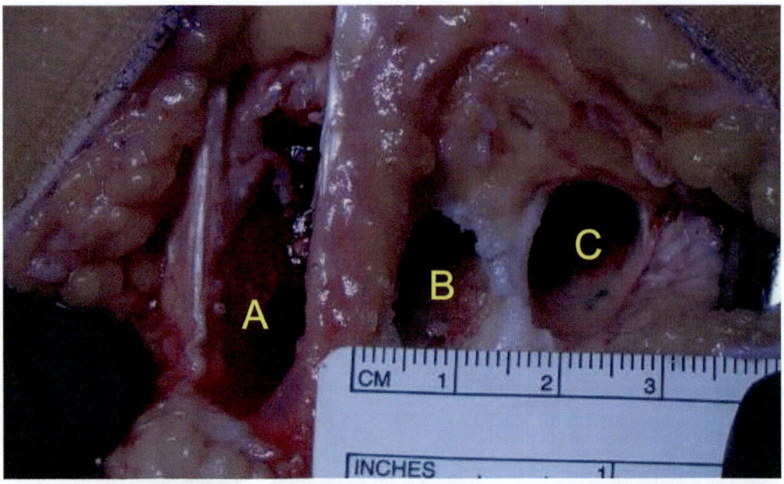

Fig. 7.16 New tunnel placed (B) in between old tunnel (C, which has been filled already with a dowel before reaming new tunnel) and the tibial tubercle harvest site (A)

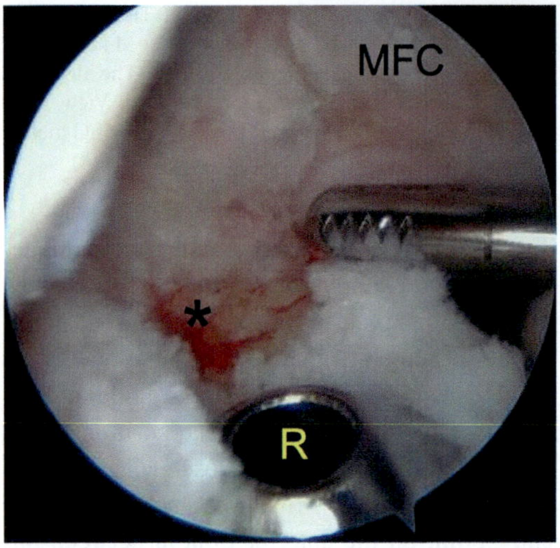

Fig. 7.17 New tibial tunnel being reamed anterior to the prior tunnel, which is now filled with an allograft dowel (LifeNet Tissue Service). There is minimal to no overlap of the tunnels. View from the anterolateral portal. (* allograft bone dowel, R reamer in new tunnel, MFC medial femoral condyle)

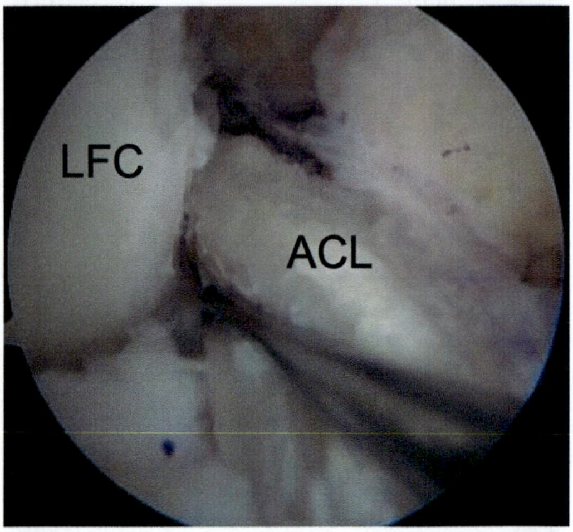

Fig. 7.18 The revised ACL bone-patellar tendon-bone autograft is tensioned and fixed with interference screws on both the femoral and tibial sides. (ACL anterior cruciate ligament, LFC lateral femoral condyle)

Case 2: Incompletely Nonanatomic Femoral Tunnel

The patient is a 21-year-old male who presented to clinic with right knee pain after feeling a "pop" while playing soccer several weeks earlier. He had his ipsilateral ACL reconstructed using hamstring tendon autograft 1 year prior at an outside hospital, and he had done well postoperatively until the recent injury. He had a positive Lachman and pivot shift exam. An MRI showed an incompetent ACL graft and a pivot shift bone contusion (Fig. 7.19). Plain imaging also revealed an excessively vertical femoral tunnel (Fig. 7.20).

A CT scan was obtained, which further characterized the tunnel size and position. The femoral tunnel measured 11 mm × 9 mm and was more vertical than the ideal position (Fig. 7.21). The tibial tunnel measured 12 mm × 10 mm with an acceptable position (Fig. 7.22). There was no malalignment. A single-stage revision ACL reconstruction was undertaken, with the plan to bone graft the prior femoral tunnel with an

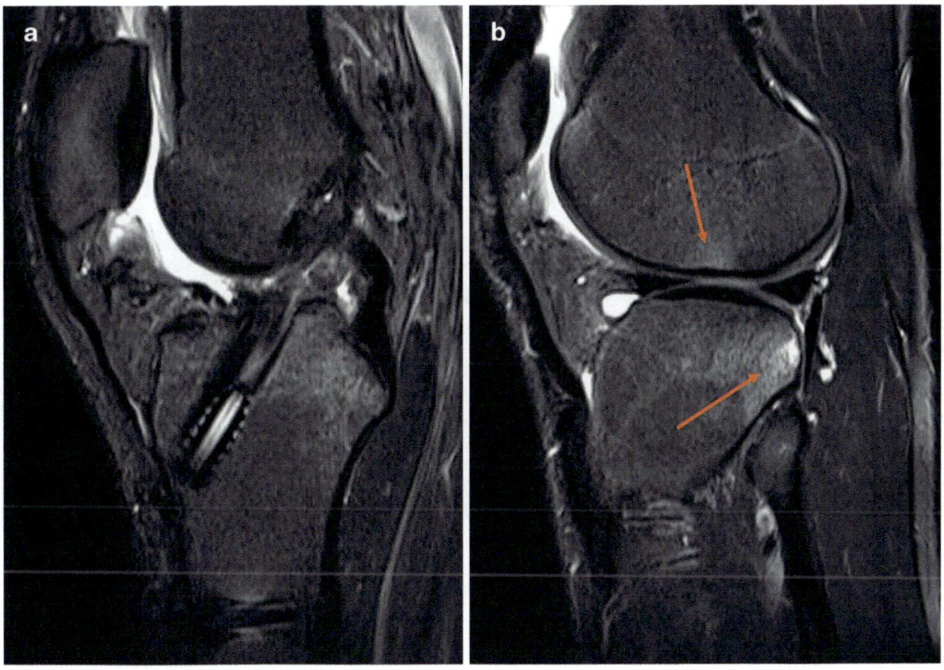

Fig. 7.19 Two sagittal cuts of the MRI of the injured knee demonstrating (**a**) a torn ACL graft and (**b**) bone edema consistent with a pivot shift contusion

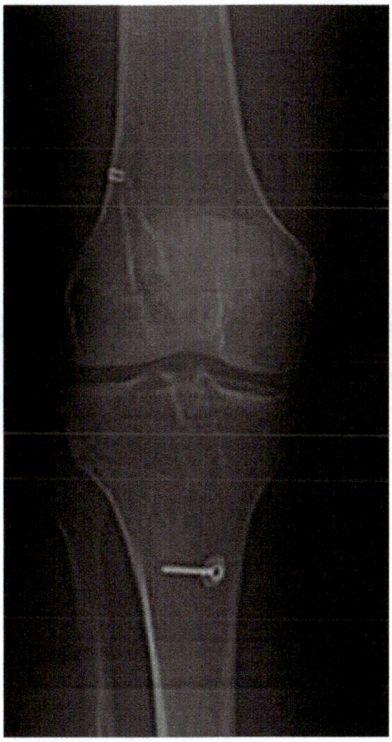

Fig. 7.20 AP radiograph taken after the twisting injury, demonstrating previous ACL reconstruction with suspensory fixation. The femoral tunnel appears vertical, and there is mild osteolysis

allograft dowel and drill the new tunnel in its anatomic location, likely with some overlap. The tibial tunnel would be reused pending intraoperative evaluation.

The case began with a BTB autograft harvest in the usual fashion, with 11-mm diameter bone plugs. Arthroscopic exam demonstrated a complete tear of the ACL graft (Fig. 7.23). After exploring the prior femoral tunnel, it was confirmed to be excessively vertical in the notch. Preparation of the tunnel for bone grafting was begun by placing a guide pin centrally in the tunnel (Fig. 7.24). Over this pin, the tunnel was reamed sequentially to 12 mm, at which point there was no additional soft tissue debris. A 12-mm diameter cannulated allograft bone dowel (LifeNet Tissue Service) was gently inserted into the tunnel. Next, a guide pin was placed into the anatomic location of the femoral ACL footprint, oriented in a divergent, more horizontal course from the previous tunnel. This pin positioning was checked with fluoroscopy before the tunnel was drilled. An 11-mm reamer was used to create the new femoral tunnel, which had about 20% overlap with the dowel (Fig. 7.25).

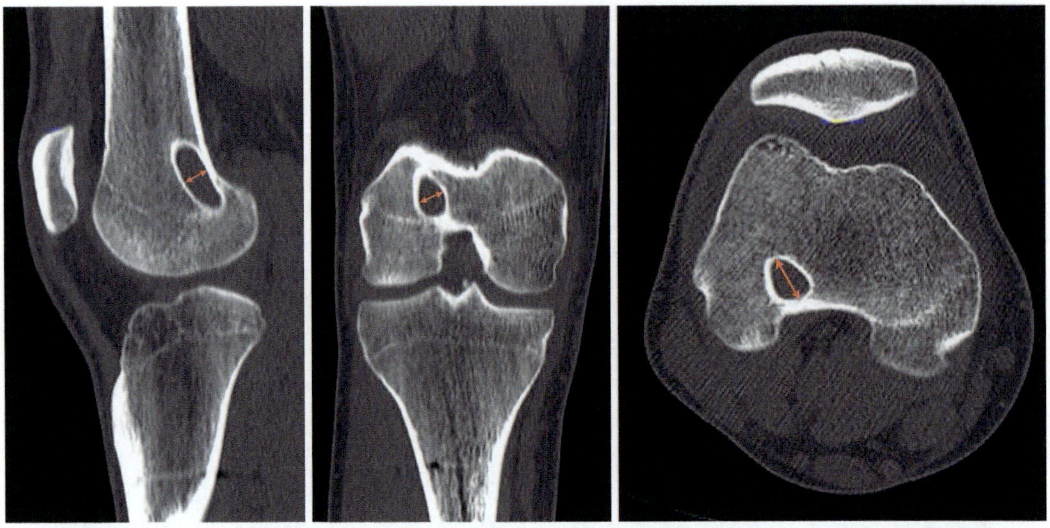

Fig. 7.21 Computed tomography (CT) of the patient's knee is obtained for preoperative planning for revision surgery. Displayed are representative sagittal, coronal, and axial (in order from left to right) cuts, demonstrating the femoral tunnel is 11 mm × 9 mm in diameter and appears excessively vertical

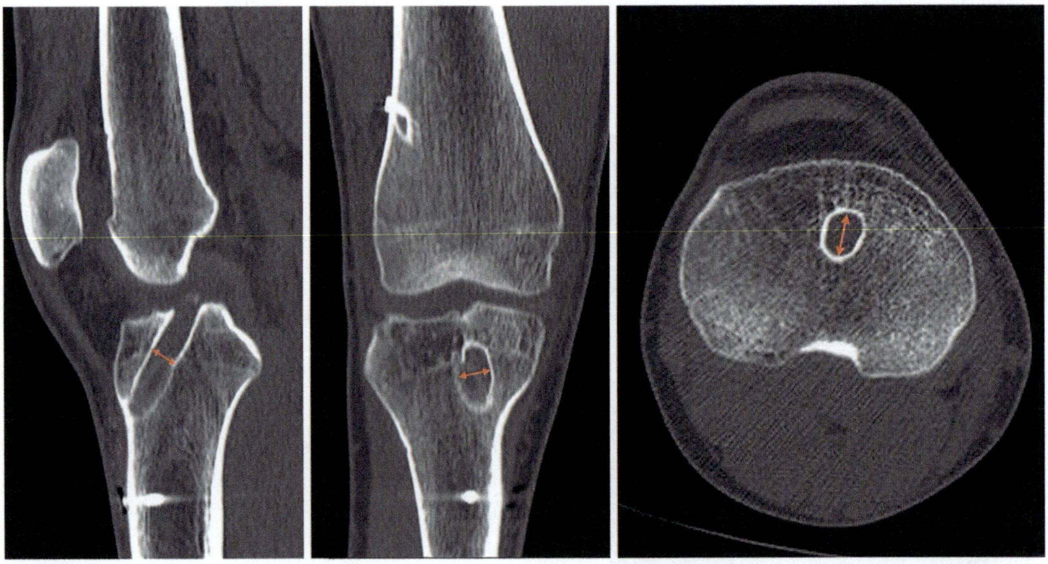

Fig. 7.22 Preoperative CT scan demonstrating the tibial tunnel is 12 mm × 10 mm in diameter, but is in acceptable position. Shown here at the representative sagittal, coronal, and axial (in order from left to right) cuts

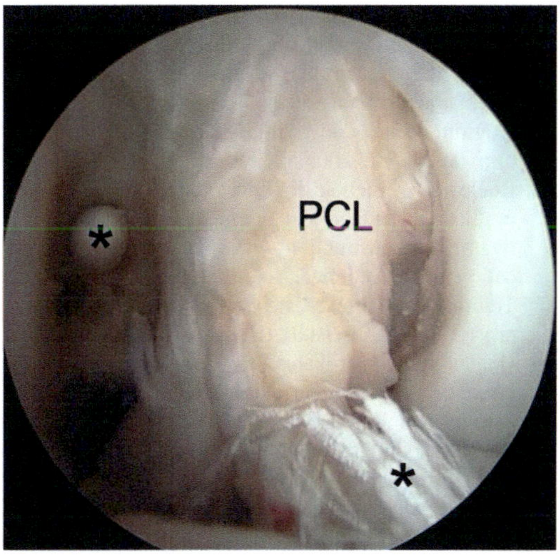

Fig. 7.23 Arthroscopic view into the notch, demonstrating a completely torn ACL graft. (* ACL graft remnant, PCL posterior cruciate ligament)

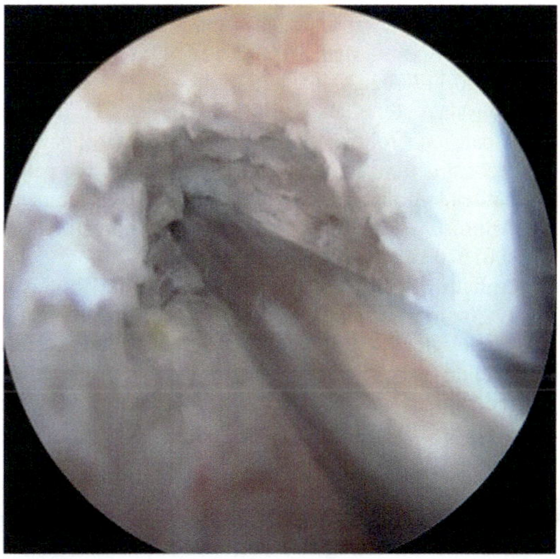

Fig. 7.24 Guide pin placed centrally in the incompletely nonanatomic (vertical) femoral tunnel

The tibial tunnel was reused, after debriding the tunnel with a reamer, shaver, and rasp. The 11-mm BTB graft was shuttled into the knee and secured on the femoral side with a 7-mm metal interference screw (Fig. 7.26). The interference screw provides fixation for both the new graft plug and the dowel when used in this manner. The knee was cycled and the graft appropriately tensioned before the insertion of a 9-mm

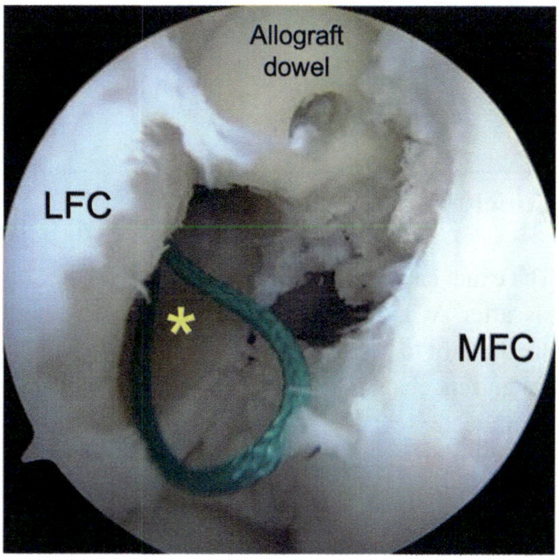

Fig. 7.25 Revision tunnel (*) drilled in improved position with slight overlap with prior tunnel aperture. Prior tunnel is now filled with an allograft bone dowel (LifeNet Tissue Supply). The tunnel trajectories laterally are divergent. A stich is in the new tunnel to facilitate graft passage (LFC lateral femoral condyle, MFC medial femoral condyle)

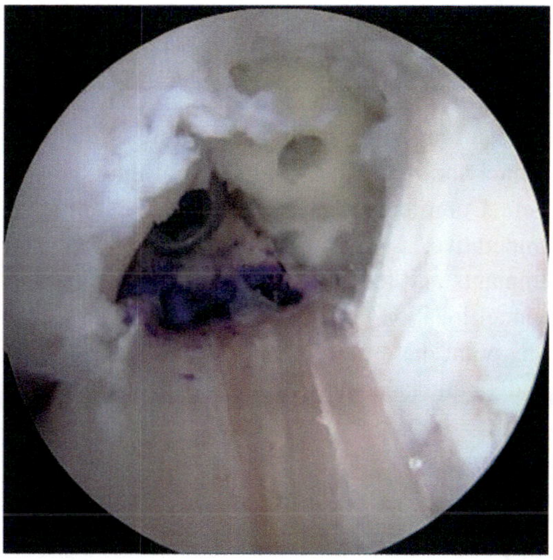

Fig. 7.26 Interference screw fixation of the new bone-patellar tendon-bone autograft adjacent to the allograft bone dowel in the prior tunnel. Note that the interference screw is providing fixation for both the dowel and the autograft bone plug

metal interference screw in the tibial tunnel. The knee exam was stable after fixation. The patient was treated postoperatively with the standard ACL rehabilitation protocol, allowing immediate weight-bearing and range of motion. He returned safely to recreational sports at 8 months postoperatively.

Conclusion

The exact causes of tunnel widening and osteolysis after ACL reconstruction are unknown, but are thought to be due to a combination of biological and mechanical factors. Widened tunnels can complicate revision ACL surgery, but can be managed effectively by having an arsenal of surgical techniques on hand. If tunnels are <14-mm wide, a single-stage revision procedure should be considered. The location of the prior tunnels dictates how bone voids can be addressed. Completely anatomic tunnels can typically be reused in the same setting, with the widened tunnel filled with either a larger graft, hardware, or bone graft. A divergent tunnel technique can also be employed. Completely nonanatomic tunnels can generally be avoided all together by the new tunnels, with or without bone grafting of the prior tunnel. Incompletely anatomic tunnels present the most challenging scenario, but can be managed successfully with bone grafting of the prior tunnel and immediate re-drilling of the new tunnel. Comprehensive preoperative planning is imperative, as thorough knowledge of the prior implants and techniques used as well as current tunnel location and size is vital to success. If at any point there is an inability to fill bony defects and obtain adequate fixation of the new ACL graft, a two-stage procedure should be performed.

References

1. Ohly NE, Murray IR, Keating JF. Revision anterior cruciate ligament reconstruction: timing of surgery and the incidence of meniscal tears and degenerative change. J Bone Joint Surg Br. 2007;89-B(8):1051–4. https://doi.org/10.1302/0301-620X.89B8.19000.
2. Mayr R, Rosenberger R, Agraharam D, Smekal V, El Attal R. Revision anterior cruciate ligament reconstruction: an update. Arch Orthop Trauma Surg. 2012;132(9):1299–313. https://doi.org/10.1007/s00402-012-1552-1.
3. Klein JP, Lintner DM, Downs D, Vavrenka K. The incidence and significance of femoral tunnel widening after quadrupled hamstring anterior cruciate ligament reconstruction using femoral cross pin fixation. Arthroscopy. 2003;19(5):470–6. https://doi.org/10.1053/jars.2003.50106.
4. Buelow J-U, Siebold R, Ellermann A. A prospective evaluation of tunnel enlargement in anterior cruciate ligament reconstruction with hamstrings: extracortical versus anatomical fixation. Knee Surg Sports Traumatol Arthrosc. 2002;10(2):80–5. https://doi.org/10.1007/s00167-001-0267-6.
5. Hantes ME, Mastrokalos DS, Yu J, Paessler HH. The effect of early motion on tibial tunnel widening after anterior cruciate ligament replacement using hamstring tendon grafts. Arthroscopy. 2004;20(6):572–80. https://doi.org/10.1016/j.arthro.2004.04.069.
6. Baumfeld JA, Diduch DR, Rubino LJ, et al. Tunnel widening following anterior cruciate ligament reconstruction using hamstring autograft: a comparison between double cross-pin and suspensory graft fixation. Knee Surg Sports Traumatol Arthrosc. 2008;16(12):1108–13. https://doi.org/10.1007/s00167-008-0606-y.
7. Wilson TC, Kantaras A, Atay A, Johnson DL. Tunnel enlargement after anterior cruciate ligament surgery. Am J Sports Med. 2004;32(2):543–9. https://doi.org/10.1177/0363546504263151.
8. L'Insalata JC, Klatt B, Fu FH, Harner CD. Tunnel expansion following anterior cruciate ligament reconstruction: a comparison of hamstring and patellar tendon autografts. Knee Surg Sports Traumatol Arthrosc. 1997;5(4):234–8. https://doi.org/10.1007/s001670050056.
9. Aglietti P, Giron F, Buzzi R, Biddau F, Sasso F. Anterior cruciate ligament reconstruction: bone-patellar tendon-bone compared with double semitendinosus and gracilis tendon grafts a prospective, randomized clinical trial. J Bone Joint Surg Am. 2004;86(10):2143–55.
10. Clatworthy MG, Annear P, Bulow JU, Bartlett RJ. Tunnel widening in anterior cruciate ligament reconstruction: a prospective evaluation of hamstring and patella tendon grafts. Knee Surg Sports Traumatol Arthrosc. 1999;7(3):138–45. https://doi.org/10.1007/s001670050138.
11. Flanigan DC, Everhart JS, DiBartola AC, et al. Bacterial DNA is associated with tunnel widening in failed ACL reconstructions. Knee Surg Sports Traumatol Arthrosc. 2019;27(11):3490–7. https://doi.org/10.1007/s00167-019-05405-6.
12. Peyrache MD, Djian P, Christel P, Witvoet J. Tibial tunnel enlargement after anterior cruciate ligament reconstruction by autogenous bone-patellar tendon-bone graft. Knee Surg Sports Traumatol Arthrosc. 1996;4(1):2–8. https://doi.org/10.1007/bf01565989.
13. Webster K, Feller J, Elliott J, Hutchison A, Payne R. A comparison of bone tunnel measurements made using computed tomography and digital plain radiography after anterior cruciate ligament reconstruc-

tion. Arthroscopy. 2004;20(9):946–50. https://doi.org/10.1016/S0749-8063(04)00655-3.
14. Wang H, Ao Y, Chen L, et al. [Measurement of bone tunnel width with computed tomography versus plain radiography after anterior cruciate ligament single-bundle reconstruction]. Zhonghua Yi Xue Za Zhi. 2013;93(41):3288–90.
15. Marchant MH, Willimon SC, Vinson E, Pietrobon R, Garrett WE, Higgins LD. Comparison of plain radiography, computed tomography, and magnetic resonance imaging in the evaluation of bone tunnel widening after anterior cruciate ligament reconstruction. Knee Surg Sports Traumatol Arthrosc. 2010;18(8):1059–64. https://doi.org/10.1007/s00167-009-0952-4.
16. Coats AC, Johnson DL. Two-stage revision anterior cruciate ligament reconstruction: indications, review, and technique demonstration. Orthopedics. 2012;35(11):958–60. https://doi.org/10.3928/01477447-20121023-08.
17. Laidlaw MS, Buyukdogan K, Werner BC, Miller MD. Management of bone deficiency in revision anterior cruciate ligament reconstruction. Ann Jt. 2017;5:1–12. https://doi.org/10.21037/aoj.2017.06.12.
18. Kamath GV, Redfern JC, Greis PE, Burks RT. Revision anterior cruciate ligament reconstruction. Am J Sports Med. 2011;39(1):199–217. https://doi.org/10.1177/0363546510370929.
19. George MS, Dunn WR, Spindler KP. Current concepts review: revision anterior cruciate ligament reconstruction. Am J Sports Med. 2006;34(12):2026–37. https://doi.org/10.1177/0363546506295026.
20. Thomas NP, Kankate R, Wandless F, Pandit H. Revision anterior cruciate ligament reconstruction using a 2-stage technique with bone grafting of the tibial tunnel. Am J Sports Med. 2005;33(11):1701–9. https://doi.org/10.1177/0363546505276759.
21. Wagner M, Strobel MJ, Weiler A. Single-staged anterior cruciate ligament revision reconstruction using autologous hamstring tendons. Tech Orthop. 2005;20(3):306–13. https://doi.org/10.1097/01.bto.0000177752.58556.af.
22. Allen CR, Anderson AF, Cooper DE, et al. Surgical predictors of clinical outcomes after revision anterior cruciate ligament reconstruction. Am J Sports Med. 2017;45(11):2586–94. https://doi.org/10.1177/0363546517712952.
23. Noyes FR, Barber-Westin SD. Anterior cruciate ligament revision reconstruction: results using a quadriceps tendon-patellar bone autograft. Am J Sports Med. 2006;34(4):553–64. https://doi.org/10.1177/0363546505281812.
24. Wilde J, Bedi A, Altchek DW. Revision anterior cruciate ligament reconstruction. Sports Health. 2014;6(6):504–18. https://doi.org/10.1177/1941738113500910.
25. Schliemann B, Treder M, Schulze M, et al. Influence of different tibial fixation techniques on initial stability in single-stage anterior cruciate ligament revision with confluent tibial tunnels: a biomechanical laboratory study. Arthroscopy. 2016;32(1):78–89. https://doi.org/10.1016/j.arthro.2015.06.044.
26. Demyttenaere J, Claes S, Bellemans J. One-stage revision anterior cruciate ligament reconstruction in cases with excessive tunnel osteolysis. Results of a new technique using impaction bone grafting. Knee. 2018;25(6):1308–17. https://doi.org/10.1016/j.knee.2018.08.015.
27. Bach BR. Revision anterior cruciate ligament surgery. Arthroscopy. 2003;19(10, Supplement 1):14–29. https://doi.org/10.1016/j.arthro.2003.09.044.
28. Werner BC, Gilmore CJ, Hamann JC, et al. Revision anterior cruciate ligament reconstruction: results of a single-stage approach using allograft dowel bone grafting for femoral defects. J Am Acad Orthop Surg. 2016;24(8):581–7. https://doi.org/10.5435/JAAOS-D-15-00572.
29. Salem HS, Axibal DP, Wolcott ML, et al. Two-stage revision anterior cruciate ligament reconstruction: a systematic review of bone graft options for tunnel augmentation. Am J Sports Med. 2020;48(3):767–77. https://doi.org/10.1177/0363546519841583.
30. Uchida R, Toritsuka Y, Mae T, Kusano M, Ohzono K. Healing of tibial bone tunnels after bone grafting for staged revision anterior cruciate ligament surgery: a prospective computed tomography analysis. Knee. 2016;23(5):830–6. https://doi.org/10.1016/j.knee.2016.04.012.
31. Franceschi F, Papalia R, Di Martino A, Rizzello G, Allaire R, Denaro V. A new harvest site for bone graft in anterior cruciate ligament revision surgery. Arthroscopy. 2007;23(5):558.e1–4. https://doi.org/10.1016/j.arthro.2006.07.054.
32. Said HG, Baloch K, Green M. A new technique for femoral and tibial tunnel bone grafting using the OATS harvesters in revision anterior cruciate ligament reconstruction. Arthroscopy. Published online 2006. https://doi.org/10.1016/j.arthro.2005.12.039.
33. Grote S, Helfen T, Mück F, Regauer M, Prall WC. Femoral marrow cavity bone harvesting used for arthroscopic refilling of misplaced or enlarged bone tunnels in revision ACL surgery: an arthroscopically supported technique with antegrade intramedullary bone harvesting by a reamer–irrigator–aspirator (RIA) system. Knee Surg Sports Traumatol Arthrosc. 2015;23(3):808–15. https://doi.org/10.1007/s00167-013-2736-0.
34. Battaglia TC, Miller MD. Management of bony deficiency in revision anterior cruciate ligament reconstruction using allograft bone dowels: surgical technique. Arthroscopy. 2005;21(6):767.e1–5. https://doi.org/10.1016/j.arthro.2005.03.029.
35. Dragoo JL, Kalisvaart M, Smith KM, Pappas G, Golish R. Single-stage revision anterior cruciate ligament reconstruction using bone grafting for posterior or widening tibial tunnels restores stability of the knee and improves clinical outcomes. Knee Surg Sports Traumatol Arthrosc. 2019;27(11):3713–21. https://doi.org/10.1007/s00167-019-05467-6.

36. Yoon KH, Kim JS, Park SY, Park SE. One-stage revision anterior cruciate ligament reconstruction: results according to preoperative bone tunnel diameter: five to fifteen-year follow-up. JBJS. 2018;100(12):993–1000. https://doi.org/10.2106/JBJS.17.01044.
37. Ra HJ, Ha JK, Kim JG. One-stage revision anterior cruciate ligament reconstruction with impacted bone graft after failed primary reconstruction. Orthopedics. 2013;36(11):860–3. https://doi.org/10.3928/01477447-20131021-07.
38. Sgaglione NA, Douglas JA. Allograft bone augmentation in anterior cruciate ligament reconstruction. Arthroscopy. 2004;20:171–7. https://doi.org/10.1016/j.arthro.2004.04.030.
39. Vaughn ZD, Schmidt J, Lindsey DP, Dragoo JL. Biomechanical evaluation of a 1-stage revision anterior cruciate ligament reconstruction technique using a structural bone void filler for femoral fixation. Arthroscopy. 2009;25(9):1011–8. https://doi.org/10.1016/j.arthro.2009.04.068.
40. Tse BK, Vaughn ZD, Lindsey DP, Dragoo JL. Evaluation of a one-stage ACL revision technique using bone void filler after cyclic loading. Knee. 2012;19(4):477–81. https://doi.org/10.1016/j.knee.2011.06.013.
41. Serbin PA, Griffin JW, Bonner KF. Single-stage revision anterior cruciate ligament reconstruction using fast-setting bone graft substitutes. Arthrosc Tech. 2020;9(2):e225–31. https://doi.org/10.1016/j.eats.2019.10.002.
42. Mitchell JJ, Cinque ME, Dornan GJ, et al. Primary versus revision anterior cruciate ligament reconstruction: patient demographics, radiographic findings, and associated lesions. Arthroscopy. Published online 2018. https://doi.org/10.1016/j.arthro.2017.08.305.

8 Management of Bone Loss/Osteolysis in Revision ACL Reconstruction: The Role of Two-Stage Reconstruction

Cort D. Lawton, Joseph D. Lamplot, Anil S. Ranawat, and Robert G. Marx

Introduction

The number of primary anterior cruciate ligament (ACL) reconstructions performed annually continues to rise at a rapid rate [1]. Failure rates following primary ACL reconstruction vary as a function of time, with rates from 2% to 5% at 2 years, compared to 11% at 15 years [2–6]. The rate of revision ACL surgery is expected to climb in parallel with the rise in primary surgery, highlighting the expanding importance of revision ACL reconstruction. Depending on the type and location of fixation, size and location of existing tunnels, and bone quality, the surgeon must plan for a two-stage reconstruction when indicated.

For a two-stage ACL reconstruction, the first stage involves removing all existing graft and hardware and filling the bony defects with bone graft. Following incorporation of the bone graft, new femoral and tibial tunnels can be created to allow for an adequate bed for fixation and incorporation of the ACL graft without compromising the location of the tunnels. A disadvantage of a staged approach includes the requirement for two surgeries and an associated prolonged rehabilitation time. Furthermore, following the first stage, the patient is left with an unstable knee that may predispose them to cartilage and meniscus injury [7, 8].

The majority of revisions can be performed in a single stage, and we avoid two-stage ACL reconstruction unless absolutely necessary because of the disadvantages stated above [7, 9, 10]. However, there are cases where single-stage revision ACL reconstruction cannot, or should not, be performed, including excessive bone loss or tunnel osteolysis that limits graft fixation, arthrofibrosis requiring surgical intervention to improve motion, infection that precludes hardware placement, and malalignment requiring deformity correction. The most common indication for a two-stage revision is tunnel osteolysis (Fig. 8.1). The Multicenter ACL Revision Study (MARS) group reported that of the 1205 patients who underwent revision ACL reconstruction 8% of the cohort required bone grafting and a two-stage revision due to bone tunnel dilation [9].

A key principle of revision ACL surgery is that the index tunnels should not compromise the accurate placement of the revision femoral and tibial tunnels [11]. Challenges of revision ACL surgery include managing previous technical errors, bone loss, and tunnel osteolysis. Malpositioned tunnels may require bone grafting to avoid tunnel convergence and allow for tunnel redirection. Bone loss from hardware removal or

C. D. Lawton (✉)
OrthoIllinois, Algonquin, IL, USA

J. D. Lamplot
Emory University, Department of Orthopedic Surgery, Atlanta, GA, USA

A. S. Ranawat · R. G. Marx
Hospital for Special Surgery, Sports Medicine Institute, New York, NY, USA

M. J. Alaia, K. J. Jones (eds.), *Revision Anterior Cruciate Ligament Reconstruction*,
https://doi.org/10.1007/978-3-030-96996-7_8

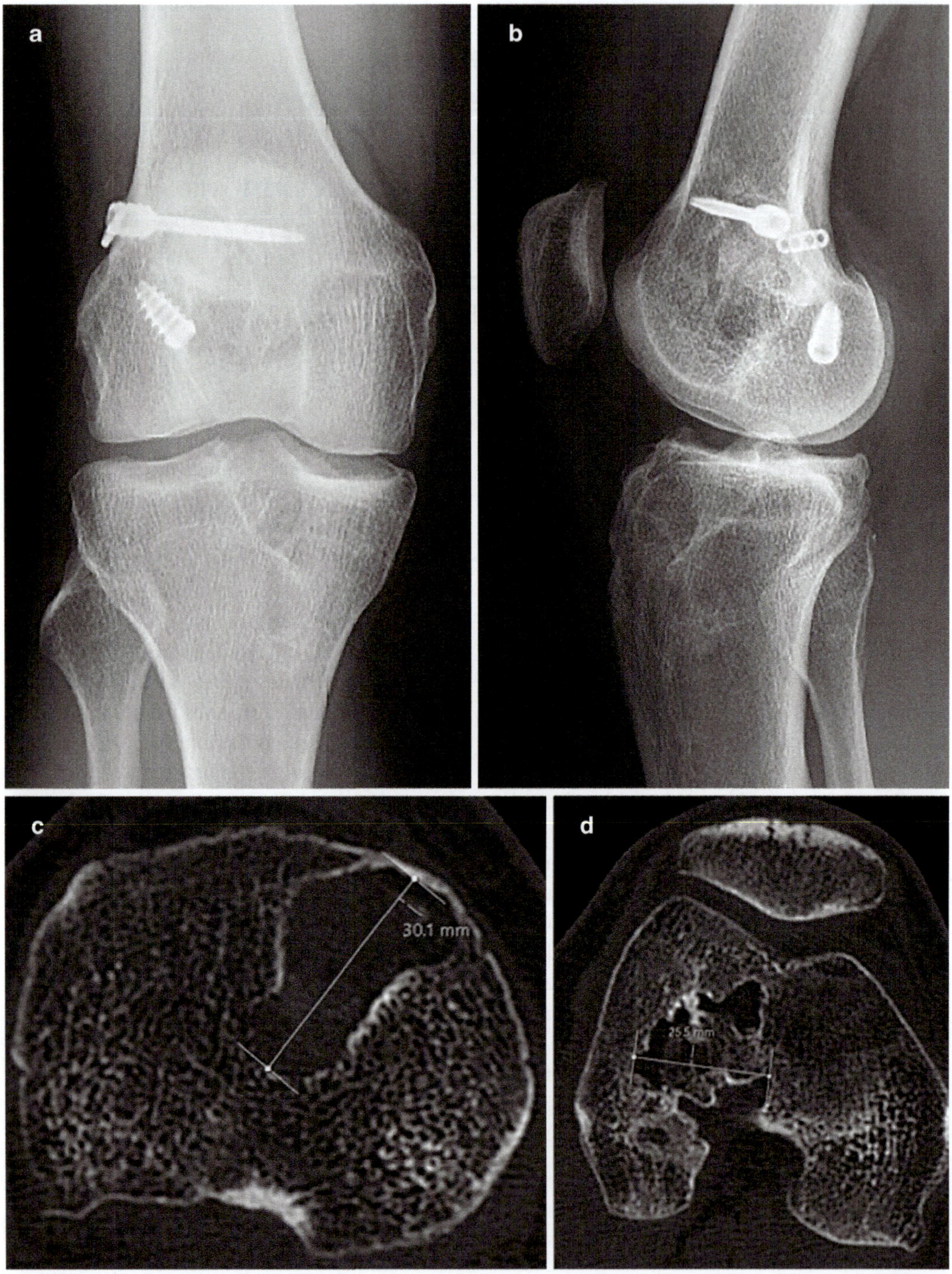

Fig. 8.1 AP (**a**) and lateral (**b**) radiograph of a right knee status post multiple failed ACL reconstructions with evidence of retained femoral-sided hardware, significant tibial tunnel osteolysis, and an anterior femoral tunnel position. Axial CT images more accurately depicting the significant tibial tunnel widening (**c**) and anterior femoral tunnel position (**d**)

tunnel osteolysis can jeopardize graft fixation and incorporation. In this chapter we discuss the role of two-stage ACL reconstruction and present cases highlighting techniques and pearls for managing bone loss and tunnel osteolysis.

Case 1

A 26-year-old male with a remote history of right knee ACL reconstruction with hamstring autograft, complicated by graft rupture, most recently 2 years status post revision ACL reconstruction with tibialis posterior allograft and partial lateral meniscectomy presented following another re-injury. He reported experiencing a non-contact pivoting injury while playing basketball. The patient reported pain, swelling, and multiple recurrent instability events. On examination, he had full range of motion from 0 to 130 degrees, medial joint line tenderness to palpation, a grade 2B Lachman, and 2+ pivot shift, and his knee was stable to varus and valgus stress at 0 and 30 degrees.

Radiographs revealed two femoral-sided buttons from prior suspensory fixation of each ACL graft and evidence of tunnel osteolysis (Fig. 8.2a, b). Magnetic resonance imaging (MRI) was obtained, confirming the diagnosis of an ACL graft rupture (Fig. 8.2c). A computed tomography (CT) scan was obtained for further evaluation of the extent of tunnel osteolysis and tunnel positioning. The CT scan showed significant tunnel osteolysis with a maximum tibial tunnel diameter of 16 mm and femoral tunnel diameter of 13 mm, with appropriate tunnel positioning (Fig. 8.3a–e).

Given the patient's pain, swelling, and recurrent instability with radiographic evidence of significant tunnel osteolysis exceeding 15 mm on the tibial side and extending over a significant length of the tunnel, the plan was to proceed with a two-stage revision ACL reconstruction. The patient was subsequently taken to the operating room, and a diagnostic arthroscopy confirmed a complete tear of the ACL graft. The graft stumps were debrided, and the previous femoral tunnel was identified. A guide wire was placed into the prior femoral tunnel, and the tunnel was reamed with a 10-mm reamer. This effectively cleared out all prior graft material, producing a bleeding cancellous bone tunnel (Fig. 8.4a). The location of the previous tibial tunnel was identified, and the PEEK interference screw was extracted. A guide

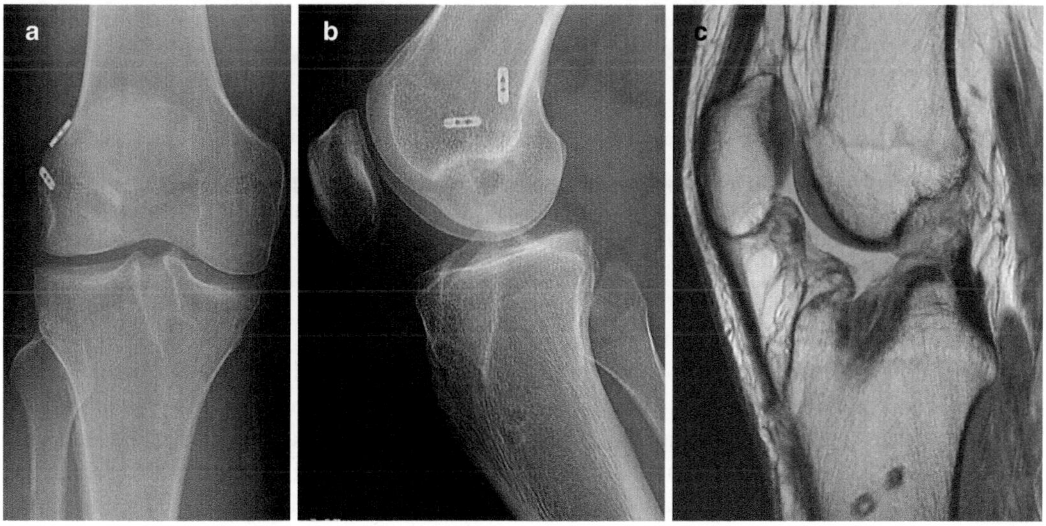

Fig. 8.2 AP (**a**) and lateral (**b**) radiograph of a right knee status post multiple failed ACL reconstructions with evidence of two retained femoral-sided buttons from prior suspensory fixation of his ACL grafts and evidence of tunnel osteolysis, more pronounced on the tibia. Sagittal proton density MRI sequence (**c**) confirming the diagnosis of an ACL graft rupture

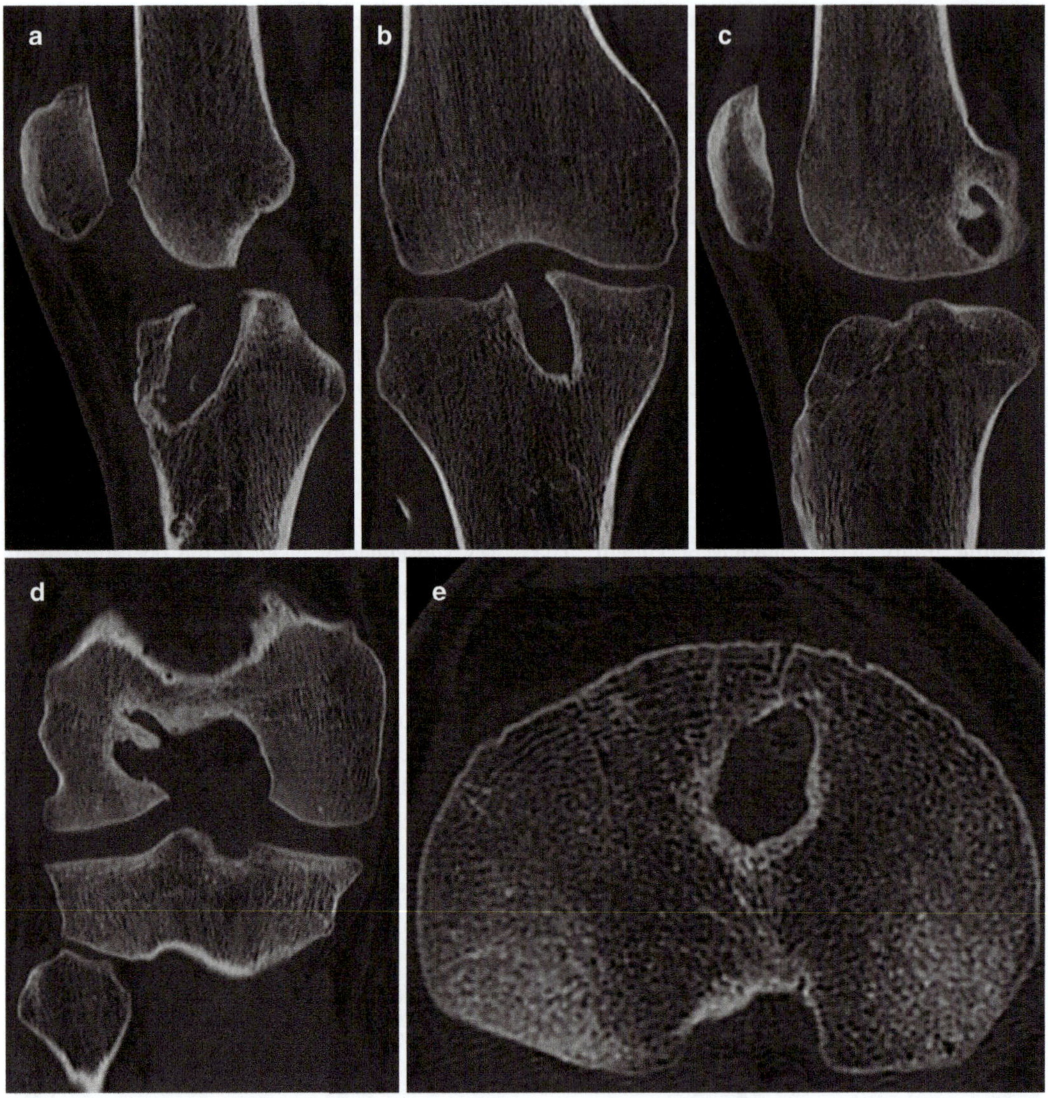

Fig. 8.3 Sagittal (**a**) and coronal (**b**) CT images demonstrating significant tunnel osteolysis with appropriate tunnel positioning. Sagittal (**c**) and coronal (**d**) CT images demonstrating femoral tunnel osteolysis measuring 13 mm with appropriate tunnel positioning. Axial CT image (**e**) showing 16 mm of tibial tunnel widening

pin was placed through the tunnel and held intra-articular with a grasper. The tunnel was sequentially reamed up to 14 mm in diameter. This effectively cleared out all prior graft material, producing a bleeding cancellous bone tunnel. A 10-mm allograft bone dowel was placed through the anteromedial portal over a guide wire into the femoral tunnel, and a 14-mm dowel was placed over a guide wire into the tibial tunnel achieving sufficient press fit fixation (Fig. 8.4c, d).

Postoperatively, the patient underwent a course of physical therapy to maintain his strength and range of motion. At 4 months postoperatively, a CT scan was obtained demonstrating adequate healing of the allograft bone dowels (Fig. 8.5a, b). The patient returned to the operating room 6 months after his bone grafting procedure for a revision ACL reconstruction with bone-patellar tendon-bone (BTB) autograft. Diagnostic arthroscopy confirmed healing of the

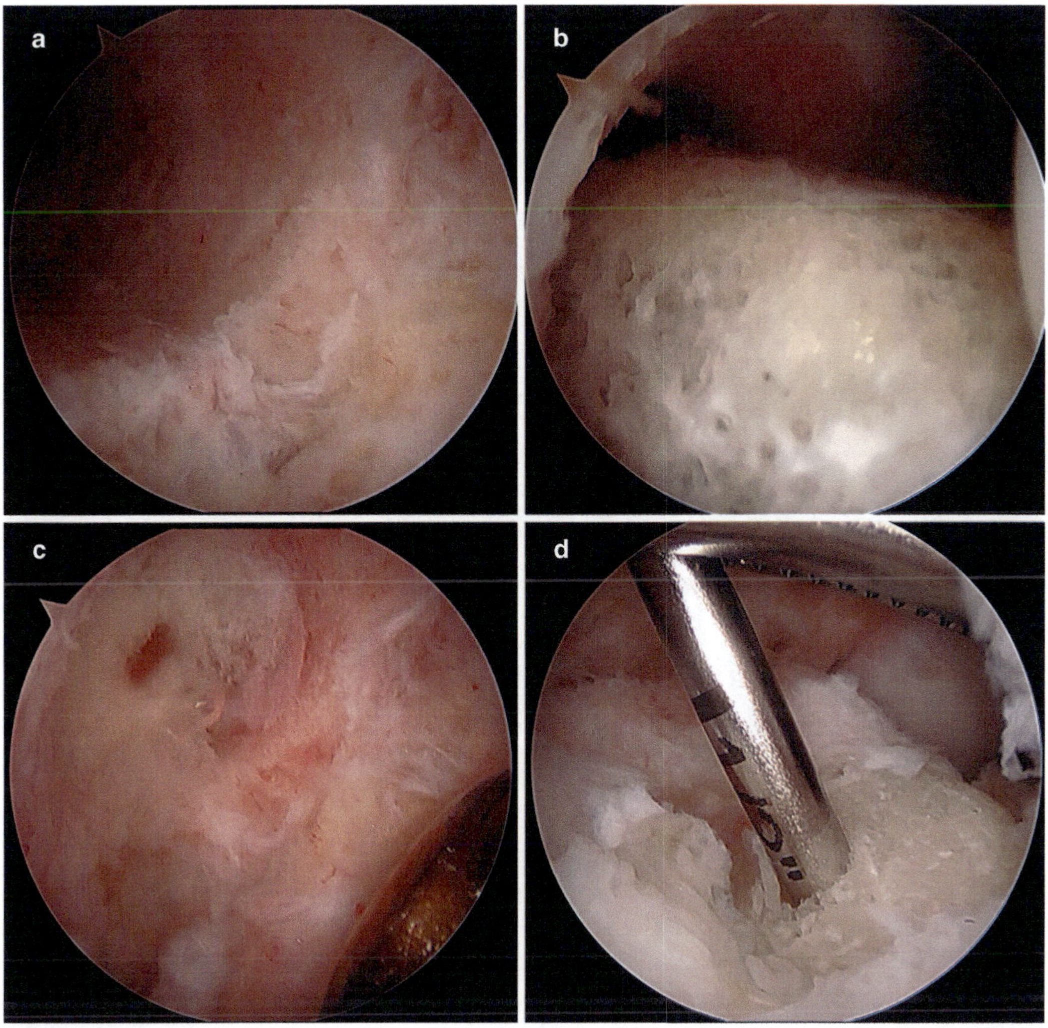

Fig. 8.4 Arthroscopic image following index femoral tunnel reaming to produce a bleeding cancellous bone tunnel (**a**) to promote healing of the allograft bone dowel (**b**, **c**). Arthroscopic imaging inserting the tibial tunnel allograft bone dowel over a guide wire (**d**)

tunnel allografts. New femoral and tibial tunnels were drilled, and the BTB autograft was passed (Fig. 8.5c, d). Aperture fixation was obtained with metal screws. At 1 year postoperatively, the patient was doing well and was cleared to return to sport (Fig. 8.5e, f).

Case-Based Discussion: Case 1

This case highlights a classic presentation of tunnel osteolysis. It is vital that osteolysis is recognized and evaluated further with CT and/or MRI. The ultimate strategy for dealing with this issue depends on tunnel location and the extent of tunnel osteolysis. When a two-stage procedure with bone grafting is indicated, multiple grafting options and surgical techniques exist to manage this problem effectively.

Causes of Tunnel Osteolysis

Osteolysis of the femoral and tibial tunnels is a well-documented problem and is believed to occur because of micro-motion at the graft-tunnel

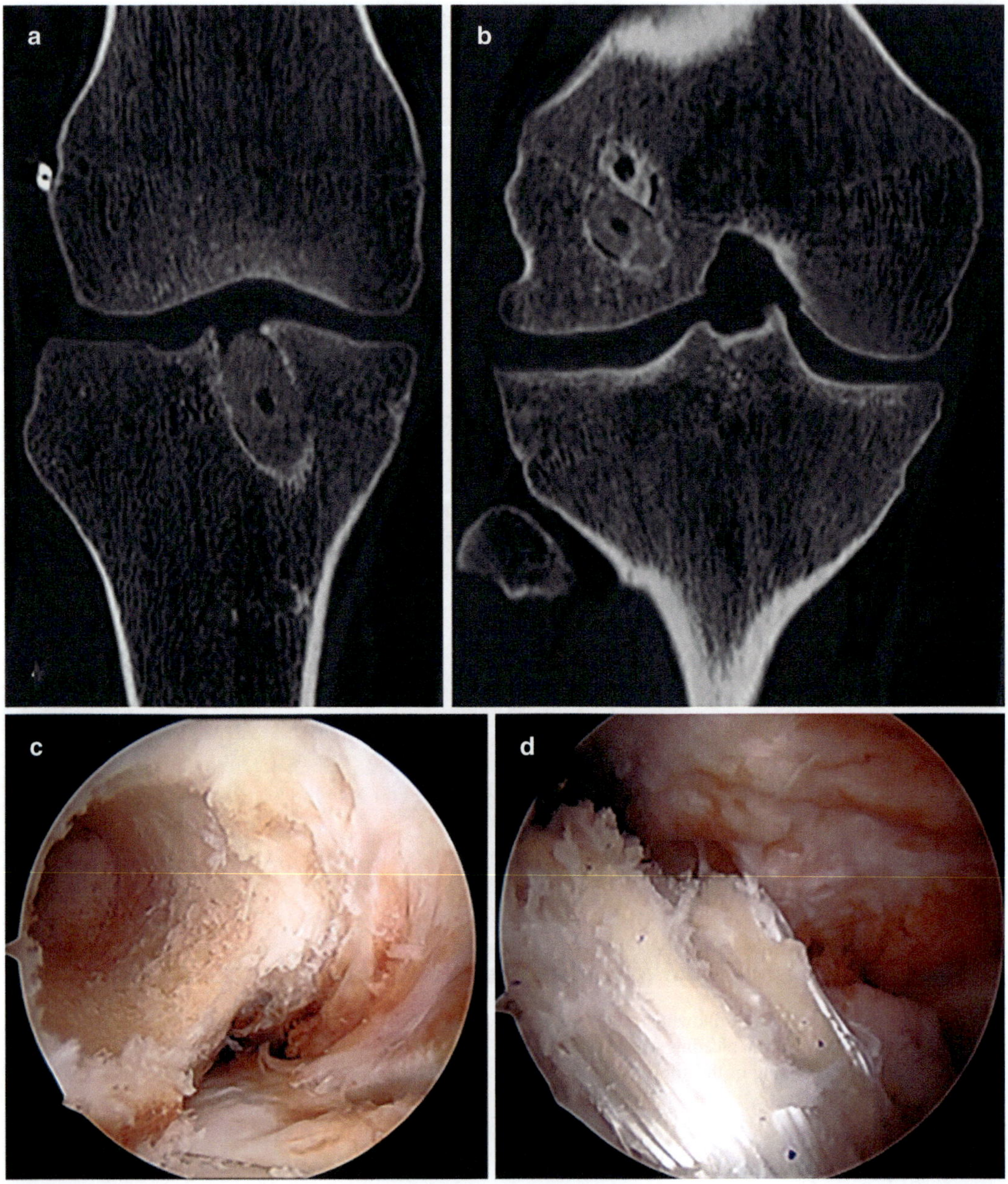

Fig. 8.5 Coronal CT image demonstrating adequate healing of the tibial (**a**) and femoral (**b**) allograft bone dowels 4 months after the grafting procedure. During the second stage, the femoral socket was drilled with evidence of healthy cancellous tunnel walls (**c**), the BTB autograft was passed (**d**), and aperture fixation was obtained with metal screws. One year postoperative AP (**e**) and lateral (**f**) radiographs demonstrated healing of the bone plugs

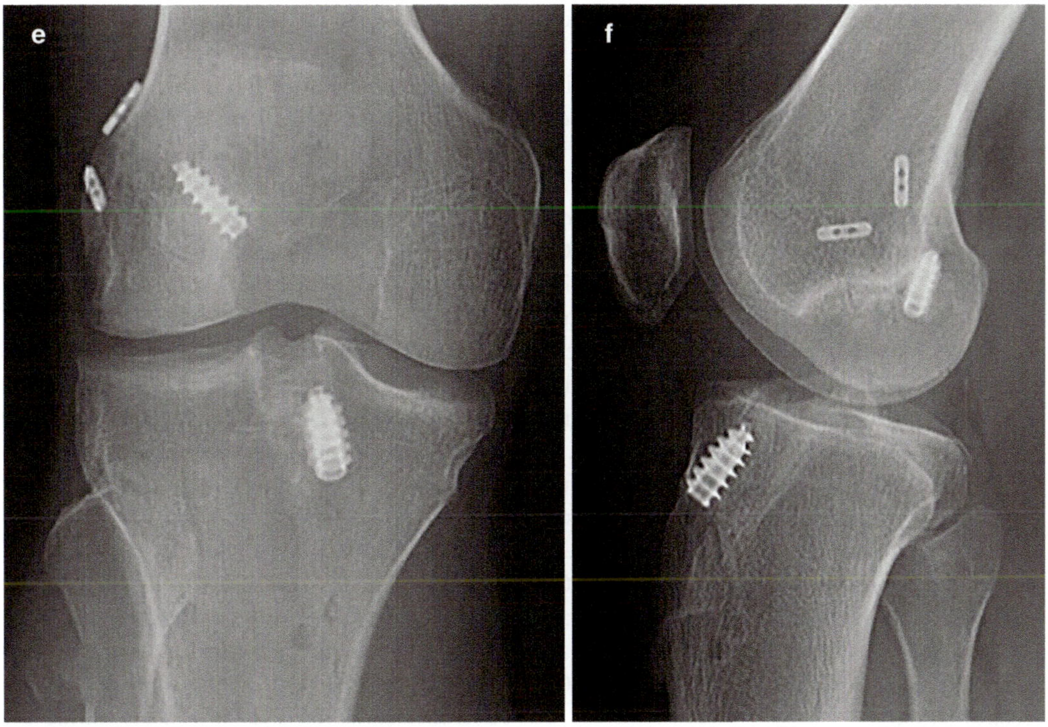

Fig. 8.5 (continued)

interface. This occurs more frequently with hamstring grafts due to the theoretical "windshield wiper" effect of the graft, especially with suspensory fixation [12–14]. It also occurs more commonly with the use of allograft, possibly related to an immunologic reaction [15]. Furthermore, osteolysis can occur with synthetic grafts and bioabsorbable fixation devices, which can cause an immune reaction from the synthetic materials. For these reasons, significant bone loss necessitating a grafting procedure to fill the defect can occur, even with properly positioned femoral and tibial tunnels.

The MARS group reported 8% of 1205 patients undergoing revision ACL reconstruction required bone grafting and a two-stage revision for tunnel dilation [9]. While the most common indication for bone grafting is tunnel osteolysis, bone defects created from hardware removal and/or tunnel convergence after attempting to reposition a tunnel may ultimately require bone grafting and staged ACL reconstruction. These alternative situations resulting in bone defects will be discussed in more detail in the case 2 discussion section.

Imaging

Plain radiographs should be obtained to determine previous tunnel position and whether tunnel osteolysis is present. Additionally, it is common practice to obtain an MRI to assess for graft integrity as well as concomitant meniscal, chondral, and ligamentous injury. If concern exists regarding bone loss after initial radiographic evaluation, a CT scan may be obtained to facilitate precise assessment of existing tunnel location, tunnel dilation, and bone quality. CT has been shown to be superior to plain radiography and MRI in identifying and measuring bone tunnel dilation and location following ACL reconstruction [16].

We recommend having a low threshold for obtaining a CT scan for the purposes of preoperative planning in the setting of suspected bone loss for revision ACL reconstruction. We find it difficult to accurately assess the degree of tunnel dilation on plain radiographs. In cases with clear evidence of osteolysis or bony defects, we routinely obtain a CT scan, as the degree of bone loss is frequently more extensive than demonstrated by radiographs alone. Furthermore, CT imaging is beneficial to assess tunnel location and to plan new tunnel placement. The tunnel locations should be scrutinized to determine if they are in acceptable locations, not requiring redirection, or an inaccurate location requiring redirection, which may require bone grafting. In the case of malpositioned tunnels, a new tunnel that converges with the index tunnel(s) can result in overlapping tunnels and a large bony defect, compromising graft location and fixation. CT imaging is often a vital tool for preoperative planning and to help determine the requirement of bone grafting and/or staging a revision ACL reconstruction.

Indications for Tunnel Bone Grafting

Although most revisions can be performed as a single-stage procedure, specific situations in which a two-stage procedure should be considered include incomplete range of motion requiring lysis of adhesions, malalignment requiring corrective osteotomy, significant tunnel widening necessitating bone grafting, and infection [17]. Tunnel expansion requiring bone grafting is the most common indication for a two-stage procedure [9]. Because increased time to revision correlates with a higher incidence of meniscal and chondral lesions, the surgeon must be judicious when deciding whether a two-stage procedure is necessary [7, 8]. A two-stage procedure generally requires a 6-month window between procedures in which the patient may continue to have instability episodes [14]. When technically feasible, we prefer to perform a single-stage ACL revision surgery, if appropriate tunnel placement and graft fixation can be achieved.

Many authors suggest that bone grafting and a staged revision should be strongly considered when tunnel widening measures greater than 15 mm in diameter [18–20]. In tunnels this size, particularly if the enlarged diameter extends over a significant length of the tunnel, graft fixation and subsequent integration may be compromised. In addition to osteolysis, tunnel expansion requiring bone grafting can result from tunnels which are close, but not ideal, resulting in tunnel confluence if redirection is attempted, and when an excessive amount of bone is removed during the hardware extraction process. Tunnel confluence is a problem wherein the tunnel made during the previous ACL reconstruction and one used at the time of revision ACL reconstruction converge along their paths to create a single larger tunnel. This can compromise fixation of the graft if the defect is too large and may result in excessive translation of the graft at the joint line, resulting in the so-called windshield wiper effect. In this case, two-stage revision reconstruction with bone grafting should be performed to avoid overlap between tunnels made at the time of revision ACL reconstruction and those made during the previous reconstruction [14].

Bone Grafting Options

Multiple grafting options exist to manage tunnel osteolysis and/or bony defects in the setting of revision ACL reconstruction, including autograft plugs, allograft dowels, and structural grafts [8, 12, 21, 22]. Autograft options can include single or multiple press fit osteochondral autograft (OAT) plugs, most commonly considered for smaller defects that require grafting. Such autograft plugs can be harvested from the proximal tibia, distal femur, or, in the setting of larger defects, the iliac crest [23, 24]. When autograft plugs are used in the setting of larger defects, cancellous allograft can be added to the autograft construct to help fill voids.

To avoid the surgical morbidity associated with autograft harvesting, we generally use allograft bone, including dowels [12, 21]. Prior tunnels can be sequentially reamed to bleeding cancellous bone and packed with premade allograft bone dowels sized to fit the dilated tunnel [25]. For larger and irregular defects, femoral head allograft may be used to allow for larger diameter plugs to be made with core reamers while also providing a source for additional graft to use for irregular and larger sized defects.

Other structural grafts include bioabsorbable interference screws or calcium phosphate cement putties. Proponents of these rigid bone void fillers advocate that they allow new tunnels to be drilled anatomically (without prior tunnels compromising location) and the graft can be securely fixed all in a single-stage procedure. No long-term results of biologic incorporation of these bone void fillers in the setting of revision ACL reconstruction are available at this time [22]. For the majority of cases, we prefer to address significant tunnel expansion in a two-stage approach with bone grafting using premade allograft bone dowels or morselized allograft, usually for the femur and tibia, respectively.

Technique Pearls

Despite the disadvantages of a two-stage procedure, there are cases where this technique is necessary. To ensure a successful first stage, a few pearls should be mentioned. Prior to grafting, a thorough debridement of any prior graft and fixation material should be performed, with the goal of producing a new tunnel with bleeding cancellous bone walls in order to facilitate new graft healing to native bone. In doing so, as little bone as possible should be removed. We recommend using sequential reaming over a guide pin, starting with a lower diameter reamer and working your way up to slowly assess the most appropriate diameter to accomplish these goals. If sclerotic bone is encountered, a curette can be used to debride the walls of the tunnel to promote graft healing.

Even with meticulous preoperative planning, the exact size of the defect is often difficult to predict. For larger and irregular defects, we prefer the use of femoral head allograft to allow for appropriate sized allograft bone dowels to be harvested as needed and allow for a source of additional allograft to use to fill irregular voids. For medium sized lesions, our preference is to use premade allograft bone dowels. It is important to preoperatively verify access to a variety of different sized dowels due to difficulties with accurately predicting tunnel size preoperatively.

Bone grafting on the tibial side can be less technically challenging, with the graft typically inserted in an inferior to superior direction directly through the tibial skin incision using a small tamp. Care should be taken not to breach the joint with the bone graft, which can be observed arthroscopically during implantation. Dry arthroscopy can be useful when grafting the femoral side to prevent washing out loose graft when used. During femoral tunnel grafting, a small arthroscopic cannula or skid can be placed through an accessory medial portal in line with the previous femoral tunnel to facilitate graft insertion. A bone tamp can be used to ensure the graft is well packed with an adequate press fit.

In a two-stage technique, the ACL reconstruction must be delayed to allow time for incorporation of the bone graft. Serial radiographs should be obtained following the bone grafting procedure to monitor the healing process. It is important to confirm complete graft incorporation prior to the second-stage procedure, which generally follows the grafting procedure by approximately 6 months [14, 20]. Prior to the second stage, we prefer to confirm incorporation of the bone graft with the use of a CT scan around 4–6 months.

Case 2

A 31-year-old male with a history of right knee ACL reconstruction with hamstring autograft complicated by graft rupture, most recently 5 years status post-revision ACL reconstruction with hamstring allograft and partial medial meniscectomy, presented for evaluation. He reported a non-contact pivoting injury while playing basketball. The patient reported a 3-year history of medial sided knee pain prior to his most recent injury and now swelling with recurrent instability episodes despite a course of physical therapy. On examination, he had full range of motion from 0 to 130 degrees, medial joint line tenderness to palpation, a grade 2B Lachman, and 2+ pivot shift, and his knee was stable to varus and valgus stress at 0 and 30 degrees.

Radiographs revealed two lateral femoral buttons from prior suspensory fixation of his ACL grafts with evidence of femoral and tibial tunnel osteolysis measuring 13 mm and 15 mm, respectively, with 13 degrees of posterior tibial slope (Fig. 8.6a, b). Standing long leg alignment radiographs showed 5 degrees of varus malalignment, with the weight-bearing axis through the lateral

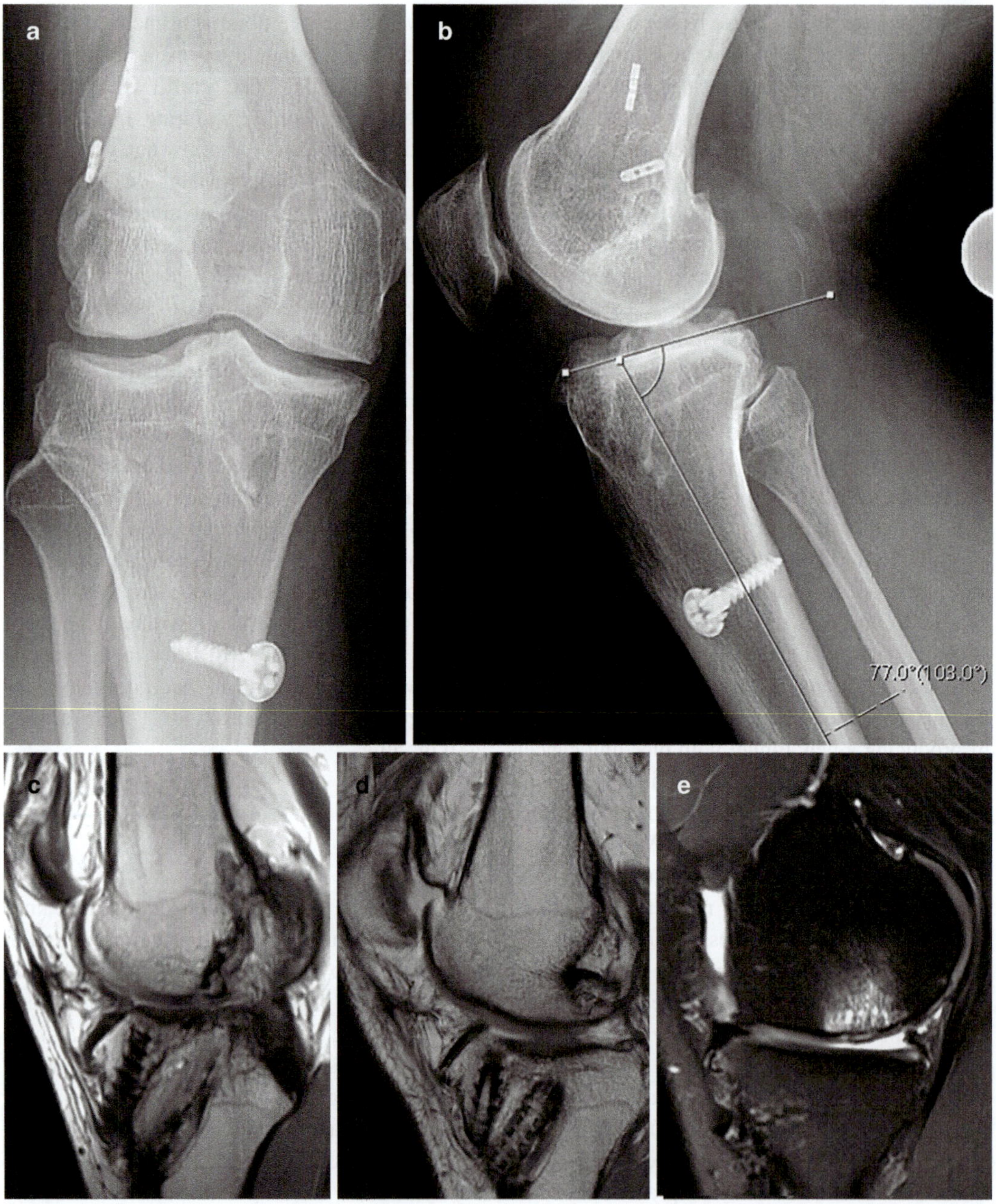

Fig. 8.6 AP (**a**) and lateral (**b**) radiograph demonstrating two lateral femoral buttons from suspensory fixation of his prior ACL grafts; screw and spiked washer in the proximal medial tibia; evidence of femoral and tibial tunnel osteolysis measuring 13 mm and 15 mm, respectively; and 13 degrees of posterior tibial slope. Sagittal proton density MRI sequence demonstrating complete ACL graft rupture (**c**), with two retained interference screws in the proximal tibial from prior ACL graft fixation (**d**). Sagittal fluid-sensitive MRI sequence demonstrating an osteochondral defect of the medial femoral condyle measuring 11 × 14 mm (**e**)

aspect of the medial tibial plateau. An MRI was obtained, which confirmed the diagnosis of an ACL graft tear (Fig. 8.6c) with two retained interference screws in the proximal tibial from prior ACL graft fixation (Fig. 8.6d), posterior horn medial meniscal deficiency from prior partial medial meniscectomy, and an osteochondral defect of the medial femoral condyle (MFC) measuring 14 × 20 mm (Fig. 8.6e).

Given the patient's pain, swelling, recurrent instability, and radiographic evidence of increased posterior slope, varus alignment, osteochondral lesion of the MFC, vertical femoral tunnel positioning, and significant tibial tunnel osteolysis, the plan was to proceed with a two-stage revision ACL reconstruction. Stage one would consist of bone grafting of his femoral and tibial tunnels, osteochondral allograft of his MFC lesion, and a high tibial osteotomy with an anterolateral hinge for correction of excessive posterior slope and varus malalignment while offloading the osteochondral allograft.

The patient was taken to the operating room, and a diagnostic arthroscopy confirmed a complete tear of the ACL graft, focal MFC osteochondral lesion measuring 20 mm in diameter, deficiency of the posterior horn of the medial meniscus, and no evidence of chondral wear in the lateral compartment. The graft stumps were debrided, and the previous femoral tunnel was identified. A guide wire was placed into the femoral tunnel. Sequential reaming of the tunnel was performed, beginning at 10 mm and advancing to a 14-mm reamer. All graft and suture debris were removed from the tunnel. A cannulated 14-mm allograft dowel was then impacted into the femoral tunnel in press fit fashion (Fig. 8.7a). The two bioabsorbable screws were identified in the tibial tunnel and removed, along with the metal screw and washer in the tibia. During removal, the distal tibial screw broke, and the tip was uneventfully left buried within the tibial shaft. A guide wire was placed into the prior tibial tunnel. Sequential reaming of the tunnel was then performed, beginning with a 10-mm and advancing to a 14-mm reamer. All graft and suture debris was removed from the tunnel. A 14-mm cannulated allograft dowel was then impacted into the tibial tunnel in press fit fashion (Fig. 8.7b). A medial parapatellar arthrotomy was then performed, and a 22-mm osteochondral allograft plug was used to address the MFC osteochondral lesion (Fig. 8.7c). A high tibial osteotomy was then performed to address the increased posterior slope and correct the varus alignment, thereby offloading the medial compartment. Our wedge was completed with a 3:1 ratio to decrease the posterior slope of the tibia, with a 2-mm anterior and 6-mm posterior opening. A medial-based plate was secured in locking fashion, and the osteotomy site was bone grafted (Fig. 8.7d, e).

Serial radiographs were obtained to monitor healing at the osteotomy site. At 8 months postoperatively, a CT scan was obtained demonstrating healing of the osteotomy, osteochondral allograft, and tunnel allografts (Fig. 8.8a–d). On examination the patient continued to have a grade 2B Lachman and 2+ pivot shift. At 10 months postoperatively, the patient underwent revision ACL reconstruction with BTB autograft, removal of osteotomy hardware, and lateral extra-articular tenodesis (Fig. 8.9a, b). At 1 year following revision ACL reconstruction, the patient was doing well and was cleared to return to sport (Fig. 8.9c, d).

Case-Based Discussion: Case 2

This case highlights the importance of preoperative planning and an inclusive workup to identify secondary causes of ACL graft failure. In addition to osteolysis, tunnel expansion requiring bone grafting can result from tunnels which are close resulting in tunnel confluence if redirection is attempted, as well as when an excessive amount of bone is removed during the hardware extraction process. For patients with multiple ACL graft ruptures, a thorough workup into the etiologies of ACL failure is important, and abnormalities should be addressed, often in a staged fashion.

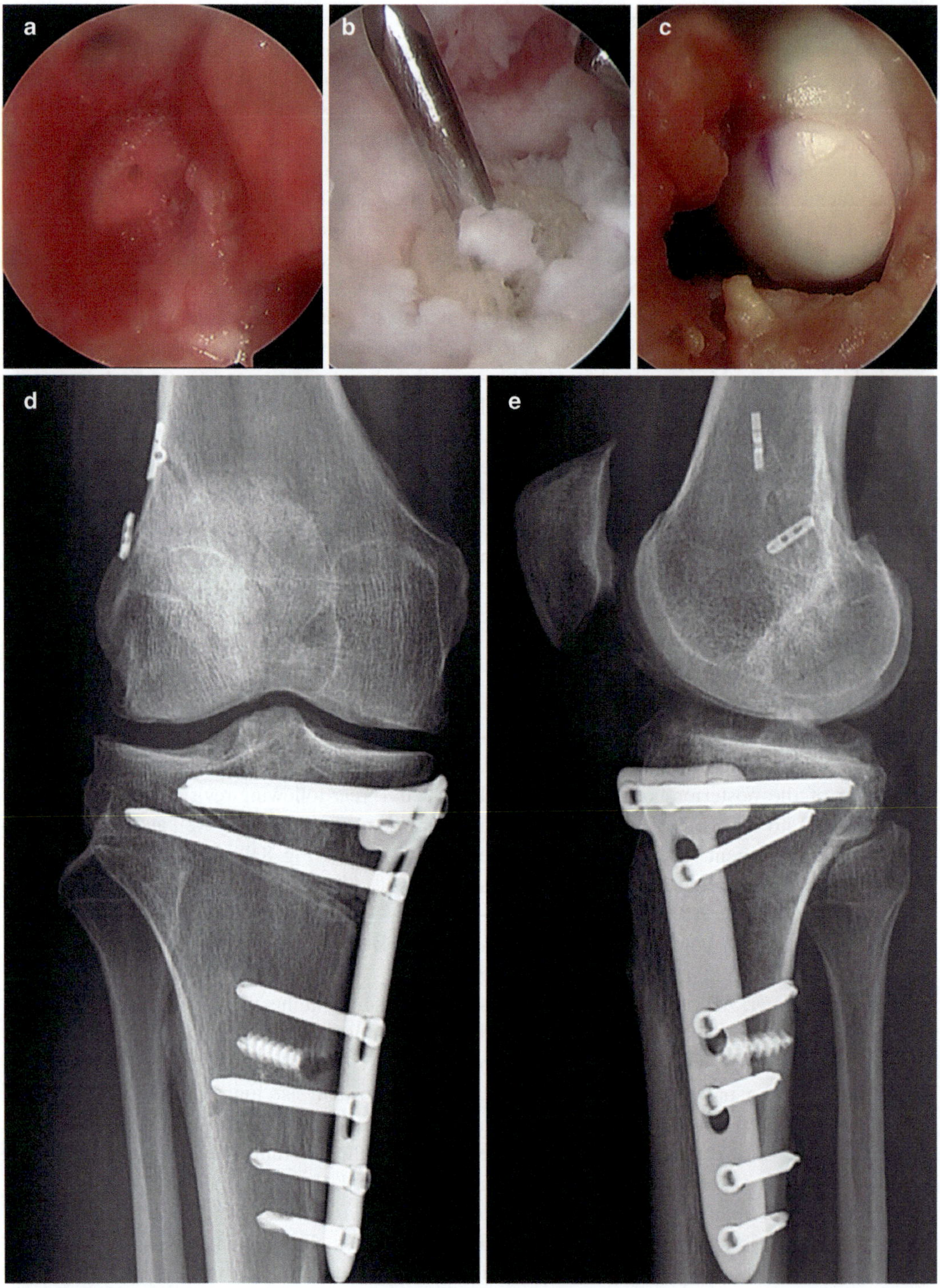

Fig. 8.7 Arthroscopic image demonstrating allograft bone dowel press fit fixation in the prior femoral (**a**) and tibial (**b**) tunnels. Arthroscopic image following osteochondral allograft plug fixation to address the MFC OCD lesion (**c**). Intraoperative AP (**d**) and lateral (**e**) radiograph demonstrating adequate bone grafting of the prior femoral and tibial tunnel, with correction of the patients varus malalignment and posterior tibial slope

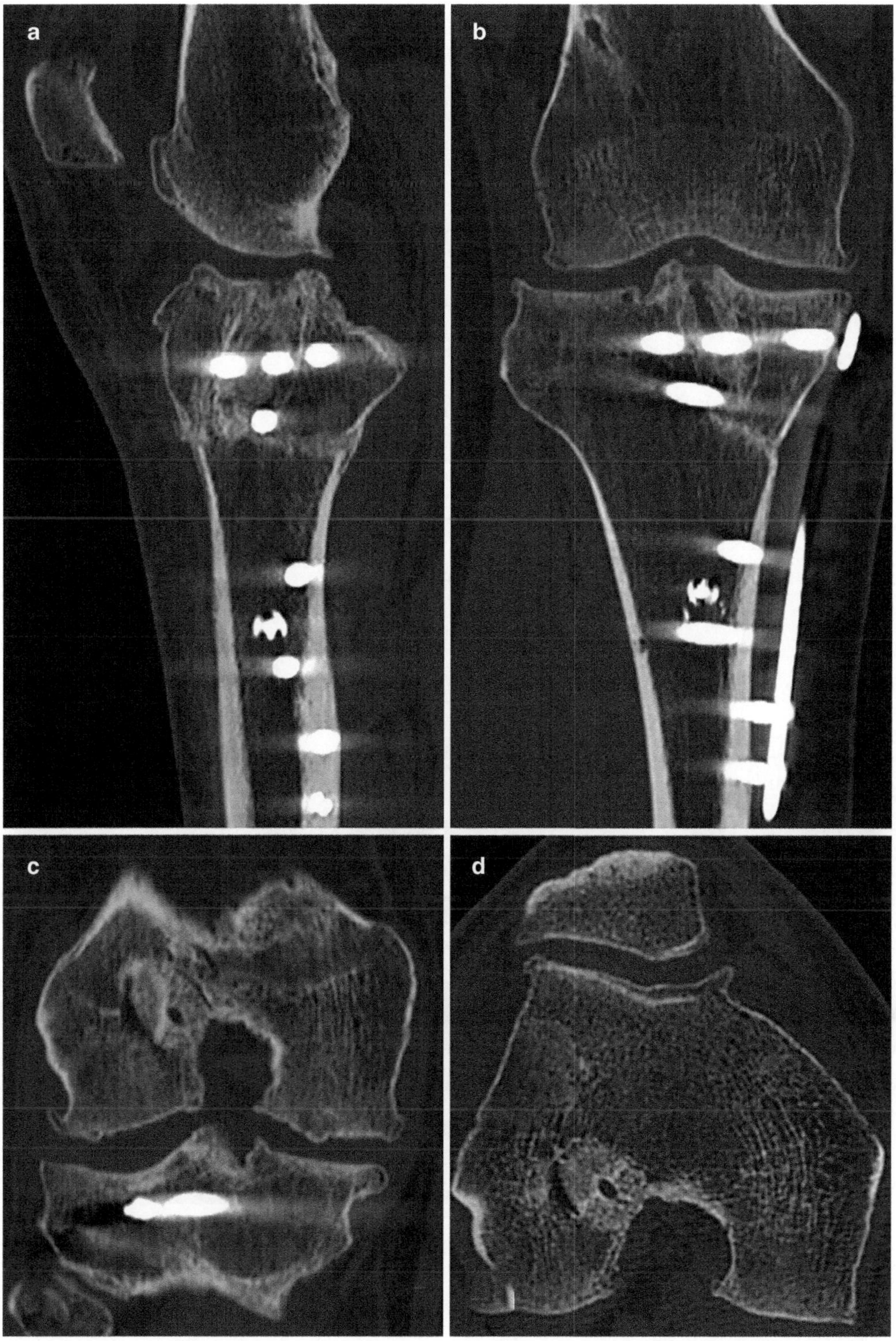

Fig. 8.8 Sagittal (**a**) and coronal (**b**) CT scan of the proximal tibia demonstrating incorporation of the tibial tunnel bone graft and healing of the high tibial osteotomy site. Coronal (**c**) and axial (**d**) CT scan of the distal femur demonstrating incorporation of the femoral tunnel bone graft

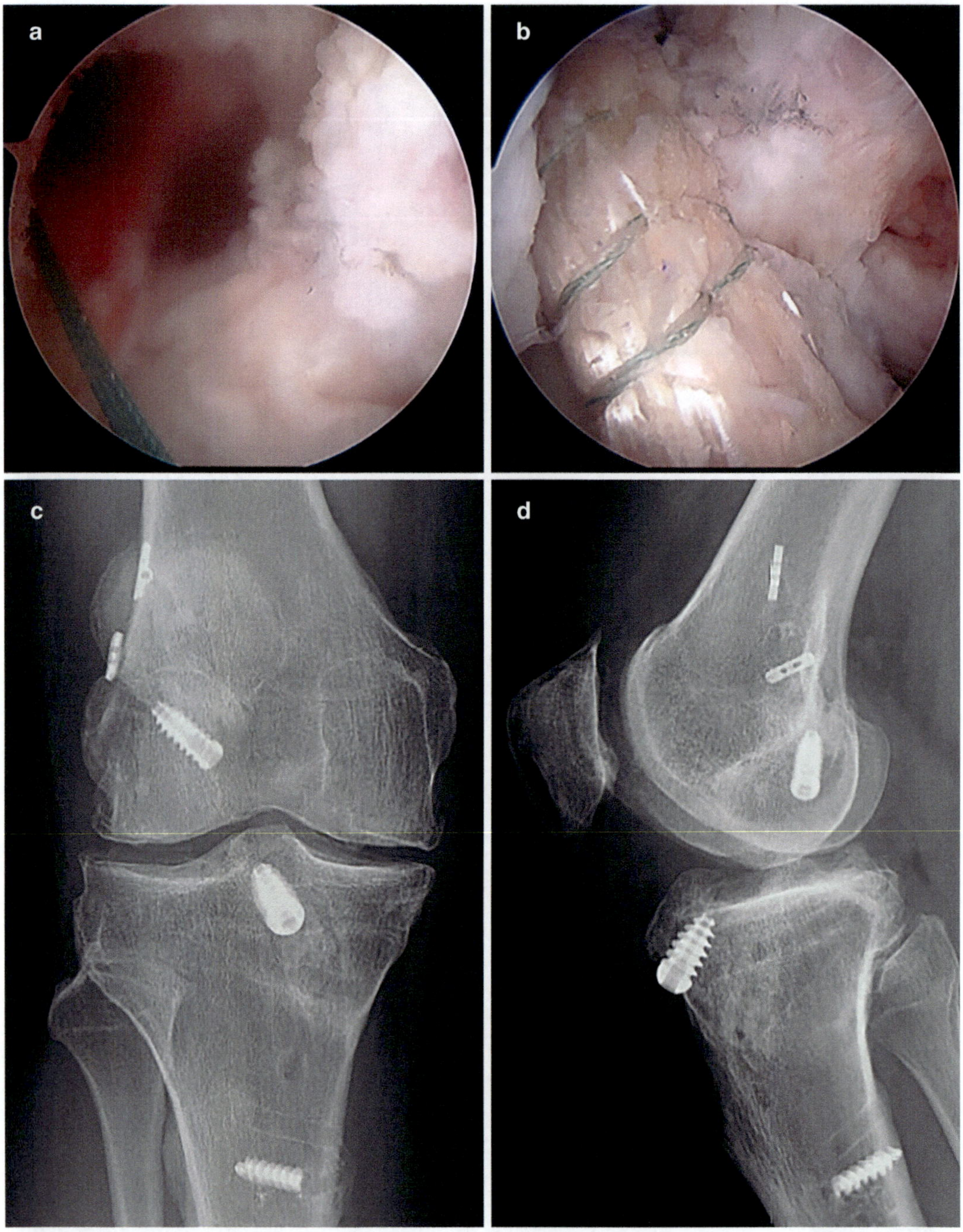

Fig. 8.9 Arthroscopic image demonstrating the femoral socket drilled during the second stage, with healthy cancellous tunnel walls (**a**), and the BTB autograft passed (**b**), and aperture fixation was obtained with metal screws. One year postoperative AP (**c**) and lateral (**d**) radiograph demonstrating healed tibial and femoral bone plugs

Bone Defects

Tunnel malpositioning is the most common technical error during primary and revision ACL reconstruction. This can result in excessive graft forces and strain resulting in inadequate graft incorporation, graft loosening, and atraumatic graft failure [26, 27]. Malpositioned tunnels are associated with increased failure rates and inferior clinic outcomes [28]. Excessive anterior placement of the femoral tunnel is the most frequent technical error [19, 20, 27]. Furthermore, excessively posterior femoral tunnel placement may result in posterior wall blowout. It is important this is identified, as this error limits fixation options at the time of revision surgery to those relying on lateral cortical fixation or requires bone grafting and a two-stage ACL reconstruction.

Prior tunnel placement may be categorized in one of three ways: (1) accurate, not requiring redirection; (2) completely inaccurate, not interfering with new tunnel creation; or (3) overlapping, such that the prior tunnel and a properly placed tunnel will partially overlap [20]. Partially overlapping tunnels are the most challenging and frequently require grafting and a two-stage procedure. If the aperture of the new tunnel would partially overlap the old tunnel leading to a large defect, depending on the situation, we recommend bone grafting the old tunnel and redirection of the revision tunnel once the bone grafting heals. Failure to identify this problem can lead to compromised fixation and excessive translation of the graft at the joint line [14].

Bone defects can be created during the hardware extraction process. As illustrated in this case, significant bone defects can result from removal of hardware. It is important to anticipate this possibility. Furthermore, care should be taken to remove as little bone as possible during the hardware extraction process as discussed in the next section. Lastly, revision cases following a primary double bundle ACL reconstruction can result in significant bone loss.

Hardware Removal

Hardware removal is frequently required in the revision setting, and the size and location of the resulting bone defect must be considered. Defects created during this process may necessitate grafting, either as part of a single-stage or two-stage revision. The requirement for hardware removal necessitates knowledge of the previous implants used and the appropriate extraction tools. Additionally, universal hardware removal trays should be available in the operating room at the time of surgery, including multiple and varied screwdrivers. Fluoroscopy should be available and can be used to facilitate removing retained hardware or to assist in tunnel placement if the decision is made to attempt to bypass the previously placed hardware.

While the goal should be to remove as little bone as possible, hardware that requires removal should be well visualized to prevent damage to adjacent healthy tissue during extraction and stripping of screws. Notch overgrowth and osteophyte formation are commonly encountered during the revision setting and may require resection of bone from the roof and lateral wall of the notch to aid in visualization for hardware removal. When extracting femoral tunnel screws, adequate soft tissue debridement should be performed for proper seating of the screwdriver and proper angle orientation to avoid stripping the screw. It is not uncommon for bone to grow into the hexagonal head. Once the screw head is located, a curette can be used to clean the hexagonal head for the screwdriver to seat properly. Additionally, bone must be removed circumferentially around the head of the screw so that it can be removed easily without breaking.

Malalignment

For revision ACL reconstruction to be successful, it is paramount to determine the underlying etiology leading to failure of the index procedure. The etiology of failure may be related to recurrent trauma, loss of motion, technical error, or failure to recognize and treat concomitant pathology, such as collateral ligament laxity. Varus malalignment and, to a greater extent, excessive posterior tibial slope have been implicated as risk factors for ACL graft failure. For this reason, in patients presenting with an ACL graft tear, radiographs that allow for evaluation of the mechanical alignment and posterior tibial slope should be obtained. In ACL-deficient knees with varus malalignment (particularly with associated lateral side laxity and a varus thrust gait) or increased posterior tibial slope, ACL reconstruction may be predisposed to gradual attenuation and eventual failure if the alignment is not first addressed with an osteotomy procedure. We generally prefer to perform a two-stage ACL reconstruction when an osteotomy is planned for alignment correction, especially in the revision setting, due to the magnitude of the surgery and recovery. However, depending on the patient and the pathoanatomy, a single-stage osteotomy and revision ACL may be appropriate. During the first stage, the tunnels are debrided and grafted and the osteotomy performed. Once healed, this allows for removal of hardware and revision ACL reconstruction with optimal tunnels for graft fixation and incorporation.

Case 3

A 17-year-old female presented 3 months after left knee ACL reconstruction with hamstring autograft, complicated by acute postoperative infection, five irrigation and debridement procedures, and removal of her graft and hardware. She had completed a 6-week course of intravenous antibiotics with daptomycin and meropenem. She reported significant instability with activities of daily living. On examination, she had 3–150 degrees of knee flexion, a grade 2B Lachman, and 3+ pivot shift, and her knee was stable to varus and valgus stress at 0 and 30 degrees. Labs were obtained and were within normal limits: white blood cell (WBC) count 8.7/nl, C-reactive protein (CRP) <0.7 mg/dl, and erythrocyte sedimentation rate (ESR) 11 mm/hr.

Radiographs revealed evidence of tibial and femoral tunnel widening (Fig. 8.10a, b). MRI showed the ACL graft to be absent with significant tibial and femoral tunnel osteolysis. A CT scan was obtained for further evaluation of the extent of tunnel osteolysis and tunnel position. The CT scan showed significant tunnel osteolysis with a tibial and femoral tunnel diameter of 15 mm (Fig. 8.10c, d).

Given the patient's instability with activities of daily living, history of infection, and radiographic evidence of significant tunnel osteolysis, the plan was to proceed with a two-stage revision ACL reconstruction. The plan during the first stage was to intraoperatively evaluate for evidence of persistent infection, obtain tissue samples and synovial fluid to send for pathology and culture, and perform bone grafting of her femoral and tibial tunnels if suspicion for ongoing infection was low. Diagnostic arthroscopy revealed some mild synovitis in the suprapatellar pouch. Synovial tissue samples were obtained and sent for culture, and a partial synovectomy was performed. The ACL was absent from the notch, with evidence of tibial and femoral tunnel widening. A guide wire was placed into the prior location of the femoral tunnel and sequentially reaming to a diameter of 12 mm. This effectively cleaned out all of the prior graft material, and bleeding cancellous bone in the femur was achieved (Fig. 8.11a). The location of the previous tibial tunnel was identified. A guide pin was then placed through the previous tibial tunnel and held intra-articular with a grasper. The tunnel was sequentially reamed to a diameter of 12 mm. This effectively cleaned out all of the prior graft material, and bleeding cancellous bone was achieved. A 12-mm diameter allograft bone dowel was placed through the anteromedial portal over a guide wire into the femoral tunnel (Fig. 8.11b, c), and a 12-mm diameter allograft bone dowel was placed over a guide wire into the tibial tunnel to achieve sufficient press fit fixation.

Intraoperative cultures were all negative. Serial radiographs were obtained to monitor healing of the bone graft. At 6 months postoperatively, a CT scan was obtained demonstrating

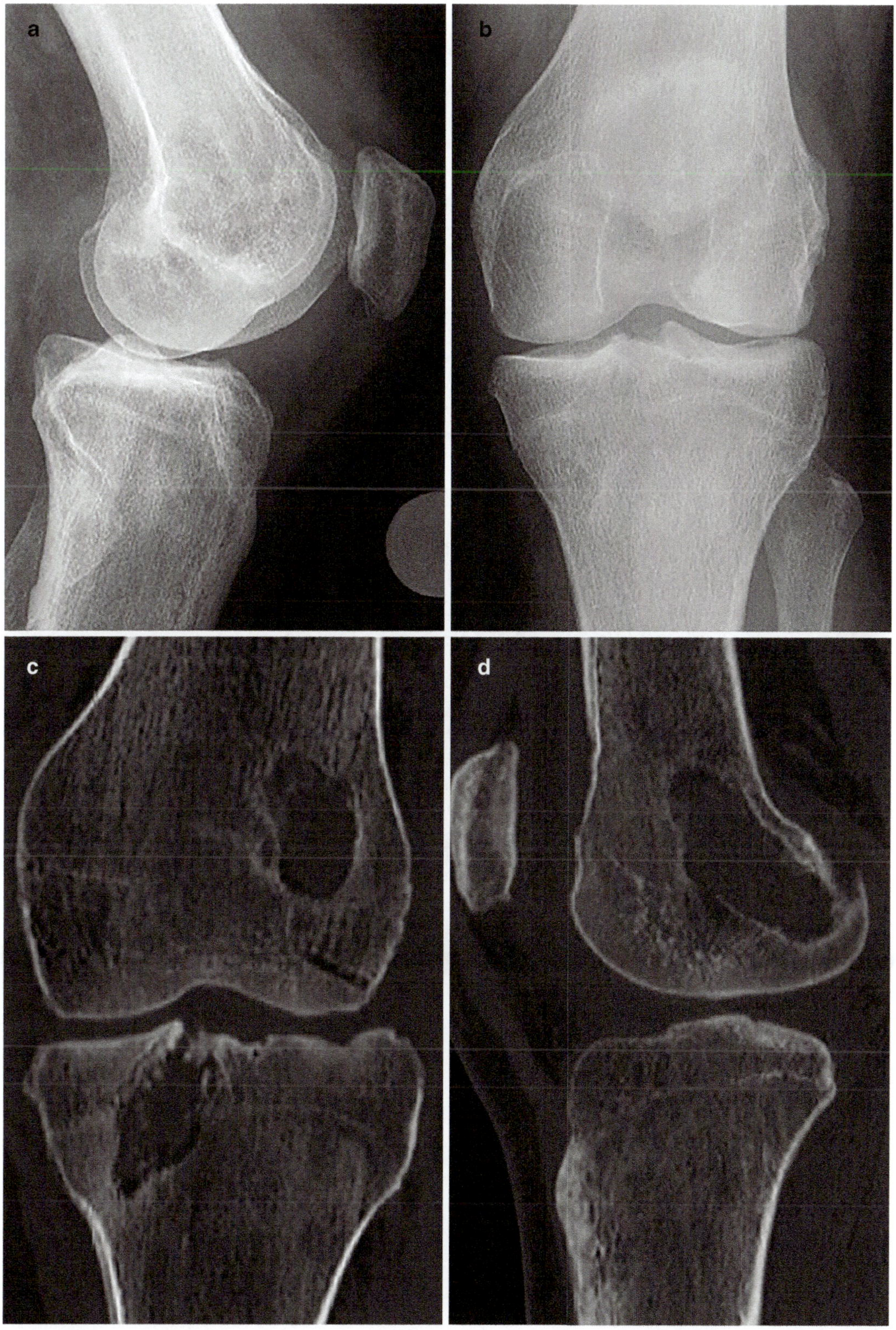

Fig. 8.10 Lateral (**a**) and AP (**b**) radiograph demonstrating evidence of tibial and femoral tunnel widening. Coronal (**c**) and sagittal (**d**) CT image demonstrating significant tibial and femoral tunnel defects measuring 15 mm in diameter

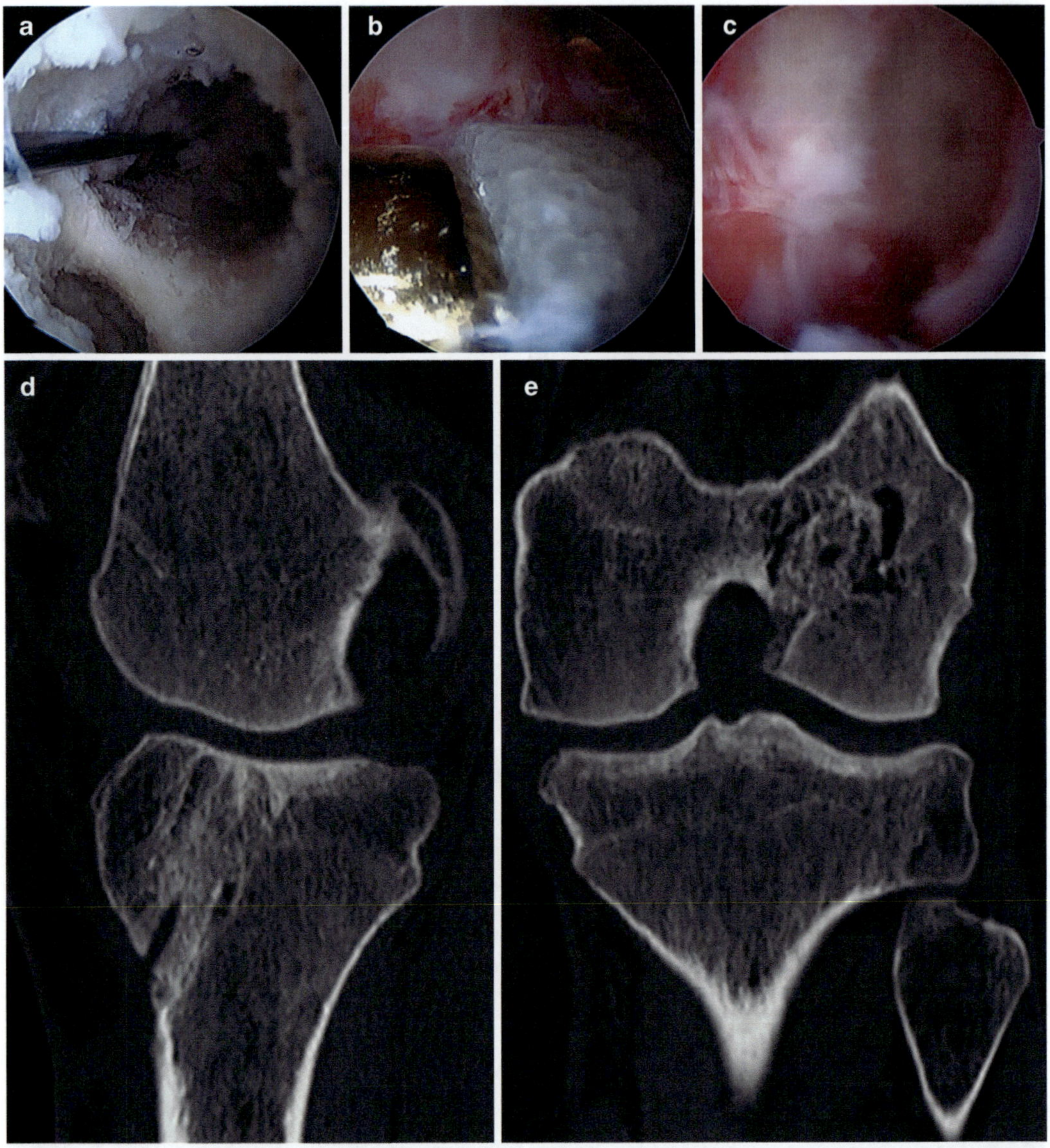

Fig. 8.11 Arthroscopic image following sequential reaming of the index femoral tunnel to produce a bleeding cancellous bone tunnel (**a**) to promote healing of the allograft bone dowel (**b**, **c**). Sagittal (**d**) and coronal (**e**) CT image obtained 6 months following the bone tunnel grafting procedure demonstrating healing of the allograft bone dowels in the tibial and femoral tunnels, respectively

healing of the tunnel allografts (Fig. 8.11d, e). On examination the patient continued to have a grade 2B Lachman and 3+ pivot shift. At 7 months postoperatively, the patient underwent revision ACL reconstruction with BTB autograft and lateral extra-articular tenodesis (Fig. 8.12a, b). At 1 year follow-up, the patient was doing well and was cleared to return to sport (Fig. 8.12c, d).

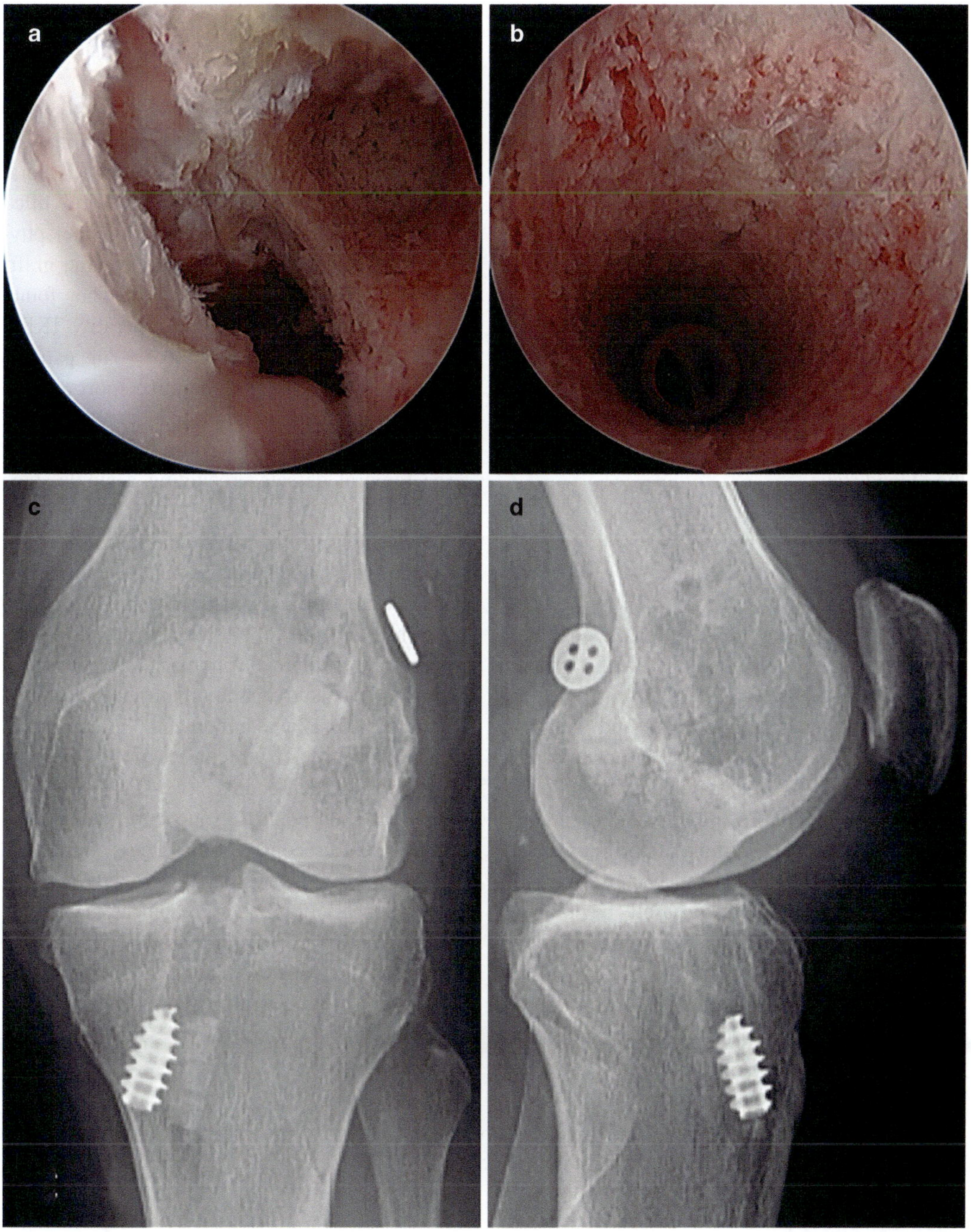

Fig. 8.12 Arthroscopic image demonstrating the femoral (**a**) and tibial (**b**) socket drilled during the second stage, with healthy cancellous tunnel walls for fixation and integration of the revision ACL graft. AP (**c**) and lateral (**d**) 6-week postoperative radiographs demonstrating ACL graft fixation with a lateral cortical button suspensory fixation on the femur and aperture fixation with a metal screw on the tibia

Case-Based Discussion: Case 3

This case highlights the use of a two-stage revision ACL reconstruction in the setting of postoperative infection. It is important to ensure the infection is eradicated prior to harvesting and fixing another ACL graft. For this reason, we feel that having a low threshold to perform a two-stage revision, especially when tunnel malposition or widening is present, is preferred. With this strategy, an intra-articular evaluation can be performed, cultures and pathology can be obtained to confirm the eradication of infection, and bone grafting of prior tunnels can be performed to ensure healthy tunnels for graft fixation during the second stage.

Infection

Infection is a rare but devastating complication following ACL reconstruction, with reported rates between 0.58% and 0.80%, typically occurring in the acute (<2 weeks) and subacute (between 2 weeks and 2 months) postoperative period [29, 30]. In cases suspicious for infection, serologic tests including a complete blood count (CBC), erythrocyte sedimentation rate (ESR), C-reactive protein (CRP), and bacterial cultures from a knee aspirate should promptly be obtained. Furthermore, in cases with significant osteolysis of previous tunnels, infection should be ruled out.

A staged revision should be performed in the setting of ACL graft failure secondary to infection. During the first stage, the intra-articular joint can be evaluated. Tissue and synovial fluid should be sent for pathology and culture, and a synovectomy of any inflamed tissues or scar should be performed. If suspicion is low for persistent infection, previous tunnels can be bone grafted. The definitive reconstruction should be delayed until it has been confirmed that the infection is eradicated and the tunnel allografts healed.

Outcomes

No current studies have directly compared outcomes following one-stage versus two-stage revision ACL reconstructions. Few studies have compared two-stage revision ACL reconstruction to primary ACL reconstruction.

Franceschi et al. reported outcomes on 30 patients who required a two-stage revision ACL reconstruction for bone grafting of large femoral defects [31]. The femoral defects were filled using autograft obtained from the tibial metaphysis, with CT scans obtained 3 months after grafting to evaluate for graft integration. They found significant improvement in postoperative IKDC and Lysholm scores, with 66.7% of patients returning to the same preoperative sport activity level. They concluded that a two-stage approach is a safe and effective procedure for patients with large femoral defects precluding a single-stage procedure.

Weiler et al. compared outcomes between patients who underwent primary versus two-stage revision ACL reconstruction and found no difference in postoperative objective IKDC scores [32]. In contrast, Thomas et al. performed a prospective study comparing outcomes in a cohort of patients who underwent two-stage revision and primary ACL reconstruction [14]. They compared 49 consecutive two-stage revisions with a matched control group that underwent a primary ACL reconstruction. They found that patients who underwent a two-stage revision ACL reconstruction had a greater degree of passive range of motion deficits, were more likely to have crepitus on exam, and had significantly worse subjective outcome scores compared to patients who underwent a primary ACL reconstruction.

Conclusion

The decision to perform a two-stage revision ACL reconstruction with bone grafting is complex and multifactorial. Tunnel osteolysis and bone defects are common, with larger defects predisposing patients to inadequate graft fixation and integration. CT imaging can be beneficial to determine the extent of tunnel malposition and tunnel dilation and to assist with decision-making for possible two-stage revision with a bone grafting procedure. Furthermore, other clinical scenarios such as index tunnel malposition, malalignment requiring a corrective osteotomy, or infection may influence the decision to perform a two-stage reconstruction. To optimize outcomes, accurate placement of the femoral and tibial tunnels should not be compromised by the index tunnels, and tunnel expansion from hardware removal or osteolysis must not jeopardize graft fixation and incorporation. As revision ACL surgery continues to become more common, ACL surgeons must be comfortable to perform a two-stage revision with bone grafting, when indicated.

References

1. Mall NA, Chalmers PN, Moric M, Tanaka MJ, Cole BJ, Bach BR Jr, Paletta GA Jr. Incidence and trends of anterior cruciate ligament reconstruction in the United States. Am J Sports Med. 2014;42:2363–70.
2. Fagelman M, Freedman KB. Revision reconstruction of the anterior cruciate ligament: evaluation and management. Am J Orthop (Belle Mead NJ). 2005;34:319–28.
3. Getelman MH, Friedman MJ. Revision anterior cruciate ligament reconstruction surgery. J Am Acad Orthop Surg. 1999;7:189–98.
4. Wright RW, Dunn WR, Amendola A, Andrish JT, Bergfeld J, Kaeding CC, Marx RG, McCarty EC, Parker RD, Wolcott M, et al. Risk of tearing the intact anterior cruciate ligament in the contralateral knee and rupturing the anterior cruciate ligament graft during the first 2 years after anterior cruciate ligament reconstruction: a prospective MOON cohort study. Am J Sports Med. 2007;35:1131–4.
5. Bourke HE, Salmon LJ, Waller A, Patterson V, Pinczewski LA. Survival of the anterior cruciate ligament graft and the contralateral ACL at a minimum of 15 years. Am J Sports Med. 2012;40:1985–92.
6. Wright RW, Magnussen RA, Dunn WR, Spindler KP. Ipsilateral graft and contralateral ACL rupture at five years or more following ACL reconstruction: a systematic review. J Bone Joint Surg Am. 2011;93:1159–65.
7. Ohly NE, Murray IR, Keating JF. Revision anterior cruciate ligament reconstruction: timing of surgery and the incidence of meniscal tears and degenerative change. J Bone Joint Surg Br. 2007;89:1051–4.
8. Diamantopoulos AP, Lorbach O, Paessler HH. Anterior cruciate ligament revision reconstruction: results in 107 patients. Am J Sports Med. 2008;36:851–60.
9. Group M, Group M. Effect of graft choice on the outcome of revision anterior cruciate ligament reconstruction in the Multicenter ACL Revision Study (MARS) Cohort. Am J Sports Med. 2014;42:2301–10.
10. Group M, Wright RW, Huston LJ, Spindler KP, Dunn WR, Haas AK, Allen CR, Cooper DE, DeBerardino TM, Lantz BB, et al. Descriptive epidemiology of the Multicenter ACL Revision Study (MARS) cohort. Am J Sports Med. 2010;38:1979–86.
11. George MS, Dunn WR, Spindler KP. Current concepts review: revision anterior cruciate ligament reconstruction. Am J Sports Med. 2006;34:2026–37.
12. Battaglia TC, Miller MD. Management of bony deficiency in revision anterior cruciate ligament reconstruction using allograft bone dowels: surgical technique. Arthroscopy. 2005;21:767.
13. Maak TG, Voos JE, Wickiewicz TL, Warren RF. Tunnel widening in revision anterior cruciate ligament reconstruction. J Am Acad Orthop Surg. 2010;18:695–706.
14. Thomas NP, Kankate R, Wandless F, Pandit H. Revision anterior cruciate ligament reconstruction using a 2-stage technique with bone grafting of the tibial tunnel. Am J Sports Med. 2005;33:1701–9.
15. Wilson TC, Kantaras A, Atay A, Johnson DL. Tunnel enlargement after anterior cruciate ligament surgery. Am J Sports Med. 2004;32:543–9.
16. Marchant MH Jr, Willimon SC, Vinson E, Pietrobon R, Garrett WE, Higgins LD. Comparison of plain radiography, computed tomography, and magnetic resonance imaging in the evaluation of bone tunnel widening after anterior cruciate ligament reconstruction. Knee Surg Sports Traumatol Arthrosc. 2010;18:1059–64.
17. Denti M, Lo Vetere D, Bait C, Schonhuber H, Melegati G, Volpi P. Revision anterior cruciate ligament reconstruction: causes of failure, surgical technique, and clinical results. Am J Sports Med. 2008;36:1896–902.
18. Allen CR, Giffin JR, Harner CD. Revision anterior cruciate ligament reconstruction. Orthop Clin North Am. 2003;34:79–98.
19. Harner CD, Giffin JR, Dunteman RC, Annunziata CC, Friedman MJ. Evaluation and treatment of recurrent instability after anterior cruciate ligament reconstruction. Instr Course Lect. 2001;50:463–74.
20. Kamath GV, Redfern JC, Greis PE, Burks RT. Revision anterior cruciate ligament reconstruction. Am J Sports Med. 2011;39:199–217.
21. Barrett GR, Brown TD. Femoral tunnel defect filled with a synthetic dowel graft for a single-staged revision anterior cruciate ligament reconstruction. Arthroscopy. 2007;23:796e791–4.
22. Vaughn ZD, Schmidt J, Lindsey DP, Dragoo JL. Biomechanical evaluation of a 1-stage revision anterior cruciate ligament reconstruction technique using a structural bone void filler for femoral fixation. Arthroscopy. 2009;25:1011–8.
23. Franceschi F, Papalia R, Di Martino A, Rizzello G, Allaire R, Denaro V. A new harvest site for bone graft in anterior cruciate ligament revision surgery. Arthroscopy. 2007;23(558):e551–4.

24. Said HG, Baloch K, Green M. A new technique for femoral and tibial tunnel bone grafting using the OATS harvesters in revision anterior cruciate ligament reconstruction. Arthroscopy. 2006;22(796):e791–3.
25. Werner BC, Gilmore CJ, Hamann JC, Gaskin CM, Carroll JJ, Hart JM, Miller MD. Revision anterior cruciate ligament reconstruction: results of a single-stage approach using allograft dowel bone grafting for femoral defects. J Am Acad Orthop Surg. 2016;24:581–7.
26. Chen JL, Allen CR, Stephens TE, Haas AK, Huston LJ, Wright RW, Feeley BT, Multicenter ACLRSG. Differences in mechanisms of failure, intraoperative findings, and surgical characteristics between single- and multiple-revision ACL reconstructions: a MARS cohort study. Am J Sports Med. 2013;41:1571–8.
27. Carson EW, Anisko EM, Restrepo C, Panariello RA, O'Brien SJ, Warren RF. Revision anterior cruciate ligament reconstruction: etiology of failures and clinical results. J Knee Surg. 2004;17:127–32.
28. Sommer C, Friederich NF, Muller W. Improperly placed anterior cruciate ligament grafts: correlation between radiological parameters and clinical results. Knee Surg Sports Traumatol Arthrosc. 2000;8:207–13.
29. Brophy RH, Wright RW, Huston LJ, Nwosu SK, Group MK, Spindler KP. Factors associated with infection following anterior cruciate ligament reconstruction. J Bone Joint Surg Am. 2015;97:450–4.
30. Barker JU, Drakos MC, Maak TG, Warren RF, Williams RJ 3rd, Allen AA. Effect of graft selection on the incidence of postoperative infection in anterior cruciate ligament reconstruction. Am J Sports Med. 2010;38:281–6.
31. Franceschi F, Papalia R, Del Buono A, Zampogna B, Diaz Balzani L, Maffulli N, Denaro V. Two-stage procedure in anterior cruciate ligament revision surgery: a five-year follow-up prospective study. Int Orthop. 2013;37:1369–74.
32. Weiler A, Schmeling A, Stohr I, Kaab MJ, Wagner M. Primary versus single-stage revision anterior cruciate ligament reconstruction using autologous hamstring tendon grafts: a prospective matched-group analysis. Am J Sports Med. 2007;35:1643–52.

Prior Femoral Implant and Tunnel Management

9

Jonathan D. Hughes, Volker Musahl, and Bryson P. Lesniak

Introduction

Although causes for anterior cruciate ligament (ACL) reconstruction failure are multifactorial, recent literature has identified femoral tunnel malposition as the most common technical error. A recent study examined the Multicenter ACL Revision Study (MARS) database and reported that femoral tunnel malposition was a cause of failure in 47.6% of cases and the only cause of failure in 25.4% of cases. Additionally, the authors reported anterior and vertical tunnel malposition as the most common error [15]. Another study reported similar findings, with anterior tunnel placement in 36% of revision cases [17]. Anterior placement of the tunnel, the most common error, results in limited flexion, while a vertical tunnel may lead to continued rotational instability and failure. However, failures occur even with well-placed tunnels. In some revision cases, the resultant widening of index tunnels may pose a challenge during revision ACL reconstruction. The complexity of revision ACL reconstruction cases can lead to reoperation rates as high as 35% in young patients [8, 20]. The following chapter will discuss management, technical considerations, and pearls to address femoral tunnel malposition and widening.

J. D. Hughes (✉) · V. Musahl · B. P. Lesniak
Department of Orthopaedic Surgery, University of Pittsburgh, UPMC Freddie Fu Sports Medicine Center, Pittsburgh, PA, USA

Preoperative Workup

Initial radiographic evaluation includes standing anterior-posterior, weight-bearing 45° flexion posterior-anterior, lateral, and Merchant views. The weight-bearing 45° flexion posterior-anterior views can be utilized to measure the angle of the prior femoral tunnel. A measurement less than 33° most likely corresponds to a nonanatomic tunnel placement [9]. The presence of fixation devices can be identified on these views, as well as tunnel position on the lateral views (Fig. 9.1). The lateral view is useful to evaluate the tibial slope, as an increased tibial slope greater than 12° can be a risk factor for ACL injury [18]. In the revision setting, this may be addressed with a tibial deflexion osteotomy [6]. The type and position of fixation devices, including interference screws, staples, and buttons, are important for operative planning, as these may need to be removed during revision surgery. Additionally, full-length standing radiographs should be obtained to evaluate overall mechanical alignment. The current magnetic resonance imaging (MRI) as well as the MRI from the initial injury should be reviewed in detail.

The authors prefer to obtain a thin-cut computed tomography (CT) scan with three-

M. J. Alaia, K. J. Jones (eds.), *Revision Anterior Cruciate Ligament Reconstruction*,
https://doi.org/10.1007/978-3-030-96996-7_9

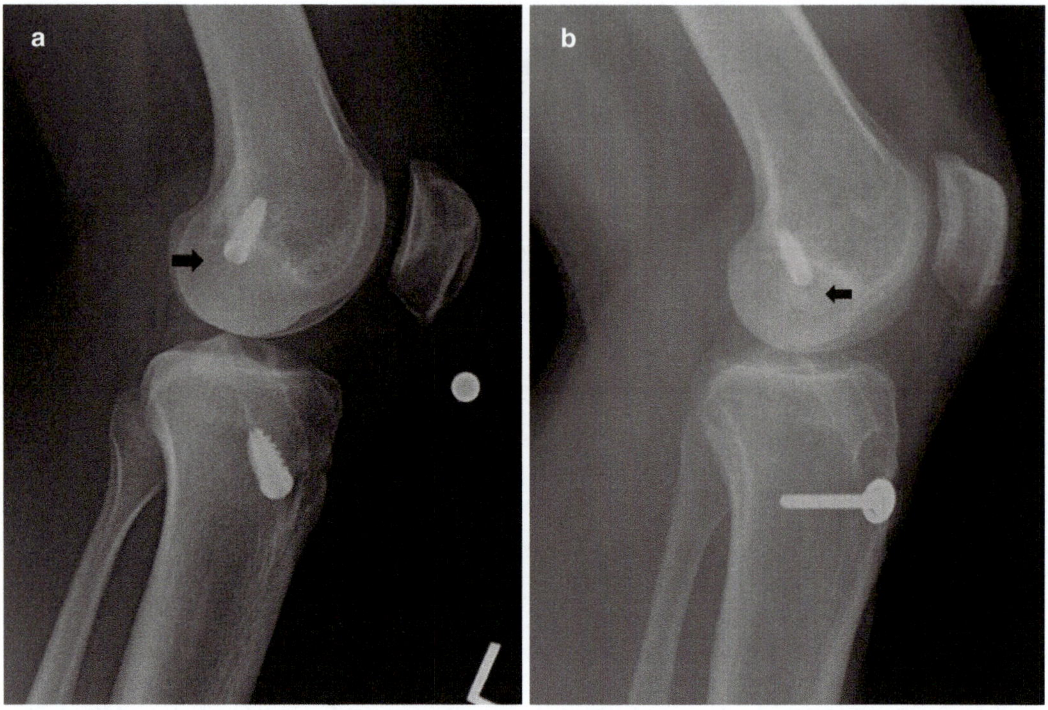

Fig. 9.1 Radiographs of tunnel position. In image (**a**), the black arrow points to a well-positioned femoral tunnel with an interference screw anterior to the tunnel. In image (**b**), the black arrow points to an anterior femoral tunnel with an interference screw within the tunnel

dimensional (3D) reconstructions in all revision settings. These images can provide crucial information on the position of the tunnels, tunnel widening, position of radiolucent fixation devices, and concomitant bony pathology (Fig. 9.2). One study reported bone tunnels seen on CT were also identified on radiographs, but there can be discrepancies in the measurements of the femoral tunnels between the imaging modalities [19]. Therefore, CT scans with 3D reconstructions can add valuable and more accurate measurements for preoperative planning, as well as understanding the spatial orientations of the tunnels [12]. Additionally, these findings may determine whether a one-stage or two-stage revision is necessary. Relative indications for two-stage revision ACL reconstruction, in regard to the femoral tunnel, include tunnel malpositioning that interferes with the placement of new anatomic tunnels or tunnel aperture ≥14 mm [4]. A recent retrospective review demonstrated similar outcomes and failure rates between one-stage and two-stage revision ACL reconstructions [14]. However, the retrospective nature of that study may make a direct comparison of those two groups difficult to interpret. The decision to perform a one-stage versus a two-stage revision should be made before proceeding with surgical intervention. If a one-stage revision is planned, the risk of converting to a two-stage procedure should be discussed with the patient in case unanticipated complications arise during the revision. As such, allograft bone graft should be available.

Surgical Planning and Technique

After a thorough review of the available imaging studies, a surgical plan can be developed that addresses mechanical alignment, any

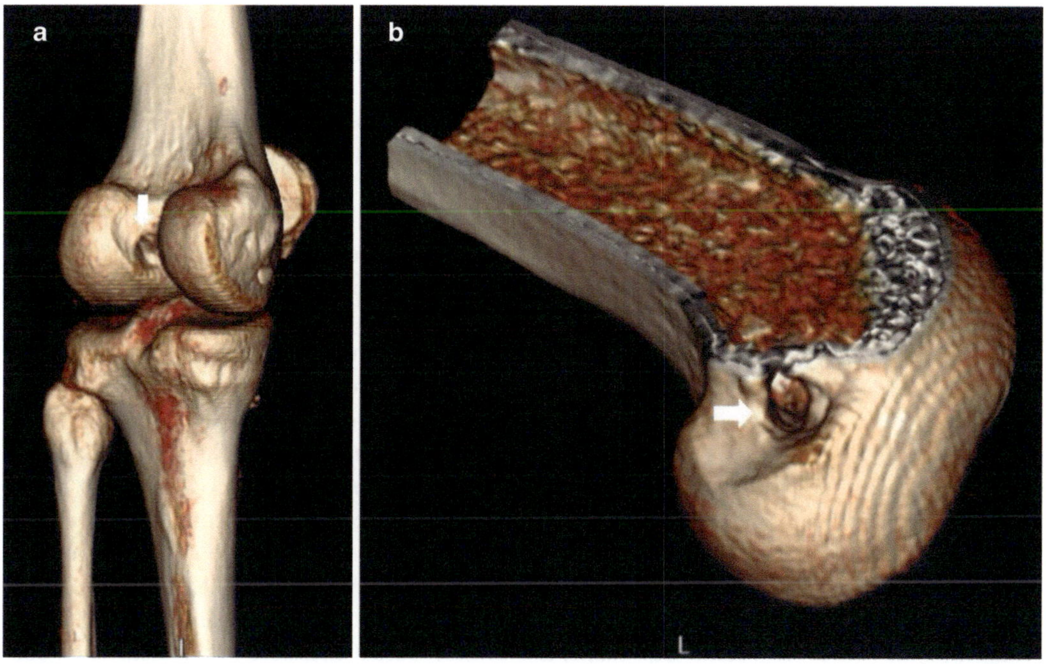

Fig. 9.2 Computed tomography (CT) scan with three-dimensional reconstructions of a distal femur. The white arrow in images (**a**) and (**b**) identify the femoral tunnel, which is placed too anterior and vertical

meniscal deficiency, tunnel position, and possible hardware removal. The prior femoral tunnel placement should be categorized according to the Revision using Imaging to guide Staging and Evaluation (REVISE) in ACL Reconstruction Classification. This classification system is as follows: type 1A in which the femoral and tibial tunnel positions are positioned well and can be used for the revision surgery without adjustment; type 1B in which the femoral and/or tibial tunnels require new drilling, but revision is one-stage; and type 2, in which a two-stage revision is required for poorly placed tunnels, bone loss tunnel widening, or infection [5]. Hardware should be left in place, if possible, to prevent the creation of bone defects, if it does not interfere with tunnel placement. One study described a technique of reaming the threads of a retained screw when a new femoral tunnel is created in order to prevent graft abrasion [13].

Type 1A

Tunnels that are appropriately placed can be used again in the revision setting, even with widening identified preoperatively. Hardware removal may be necessary if interference screws were utilized previously. Cortical fixation devices, staples, and cortical screws do not need to be removed unless they are an obstruction to the revision procedure. During screw removal, any bone around the screw should be removed first with a curette or burr. Be sure to have various screw removal sets available if the prior implant is not known. The remaining soft tissue in the tunnel is removed, and the tunnel is dilated to the appropriate size to ensure a healthy, bleeding bone interface for a graft. A larger soft tissue graft can be used with adjustable or continuous loop cortical fixation devices, especially if the posterior wall is incompetent. If the tunnel remains larger than the graft after cortical fixation, or a defect remains from the screw removal, an interference screw or bone graft can also be placed into the tunnel. Grafts with bone blocks can also be used, either autograft or allograft, with allograft providing the ability to obtain a larger bone block if needed to fill the prior tunnel. However, the authors' preferred method is to avoid the use of allograft in primary or revision ACL reconstructions given the recent studies demonstrated increased failure rates with allograft tissues [7, 10, 11].

Type 1B

In many instances, the prior tunnel is placed so far anteriorly or vertically that a new tunnel can be placed without addressing the prior tunnel (Fig. 9.3). A recent case series of the MARS cohort detailed drilling an entirely new femoral tunnel in 82% of cases [15]. If the prior tunnel is widened or enlarged, bone graft or an interference screw can be placed into the tunnel to fill the void and avoid collapse between the two tunnels.

A very common scenario in revision cases occurs when the prior tunnel is not quite anatomic and will overlap with the new tunnel. In this situation, the "divergent tunnel" technique should be employed. This involves drilling the new tunnel in a divergent angle to the previous tunnel to minimize tunnel overlap [1]. If the tunnel aperture becomes significantly widened due to the overlap, several options exist intraoperatively to address this issue. One option includes bone grafting the previous tunnel with autograft, allograft bone chips, allograft bone graft substitute, or allograft bone dowels. This option provides stability of the bone graft with the ability to drill a new tunnel through the bone graft [2, 3]. Another option includes placing a large interference screw in the anterior aspect of the widened tunnel and diverging its trajectory from the tunnels to allow bony fixation of the screw.

If significant widening of the tunnel is present, there are three options: the over-the-top (OTT) procedure, one-stage bone grafting, or two-stage bone grafting. The definition of "significant tunnel widening" is up for debate. While some authors suggest greater than 14 mm as a "rule of thumb," recent literature has demonstrated concern for inferior results with single-stage revisions with index tunnels greater than 12.5-mm diameter [21]. The OTT procedure can be an effective single-stage option in these cases and includes creating a trench in the anatomic footprint of the femur to allow graft healing. The graft is passed from the tibia to posterior to the lateral femoral condyle and through the posterolateral capsule and secured to the lateral femoral condyle with a staple, bicortical screw, or another

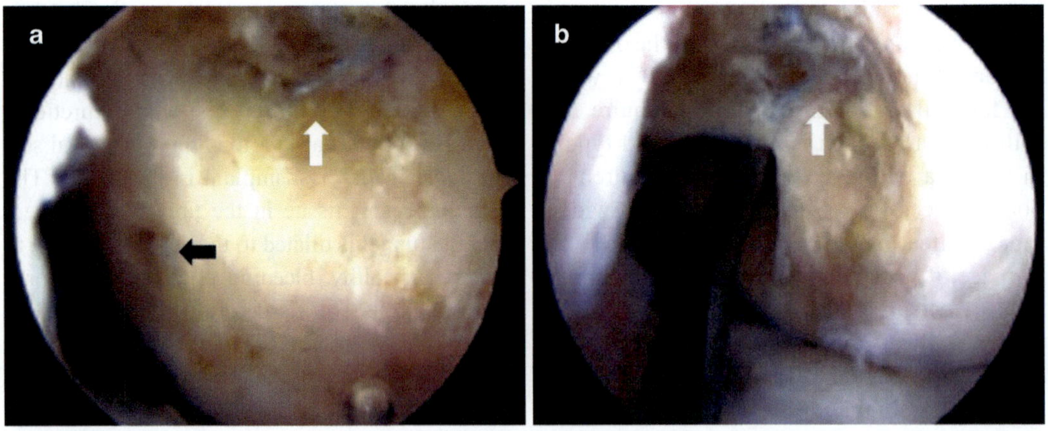

Fig. 9.3 Intraoperative photos of an incorrect tunnel position. In image (**a**), the white arrow identifies the prior tunnel that was placed anterior and vertical, while the black arrow demonstrates the planned position of the new, anatomic femoral tunnel. In image (**b**), the white arrow points to the prior tunnel, which does not diverge nor overlap with the new anatomic femoral tunnel

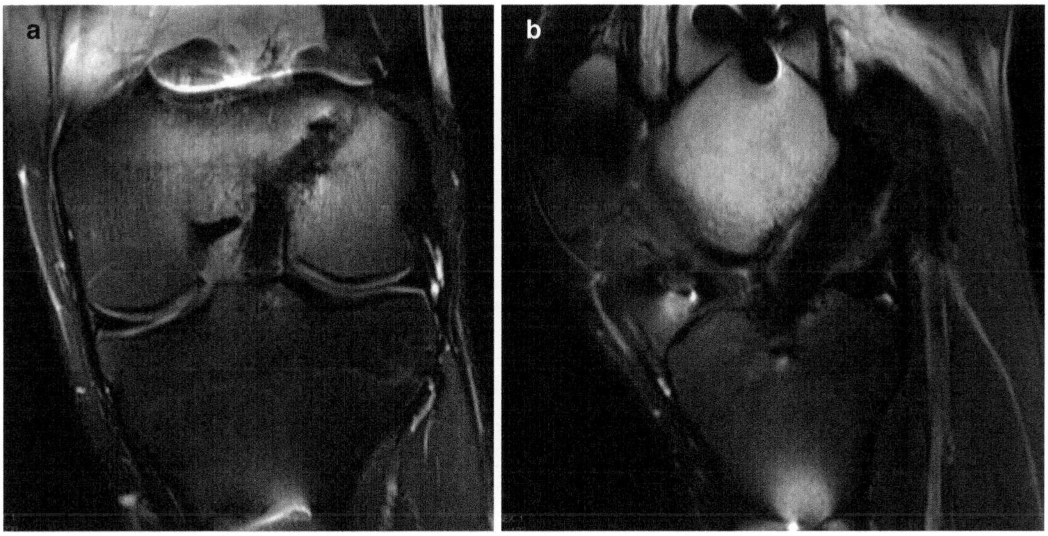

Fig. 9.4 Magnetic resonance imaging (MRI) of over-the-top (OTT) anterior cruciate ligament (ACL) reconstruction. Images (**a**) and (**b**) are coronal and sagittal images, respectively, of a healed OTT ACL reconstruction

suspensory fixation device. This technique avoids the need for a femoral tunnel and allows the graft to heal along the trench in the femur along the posterior cortex of the lateral femoral condyle (Fig. 9.4). A recent systematic review demonstrated comparable outcomes between OTT ACL reconstruction and traditional ACL reconstruction in the primary and revision setting [16].

Type 2

A two-stage procedure is indicated for poorly placed tunnels that don't allow a new, anatomic tunnel to be created, tunnel widening is so significant on both the tibia and femur that over-the-top procedure or one-stage bone grafting are not feasible, or significant infection. The two-stage procedure involves an initial bone grafting procedure, or in the case of infection multiple debridements followed by bone grafting, and allowing the bone graft to fully heal before the subsequent revision ACL-R. At the initial surgery, hardware is removed from the tunnels, and the tunnels are debrided of all soft tissue and sclerotic bone. Bone graft is impacted into the tunnels. The source of bone graft can be autograft from the tibia or iliac crest, allograft, or synthetic graft. Following the primary bone grafting procedure, the patient is followed clinically for 3–4 months to allow the bone graft to fully incorporate. Repeat radiographs and CT scan are taken at the 3–4-month mark to ensure adequate healing and incorporation. If the bone grafts have not fully incorporated, the patient should continue to be followed clinically with repeat imaging studies in 1–2 months to ensure adequate incorporation.

Conclusion

Managing femoral tunnels and hardware in the ACL revision setting can be challenging and requires meticulous preoperative planning and surgical technique. The combination of a full series of radiographs, a CT scan with 3D reconstructions, and both current and prior MRIs will facilitate the revision surgery. This includes identification of prior tunnel placement and hardware, as malposition or widening of the femoral tunnel may alter surgical technique. Hardware in many cases can be left in place, but one must always have hardware removal sets available for every surgery. The treating surgeon should attempt a single-stage revision when possible. Lastly, the revision surgery should possess the necessary repertoire of surgical techniques to address any pathology they may encounter during revision surgery, including bone grafting, over-the-top technique, and utilizing various fixation techniques.

References

1. Bach BR. Revision anterior cruciate ligament surgery. Arthroscopy. 2003;19:14–29.
2. Barrett GR, Brown TD. Femoral tunnel defect filled with a synthetic dowel graft for a single-staged revision anterior cruciate ligament reconstruction. Arthroscopy. 2007;23:796.e791–4.
3. Battaglia TC, Miller MD. Management of bony deficiency in revision anterior cruciate ligament reconstruction using allograft bone dowels: surgical technique. Arthroscopy. 2005;21:767. e761–5.
4. Chahla J, Dean CS, Cram TR, Civitarese D, O'Brien L, Moulton SG, et al. Two-stage revision anterior cruciate ligament reconstruction: bone grafting technique using an allograft bone matrix. Arthrosc Tech. 2016;5:e189–95.
5. Crum RJ, Rabuck S, Ayeni O, Bedi A, Baraga M, Getgood A, et al. The REVision using imaging to guide staging and evaluation (REVISE) in ACL reconstruction classification. J Knee Surg. 2021;34(5):509–19.
6. Dejour D, Saffarini M, Demey G, Baverel L. Tibial slope correction combined with second revision ACL produces good knee stability and prevents graft rupture. Knee Surg Sports Traumatol Arthrosc. 2015;23:2846–52.
7. Group M. Effect of graft choice on the outcome of revision anterior cruciate ligament reconstruction in the Multicenter ACL Revision Study (MARS) Cohort. Am J Sports Med. 2014;42:2301–10.
8. Group M, Ding DY, Zhang AL, Allen CR, Anderson AF, Cooper DE, et al. Subsequent surgery after revision anterior cruciate ligament reconstruction: rates and risk factors from a multicenter cohort. Am J Sports Med. 2017;45:2068–76.
9. Illingworth KD, Hensler D, Working ZM, Macalena JA, Tashman S, Fu FH. A simple evaluation of anterior cruciate ligament femoral tunnel position: the inclination angle and femoral tunnel angle. Am J Sports Med. 2011;39:2611–8.
10. Kaeding CC, Aros B, Pedroza A, Pifel E, Amendola A, Andrish JT, et al. Allograft versus autograft anterior cruciate ligament reconstruction: predictors of failure from a MOON prospective longitudinal cohort. Sports Health. 2011;3:73–81.
11. Kaeding CC, Pedroza AD, Reinke EK, Huston LJ, Spindler KP. Risk factors and predictors of subsequent ACL injury in either knee after ACL reconstruction: prospective analysis of 2488 primary ACL reconstructions from the MOON cohort. Am J Sports Med. 2015;43:1583–90.
12. Kitamura G, Albers MBV, Lesniak BP, Rabuck SJ, Musahl V, Andrews CL, et al. 3-dimensional printed models may be a useful tool when planning revision anterior cruciate ligament reconstruction. Arthrosc Sports Med Rehabil. 2019;1:e41–6.
13. Miller MD. Revision cruciate ligament surgery with retention of femoral interference screws. Arthroscopy. 1998;14:111–4.
14. Mitchell JJ, Chahla J, Dean CS, Cinque M, Matheny LM, LaPrade RF. Outcomes after 1-stage versus 2-stage revision anterior cruciate ligament reconstruction. Am J Sports Med. 2017;45:1790–8.
15. Morgan JA, Dahm D, Levy B, Stuart MJ. Femoral tunnel malposition in ACL revision reconstruction. J Knee Surg. 2012;25:361–8.
16. Sarraj M, Shanmugaraj A, Musahl V, Lesniak BP. Over-the-top ACL reconstruction yields comparable outcomes to traditional ACL reconstruction in primary and revision settings: a systematic review. Knee Surg Sports Traumatol Arthrosc. 2019;27:427–44.
17. Trojani C, Sbihi A, Djian P, Potel J-F, Hulet C, Jouve F, et al. Causes for failure of ACL reconstruction and influence of meniscectomies after revision. Knee Surg Sports Traumatol Arthrosc. 2011;19:196–201.
18. Webb JM, Salmon LJ, Leclerc E, Pinczewski LA, Roe JP. Posterior tibial slope and further anterior cruciate ligament injuries in the anterior cruciate ligament–reconstructed patient. Am J Sports Med. 2013;41:2800–4.
19. Webster KE, Feller JA, Elliott J, Hutchison A, Payne R. A comparison of bone tunnel measurements made using computed tomography and digital plain radiography after anterior cruciate ligament reconstruction. Arthroscopy. 2004;20:946–50.
20. Wright RW, Dunn WR, Amendola A, Andrish JT, Flanigan DC, Jones M, et al. Anterior cruciate ligament revision reconstruction: two-year results from the MOON cohort. J Knee Surg. 2007;20:308–11.
21. Yoon KH, Kim JS, Park SY, Park SE. One-stage revision anterior cruciate ligament reconstruction: results according to preoperative bone tunnel diameter: five to fifteen-year follow-up. JBJS. 2018;100:993–1000.

Managing the Tibial Tunnel in Revision Anterior Cruciate Ligament (ACL) Reconstruction

10

Matthew J. Craig and Travis G. Maak

When evaluating preoperative imaging, tunnels should be evaluated for both appropriateness of their position and widening. When viewed on plain lateral X-ray, the tibial tunnel should be roughly parallel to the slope of the intercondylar roof, and the aperture should be just posterior to the intersection of Blumensaat's line and the tibia (Fig. 10.1) [1, 2]. The tibial aperture of the ACL should be located at 43% of the distance of the Amis and Jakob line [3–5]. A tibial tunnel placed too anteriorly may result in graft impingement in the intercondylar notch in full extension which can result in loss of extension, development of a cyclops lesion, and graft injury [6]. A tibial tunnel placed too posteriorly may impinge on the PCL and cause loss of knee flexion. This posterior position may also result in a vertical graft orientation and rotational instability with a positive pivot shift. Excessive medial or lateral placement of the tibial tunnel may result in notch impingement and damage to the chondral surfaces of the medial and lateral tibial plateaus. Excessive lateral placement of the guide pin during tibial tunnel reaming may also result in a significant decrease in the attachment area and ultimate failure strength of the lateral meniscus anterior root [7].

M. J. Craig · T. G. Maak (✉)
Department of Orthopedic Surgery – Hip and Knee Preservation, University of Utah, Salt Lake City, UT, USA

Grossly malpositioned tunnels can often allow for new independent tunnel drilling. While this is commonly performed with femoral tunnels, it is less common for the tibia, as gross tibial tunnel malposition is restricted by tibial cartilage and anterior and posterior meniscal roots. Nevertheless, a partially malpositioned tibial tunnel presents a significant challenge for a single-stage revision ACL reconstruction [8].

If the tibial tunnel is anatomically positioned with minimal tunnel widening (<100% of the original tunnel with the tunnel measuring <16–20 mm in all directions) and good bone quality, a single-stage revision can be considered [9]. In this setting, prior fixation hardware can be removed directly or with a through-reaming technique. The tunnel can then be reused. Fluoroscopic imaging can help identify the location of metal implants which can then be removed, while absorbable implants may need to be removed or reamed though to facilitate tunnel preparation and graft passage. A complete debridement of old graft material, implants, and fibrotic debris should be performed to establish a circumferential healthy bone interface to facilitate optimal graft incorporation.

If preoperative imaging demonstrates an anatomic intra-articular tibial tunnel aperture, but the tunnel is too short, a funnel technique can be considered. This technique creates a new tunnel by utilizing the original intra-articular footprint of the index reconstruction while creating a new

M. J. Alaia, K. J. Jones (eds.), *Revision Anterior Cruciate Ligament Reconstruction*,
https://doi.org/10.1007/978-3-030-96996-7_10

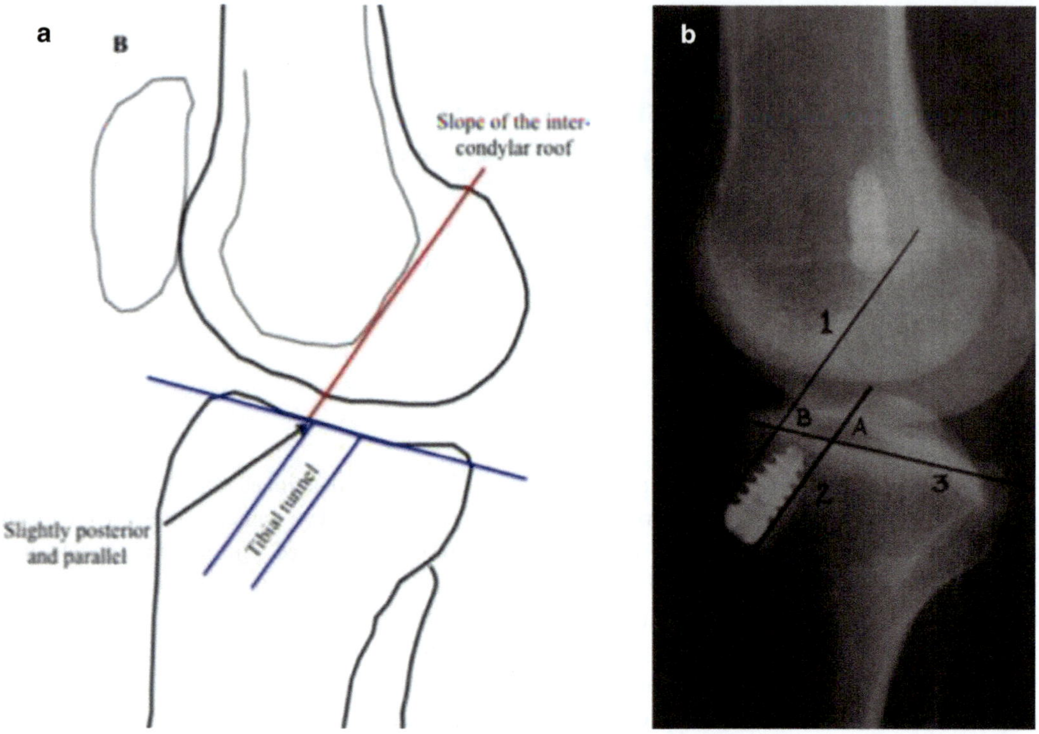

Fig. 10.1 Schematic (**a**) and plain lateral radiograph (**b**) demonstrating the optimal tibial tunnel parallel to the slope of the intercondylar roof with the aperture just posterior to the intersection of Blumensaat's line and the tibial plateau

extra-articular orientation. The tibia offers a significant amount of anteromedial bone that allows for drilling this new tunnel. The outside in technique used on the tibial side also allows for precise control when setting your new extra-articular entry point. The new extra-articular starting point on the tibia should ideally be at least 2.5 cm distal to the joint line and halfway between the tibial tubercle and posteromedial corner of the tibia [10]. However, this ideal point may be modified depending on the prior reconstruction entry point and the graft type selected for the revision reconstruction. The angle of the tibial ACL guide should be adjusted to ensure optimal graft-tunnel length matching, particularly in the setting of bone-patellar tendon-bone revision graft selection.

Technical note Tibial tunnel position and length are crucial when considering revision graft selection, as graft-tunnel mismatch is a significant concern when selecting bone-patellar tendon-bone (BTB) as a revision graft choice. While the benefits of low re-rupture rates have been well documented when revision ACL reconstruction is performed with BTB autograft, this selection affords less surgical flexibility regarding tibial tunnel length. Graft selection such as hamstring autograft or allograft in which the soft tissue component of the graft is present in the tibial tunnel provides increased flexibility for tibial tunnel length, but this flexibility must be balanced with a potentially increased risk of graft selection related re-rupture.

Once the ACL tibial guide is appropriately positioned to ensure adequate tunnel length and aperture entry, the guide pin should be introduced. Notably, when employing the funnel technique, the previous tunnel aperture is maintained, and thus the guide pin may not be adequately controlled during reaming when tunnel convergence occurs at the aperture. To prevent reamer migration, a clamp can be used to secure the pin while reaming the new tunnel.

Technical Note Tibial tunnel reaming may be achieved with a variety of different reamer types including straight and acorn reamers. It is the senior author's preference to utilize straight reamers during revision ACL reconstruction as the shaft of the straight reamer affords more stability to the reamer and minimizes asymmetric reaming that may occur with acorn reamers when they encounter convergence with the prior tibial tunnel.

Occasionally, pre-existing hardware may be encountered during reaming and can be removed at this time. Otherwise, prior hardware can often be left in place. The bone bridge created between the two tunnels may allow for aperture fixation; however, if there are concerns about fixation quality, secondary post fixation should be considered.

In situations where the tibial tunnel is positioned too anteriorly, it is often possible to drill a new tibial tunnel that is posterior to the malpositioned tunnel. If convergence of the tunnel sites occur at the aperture, it is often acceptable provided the posterior aspect of your new tunnel is located anatomically. The intra-articular trajectory of the graft ensures that the graft will position posteriorly in the tunnel and into an anatomic position.

A tibial tunnel that is located too posteriorly is more challenging. Creation of a new tunnel anterior to the malpositioned tunnel with a separate aperture may result in anterior tunnel malposition and subsequent graft impingement and failure. Utilizing the funnel technique will result in convergence of the tunnel sites at the aperture. Unlike an anteriorly malpositioned tunnel, in this case, the graft will fall posterior into the malpositioned tunnel and thus remain malpositioned. If desired, a single-stage reconstruction can be performed in this situation using structural allograft. In this setting, the index malpositioned tibial tunnel should first be identified. A complete debridement and tunnel preparation should occur. Following this, the malpositioned tunnel should be filled with structural bone graft, such as femoral head allograft dowel, with a secure press fit technique. Once bone grafting is completed, a new anatomic tibial tunnel can be drilled in an anterior, anatomic position. A new extra-articular starting point should be found, and the guide pin can be advanced to an anatomic position intra-articularly, and the new tunnel can then be created. The structural bone graft serves as a bony block, preventing the graft from falling posterior into the previously drilled malpositioned tunnel. Alternatively, a two-stage procedure with bone grafting of the tibial tunnel followed by delayed reconstruction of the ACL can be performed (Fig. 10.2).

Tibial Tunnel Widening in Revision Anterior Cruciate Ligament (ACL) Reconstruction

Multiple factors are thought to contribute to tunnel widening including mechanical factors such as improper graft placement, graft motion at the tunnel edge, and the bungee cord effect, while biological factors such as sterilization techniques, graft choice, implant material, and synovial fluid propagation have also been implicated [9, 11]. While the clinical implications of tunnel widening are not clear, enlarged tunnel management can present a significant challenge when proceeding with revision ACL surgery.

Widening may be underappreciated on X-rays. Given this, advanced imaging such as magnetic resonance imaging (MRI) or a computed tomographic (CT) scan should be considered to further evaluate multiplanar tunnel characteristics. If the MRI does not allow for sufficient assessment of tunnel positioning and widening, a supplementary CT scan should be considered, as this will provide an optimal assessment of bony anatomy, the cross sectional area of the tunnels, and the amount of sclerosis [9, 12, 13].

Tunnel widening may also influence the graft choices in revision ACL reconstruction. Tunnel widening and poor bone stock can make it difficult to achieve the fit and fill fixation that hamstring autograft and allografts require for optimal healing. However, soft tissue only graft options should be used cautiously in this case as they

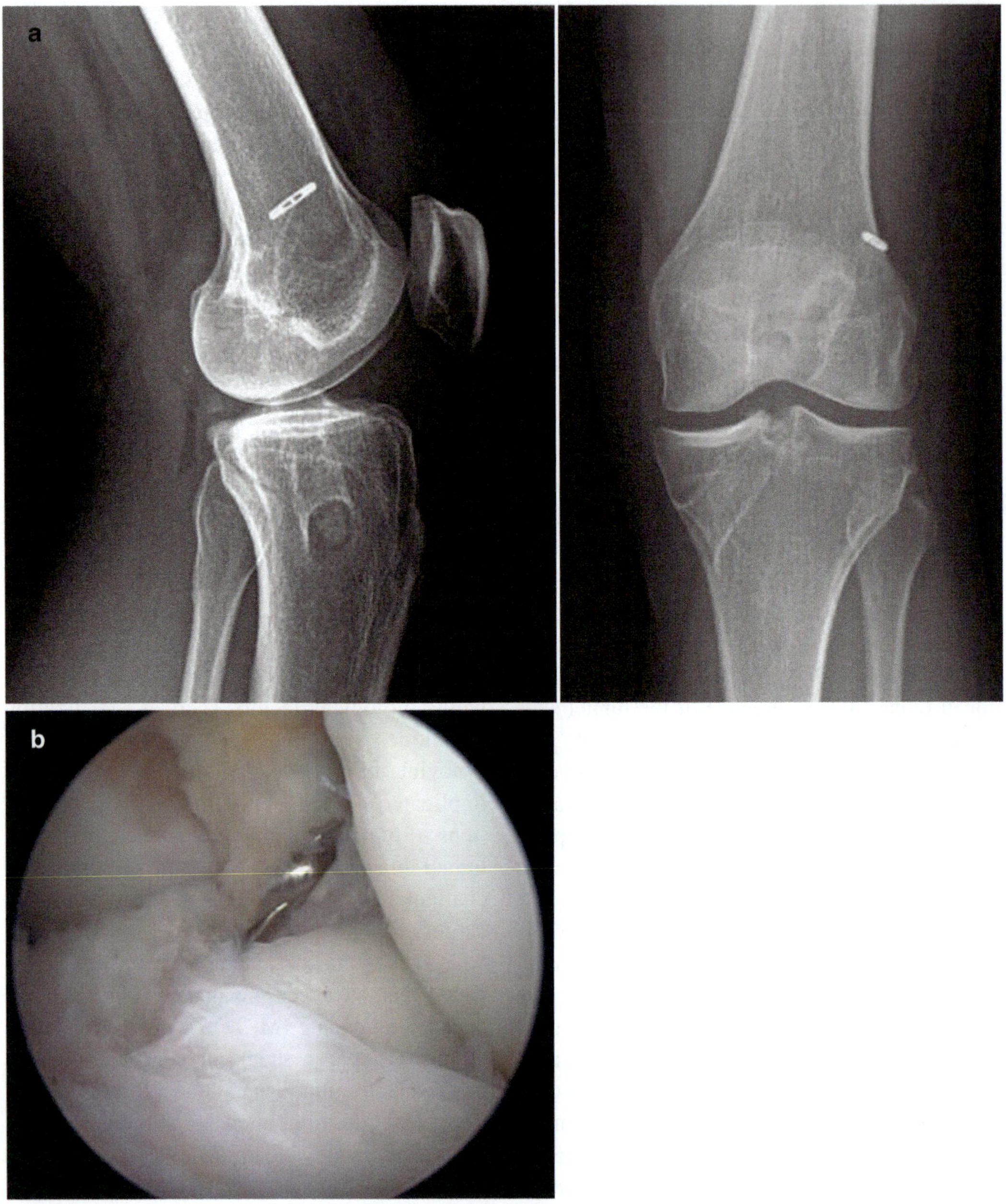

Fig. 10.2 Anteroposterior and lateral plain radiographs (**a**) demonstrating a two-stage ACL reconstruction due to tunnel widening and posterior tibial tunnel position. Bone grafting of both femoral and tibial tunnels was performed followed by revision with BTB Autograft. Arthroscopic image (**b**) demonstrates an intra-articular aperture of the original tunnel in a far posterior position

have been associated with increased tunnel widening in some studies [9]. As an alternative, a bone-patellar tendon-bone (BTB) autograft (ipsilateral or contralateral), Achilles tendon allograft, or BTB allograft could be considered. Revision surgery with autograft has been demonstrated to have a lower re-rupture rate and should be considered whenever possible [14–16].

The clinical scenario of mild tunnel widening (<100% of tunnel width or under 10–15 mm in all planes) and an anatomic tunnel can often be managed with a large graft and/or suspensory fixation. If using a hamstring autograft, supplementation with allograft can be considered to help increase the size of the graft and allow for a better fill of the widened tunnel. Hybrid grafts like this have been shown to have a lower re-rupture rate, 3.8%, than soft tissue allografts, 5.4% (in a primary ACL setting) [17]. In this scenario, aperture fixation should ideally be performed with metal implants, as bioabsorbable implants have been associated with tunnel widening. However, if there is a concern about the quality of aperture fixation, a suspensory method of fixation can be used. While Achilles allografts have been well described in the management of widened femoral tunnels, they also offer an advantage when managing tibial tunnel widening given the large diameter of the tendinous portion of the graft and the ability to select a larger allograft size when necessary.

Multiple strategies have been described for the management of the mildly widened anatomic tunnel on the femoral side. The principles of these strategies can also be employed on the tibial side, especially in scenarios where there are concerns about bone quality. The stacking interference screw technique involves removing the primary interference screw and drilling a new tunnel. Following this, the surgeon can then insert two interference screws into the widened tunnel to obtain appropriate fixation. Another alternative in this scenario is matchstick bone grafting which requires stacking of cortical allograft "matchsticks" in a widened tunnel prior to graft placement. A third option, and one frequently employed by the senior author, includes the jumbo plug technique, in which a large structural allograft dowel is utilized to fill the prior tibial tunnel followed by new tunnel creation. This is followed by passage of the graft and interference screw placement. However, if there are any concerns about graft fixation using these techniques, a two-stage technique should be used as a poorly performed single-stage technique will have an increased failure rate.

Anteriorly malpositioned tunnel placement with or without expansion can often be managed with a single-stage technique with divergent drilling, a large graft, and/or suspensory tibial fixation (Fig. 10.3). A posteriorly malpositioned tibial tunnel with significant widening is most often optimally addressed with bone tunnel grafting and staged reconstruction. In this scenario, the first stage involves removal of implants and debridement of the old graft and any fibrotic material within the tunnels. Multiple techniques for bone grafting have been described using morselized autograft iliac crest, allograft bone chips, allograft bone matrix, and demineralized bone matrix. Structural bone grafting is another alternative that can be performed with the use of dowels from a femoral head allograft. The prior tunnels are sequentially reamed and debrided until good bleeding bone is seen, and the bone graft is then placed into the tunnels. The second stage of the procedure can occur 3–4 months after the first provided X-rays show good incorporation of the bone.

Graft-Tunnel Mismatch with Revision Autograft BTB

In the revision ACL setting, allografts have been shown to have a higher re-rupture rate than autografts [14]. Autograft BTB has been shown in some studies to have the lowest re-rupture rate in the primary and revision setting and is the ideal graft choice when planning a revision ACL to minimize the risk of re-rupture [18–21].

When using a BTB graft, graft-tunnel mismatch is an important issue that must be considered. Graft-tunnel mismatch may occur when in settings of patella alta or short tunnels due to a fixed BTB graft length. The transition to using a more anatomic femoral side tunnel has also resulted in shorter femoral tunnels compared to a transtibial technique which may also contribute to the mismatch problem [22]. This mismatch results in a prominent tibial bone plug that can compromise interference screw fixation, while a graft that is too short results in blind placement of the tibial interference screw which can result in

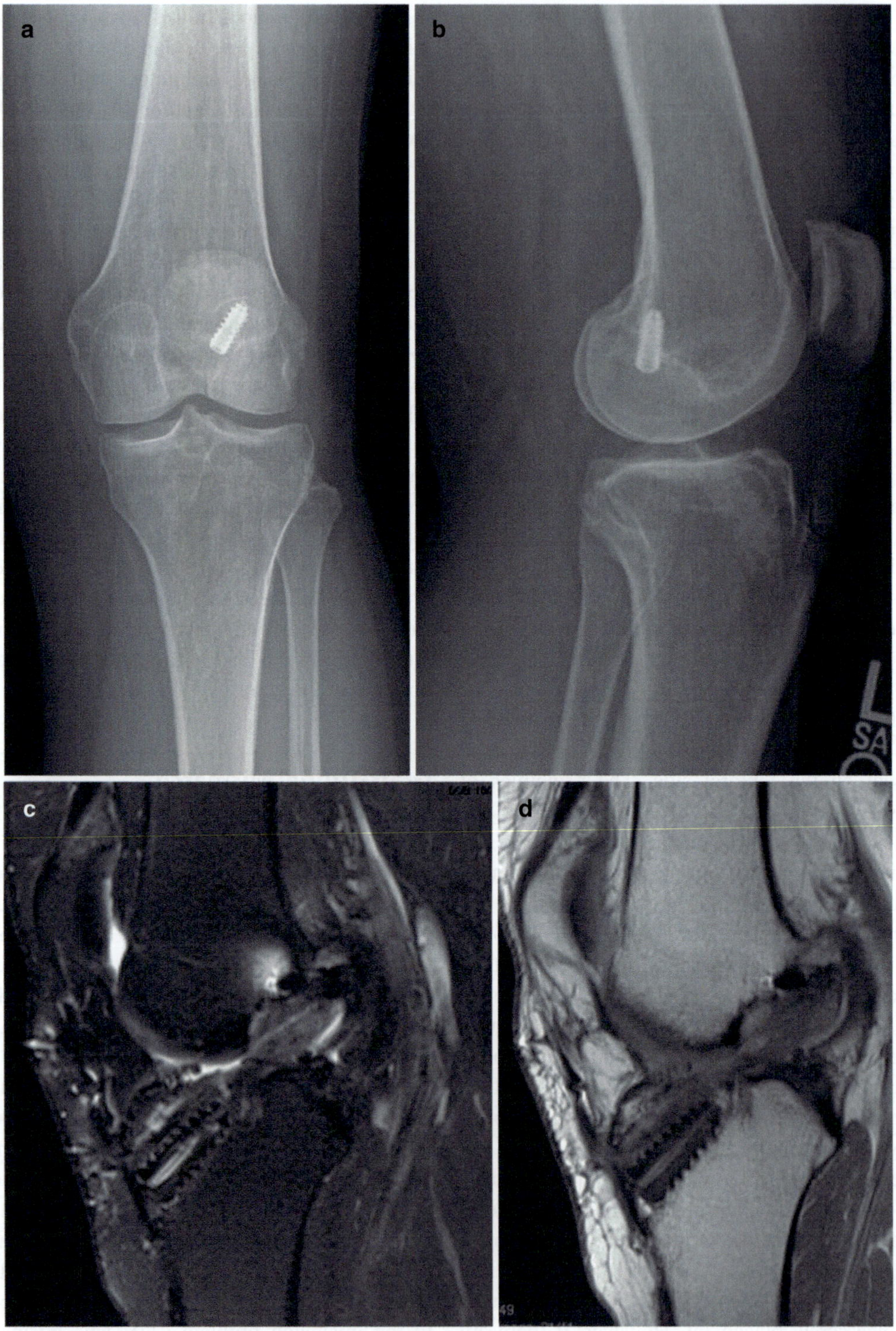

Fig. 10.3 Anteroposterior and lateral plain radiographs (**a**, **b**) and sagittal plane T2 and T1 magnetic resonance images (**c**, **d**) demonstrate an ACL graft rupture with tunnel positions that allowed a single-stage revision ACL. The index tibial tunnel is positioned anterior but can be modified with single-stage bone grafting and convergent reaming into a more anatomic position. The femoral hardware may be removed, and a divergent tunnel technique was employed to create an anatomic femoral tunnel. Anteroposterior and lateral postoperative plain radiographs demonstrate revision of an allograft ACL rupture with hamstring autograft using interference screw and backup post tibial fixation given the convergent tibial tunnel technique (**e**, **f**)

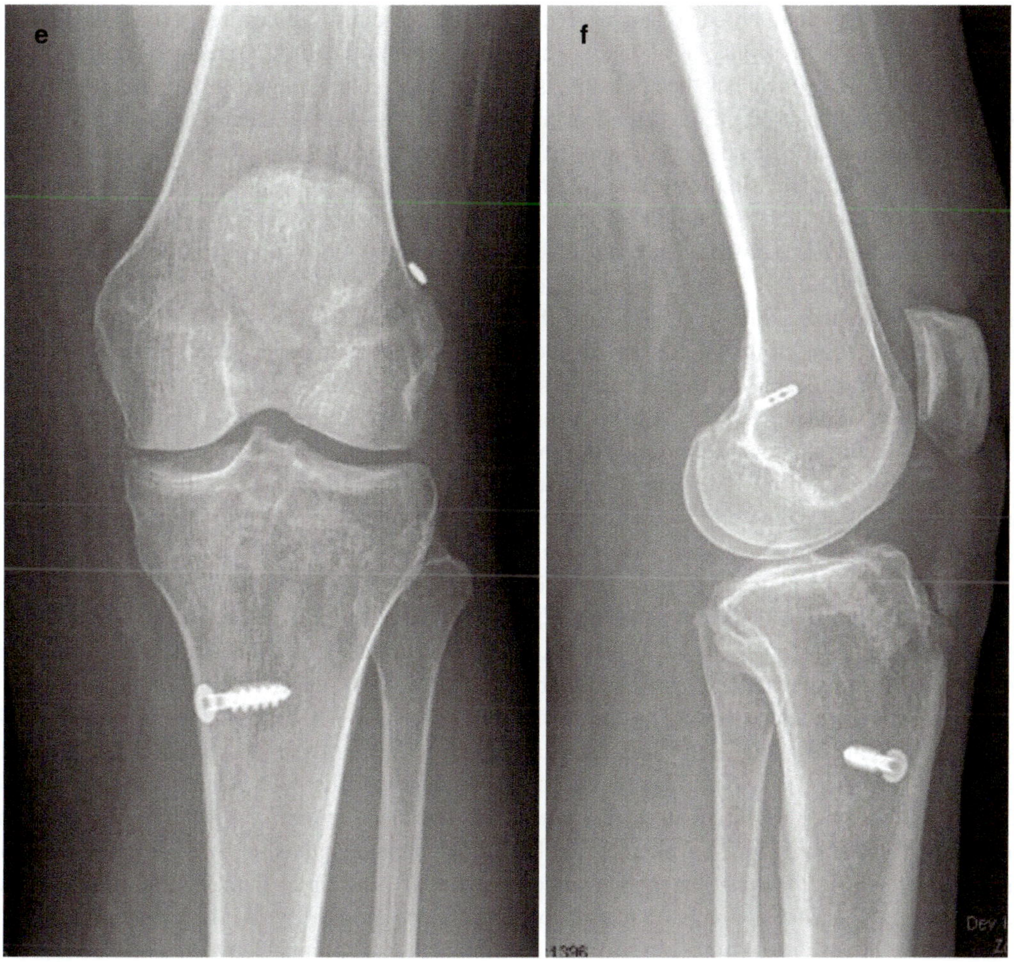

Fig. 10.3 (continued)

screw divergence, graft laceration, or intra-articular penetration. Soft tissue grafts, such as hamstrings, quad tendon, and Achilles allograft, are not susceptible to this problem as they are not fixed length grafts and can be shortened to the desired length.

The issue of graft-tunnel mismatch is further complicated in the revision setting as the tibial tunnel that is placed during the index ACL must be adequate in length and position to support a BTB graft. The length of the tunnel has already been set, and there is less flexibility so more careful preoperative and intraoperative planning is essential. Preoperatively, a careful examination of imaging should evaluate the position and length of the tibial tunnel. It is also important to use the Insall-Salvati and Blackburne-Peel methods and evaluate for patella alta and baja. Patella alta may result in a longer graft, while patella baja may result in a shorter graft that may have inadequate intra-articular length. The preoperative MRI can also be used to measure the length of the central third of the patella tendon. If the patient has significant patella baja, an alternative graft may need to be considered.

While imaging may give you an approximate length, it is critical to re-evaluate the length of the tunnel and patella tendon graft intraoperatively before proceeding with any graft harvest. If considering using an BTB allograft, a positive correlation between height and intra-articular length of the graft has been seen, so matching the allograft to the patient's height and sex may help decrease the risk of graft-tunnel mismatch [23, 24]. If the existing tibia tunnel appears to be inadequate to support a BTB graft, a two-stage revision with bone grafting is required if a BTB graft is the graft of choice. Alternatively, a soft tissue graft can be used.

The length of the BTB graft is composed of the femoral bone plug, tibial bone plug, and the patellar tendon connecting soft tissue component. The femoral bone plug should ideally sit flush with the femoral tunnel aperture when using interference screw fixation. Recessing the graft up to 15 mm has shown no significant differences in KT-1000 measurements at 12 months, while others have shown in a cadaveric model that 10 mm of recession may lead to impingement of the graft, graft abrasion, and eventual failure [25, 26]. Therefore, the length of the tibial bone plug and soft tissue component of the graft should be equal to the intra-articular length of the graft and the length of the tibial tunnel. The intra-articular distance of the graft is approximately 30 mm [27–29]. When trying to anticipate graft-tunnel mismatch, the following pre-op planning technique is useful [30]. If the patella tendon component of the graft measures 45 mm, 15 mm of soft tissue will be in your tibial tunnel in addition to the tibial bone plug. A 20–25-mm interference screw should be used on the tibial side to obtain adequate interference fixation [30]. Using a patella tendon length of 45 mm, if we use a 25-mm femoral bone plug with 30 mm of intra-articular soft tissue graft, we need a tibial tunnel length of at least 40–15 mm of residual patella tendon graft +25 mm of tibial bone plug for an interference fit [30].

However, it is important to remember that in the revision setting, the length of the graft will be unique to the individual and you will not have the ability to alter the tibial tunnel length. A careful preoperative estimate of the patella tendon length should be performed, and the above formula can then be used to estimate the length of the needed tibial tunnel which can then be compared to the patient's tunnel. This process should be repeated intraoperatively before the graft is harvested. The senior author recommends identifying the tibial tunnel, placing a guidewire up the tunnel until it is flush with the intra-articular surface, and measuring the actual length of the tibial tunnel. The length of the patella tendon graft should then be measured, and an appropriate fit should be confirmed prior to harvest.

If proceeding with a two-stage ACL revision, there will be more control over the length of the tibial tunnel as you will be drilling a new, independent tunnel. In this setting, there are strategies that have been described for a primary ACL that may help avoid graft-tunnel mismatch. The "graft – 50" formula described by Kenna estimates the tibial tunnel length by measuring the total graft length and subtracting 50 mm (20 mm femoral bone plug +30 mm intra-articular graft) to give the ideal tibial tunnel length [31]. Another popular method is the "N+" class. The N+ 7 formula describes adding 7 to the length of the soft tissue component of the graft to determine the angle of tibial tunnel drilling, while others have proposed a N + 10 formula for tibial tunnel guide angle [32, 33]. The N + 2 formula adds 2 mm to the length of the patella tendon to estimate the tibial tunnel length [34]. Intraoperatively, the tibial tunnel length is set by the tibial ACL guide. Generally, the tibial tunnel guide should be set between 45° and 65°. With each added degree of inclination, the tunnel lengthens by 0.68 mm [30, 35]. On average, setting the tibial tunnel guide to 55° results in a tunnel length of approximately 45–50 mm [35, 36]. At angles lower than 45°, there is a significant risk of having too short a tunnel with bone block protrusion. Angles greater than 65° may result in posterior tibial tunnel placement and failure [37].

The decision to use a BTB graft for the revision ACL results in significantly less flexibility in accepting varied tunnel and socket lengths. If preoperative or intraoperative assessment of graft and tunnel length suggests the potential for a significant graft tendon mismatch, it may be more optimal to proceed with a two-stage revision than risk poor graft placement and fixation. Another alternative is to change your graft choice to a soft tissue graft as this offers more flexibility with graft and tunnel length.

Intraoperatively, if you find yourself encountering graft-tunnel mismatch, the following strategies are options to help navigate this problem. A deeper femoral socket can be drilled and fixed, or adjustable loop suspensory fixation on the femoral side can be used. Biomechanical data has shown similar tensile strength and failure load, while clinical data has shown good outcomes with suspensory fixation with BTB grafts [38–42]. Another strategy in this setting is to proceed with two incisions outside in fixation on the femoral side using aperture fixation or post fixation. If considering an extra-articular tenodesis, such as a Lemaire, it's important to consider that a two-incision technique may also compromise the starting point or fixation for the tenodesis.

If the tibial bone plug is larger than the femoral bone plug by an amount greater or equal to the amount of prominent tibial plug distally, and the intra-articular portion of the graft is equal to the soft tissue component, the orientation of the plugs can be reversed [30]. An additional method to consider is rotation of the graft. Rotation between 540° and 630° has been shown to decrease graft length by 10–25%, but there is concern this may increase graft strain and lead to eventual failure [43–45]. Trimming the remaining tibial bone block and using a shorter interference screw is another alternative. Fixation strength of an interference screw can be preserved as long as there is at least 10 mm of bone in the tunnel.

If there is a more significant mismatch >12 mm, the free bone block transfer technique can be considered. The tibial bone plug is removed from the graft and slid proximally. A running locking stitch is then placed in the distal graft to pull tension while an interference screw is placed. Another alternative, the screw and post, is to use the same construct, but distal fixation is achieved via a screw and washer. Finally, a trough technique can also be considered. The bone plug is left in place and a distal osseous trough is created. Staples are then used to fix the plug into the trough.

If preoperative evaluation of the MRI suggests a patella tendon length greater than 60 mm, a single tibial plug technique can be considered. A tibial bone plug of 20–25 mm is harvested from the tibia, while on the patella, the tendon is removed from the inferior pole with a 10–15-mm periosteal strip. Aperture interference screw fixation is achieved on the femoral side, while a soft tissue screw is used for fixation on the tibial side. This fixation can be backed up with an anchor or screw and washer [46]. Care must be taken to appropriately evaluate the length of the patella tendon as there is a risk of having too short of a graft with a tendon length <60 mm.

While less common, there are occasions where the graft may be too short. In these situations, a nonmetallic screw can be used and inserted deeper. However, there is a risk of divergent screw placement or injury to the graft with this technique. An alternative is to use post fixation on the tibial side.

Tibial tunnel management in revision ACL frequently presents unique challenges. For tunnels with anatomic apertures with short or long lengths, funnel drilling techniques can be employed with good success. Anteriorly placed tunnels can often be managed with a new, more posteriorly directed tunnel, while posteriorly placed tunnels represent a greater challenge that may require single- or two-stage revision with bone graft. Slightly widened tunnels that are anatomic can often be managed with a larger graft, while malpositioned tunnels may need a two-stage procedure. When using a BTB graft, the existing tibial tunnel must be adequate in length to accept a graft, otherwise a two-stage procedure or alternative graft choice is recommended.

Example Cases

Case #1

A 31-year-old female soccer player presented to clinic with right knee pain, instability, and an effusion after a soccer injury. She had a history of a right knee ACL reconstruction done 14 years prior to her recent injury. Her physical exam demonstrated a 1+ effusion, range of motion −5/0/100, a 2B Lachman, 1+ anterior drawer, 1+ pivot shift, negative posterior drawer, and negative posterior sag. Initial X-rays demonstrated an anteriorly placed femoral tunnel and a posteriorly positioned tibial tunnel (Fig. 10.4a, b). Slight widening of the tibial tunnel and the posterior position are demonstrated on the CT scan (Fig. 10.5). Given the position of the tibial tun-

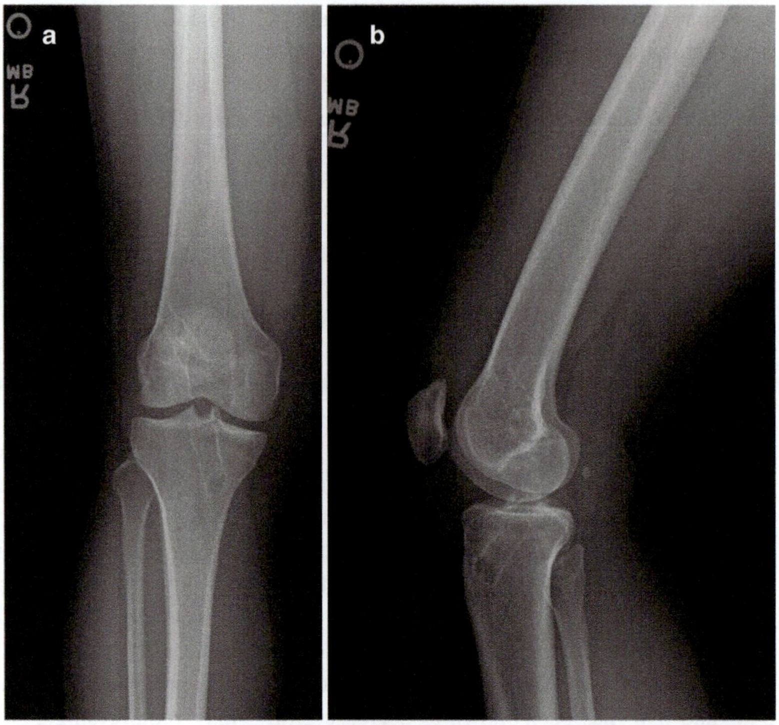

Fig. 10.4 Anteroposterior and lateral plain radiographs (**a**, **b**) demonstrate ACL graft rupture with significant posterior tibial tunnel positioning and vertical femoral tunnel position

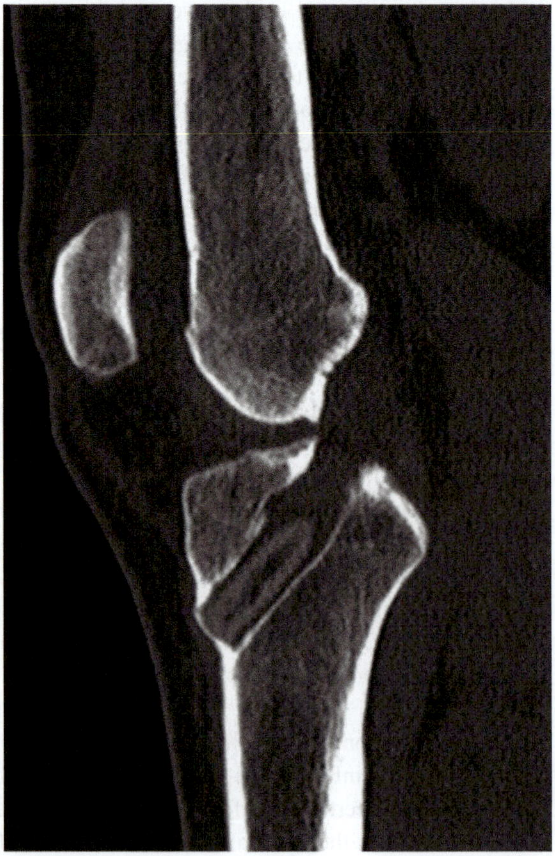

Fig. 10.5 Sagittal computed tomographic scan demonstrates the significant posterior tibial tunnel position of the ACL almost to the level of the PCL insertion with anterior tibial subluxation

nel, a single-stage bone grafting with femoral head allograft was performed for the tibial tunnel followed by funnel technique drilling of a new tibial tunnel, a new anatomic femoral tunnel was drilled with a divergent technique, and an Achilles allograft was selected due to tunnel widening. Postoperative X-rays are seen in Fig. 10.6a, b.

Case #2

A 20-year-old female soccer player presented to clinic with continued right knee pain, instability, and decreased motion after an ACL reconstruction performed using hamstring autograft supplemented with allograft 2 years ago. Her physical exam demonstrated no effusion, ROM 5/0/145, a

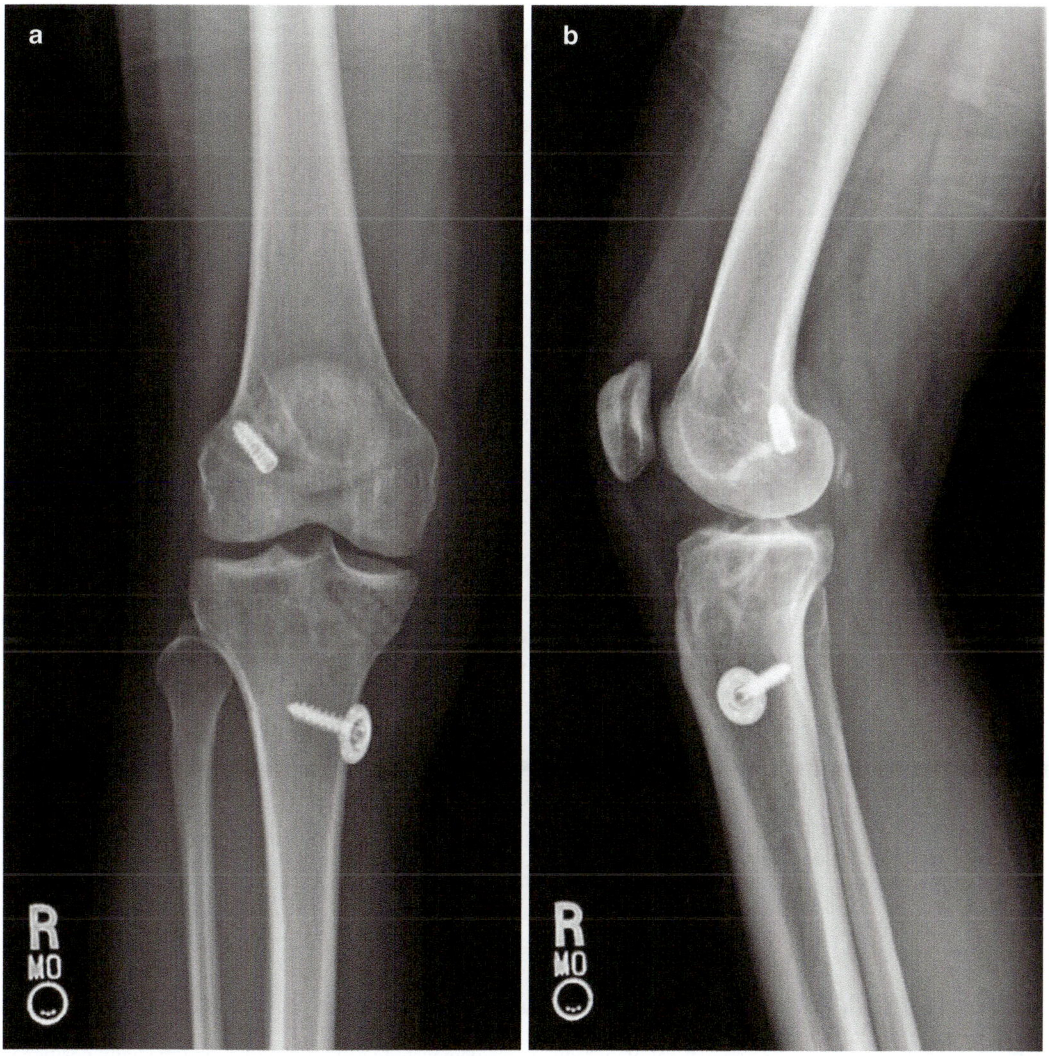

Fig. 10.6 (**a**, **b**) Anteroposterior and lateral postoperative plain radiographs demonstrate a single-stage tibial and femoral tunnel bone grafting followed by convergent tibial tunnel and divergent femoral tunnel reaming technique. Notably, in this case a concomitant MCL reconstruction was performed using interference femoral fixation and spiked soft tissue washer tibial fixation. Aperture fixation was utilized in isolation for the ACL revision reconstruction

2A Lachman, 2+ pivot shift, negative posterior drawer, and negative posterior sag. Initial X-rays demonstrated a short, anterior, and medially positioned tibial tunnel and a slightly vertical anteriorly placed femoral tunnel (Fig. 10.7a, b). Intraoperatively, the tibial tunnel was found to involve the anteromedial aspect of the tibial plateau (Fig. 10.8a), while the femoral tunnel was anteriorly placed, and the decision was made to proceed with a two-stage ACL revision. Extensive debridement of the prior tunnels was performed, and femoral head allograft dowels were used for bone grafting (Fig. 10.8b). Four months later, a second-stage revision was performed with BTB autograft. A significant amount of fibrocartilage fill was seen at the site of the grafted tibial tunnel (Fig. 10.9). Postoperative X-rays are seen in Fig. 10.10.

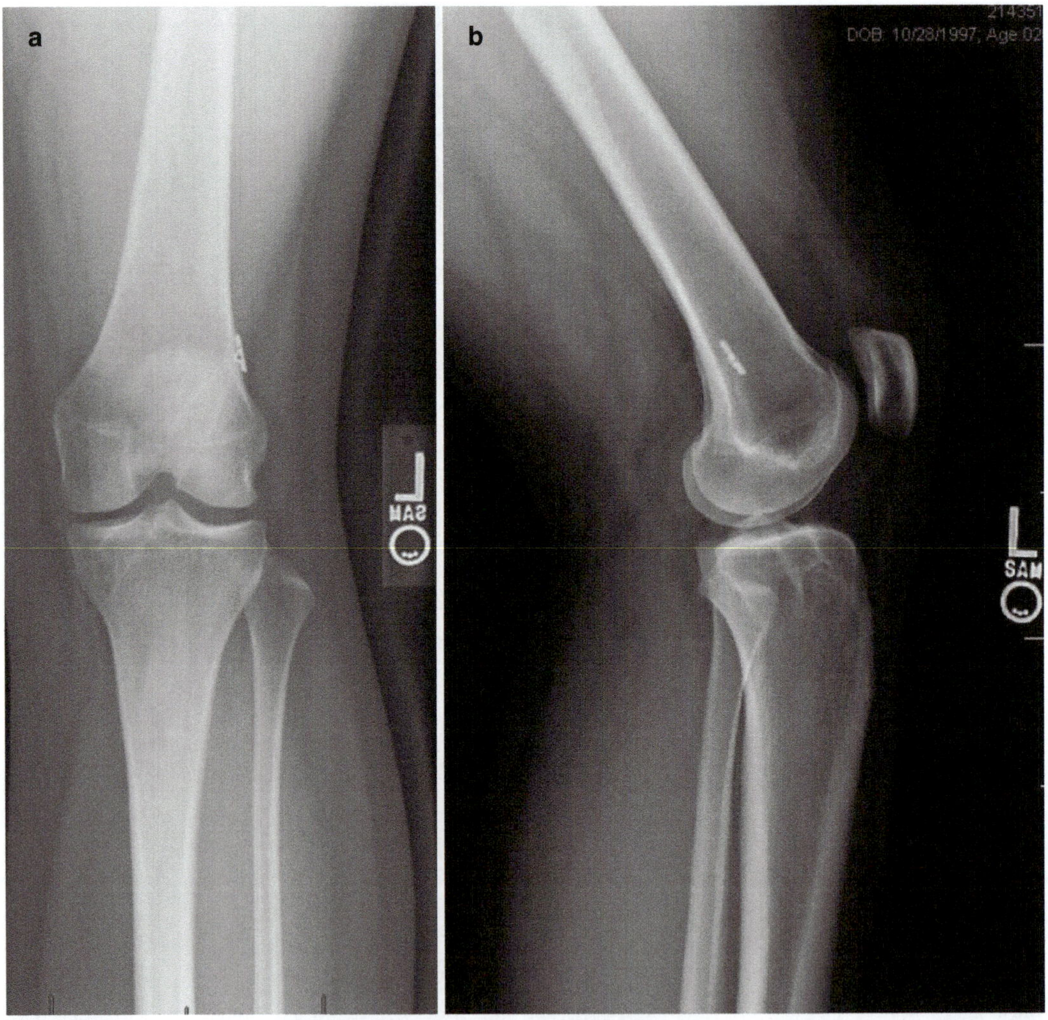

Fig. 10.7 (**a**, **b**) Anteroposterior and lateral plain radiographs demonstrate a short, anterior, and medially positioned tibial tunnel

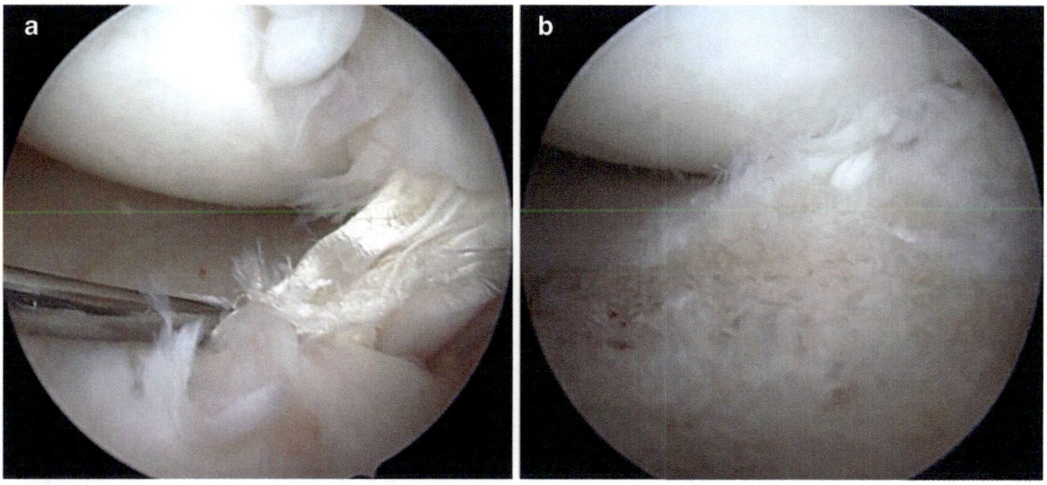

Fig. 10.8 (**a**, **b**) Arthroscopic images demonstrate a tibial tunnel aperture positioned through the anteromedial tibial plateau articular cartilage medial to the medial tibial spine (**a**). Bone grafting of the tibial tunnel with femoral head allograft dowels was utilized (**b**)

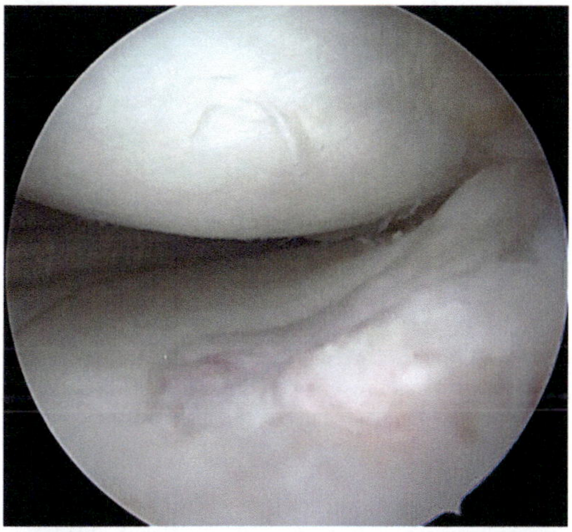

Fig. 10.9 Arthroscopic image obtained 5 months post bone grafting at the time of staged revision ACL reconstruction demonstrates excellent fibrocartilaginous fill of the medial tibial plateau at the location of the prior tibial tunnel aperture

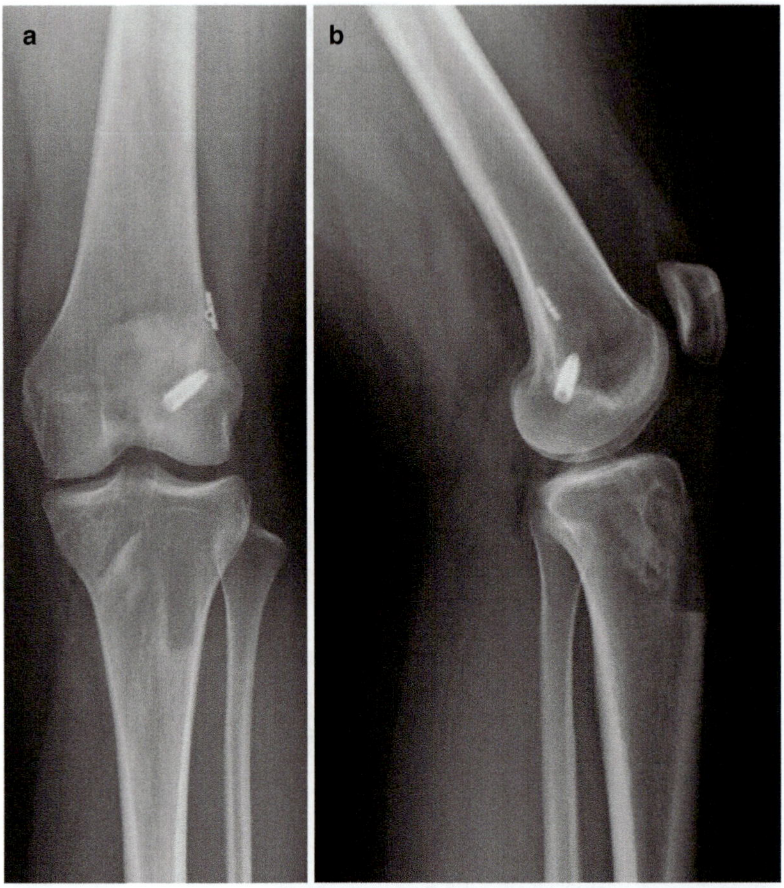

Fig. 10.10 (**a**, **b**) Anteroposterior and lateral postoperative plain radiographs obtained following revision ACL reconstruction with bone-patella tendon-bone autograft demonstrate an anatomic tibial tunnel positioned posterior and lateral to the index tunnel with anatomic femoral tunnel position. Metal interference screw fixation was utilized in the femoral tunnel with biocomposite interference screw fixation in the tibial tunnel

References

1. Morgan CD, Kalman VR, Grawl DM. Definitive landmarks for reproducible tibial tunnel placement in anterior cruciate ligament reconstruction. Arthroscopy. 1995;11(3):275–88.
2. Kirwan G, Bourke MG, Chipchase L, Dalton PA, Russell TG. Graft tensioning practices in anterior cruciate ligament reconstruction amongst orthopaedic surgeons in Australia: a national survey. Arch Orthop Trauma Surg. 2015;135(12):1733–41.
3. Howell SM, Clark JA, Farley TE. Serial magnetic resonance study assessing the effects of impingement on the MR image of the patellar tendon graft. Arthroscopy. 1992.
4. Howell SM, Wallace MP, Hull ML, Deutsch ML. Evaluation of the single-incision arthroscopic technique for anterior cruciate ligament replacement. Am J Sports Med. 1999.
5. Sullivan JP, Cook S, Gao Y, Wolf BR. Radiographic anatomy of the native anterior cruciate ligament: a systematic review. HSS J. 2015.
6. Howell SM, Hull ML. Checkpoints for judging tunnel and anterior cruciate ligament graft placement. J Knee Surg. 2009.
7. Laprade CM, Smith SD, Rasmussen MT, Hamming MG, Wijdicks CA, Engebretsen L, et al. Consequences of tibial tunnel reaming on the meniscal roots during cruciate ligament reconstruction in a cadaveric model, part 1: the anterior cruciate ligament. Am J Sports Med. 2015.
8. Wilde J, Bedi A, Altchek DW. Revision anterior cruciate ligament reconstruction. Sports Health. 2014.
9. Maak TG, Voos JE, Wickiewicz TL, Warren RE. Tunnel widening in revision anterior cruciate ligament reconstruction. J Am Acad Orthop Surg. 2010.
10. Gomoll AH, Bach BR. Managing tunnel malposition and widening in revision anterior cruciate ligament surgery. Oper Tech Sports Med. 2006.
11. Demyttenaere J, Claes S, Bellemans J. One-stage revision anterior cruciate ligament reconstruction in cases with excessive tunnel osteolysis. Results of a new technique using impaction bone grafting. Knee. 2018.
12. Getelman MH, Friedman MJ. Revision anterior cruciate ligament reconstruction surgery. J Am Acad Orthop Surg. 1999.
13. Iorio R, Vadalà A, Argento G, Di Sanzo V, Ferretti A. Bone tunnel enlargement after ACL reconstruction using autologous hamstring tendons: a CT study. Int Orthop. 2007.

14. Wright RW. Effect of graft choice on the outcome of revision anterior cruciate ligament reconstruction in the multicenter ACL revision study (MARS) cohort. Am J Sports Med. 2014.
15. Nissen KA, Eysturoy NH, Nielsen TG, Lind M. Allograft use results in higher re-revision rate for revision anterior cruciate ligament reconstruction. Orthop J Sports Med. 2018.
16. Tejwani SG, Chen J, Funahashi TT, Love R, Maletis GB. Revision risk after allograft anterior cruciate ligament reconstruction. Am J Sports Med. 2015.
17. Mirzayan R, Prentice HA, Essilfie A, Burfeind WE, Ding DY, Maletis GB. Revision risk of soft tissue allograft versus hybrid graft after anterior cruciate ligament reconstruction. Am J Sports Med. 2020.
18. Kaeding CC, Spindler KP, Huston LJ, Zajichek A. ACL reconstruction in high school and college-aged athletes: does autograft choice affect recurrent ACL revision rates? Orthop J Sports Med. 2019.
19. Erickson BJ, Cvetanovich GL, Frank RM, Riff AJ, Bach BR. Revision ACL reconstruction: a critical analysis review. JBJS Rev. 2017.
20. Reinhardt KR, Hetsroni I, Marx RG. Graft selection for anterior cruciate ligament reconstruction: a level I systematic review comparing failure rates and functional outcomes. Orthop Clin N Am. 2010.
21. Persson A, Fjeldsgaard K, Gjertsen JE, Kjellsen AB, Engebretsen L, Hole RM, et al. Increased risk of revision with hamstring tendon grafts compared with patellar tendon grafts after anterior cruciate ligament reconstruction: a study of 12,643 patients from the Norwegian Cruciate Ligament Registry, 2004-2012. Am J Sports Med. 2014.
22. Hensler D, Working ZM, Illingworth KD, Tashman S, Fu FH. Correlation between femoral tunnel length and tunnel position in ACL reconstruction. J Bone Joint Surg Am. 2013.
23. Goldstein JL, Verma N, McNickle AG, Zelazny A, Ghodadra N, Bach BR. Avoiding mismatch in allograft anterior cruciate ligament reconstruction: correlation between patient height and patellar tendon length. Arthroscopy. 2010.
24. Brown JA, Brophy RH, Franco J, Marquand A, Solomon TC, Watanabe D, et al. Avoiding allograft length mismatch during anterior cruciate ligament reconstruction: patient height as an indicator of appropriate graft length. Am J Sports Med. 2007.
25. Shah AA, Heckman MM, Gilley JS. Recessed femoral interference screws in anterior cruciate ligament reconstruction. Am J Orthop (Belle Mead NJ). 2009.
26. Taylor DE, Dervin GF, Keene GCR. Femoral bone plug recession in endoscopic anterior cruciate ligament reconstruction. Arthroscopy. 1996.
27. Duthon VB, Barea C, Abrassart S, Fasel JH, Fritschy D, Ménétrey J. Anatomy of the anterior cruciate ligament. Knee Surg Sports Traumatol Arthrosc. 2006.
28. Amis AA, Dawkins GPC. Functional anatomy of the anterior cruciate ligament. Fibre bundle actions related to ligament replacements and injuries. J Bone Joint Surg Br. 1991.
29. Miller MD, Olszewski AD. Cruciate ligament graft intra-articular distances. Arthroscopy. 1997.
30. Yanke A, Ellman MB, Sherman SL, Bach BR. Graft-tunnel mismatch in bone-tendon-bone ACL reconstruction: prevention and treatment. Tech Orthop. 2012.
31. Kenna B, Simon TM, Jackson DW, Kurzweil PR. Endoscopic ACL reconstruction: a technical note on tunnel length for interference fixation. Arthroscopy. 1993.
32. Verma NN, Dennis MG, Carreira DS, Bojchuk J, Hayden JK, Bach BR. Preliminary clinical results of two techniques for addressing graft tunnel mismatch in endoscopic anterior cruciate ligament reconstruction. J Knee Surg. 2005.
33. Miller MD, Hinkin DT. The "N + 7 rule" for tibial tunnel placement in endoscopic anterior cruciate ligament reconstruction. Arthroscopy. 1996.
34. Olszewski AD, Miller MD, Ritchie JR. Ideal tibial tunnel length for endoscopic anterior cruciate ligament reconstruction. Arthroscopy. 1998.
35. Denti M, Bigoni M, Randelli P, Monteleone M, Cevenini A, Ghezzi A, et al. Graft-tunnel mismatch in endoscopic anterior cruciate ligament reconstruction: intraoperative and cadaver measurement of the intra-articular graft length and the length of the patellar tendon. Knee Surg Sports Traumatol Arthrosc. 1998.
36. Wallace M, Bedi A, Lesniak BP, Farrow LD, Ajibade D, Israel HA, et al. What effect does anterior cruciate ligament tibial guide orientation have on tibial tunnel length? Arthroscopy. 2011.
37. Inderhaug E, Raknes S, Østvold T, Solheim E, Strand T. Increased revision rate with posterior tibial tunnel placement after using the 70-degree tibial guide in ACL reconstruction. Knee Surg Sports Traumatol Arthrosc. 2017.
38. Smith PA, Stannard JP, Pfeiffer FM, Kuroki K, Bozynski CC, Cook JL. Suspensory versus interference screw fixation for arthroscopic anterior cruciate ligament reconstruction in a translational large-animal model. Arthroscopy. 2016.
39. Chen W, Li H, Chen Y, Jiang F, Wu Y, Chen S. Bone–patellar tendon–bone autografts versus hamstring autografts using the same suspensory fixations in ACL reconstruction: a systematic review and meta-analysis. Orthop J Sports Med. 2019.
40. Mirzatolooei F, Tabrizi A, Bagheri F, Mokaram Gargari MS. Bone-patellar tendon-bone graft preparation for fixation with suspensory method in anterior cruciate reconstruction: a biomechanical study. Asian J Sports Med. 2018.
41. Mickelson DT, Lefebvre T, Gall K, Riboh JC. Adjustable-loop femoral cortical suspensory fixation for patellar tendon anterior cruciate ligament reconstruction: a time zero biomechanical comparison with interference screw fixation. Am J Sports Med. 2018.
42. Kusano M, Kazui A, Uchida R, Mae T, Tsuda T, Toritsuka Y. Loop length change of an adjustable-

length femoral cortical suspension device in anatomic rectangular tunnel anterior cruciate ligament reconstruction with a bone–patellar tendon–bone graft and associated clinical outcomes. Arthroscopy. 2018.

43. Augé WK, Yifan K. A technique for resolution of graft-tunnel length mismatch in central third bone-patellar tendon-bone anterior cruciate ligament reconstruction. Arthroscopy. 1999.
44. Verma N, Noerdlinger MA, Hallab N, Bush-Joseph CA, Bach BR. Effects of graft rotation on initial biomechanical failure characteristics of bone-patellar tendon-bone constructs. Am J Sports Med. 2003.
45. Oliveira DRO de, Garcia ET, Fuso FAF, Pereira CAM, Lages MM, Almeida AM de, et al. The biomechanical effects of graft rotation on ACL reconstruction tunnel mismatch. Knee Surg Sports Traumatol Arthrosc. 2017.
46. Grawe B, Smerina A, Allen A. Avoiding graft-tunnel length mismatch in anterior cruciate ligament reconstruction: the single-bone plug technique. Arthrosc Tech. 2014.

Management of Medial-Sided Ligamentous Laxity and Posteromedial Corner

11

Robert S. Dean, Jorge Chahla, Nicholas N. DePhillipo, Jill K. Monson, and Robert F. LaPrade

Anatomy and Function

Medial collateral ligament (MCL) knee injuries are closely linked to participation in sports such as soccer, American football, ice hockey, and skiing. Because participation in these activities continues to increase, the incidence of MCL injuries continues to grow [1, 2]. In order to understand injuries to the medial aspect and posteromedial corner (PMC) of the knee, it is important to appreciate the local anatomy.

The medial and PMC primarily act to prevent valgus motion of the knee. The PMC extends from the medial aspect of the patellar tendon to the medial border of the gastrocnemius tendon. It has five major structures, the superficial MCL (sMCL), deep MCL (dMCL), posterior oblique ligament (POL), oblique popliteal ligament (OPL), and posterior horn of the medial meniscus (PHMM) [3]. Additionally, the semimembranosus and its respective expansions provide dynamic stability to the PMC. The bony anatomy of the medial aspect of the knee is formed by the medial femoral condyle and the medial tibial plateau, which articulate in a convex on concave fashion (Fig. 11.1). This inherently stable articulation helps facilitate healing of the MCL concurrent with its dense vascularization [3].

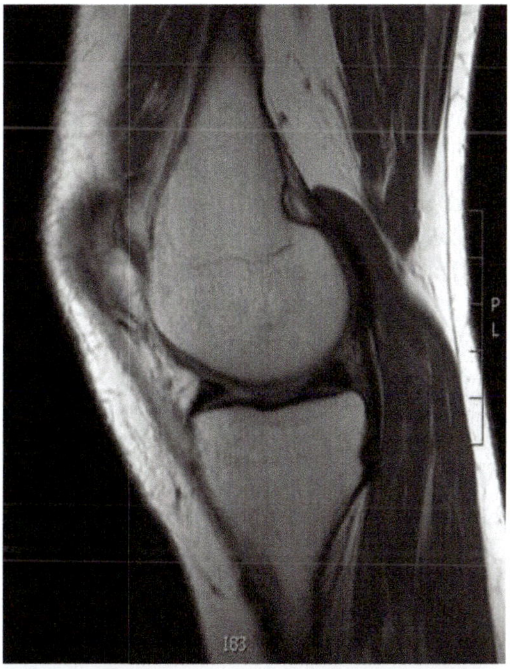

Fig. 11.1 Sagittal magnetic resonance image depicting the convex on concave articulation of the medial knee

The *superficial medial collateral ligament* (sMCL) is the largest structure of the medial aspect of the knee and serves as the primary restraint to valgus forces. The femoral attach-

R. S. Dean · J. K. Monson · R. F. LaPrade (✉)
Twin Cities Orthopedics, Edina, MN, USA

J. Chahla
Midwest Orthopaedics at RUSH, Chicago, IL, USA

N. N. DePhillipo
Twin Cities Orthopedics, Edina, MN, USA

Oslo Sports Trauma Research Center, Oslo, Norway

M. J. Alaia, K. J. Jones (eds.), *Revision Anterior Cruciate Ligament Reconstruction*,
https://doi.org/10.1007/978-3-030-96996-7_11

ment is centered approximately 3.2 mm proximal and 4.8 mm posterior to the medial epicondyle. These landmarks are particularly important during reconstructive procedures. There are two distinct tibial attachments. The proximal tibial attachment is found directly over the anterior arm of the semimembranosus, approximately 11.2 mm distal to the joint line. The distal tibial insertion attaches directly to the medial aspect of the tibia, 61.2 mm distal to the joint line. In total, the sMCL is approximately 9–10 cm in length and is the largest structure on the medial aspect of the knee (Figs. 11.2 and 11.3) [3].

The *deep medial collateral ligament* (dMCL) is essentially a thickening of the medial joint capsule. It is deep and mildly adherent to the sMCL. The dMCL has a distinct meniscofemoral portion that attaches distal and deep to the femoral attachment of the sMCL. It also has a meniscotibial portion that is much shorter and thicker, which attaches just distal to the edge of the articular cartilage of the medial tibial plateau [3].

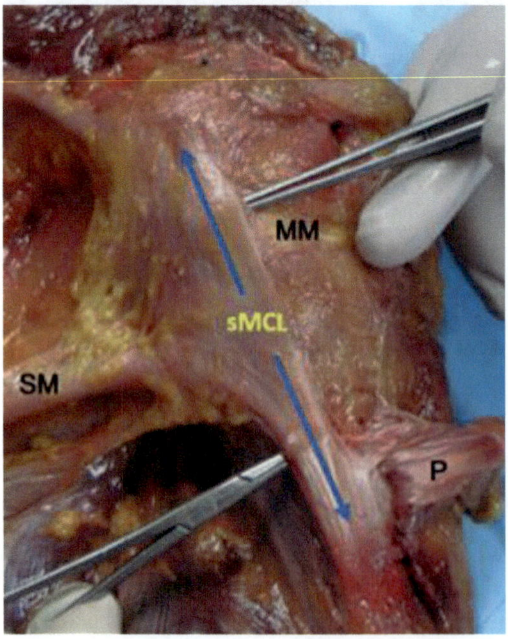

Fig. 11.2 Dissection of the major structures of the medial knee with the pes tendons reflected. *sMCL* superficial medial collateral ligament, *MM* medial meniscus, *SM* semimembranosus, *P* pes tendons

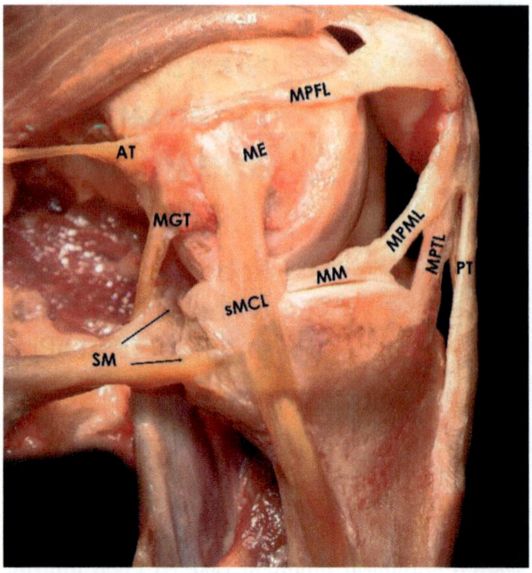

Fig. 11.3 Dissection of the major structures of the medial knee. *AT* adductor magnus tendon, *MPFL* medial patellofemoral ligament, *ME* medial epicondyle, *MGT* medial gastrocnemius tendon, *SM* semimembranosus, *sMCL* superficial medial collateral ligament, *MM* medial meniscus, *MPML* medial patellomeniscal ligament, *MPTL* medial patellotibial ligament, *PT* patellar tendon

The *posterior oblique ligament* (POL) consists of three fascial attachments: the superficial, central, and capsular arms. They course from the distal aspect of the semimembranosus tendon and travel longitudinally across the joint line. The POL attaches on the femur 7.7 mm distal and 6.4 posterior to the adductor tubercle and 1.4 mm distal and 2.9 mm anterior to the gastrocnemius tubercle [3–5]. These anatomical landmarks are particularly important as the POL is reconstructed during anatomic reconstruction of the PMC. The superficial arm of the POL blends with the central arm proximally, and distally it courses parallel to the posterior aspect of the sMCL until it blends with the distal tibial expansion of the semimembranosus and its respective tibial attachment [3, 6]. The central arm of the POL is the largest and strongest of the fascicles and originates from the distal aspect of the semimembranosus tendon. During its course, the central arm provides reinforcement for both the meniscofemoral and meniscotibial portions of the posteromedial capsule, with a robust attachment to the medial meniscus. Anteriorly, the central arm merges with the sMCL. The capsular arm of the POL originates off the distal aspect of the semimembranosus tendon, just posterior and lateral to the meniscofemoral capsular attachments of the central arm. This arm primarily blends with the posteromedial joint capsule and the medial aspect of the OPL. Moreover, it has lesser attachments to the medial gastrocnemius tendon, the adductor magnus tendon expansion, and the adductor magnus tendon femoral attachment site. Of note the capsular arm has no osseous attachment site. Functionally, the POL provides both static and dynamic resistance to valgus forces and has a secondary role to prevent posterior tibial translation (Fig. 11.4) [3].

The *semimembranosus tendon* bifurcates just distal to the joint line and forms anterior and direct arms. The direct arm inserts distally into a small groove just distal to the tuberculum tendinis, which lies posterior to the medial tibial crest. The anterior arm passes deep to the POL and attaches to the tibia in an oval fashion, just distal to the joint line and deep to the proximal tibial attachment of the sMCL. The anterior branch of the tendon blends with the capsular arm of the POL, which then merges with the posteromedial joint capsule with a reported attachment to the posterior inferior margin of the PHMM [3, 7, 8]. The distal border of the semimembranosus bursa can be found along the proximal edge of the tibial attachment site of the direct arm. The semimembranosus bursa is found medial to the anterior arm of the semimembranosus tendon, until the anterior arm attaches to the posteromedial aspect of the tibia.

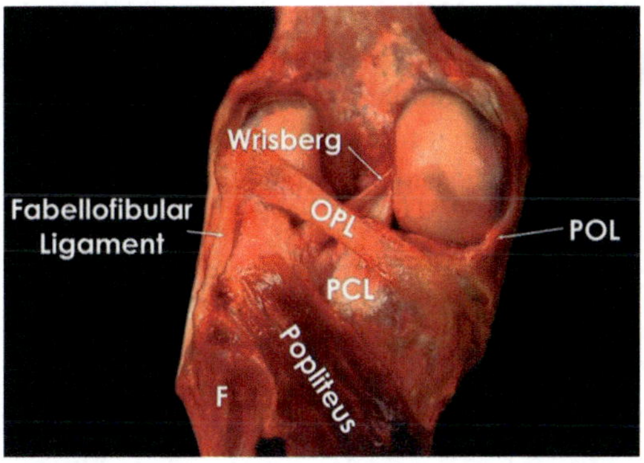

Fig. 11.4 Dissection of the posterior knee. One can visualize the course of the posterior oblique ligament (POL) along the posterior aspect of the knee. *OPL* oblique popliteus ligament, *PCL* posterior cruciate ligament, *F* fibula; Wrisberg, ligament of Wrisberg

The *oblique popliteal ligament* (OPL) is a broad fascial band that courses longitudinally across the posterior aspect of the knee. It arises from the capsular arm of the POL and the lateral expansion of the semimembranosus tendon and extends laterally until reaching its two attachment sites. The proximal and lateral attachment site is to an osseous or cartilaginous fabella, the meniscofemoral portion of the posterolateral joint capsule and the plantaris muscle. The distal and lateral attachment location is just lateral to the posterior cruciate ligament and distal to the posterior root attachment of the lateral meniscus on the tibia. The average length of the OPL has been reported to be 48 mm (Fig. 11.4) [3].

The *posterior horn of the medial meniscus* (PHMM) is intimately associated with the posteromedial capsule, the POL, and the semimembranosus tendon expansion. Together, these structures form a cascade-type system in which the function of each structure is dependent on the neighboring structures. The posteromedial capsule has an average reported length of 21.3 mm, whereas the PHMM has an average length of 20.2 mm and is essentially confluent with the entire length of the posterior capsule [8]. The posterior horn is stabilized further by the meniscotibial portion of the dMCL which helps prevent anterior tibial translation. The PHMM is the most important weightbearing portion of the meniscus [3].

The *medial gastrocnemius tendon* is rarely injured, which makes it an important surgical landmark. The medial gastrocnemius originates from a small depression just proximal and adjacent to the gastrocnemius tubercle at an osseous prominence located over the posteromedial edge of the medial femoral condyle [3]. The tendon courses posterior to the sMCL and deep to the semimembranosus tendon. Distally, this tendon extends to form the muscle belly of the medial gastrocnemius muscle (Fig. 11.5) [3].

The *adductor magnus tendon* attaches at a small bony depression 3 mm posterior and

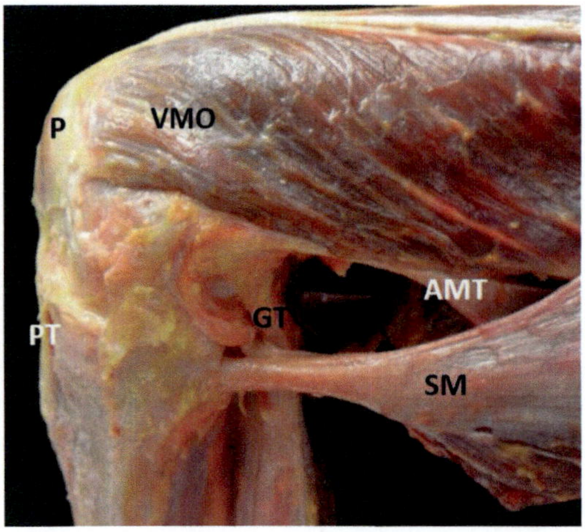

Fig. 11.5 Dissection of medial knee with knee flexed. *P* patella, *PT* patellar tendon, *VMO* vastus medius obliquus, *GT* medial gastrocnemius tendon, *AMT* adductor magnus tendon, *SM* semimembranosus

2.7 mm proximal to the adductor tubercle. This is rarely injured, and thus it is usually used as an anatomical reference for medial-sided reconstructions. Additionally, it has a thick fascial attachment which extends posteriorly from the distal aspect of the tendon to attach to the proximal aspect of the medial gastrocnemius tendon and posteromedial joint capsule [3].

The *vastus medius obliquus* (VMO) has its primary origin from the adductor tubercle in addition to lesser origins from the adductor magnus tendon and the medial intermuscular septum. The distal border of the VMO has an intimate relationship with the proximal edge of the medial patellofemoral ligament (MPFL) as they course together until reaching the patella at which point the fibers of the VMO begin to merge into the quadriceps tendon (Fig. 11.5).

The *pes anserinus* tendons attach at the anteromedial aspect of the proximal tibia. From proximal to distal, the tendons attach in the following order: sartorius, gracilis, and semitendinosus. Collectively, they form the roof of the pes anserine bursa, which can be implicated in a variety of pathologies (Fig. 11.6) [9].

The *saphenous nerve* is the largest cutaneous branch of the femoral nerve and arises from the femoral nerve between the gracilis and semitendinosus tendons. The saphenous nerve further

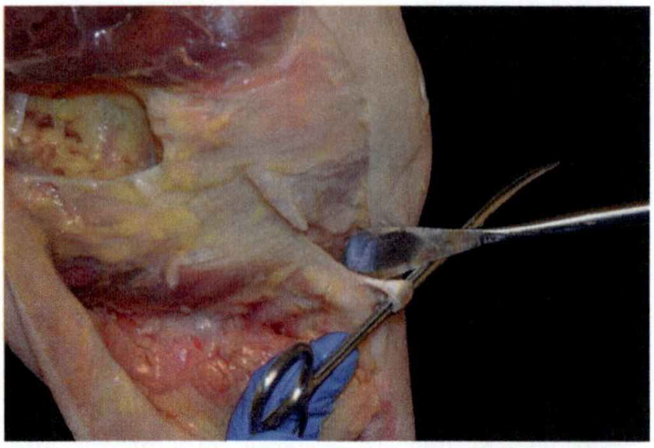

Fig. 11.6 Medial dissection of a left knee demonstrating the anatomical location of the pes tendons (hamstring tendons)

branches into the *infrapatellar branch* just distal to the adductor canal [10, 11]. The infrapatellar branch of the saphenous nerve provides sensory innervation to the proximal part of the lower leg, the anteroinferior part of the knee joint capsule, and the anterior aspect of the knee. It courses either posterior or anterior or through the main saphenous nerve [12].

The *medial superior and inferior genicular arteries* are both found on the medial aspect of the knee. The superior medial genicular artery originates from either the superficial femoral artery or popliteal artery and joins with the superior lateral genicular artery slightly superior to the patella and just anterior to the quadriceps tendon [13, 14]. The inferior medial genicular artery originates from the popliteal artery and courses deep to the sMCL between its two tibial attachment sites below the medial tibial plateau. From there, it rises on the anterior aspect of the tibial plateau where it forms and anastomoses with the peripatellar anastomotic ring [14].

Biomechanics

Although the medial aspect of the knee contains numerous structures, the sMCL, dMCL, and POL serve as the primary functional static stabilizers. Collectively, their main function is to resist valgus forces, with secondary roles in resisting internal and external rotation and resisting anterior and posterior tibial translation [15, 16].

Biomechanical studies have shown that in a MCL-deficient knee, the ACL has secondary valgus stabilizing responsibilities and faces a 185% increase in tension with the application of a valgus force [17]. As such, MCL stability and functionality have an integral role in preventing ACL graft failure following reconstruction [18].

The proximal division of the sMCL is the primary static stabilizer to valgus rotation at 0–90°. Further, at 90° of flexion, it acts as a secondary stabilizer to external rotation, and at 0–90°, the proximal aspect of the sMCL is a secondary stabilizer against internal rotation [15, 19]. The distal division acts primarily on rotational stabilization, as it is the primary stabilizer against external rotation when the knee is at 30° of flexion, and internal rotation at 20–90° of flexion [15]. Previous literature has reported that the mean load at failure for the sMCL with the intact femoral and distal tibial attachments is 557 N. Mean load at failure is 88 N for the intact femoral and proximal tibial divisions of the superficial MCL.

The meniscofemoral division of the dMCL, which is the most common location for structural failure of the dMCL, provides primary stability against internal rotation at 20–90° and secondary external rotational stability at 30° and 90° [4, 19]. Further, the meniscofemoral division provides valgus stabilization at 0–90° and secondary internal rotational stability at 0–30°. The meniscotibial arm of the dMCL functions as a secondary valgus stabilizer at 60° of flexion and a stabilizer against internal rotation at 0–90° of flexion. Collectively, the average load at failure for the dMCL was 100.5 N [19].

The POL is the primary restraint to internal rotation and acts as a secondary stabilizer against valgus force [15]. Further, the POL has a minor role in resisting anterior and posterior tibial rotation [15]. In sectioning studies, the average load at failure for the POL was 256.2 N [19].

Case Presentation: Subjective

Patient is a 65-year-old female that presented to clinic with chronic right knee pain and instability. The patient has a past medical history significant for right knee ACL reconstruction 2 years prior with a different surgeon. The patient notes that at that time she fell off a ladder and her right leg got caught in the ladder; she felt her knee bend inward. At that time, she was diagnosed with a combined ACL and MCL tear. Her ACL was reconstructed acutely, and her MCL tear was managed conservatively with a hinged knee brace. Upon current presentation, she reports significant functional limitations when not wearing the knee brace. Her pain and side-to-side instability are significantly impacting her ability to do work around the house and attend fitness classes.

Mechanism of Injury and Clinical Presentation

Patients with medial knee injuries usually present after having sustained a valgus stress to the knee, typically in the setting of contact or sport. As such, it is essential to obtain a thorough injury history, including inciting events, chronicity, and the reported localization of the symptoms. They typically have localized pain and swelling along the meniscofemoral or meniscotibial division of the MCL. For patients with severe, grade III, full-thickness sMCL ruptures, they typically have side-to-side instability with a valgus thrust on gait analysis and may have difficulty with physical activity [20].

The physical exam can be highly diagnostic for a MCL tear, particularly in the acute setting. Care should be taken to inspect the skin for any signs of abrasions, lacerations, contusions, or localized swelling [3]. Next, the clinician should palpate the joint, making sure to individually palpate the meniscofemoral and meniscotibial divisions of the medial structures of the knee. In addition to the classic knee exam to rule out concomitant injury, there are several medial knee-specific clinical exam maneuvers to consider. The valgus stress test is performed when a valgus force is applied to the knee in full extension and also at 20°. The medial joint line should be palpated to help estimate the amount of medial compartment gapping. Typically, increased medial compartment gapping in full extension is characteristic of a more significant injury with a possible cruciate ligament tear. Valgus stress testing at 20° predominately isolates the sMCL. The anteromedial drawer test is performed with the knee flexed to 90° and the foot external rotated 10°. In this position, a coupled anterior and external rotary force is applied to the knee. An increased amount of anteromedial rotation during this test heightens the suspicion for an injury to the distal aspect of the sMCL, POL, and meniscotibial portion of the dMCL. Finally, the dial test should also be performed at both 30° and 90° of knee flexion. The dial test is considered positive when there is greater than 15° of increased external rotation compared to the contralateral limb at both 30° and 90°. Of note, it is important for the clinician to perform this test while palpating the joint and with the patient in both the supine and prone positions to help differentiate between a posterolateral corner injury, posteromedial corner injury, and meniscal root tear [20]. It is also essential to assess gait on patients with suspected medial-sided instability.

Further, medial-sided knee injuries can present secondary to ACL deficiency. In sectioning studies, Lujan et al. [21] reported that after sectioning the ACL, the load on the MCL was significantly larger at peak anterior translation, while the tension was not significantly affected after a valgus applied force [21]. Specifically, at 30° of flexion with anterior translation, the load on the MCL was significantly greater. This conclusion suggests that ACL deficiency can contribute to medial-sided laxity and should be addressed in order to prevent increased load on the MCL.

Case Presentation: Physical Exam

On physical examination, the patient had a 1+ Lachman's test. Her valgus stress test at 30° was a 3+, and at full extension, she had 2+ valgus gapping. Her anteromedial drawer test was normal. Her dial test demonstrated approximately 20° of side-to-side difference at both 30 and 90°. The patient had an obvious valgus thrust gait when not wearing a hinged knee brace.

Diagnosis and Imaging

Any suspicion for medial knee injury, either acute or chronic, warrants bilateral physician-applied valgus stress radiographs. Typically, these are performed with the knee at 20° flexion with a foam bolster under the knee. With a 10 N clinician-applied valgus stress, the radiographs are assessed for side-to-side differences compared to the normal contralateral knee in medial compartment gapping [20]. LaPrade et al. [22] reported that at 20° an isolated grade III sMCL tear results in 3.2 mm of increased side-to-side medial compartment gapping. A complete tear of the sMCL, dMCL, and POL resulted in 9.8 mm of increased side-to-side medial compartment gapping at 20° [22]. Valgus stress radiographs are particularly valuable in the chronic setting when the results of the clinical exam are unclear [20]. Further, they are particularly of value as the results are both objective and reproducible (Fig. 11.7).

Standard anteroposterior and lateral radiographs should also be obtained to assess for concomitant fracture or avulsions. Avulsions near the native attachment sites of the sMCL should increase the clinical suspicion for medial-sided instability. Additionally, the Pellegrini-Stieda syndrome, which is characterized by intraligamentous calcification in the region of the attachment sites of the sMCL, can be identified radiographically and addressed with either observation or surgical excision [23–25]. Further, full-length weightbearing radiographs should be obtained to assess for coronal plane limb alignment for chronic MCL tears because valgus alignment leads to an increased risk for medial instability. If valgus alignment is identified in chronic cases, alignment correction via osteotomy should be considered prior to or concurrent with surgical intervention for the medial soft tissues because the grafts would otherwise be at risk of stretching out [26].

Magnetic resonance imaging (MRI) is also useful to help diagnose injuries to the medial knee, particularly in the acute setting. Generally, MR images have been reported to have an accuracy and sensitivity of 86% for diagnosing acute

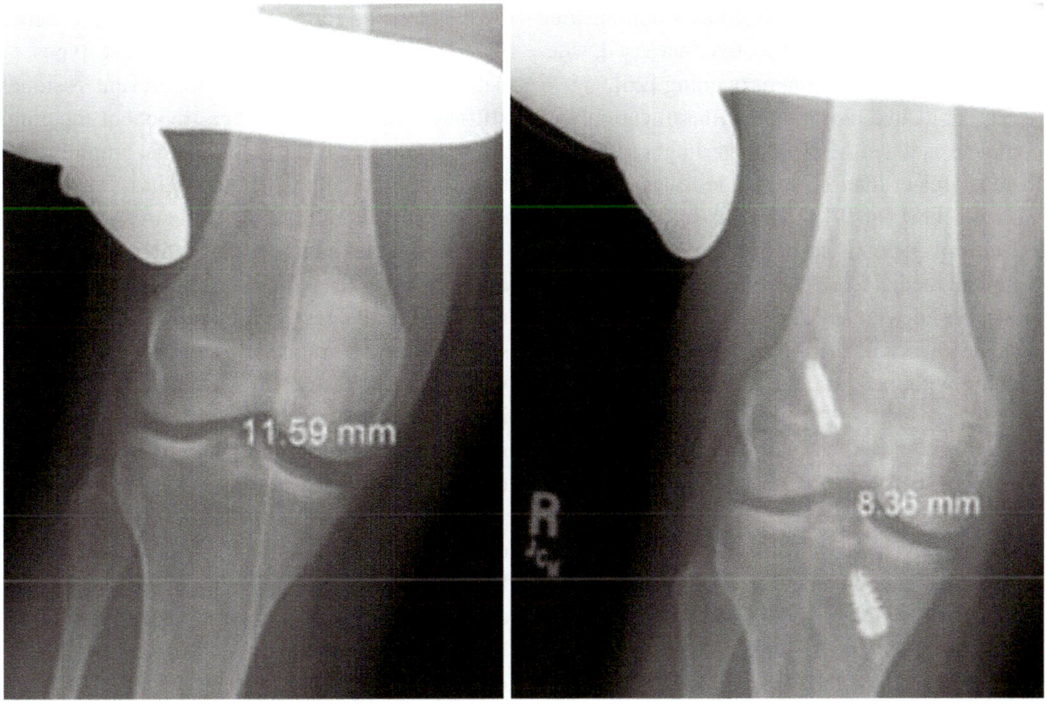

Fig. 11.7 Stress radiographs used to identify medial knee laxity. The left image demonstrates 11.59 mm of medial gapping on pre-operative valgus stress testing. The image on the right is at 6 months post-operation and demonstrates 8.36 mm of medial gapping on valgus stress radiographs

grade III sMCL injures [27, 28]. Besides sMCL attenuation or increased signal intensities, clinicians should look for the presence of lateral compartment bone bruises which have been reported to be present in 45% of isolated sMCL tears [29]. Further, MRI can help diagnose concomitant knee injuries that may have a significant impact on medial-sided laxity and will compromise any potential surgical intervention (i.e., cruciate or meniscal pathology).

Case Presentation: Imaging

On valgus stress radiographs at 20° of knee flexion (Fig. 11.7), the patient had 11.6 mm of medial compartment gapping and 6.8 mm of increased side-to-side difference. Further, MRI results revealed the ACL graft was intact with mild widening of both femoral and tibial tunnels, there was mild lateral compartment osteoarthritis, she had a moderate knee effusion, and a chronic tear of the MCL was evident. Full-length weightbearing radiographs demonstrated that the patient was in neutral alignment.

Classification

The degree of MCL injury is most commonly classified by the amount of medial compartment gapping noted with the application of valgus stress, either subjectively on clinical exam or objectively on valgus stress radiographs. Subjectively, grade I injuries have medial knee tenderness with mild soft tissue swelling and no instability; grade I injuries have 1–5 mm of increased, side-to-side medial compartment opening. Grade II injuries have broad tenderness and partially torn medial structures; they have 5–10 mm of increased, side-to-side medial compartment opening. Grade III injuries have complete medial knee disruption with no clear endpoint on valgus stress examination with the knee at 20° of flexion; these injuries demonstrate greater than 10 mm of subjective increased, side-to-side medial compartment opening [26].

The objective radiographic classification of a complete isolated MCL tear is diagnosed when there is greater than 1.7 mm side-to-side gapping with the knee at 0° of flexion or greater than 3.2 mm of gapping at 20° of flexion. Further, a complete medial knee tear (sMCL, POL, dMCL) is diagnosed with greater than 6.5 mm gapping with the knee at 0° flexion or greater than 9.8 mm gapping with the knee at 20° flexion [22].

Case Presentation: Classification

Given the physical exam and corroborating imaging results, the patient was diagnosed with a grade III, or complete, medial-sided injury. Given the literature and the findings on her stress radiographs, it is likely that her sMCL, POL, and dMCL are each involved.

Treatment Options

Precise identification of the tear location is imperative in the treatment decision process. Recognizing the specific injury location becomes important because tears involving the distal tibial attachment site of the sMCL have been reported to be less likely to heal with conservative management [30–32]. Further, injuries that present with medial compartment gapping when the knee is in full extension are likely more significant with either grade III sMCL or concomitant cruciate or meniscal injury. These injuries are less likely to heal with conservative management [15, 22].

Conservative Management

Almost all isolated grade I or II sMCL injuries can initially be treated conservatively, particularly those that occur in the acute setting [5, 33]. Furthermore, treatment of isolated sMCL tears has been reported to provide good or excellent subjective patient-reported outcomes as defined by the Hospital for Special Surgeries Knee Score [34–38]. Cast immobilization in these types of patients should be avoided to prevent residual stiffness and to encourage ligament healing. Animal models have reported that immobilization of the collateral ligaments has detrimental effects on their cellular metabolism [39, 40].

Non-operative intervention with physical therapy begins with symptom management, which includes relative rest, cryotherapy, joint compression, and early range of motion (ROM) in a varus-valgus constrained knee brace. Early ROM is desirable because it has been found to promote increased collagen proliferation and organization that contribute to increased tissue strength while simultaneously avoiding the deleterious effects of immobilization (ground substance leaching at ligament attachment sites and decreased biomechanical properties of the ligament) [41, 42]. Patients may be restricted to partial weightbearing in the early stages of treatment if they are unable to walk without a limp or experience increased symptoms of joint pain and/or swelling with gait. The brace is worn with gait to minimize valgus or rotational stress through the medial knee. Early goals are to create a protective environment for healing, reduce joint irritability (pain and swelling), and gradually restore full joint range of motion, a strong volitional quadriceps activation, and normal functional movement patterns. Electrical stimulation to the quadriceps muscle is beneficial early on, because it is effective in over-riding the volitional quadriceps activation deficit that occurs secondary to knee ligament injury [43, 44]. Hamstring muscle activation and strengthening should be phased in gradually, as the medial hamstring's insertion proximity to the zone of injury may contribute to pain and irritation with heavy resisted training. A gradual and progressive muscle training program for quadriceps and hamstring muscles, as well as the other large muscle groups of the hip and lower limb, should be conducted, graduating from muscular activation to endurance, hypertrophy, strength, and finally power exercises. Postural stability and balance should be addressed to improve limb and trunk motor control and reduce the risk of reinjury [45]. Sport-specific training progressions may be implemented as individual muscle strength testing and athletic performance measures (Y-balance, hop testing) demonstrate first >80% limb symmetry index (LSI) and eventually >90% LSI. Objective testing should guide decision-making for progressions through higher levels of physical therapy as well as decision-making regarding return to sport participation and competition [46–48]. Studies have reported that a structured, progressive, and goal-based rehabilitation protocol results in excellent long-term subjective results in patients [48]. Conservative treatment can also be considered in patients with grade III tears that reside in neutral or slightly varus alignment [5]. However, more severe injuries, particularly those distal to the joint line, are less likely to succeed with conservative management.

Biological Augmentation

The literature regarding the use of biological agent augmentation in the setting of MCL injury is controversial. Yoshioka et al. reported significantly increased ultimate load and a trend toward improved stiffness in unrepaired rabbit MCLs at 6 weeks post-injury treated with a single PRP injection when compared to a no PRP control group. Of note, this study included only three subjects per cohort, and the control group included separate subjects rather than the contralateral limb [49]. Similarly, da Costa et al. reported significant increases in tensile strength following PRP injection compared to saline injection at either 3 or 6 weeks in rats with grade III MCL tears [50]. Further, two clinical case reports describe positive outcomes for the treatment of acute isolated MCL tears following three sequentially spaced PRP injections within 1 month. The patients reported return to sport at 18 days and 31 days post-injury [51, 52].

Conversely, LaPrade et al. demonstrated no significant improvement in healing of 160 rabbit MCLs following experimentation with varying concentrations of platelets. This study demonstrated that PRP at four times blood concentration levels negatively affected both strength and histological appearance of the damaged tendon at 6 weeks post-injury [53]. Similarly, Amar et al. reported no significant difference with the use of PRP in acute MCL injury after analysis at 3 weeks post-operation in rats [54].

Operative Treatment

Failed conservative management of sMCL tears, or chronic medial-sided laxity, can result in debilitating, persistent instability, ACL dysfunction, weakness, and progression/development of osteoarthritis. In these cases, surgical intervention is usually the most appropriate next option. A number of surgical techniques have been described: direct suture repair of the sMCL and POL [55], primary repair with augmentation [56], advancement of the tibial insertion site of the superficial medial collateral ligament [57], pes anserinus transfer [58], proximal advancement of the superficial medial collateral ligament [59], non-anatomic reconstruction techniques [60], and anatomic reconstruction techniques [61]. The surgical options discussed in the current chapter will focus on the current authors' preferred technique.

Case Presentation: Treatment Decision

Given the patient's severe instability and 2 years of failed conservative management, the current authors recommended surgical reconstruction of the PMC. This involved reconstruction of the sMCL and POL using the surgical technique described in the current chapter.

Authors Preferred Operative Treatment

Anatomic Reconstruction, Double Bundle

Coobs et al. [61] developed, and biomechanically validated, an anatomical reconstruction of the PMC by reconstructing the proximal and distal fascicles of the sMCL and POL using two independent grafts and four total bone tunnels: two femoral and two tibial tunnels [61]. Soft tissue (hamstrings or anterior tibialis) allografts or gracilis and semitendinosus autografts are the preferred graft choices for this technique. On average, the sMCL graft should be 16 cm in length, and the POL graft should be 12 cm in length. The original technique describes a single anteromedial incision, but other adaptations use three smaller incisions for this procedure. The first step is to identify the distal insertion of the sMCL on the tibia. It can be found deep to the pes anserinus bursa, approximately 6 cm distal to the joint line. Once the tibial footprint is identified, the hamstring tendons can be harvested if desired. After graft harvesting, a pin is placed transversely across the tibia 6 cm distal to the joint line, and a 7 mm tunnel is reamed to a depth of 25 mm. Next the central arm of the POL is located at the posteromedial tibia, slightly anterior to the insertion of the semimembranosus tendon and at the posterior margin of the anterior arm. With the footprint located, a pin is placed in an oblique direction toward Gerdy's tubercle, followed by a 7 mm tunnel reamed to a depth of 25 mm.

Next, attention is turned to the femur. Identification of key anatomic landmarks on the femur may require fluoroscopy to assist with proper identification [62]. In order to accurately identify the femoral landmarks, one should first identify the distal attachment of the adductor magnus tendon. The adductor magnus tendon is utilized to dissect down to and identify the adductor tubercle, and because it is rarely injured, it has been called "the lighthouse of the medial aspect of the knee." From there, the medial epicondyle can be identified 12.6 mm distal and 8.3 mm anterior to the adductor tubercle. The sMCL attachment site is 3.2 mm proximal and 4.8 posterior to the medial epicondyle (Fig. 11.8). Once identified, an eyelet pin is placed anterolaterally across the distal thigh, but the tunnel should not be reamed until the femoral footprint of the POL is also identified in order to avoid tunnel convergence. The POL attachment site is 7.7 mm distal and 2.9 mm anterior to the gastrocnemius tubercle. This can be more easily identified if the posteromedial capsule is torn off the femur, but if this is still intact, a small incision can be made just posterior to the remnants of the sMCL, vertically and into the joint to identify its femoral attachment site. Once the POL attachment site is identified, an eyelet passing pin can be placed, and both femoral tunnels can be reamed with a 7 mm reamer to a depth of 25 mm.

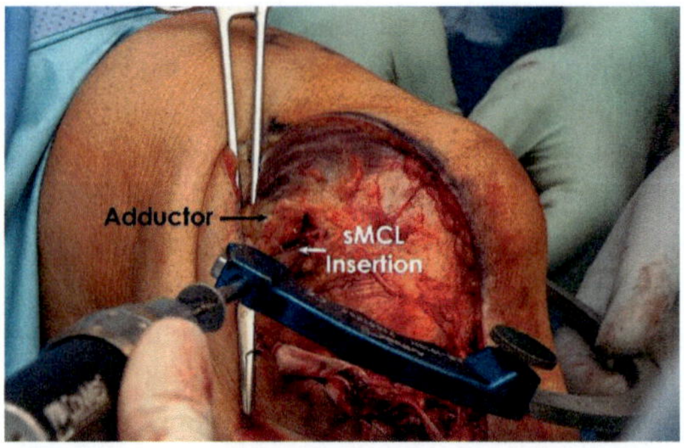

Fig. 11.8 Image showing the anatomical location of the femoral insertion of the superficial medial collateral ligament identified during reconstruction

Anatomic Augmented Surgical Repair with Semitendinosus Tendon Autograft

For the sMCL augmentation repair technique alone, after superficial medial dissection, the semitendinosus tendon is identified at its tibial attachment for graft harvesting. The tendon is then anchored to the tibia at the dMCL distal attachment site (approximately 6 cm distal to the joint line) [3] using both suture anchors and additional sutures to reattach the graft to the underlying remnant of the distal sMCL. The graft is then passed proximally, deep to the intact sartorius fascia, to the femoral attachment site of the sMCL. At this anatomic footprint, a femoral tunnel is reamed with a 7 mm reamer to a depth of 25 mm. The free end of the graft is then measured, and 3 cm of the graft is whipstitched to fit this tunnel. The graft is then fixed using screw fixation, while a 60 N traction force is applied with the knee at 20° of flexion, in neutral rotation, and a slight varus force. Finally, a suture anchor is used to anatomically restore the proximal tibial division of the sMCL, 12 mm distal to the joint line, directly over the anterior arm of the semimembranosus [3, 61–64].

Multistage Surgical Management

When valgus alignment is identified on full-length weightbearing radiographs for chronic PMC tears, surgeons should consider a two-stage intervention, with an osteotomy prior to surgical intervention for the soft tissue laxity to correct the alignment to neutral [65]. One biomechanical study demonstrated a 36% reduction in the amount of medial compartment gapping with the application of a valgus force following a lateral, opening-wedge distal femoral osteotomy for the correction of a valgus deformity [66].

Rehabilitation

Early post-operative range of motion with physical therapy has been shown to decrease stiffness [20, 45]. Specific rehabilitation protocols are dependent on the concomitant surgical procedures, but isolated PMC reconstruction rehabilitation entails non-weightbearing with crutches and the use of a stabilizing knee brace for the first 6 weeks post-operatively. During this time, patients should undergo intensive physical therapy with focus on pain and swelling reduction, passive to active assisted knee range of motion, and quadriceps activation exercises [67–70]. Compared to non-operative management, post-operative rehabilitation is more restricted in the early recovery period to honor soft tissue trauma associated with surgery and protect the joint for adequate healing at bone tunnel and suture graft fixation sites. Goals for therapy progression and return to activity/sport are similar to those of the non-operative management pathway, but with delayed timeframes. Assuming progressive functional milestones are met, including passing the Sport Performance TRAC Testing (Testing for Return to Athletic Competition), patients with isolated PMC injuries are expected to return to sport 6–9 months following PMC reconstruction. The step-by-step milestones for MCL rehabilitation are provided in Fig. 11.9.

Outcomes

Historically, repairs were the preferred surgical technique, but recently it has been recognized that reconstructions are associated with less failures and allow for earlier knee motion which reduces the subsequent risk of arthrofibrosis. Clinical outcomes following surgical repair of PMC injuries in the setting of multiligament knee injuries have been reported to demonstrate a failure rate of 20%, compared to a failure rate of 4% with reconstruction techniques [71].

Kim et al. [72] described clinical outcomes of non-anatomic reconstructions of the PMC using a semitendinosus autograft with a preserved tibial attachment in a 24-patient case series. They reported a reduction from 7.8 mm of medial compartment opening on valgus stress radiographs to less than 2 mm post-operatively in 91.7% (22/24) of patients. Further, they reported IKDC scores graded as normal or nearly normal (IKDC grade A or B) in 92% of patients and mean post-operative Lysholm score of 91.9 [72]. Ibrahim et al. [73] also performed non-anatomic reconstructions of the sMCL in 15 patients, 5 of which demonstrated 1+ residual valgus laxity at average 43-month follow-up [73]. In 61 patients with grade III or IV medial instability at the time of surgery, Lind et al. [74] reported a 98% normal or nearly normal medial stability and reported a 91% satisfaction rating with non-anatomic reconstruction at 2-year follow-up [74].

Other studies used a non-anatomic double bundle technique to reconstruct isolated sMCL injuries. Post-operatively, Liu et al. [75] reported a relative increase of 1.1 mm in side-to-side difference on stress radiographs, but excellent subjective patient-reported outcomes scores post-operatively, and Dong et al. [76] reported anteromedial rotary instability in 9.4% of patients, with an average of 2.9 mm of residual side-to-side medial compartment opening on stress radiographs [73, 74].

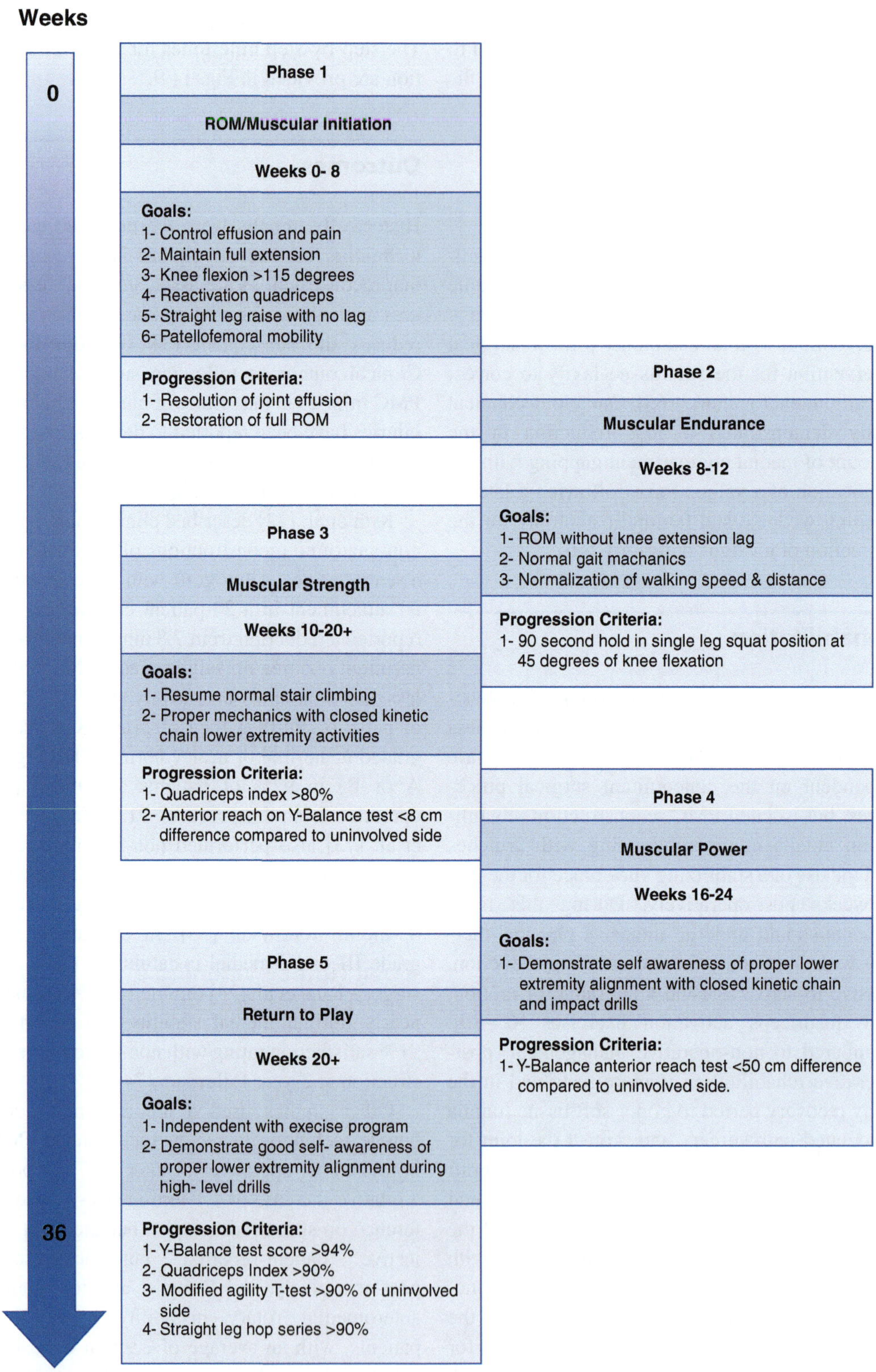

Fig. 11.9 Step-by-step rehabilitation milestones

Outcomes for biomechanically validated anatomic reconstruction techniques [61] have been generally very positive. LaPrade and Wijdicks reported on 28 patients who had single-stage anatomic reconstructions of the PMC (POL and sMCL), with concurrent cruciate ligament reconstruction. Patients reported improved subjective IKDC scores, and all patients demonstrated resolution of side-to-side medial instability at 2-year follow-up. On valgus stress radiographs, there was improvement from 6.3 mm to 1.3 mm in side-to-side medial compartment gapping [20]. The most common reported complications for anatomic reconstruction techniques include deep implant removal, persistent pain, superficial wound infection, joint stiffness, and arthrofibrosis [67, 77, 75].

Case Presentation: Follow-Up

At her most recent 3-month follow-up, the patient reported being able to walk without a limp. Her follow-up stress radiographs demonstrated 0.7 mm of side-to-side difference in medial compartment gapping. Her physical examination was significant only for a mild effusion in her right knee. The patient was instructed to return to clinic in 3 months.

Management in Concomitant Cruciate Injury

Management for patients with medial knee injuries and concomitant cruciate injury is controversial. Moreover, this is a particularly important topic as it has been reported that 78% of patients with grade III MCL injuries have a concomitant cruciate injury [76, 78]. Of note, a previous study reported that in patients with combined sMCL and ACL tears, confirmed operatively, 95.7% (22/23) of patients were also found to have a POL injury [79].

Previous studies report positive outcomes following delayed ACL reconstruction with early MCL surgical management and subsequent rehabilitation to regain valgus stability [80]. Conversely, biomechanical analysis suggests that in the ACL-deficient knee, there is increased tension on the MCL with 30° of flexion and anterior translation suggesting that ACL deficiency may compromise the MCL graft [21]. Further analysis demonstrates that both persistent anteromedial rotatory instability and valgus instability lead to increased forces on the ACL suggesting that reconstructing the ACL in isolation with a deficient MCL may compromise the ACL graft. As such, the majority of literature supports operative treatment of complete PMC injuries at the time of cruciate ligament reconstruction, especially for those patients with residual valgus laxity after non-operative management of medial knee injury [19, 80–85].

In the case of combined PCL and MCL injury, it is important to surgically reconstruct all damaged ligaments in the acute setting, with thorough exploration of the PMC structures [16]. Specifically, the POL plays an important role in the stability of the PCL, and failure to address any injury to this structure of the PMC could compromise the PCL reconstruction [86].

Conclusion

Management of medial-sided ligamentous knee injuries includes both conservative and operative treatment, with anatomic reconstruction demonstrating both biomechanical validation and favorable clinical outcomes. Clinical examination and including the use of valgus stress radiographs and MRI allow for an appropriate diagnosis and classification of medial-sided knee ligament injuries. Despite the complexity of posteromedial corner injuries, relying on surgically relevant anatomical landmarks is key for a successful surgical reconstruction.

References

1. Chen L, Kim PD, Ahmad CS, Levine WN. Medial collateral ligament injuries of the knee: current treatment concepts. Curr Rev Musculoskelet Med [Internet]. 2008 [cited 2019 Sep 23];1(2):108–13. Available from.: http://www.ncbi.nlm.nih.gov/pubmed/19468882.

2. Phisitkul P, James SL, Wolf BR, Amendola A. MCL injuries of the knee: current concepts review. Iowa Orthop J [Internet]. 2006; [cited 2019 Sep 23];26:77–90. Available from: http://www.ncbi.nlm.nih.gov/pubmed/16789454
3. LaPrade RF, Engebretsen AH, Ly TV, Johansen S, Wentorf FA, Engebretsen L. The anatomy of the medial part of the knee. J Bone Jt Surg [Internet]. 2007; [cited 2019 Sep 23];89(9):2000. Available from: http://www.ncbi.nlm.nih.gov/pubmed/17768198
4. Robinson JR, Sanchez-Ballester J, Bull AMJ, Thomas R de WM, Amis AA. The posteromedial corner revisited. An anatomical description of the passive restraining structures of the medial aspect of the human knee. J Bone Joint Surg Br [Internet]. 2004 [cited 2019 Sep 23];86(5):674–81. Available from: http://www.ncbi.nlm.nih.gov/pubmed/15274262.
5. Bonasia DE, Bruzzone M, Dettoni F, Marmotti A, Blonna D, Castoldi F, et al. Treatment of medial and posteromedial knee instability: indications, techniques, and review of the results. Iowa Orthop J [Internet]. 2012; [cited 2019 Sep 23];32:173–83. Available from: http://www.ncbi.nlm.nih.gov/pubmed/23576938
6. LaPrade RF, Morgan PM, Wentorf FA, Johansen S, Engebretsen L. The anatomy of the posterior aspect of the knee: an anatomic study; J Bone Jt Surg [Internet]. 2007. [cited 2019 Sep 23];89(4):758. Available from: http://www.ncbi.nlm.nih.gov/pubmed/17403797.
7. Dold AP, Swensen S, Strauss E, Alaia M. The posteromedial corner of the knee. J Am Acad Orthop Surg [Internet]. 2017 [cited 2019 Sep 23];25(11):752–61. Available from: http://www.ncbi.nlm.nih.gov/pubmed/29059112.
8. DePhillipo NN, Moatshe G, Chahla J, Aman ZS, Storaci HW, Morris ER, et al. Quantitative and qualitative assessment of the posterior medial meniscus anatomy: defining meniscal ramp lesions. Am J Sports Med [Internet]. 2019 [cited 2019 Oct 2];47(2):372–8. Available from: http://www.ncbi.nlm.nih.gov/pubmed/30525875.
9. LaPrade MD, Kennedy MI, Wijdicks CA, LaPrade RF. Anatomy and biomechanics of the medial side of the knee and their surgical implications. Sports Med Arthrosc [Internet]. 2015 [cited 2019 Sep 24];23(2):63–70. Available from: http://www.ncbi.nlm.nih.gov/pubmed/25932874.
10. Tennent TD, Birch NC, Holmes MJ, Birch R, Goddard NJ. Knee pain and the infrapatellar branch of the saphenous nerve. J R Soc Med [Internet]. 1998 [cited 2019 Sep 23];91(11):573–5. Available from: http://www.ncbi.nlm.nih.gov/pubmed/10325872.
11. Frank Netter H, Colacino S. Atlas of human anatomy [internet]. Ther Nova. 1997; [cited 2019 Sep 23]. 525 p. Available from: https://cmc.marmot.org/Record/.b10969123
12. Kerver ALA, Leliveld MS, den Hartog D, Verhofstad MHJ, Kleinrensink GJ. The surgical anatomy of the infrapatellar branch of the saphenous nerve in relation to incisions for anteromedial knee surgery. J Bone Jt Surg [Internet]. 2013 [cited 2019 Sep 17];95(23):2119–25. Available from: http://insights.ovid.com/crossref?an=00004623-201312040-00006.
13. Fox AJS, Wanivenhaus F, Rodeo SA. The basic science of the patella: structure, composition, and function. J Knee Surg [Internet]. 2012 [cited 2019 Sep 23];25(2):127–41. Available from: http://www.ncbi.nlm.nih.gov/pubmed/22928430.
14. Lazaro LE, Cross MB, Lorich DG. Vascular anatomy of the patella: Implications for total knee arthroplasty surgical approaches. Knee [Internet]. 2014 [cited 2019 Sep 23];21(3):655–60. Available from: http://www.ncbi.nlm.nih.gov/pubmed/24767718.
15. Griffith CJ, LaPrade RF, Johansen S, Armitage B, Wijdicks C, Engebretsen L. Medial knee injury: part 1, static function of the individual components of the main medial knee structures. Am J Sports Med [Internet]. 2009 [cited 2019 Sep 17];37(9):1762–70. Available from: http://journals.sagepub.com/doi/10.1177/0363546509333852.
16. Tandogan NR, Kayaalp A. Surgical treatment of medial knee ligament injuries: current indications and techniques. EFORT open Rev [Internet]. 2016 [cited 2019 Sep 22];1(2):27–33. Available from: http://www.ncbi.nlm.nih.gov/pubmed/28461925.
17. Battaglia MJ, Lenhoff MW, Ehteshami JR, Lyman S, Provencher MT, Wickiewicz TL, et al. Medial collateral ligament injuries and subsequent load on the anterior cruciate ligament. Am J Sports Med [Internet]. 2009 [cited 2019 Oct 3];37(2):305–11. Available from: http://journals.sagepub.com/doi/10.1177/0363546508324969.
18. Johnson DL, Swenson TM, Irrgang JJ, Fu FH, Harner CD. Revision anterior cruciate ligament surgery: experience from Pittsburgh. Clin Orthop Relat Res [Internet]. 1996 [cited 2019 Oct 3];325(325):100–9. Available from: http://www.ncbi.nlm.nih.gov/pubmed/8998862.
19. Wijdicks CA, Ewart DT, Nuckley DJ, Johansen S, Engebretsen L, LaPrade RF. Structural properties of the primary medial knee ligaments. Am J Sports Med [Internet]. 2010 [cited 2019 Sep 23];38(8):1638–46. Available from: http://www.ncbi.nlm.nih.gov/pubmed/20675650.
20. Laprade RF, Wijdicks CA. The management of injuries to the medial side of the knee. J Orthop Sport Phys Ther [Internet]. 2012 [cited 2019 Aug 24];42(3):221–33. Available from: http://www.jospt.org/doi/10.2519/jospt.2012.3624.
21. Lujan TJ, Dalton MS, Thompson BM, Ellis BJ, Weiss JA. Effect of ACL deficiency on MCL strains and joint kinematics. J Biomech Eng [Internet]. 2006 [cited 2019 Sep 24];129(3):386–92. Available from: http://www.ncbi.nlm.nih.gov/pubmed/17536905.
22. LaPrade RF, Bernhardson AS, Griffith CJ, Macalena JA, Wijdicks CA. Correlation of valgus stress radiographs with medial knee ligament injuries. Am J Sports Med [Internet]. 2010 [cited 2019 Sep 17];38(2):330–8. Available from: http://www.ncbi.nlm.nih.gov/pubmed/19966093.

23. Altschuler EL, Bryce TN. Pellegrini–Stieda syndrome. N Engl J Med [Internet]. 2006. [cited 2019 Sep 23];354(1):e1. Available from: http://www.ncbi.nlm.nih.gov/pubmed/16394294.
24. Muschol M, Müller I, Petersen W, Hassenpflug J. Symptomatic calcification of the medial collateral ligament of the knee joint: a report about five cases. Knee Surg Sport Traumatol Arthrosc [Internet]. 2005 [cited 2019 Sep 23];13(7):598–602. Available from: http://www.ncbi.nlm.nih.gov/pubmed/15726327.
25. Chang W-C, Huang G-S, Lee C-H, Kao H-W, Chen C-Y. Calcification of medial collateral ligament of the knee. JCR J Clin Rheumatol [Internet]. 2006 [cited 2019 Sep 23];12(4):204–5. Available from: http://www.ncbi.nlm.nih.gov/pubmed/16891928.
26. Gelber PE, Perelli S. Treatment of the medial collateral ligament injuries. Ann Jt [Internet]. 2018; [cited 2019 Sep 22];3:78–78. Available from: http://aoj.amegroups.com/article/view/4615/5178
27. Yao L, Dungan D, Seeger LL. MR imaging of tibial collateral ligament injury: comparison with clinical examination. Skeletal Radiol [Internet]. 1994 [cited 2019 Sep 17];23(7):521–4. Available from: http://www.ncbi.nlm.nih.gov/pubmed/7824979.
28. Halinen J, Koivikko M, Lindahl J, Hirvensalo E. The efficacy of magnetic resonance imaging in acute multi-ligament injuries. Int Orthop [Internet]. 2009 [cited 2019 Oct 3];33(6):1733–8. Available from: http://www.ncbi.nlm.nih.gov/pubmed/19050885.
29. Miller MD, Osborne JR, Gordon WT, Hinkin DT, Brinker MR. The natural history of bone bruises. Am J Sports Med [Internet]. 1998 [cited 2019 Sep 17];26(1):15–9. Available from: http://www.ncbi.nlm.nih.gov/pubmed/9474396.
30. Wilson TC, Satterfield WH, Johnson DL. Medial collateral ligament "tibial"; injuries: indication for acute repair. Orthopedics [Internet]. 2004 [cited 2019 Sep 22];27(4):389–93. Available from: http://www.ncbi.nlm.nih.gov/pubmed/15101482.
31. Azar FM. Evaluation and treatment of chronic medial collateral ligament injuries of the knee. Sports Med Arthrosc [Internet]. 2006 [cited 2019 Oct 3];14(2):84–90. Available from: https://insights.ovid.com/crossref?an=00132585-200606000-00006.
32. Shelbourne KD, Klootwyk TE. Low-velocity knee dislocation with sports injuries. Treatment principles. Clin Sports Med [Internet]. 2000 [cited 2019 Oct 3];19(3):443–56. Available from: http://www.ncbi.nlm.nih.gov/pubmed/10918959.
33. Bonasia DE, Bruzzone M, Dettoni F, Marmotti A, Blonna D, Castoldi F, et al. Treatment of medial and posteromedial knee instability: indications, techniques, and review of the results. Iowa Orthop J [Internet]. 2012; [cited 2019 Sep 16];32:173–83. Available from: http://www.ncbi.nlm.nih.gov/pubmed/23576938
34. Reider B, Sathy MR, Talkington J, Blyznak N, Kollias S. Treatment of isolated medial collateral ligament injuries in athletes with early functional rehabilitation. A five-year follow-up study. Am J Sports Med [Internet]. 1994 [cited 2019 Sep 19];22(4):470–7. Available from: http://journals.sagepub.com/doi/10.1177/036354659402200406.
35. Indelicato PA, Hermansdorfer J, Huegel M. Nonoperative management of complete tears of the medial collateral ligament of the knee in intercollegiate football players. Clin Orthop Relat Res [Internet]. 1990; [cited 2019 Sep 19];(256):174–7. Available from: http://www.ncbi.nlm.nih.gov/pubmed/2364606
36. Ballmer PM, Jakob RP. The non operative treatment of isolated complete tears of the medial collateral ligament of the knee. A prospective study. Arch Orthop Trauma Surg [Internet]. 1988 [cited 2019 Sep 19];107(5):273–6. Available from: http://www.ncbi.nlm.nih.gov/pubmed/3178440.
37. Sandberg R, Balkfors B, Nilsson B, Westlin N. Operative versus non-operative treatment of recent injuries to the ligaments of the knee. A prospective randomized study. J Bone Joint Surg Am [Internet]. 1987 [cited 2019 Sep 19];69(8):1120–6. Available from: http://www.ncbi.nlm.nih.gov/pubmed/3312204.
38. Petermann J, von Garrel T, Gotzen L. Non-operative treatment of acute medial collateral ligament lesions of the knee joint. Knee Surg Sports Traumatol Arthrosc [Internet]. 1993 [cited 2019 Sep 24];1(2):93–6. Available from: http://www.ncbi.nlm.nih.gov/pubmed/8536015.
39. Walsh S, Frank C, Hart D. Immobilization alters cell metabolism in an immature ligament. Clin Orthop Relat Res [Internet]. 1992; [cited 2019 Oct 3];(277):277–88. Available from: http://www.ncbi.nlm.nih.gov/pubmed/1555352
40. Padgett LR, Dahners LE. Rigid immobilization alters matrix organization in the injured rat medial collateral ligament. J Orthop Res [Internet]. 1992 [cited 2019 Oct 3];10(6):895–900. Available from: http://www.ncbi.nlm.nih.gov/pubmed/1403304.
41. Woo SL, Gomez MA, Sites TJ, Newton PO, Orlando CA, Akeson WH. The biomechanical and morphological changes in the medial collateral ligament of the rabbit after immobilization and remobilization. J Bone Joint Surg Am [Internet]. 1987 [cited 2019 Oct 16];69(8):1200–11. Available from: http://www.ncbi.nlm.nih.gov/pubmed/3667649.
42. Newton PO, Woo SL, Kitabayashi LR, Lyon RM, Anderson DR, Akeson WH. Ultrastructural changes in knee ligaments following immobilization. Matrix [Internet]. 1990 [cited 2019 Oct 16];10(5):314–9. Available from: http://www.ncbi.nlm.nih.gov/pubmed/2084512.
43. Hart JM, Pietrosimone B, Hertel J, Ingersoll CD. Quadriceps activation following knee injuries: a systematic review. J Athl Train [Internet]. 2010 [cited 2019 Oct 16];45(1):87–97. Available from: http://www.ncbi.nlm.nih.gov/pubmed/20064053.
44. Kim K-M, Croy T, Hertel J, Saliba S. Effects of neuromuscular electrical stimulation after anterior cruciate ligament reconstruction on quadriceps strength, function, and patient-oriented outcomes: a systematic

review. J Orthop Sport Phys Ther [Internet]. 2010 [cited 2019 Oct 16];40(7):383–91. Available from: http://www.ncbi.nlm.nih.gov/pubmed/20592480.

45. Arundale AJH, Bizzini M, Giordano A, Hewett TE, Logerstedt DS, Mandelbaum B, et al. Exercise-based knee and anterior cruciate ligament injury prevention. J Orthop Sports Phys Ther. 2018;48(9):A1–25.
46. Logan CA, O'Brien LT, LaPrade RF. Post operative rehabilitation of grade iii medial collateral ligament injuries: evidence based rehabilitation and return to play. Int J Sports Phys Ther [Internet]. 2016 [cited 2019 Sep 23];11(7):1177–90. Available from: http://www.ncbi.nlm.nih.gov/pubmed/27999730.
47. Logerstedt DS, Scalzitti D, Risberg MA, Engebretsen L, Webster KE, Feller J, et al. Knee stability and movement coordination impairments: knee ligament sprain revision 2017. J Orthop Sports Phys Ther Movement Science Media. 2017;47:A1–47.
48. Lundberg M, Messner K. Long-term prognosis of isolated partial medial collateral ligament ruptures. Am J Sports Med [Internet]. 1996 [cited 2019 Sep 18];24(2):160–3. Available from: http://www.ncbi.nlm.nih.gov/pubmed/8775113.
49. Yoshioka T, Kanamori A, Washio T, Aoto K, Uemura K, Sakane M, et al. The effects of plasma rich in growth factors (PRGF-Endoret) on healing of medial collateral ligament of the knee. Knee Surgery, Sport Traumatol Arthrosc [Internet]. 2013 [cited 2019 Sep 8];21(8):1763–9. Available from: http://www.ncbi.nlm.nih.gov/pubmed/22527414.
50. Costa EL da, Teixeira LEM, Pádua BJ, Araújo ID de, Vasconcellos L de S, Dias LSB, et al. Biomechanical study of the effect of platelet rich plasma on the treatment of medial collateral ligament lesion in rabbits. Acta Cir Bras [Internet]. 2017 [cited 2019 Aug 7];32(10):827–35. Available from: http://www.scielo.br/scielo.php?script=sci_arttext&pid=S0102-86502017001000827&lng=en&tlng=en.
51. Bagwell MS, Wilk KE, Colberg RE, Dugas JR. The use of serial platelet rich plasma injections with early rehabilitation to expedite grade iii medial collateral ligament injury in a professional athlete: a case report. Int J Sports Phys Ther [Internet]. 2018 [cited 2019 Aug 9];13(3):520–5. Available from: http://www.ncbi.nlm.nih.gov/pubmed/30038838.
52. Eirale C, Mauri E, Hamilton B. Use of platelet rich plasma in an isolated complete medial collateral ligament lesion in a professional football (soccer) player: a case report. Asian J Sports Med [Internet]. 2013 [cited 2019 Aug 26];4(2):158–62. Available from: http://www.ncbi.nlm.nih.gov/pubmed/23802059.
53. LaPrade RF, Goodrich LR, Phillips J, Dornan GJ, Turnbull TL, Hawes ML, et al. Use of Platelet-Rich Plasma Immediately After an Injury Did Not Improve Ligament Healing, and Increasing Platelet Concentrations Was Detrimental in an In Vivo Animal Model. Am J Sports Med [Internet]. 2018 [cited 2019 Aug 7];46(3):702–12. Available from: http://journals.sagepub.com/doi/10.1177/0363546517741135.
54. Amar E, Snir N, Sher O, Brosh T, Khashan M, Salai M, et al. Platelet-rich plasma did not improve early healing of medial collateral ligament in rats. Arch Orthop Trauma Surg [Internet]. 2015 [cited 2019 Aug 26];135(11):1571–7. Available from: http://link.springer.com/10.1007/s00402-015-2306-7.
55. Hughston JC, Eilers AF. The role of the posterior oblique ligament in repairs of acute medial (collateral) ligament tears of the knee. J Bone Joint Surg Am [Internet]. 1973 [cited 2019 Sep 23];55(5):923–40. Available from: http://www.ncbi.nlm.nih.gov/pubmed/4760100.
56. Gorin S, Paul DD, Wilkinson EJ. An anterior cruciate ligament and medial collateral ligament tear in a skeletally immature patient: a new technique to augment primary repair of the medial collateral ligament and an allograft reconstruction of the anterior cruciate ligament. Arthrosc J Arthrosc Relat Surg [Internet]. 2003 [cited 2019 Sep 23];19(10):e159–64. Available from: http://www.ncbi.nlm.nih.gov/pubmed/14673466.
57. O'Donoghue DH. Reconstruction for medial instability of the knee. In: Late reconstructions of injured ligaments of the knee [Internet]. Berlin, Heidelberg: Springer Berlin Heidelberg; 1978 [cited 2019 Sep 23]. p. 66–75. Available from: http://www.springerlink.com/index/10.1007/978-3-642-87274-7_9.
58. Slocum DB, Larson RL. The classic: rotatory instability of the knee. Clin Orthop Relat Res [Internet]. 2007. [cited 2019 Sep 23];454:5–13. Available from: http://www.ncbi.nlm.nih.gov/pubmed/17202912.
59. Shahane SA, Bickerstaff DR. Proximal advancement of the medial collateral ligament for chronic medial instability of the knee joint. Knee [Internet]. 1998 [cited 2019 Sep 24];5(3):191–7. Available from: https://linkinghub.elsevier.com/retrieve/pii/S0968016097100230.
60. Dong J, Ji G, Zhang Y, Gao S, Wang F, Chen B. Single allograft medial collateral ligament and posterior oblique ligament reconstruction: a technique to improve valgus and rotational stability. Eur J Orthop Surg Traumatol [Internet]. 2014 [cited 2019 Sep 24];24(6):1025–9. Available from: http://www.ncbi.nlm.nih.gov/pubmed/23807396.
61. Coobs BR, Wijdicks CA, Armitage BM, Spiridonov SI, Westerhaus BD, Johansen S, et al. An in Vitro Analysis of an Anatomical Medial Knee Reconstruction. Am J Sports Med [Internet]. 2010 [cited 2019 Sep 20];38(2):339–47. Available from: http://www.ncbi.nlm.nih.gov/pubmed/19966100.
62. Wijdicks CA, Griffith CJ, LaPrade RF, Johansen S, Sunderland A, Arendt EA, et al. Radiographic identification of the primary medial knee structures. J Bone Jt Surgery-American Vol [Internet]. 2009 [cited 2019 Sep 24];91(3):521–9. Available from: http://www.ncbi.nlm.nih.gov/pubmed/19255211.
63. Wijdicks CA, Michalski MP, Rasmussen MT, Goldsmith MT, Kennedy NI, Lind M, et al. Superficial Medial Collateral Ligament Anatomic Augmented Repair Versus Anatomic Reconstruction. Am J Sports Med [Internet]. 2013 [cited 2019 Sep

24];41(12):2858–66. Available from: http://journals.sagepub.com/doi/10.1177/0363546513503289.
64. Wijdicks CA, Brand EJ, Nuckley DJ, Johansen S, LaPrade RF, Engebretsen L. Biomechanical evaluation of a medial knee reconstruction with comparison of bioabsorbable interference screw constructs and optimization with a cortical button. Knee Surgery, Sport Traumatol Arthrosc [Internet]. 2010 [cited 2019 Oct 3];18(11):1532–41. Available from: http://www.ncbi.nlm.nih.gov/pubmed/20563561.
65. Encinas-Ullán CA, Rodríguez-Merchán EC. Isolated medial collateral ligament tears. EFORT Open Rev [Internet]. 2018 [cited 2019 Sep 24];3(7):398–407. Available from: http://www.ncbi.nlm.nih.gov/pubmed/30233815.
66. Hetsroni I, Lyman S, Pearle AD, Marx RG. The effect of lateral opening wedge distal femoral osteotomy on medial knee opening: clinical and biomechanical factors. Knee Surg Sports Traumatol Arthrosc [Internet]. 2014 [cited 2019 Sep 23];22(7):1659–65. Available from: http://link.springer.com/10.1007/s00167-013-2405-3.
67. Fanelli GC, Harris JD. Surgical treatment of acute medial collateral ligament and posteromedial corner injuries of the knee. Sports Med Arthrosc [Internet]. 2006 [cited 2019 Sep 23];14(2):78–83. Available from: http://www.ncbi.nlm.nih.gov/pubmed/17135951.
68. Vaughn ZD, Schmidt J, Lindsey DP, Dragoo JL. Biomechanical evaluation of a 1-stage revision anterior cruciate ligament reconstruction technique using a structural bone void filler for femoral fixation. Arthrosc J Arthrosc Relat Surg [Internet]. 2009 [cited 2019 Sep 23];25(9):1011–8. Available from: http://www.ncbi.nlm.nih.gov/pubmed/19732640.
69. Tardy N, Boisrenoult P, Teissier P, Steltzlen C, Beaufils P, Pujol N. Clinical outcomes after multiligament injured knees: medial versus lateral reconstructions. Knee Surgery, Sport Traumatol Arthrosc [Internet]. 2017 [cited 2019 Sep 23];25(2):524–31. Available from: http://www.ncbi.nlm.nih.gov/pubmed/27000392.
70. Koga H, Muneta T, Yagishita K, Ju Y-J, Sekiya I. Surgical management of grade 3 medial knee injuries combined with cruciate ligament injuries. Knee Surg Sport Traumatol Arthrosc [Internet]. 2012 [cited 2019 Sep 23];20(1):88–94. Available from: http://www.ncbi.nlm.nih.gov/pubmed/21556825.
71. Stannard J, Black B, Azbell C, Volgas D. Posteromedial corner injury in knee dislocations. J Knee Surg [Internet]. 2012 [cited 2019 Sep 24];25(05):429–34. Available from: http://www.ncbi.nlm.nih.gov/pubmed/23150355.
72. Kim S-J, Lee D-H, Kim T-E, Choi N-H. Concomitant reconstruction of the medial collateral and posterior oblique ligaments for medial instability of the knee. J Bone Joint Surg Br [Internet]. 2008; [cited 2019 Sep 24];90-B(10):1323–7. Available from: http://online.boneandjoint.org.uk/doi/10.1302/0301-620X.90B10.20781
73. Ibrahim SAR, Ahmad FHF, Salah M, Al Misfer ARK, Ghaffer SA, Khirat S. Surgical management of traumatic knee dislocation. Arthrosc J Arthrosc Relat Surg [Internet]. 2008 [cited 2019 Sep 24];24(2):178–87. Available from: http://www.ncbi.nlm.nih.gov/pubmed/18237702.
74. Lind M, Jakobsen BW, Lund B, Hansen MS, Abdallah O, Christiansen SE. Anatomical reconstruction of the medial collateral ligament and posteromedial corner of the knee in patients with chronic medial collateral ligament instability. Am J Sports Med [Internet]. 2009 [cited 2019 Oct 3];37(6):1116–22. Available from: http://journals.sagepub.com/doi/10.1177/0363546509332498.
75. Liu X, Feng H, Zhang H, Hong L, Wang XS, Zhang J, et al. Surgical treatment of subacute and chronic valgus instability in multiligament-injured knees with superficial medial collateral ligament reconstruction using achilles allografts. Am J Sports Med [Internet]. 2013 [cited 2019 Sep 24];41(5):1044–50. Available from: http://www.ncbi.nlm.nih.gov/pubmed/23467556.
76. Dong JT, Chen BC, Men XQ, Wang F, Hao JD, Zhao JN, et al. Application of triangular vector to functionally reconstruct the medial collateral ligament with double-bundle allograft technique. Arthrosc J Arthrosc Relat Surg [Internet]. 2012 [cited 2019 Sep 24];28(10):1445–53. Available from: http://www.ncbi.nlm.nih.gov/pubmed/22796140.
77. Lind M, Menhert F, Pedersen AB. The first results from the Danish ACL reconstruction registry: epidemiologic and 2 year follow-up results from 5,818 knee ligament reconstructions. Knee Surg Sport Traumatol Arthrosc [Internet]. 2009 [cited 2019 Sep 23];17(2):117–24. Available from: http://www.ncbi.nlm.nih.gov/pubmed/18974970.
78. Stannard J, Bauer K. Current concepts in knee dislocations: PCL, ACL, and medial sided injuries. J Knee Surg [Internet]. 2012 [cited 2019 Sep 24];25(04):287–94. Available from: http://www.ncbi.nlm.nih.gov/pubmed/23150156.
79. Halinen J, Lindahl J, Hirvensalo E, Santavirta S. Operative and nonoperative treatments of medial collateral ligament rupture with early anterior cruciate ligament reconstruction. Am J Sports Med [Internet]. 2006 [cited 2019 Sep 24];34(7):1134–40. Available from: http://www.ncbi.nlm.nih.gov/pubmed/16452264.
80. Grant JA, Tannenbaum E, Miller BS, Bedi A. Treatment of combined complete tears of the anterior cruciate and medial collateral ligaments. Arthrosc J Arthrosc Relat Surg [Internet]. 2012 [cited 2019 Oct 3];28(1):110–22. Available from: http://www.ncbi.nlm.nih.gov/pubmed/22119290.
81. Fetto JF, Marshall JL. Medial collateral ligament injuries of the knee: a rationale for treatment. Clin Orthop Relat Res [Internet]. 1978 [cited 2019 Oct 3];(132):206–18. Available from: http://www.ncbi.nlm.nih.gov/pubmed/679543.
82. Fanelli GC. Evaluation and treatment of medial instability of the knee. Sports Med Arthrosc [Internet].

2015 [cited 2019 Sep 24];23(2):61–2. Available from: http://www.ncbi.nlm.nih.gov/pubmed/25932873.
83. Bollier M, Smith P. Anterior cruciate ligament and medial collateral ligament injuries. J Knee Surg [Internet]. 2014 [cited 2019 Sep 24];27(05):359–68. Available from: http://www.ncbi.nlm.nih.gov/pubmed/24949985.
84. Fanelli GC, Harris JD. Surgical treatment of acute medial collateral ligament and posteromedial corner injuries of the knee. Sports Med Arthrosc [Internet]. 2006 [cited 2019 Sep 24];14(2):78–83. Available from: https://insights.ovid.com/crossref?an=00132585-200606000-00005.
85. LaPrade RF, Moulton SG, Nitri M, Mueller W, Engebretsen L. Clinically relevant anatomy and what anatomic reconstruction means. Knee Surgery, Sport Traumatol Arthrosc [Internet]. 2015 [cited 2019 Sep 24];23(10):2950–9. Available from: http://www.ncbi.nlm.nih.gov/pubmed/25957611.
86. Weimann A, Schatka I, Herbort M, Achtnich A, Zantop T, Raschke M, et al. Reconstruction of the posterior oblique ligament and the posterior cruciate ligament in knees with posteromedial instability. Arthrosc J Arthrosc Relat Surg [Internet]. 2012 [cited 2019 Oct 3];28(9):1283–9. Available from: http://www.ncbi.nlm.nih.gov/pubmed/22541643.

Management of Lateral-Sided Ligamentous Laxity and Posterolateral Corner

12

Gregory C. Fanelli, Matthew G. Fanelli, David G. Fanelli, and Michael G. Doran

Introduction

Combined anterior cruciate ligament and posterolateral injury of the knee can result in significant functional instability for the affected individual. Both components of the instability must be treated to maximize the probability of success for the surgical procedure. Higher failure rates of anterior cruciate ligament reconstruction have been reported when the posterolateral instability has been left untreated. There are varying degrees of posterolateral instability with respect to pathologic external tibial rotation and varus laxity. Surgical treatment of posterolateral instability (PLI) must address all components of the PLI (popliteus tendon, popliteofibular ligament, lateral collateral ligament, and the lateral-posterolateral capsule), the abnormal planes of motion, as well as other structural injuries [1–8]. Successful anterior cruciate ligament surgery depends upon recognition and treatment of concomitant posterolateral corner injuries.

Surgical Anatomy

The function of the posterolateral corner is to resist varus stress, to resist posterior tibial translation near full extension, and to resist external tibial rotation. The important structures responsible for posterolateral stability include the complex interaction of the fibular collateral ligament, the popliteus tendon, the popliteofibular ligament, the midlateral capsule, and the posterolateral capsule. The goal of posterolateral reconstruction surgery is to correct the abnormal patterns of motion about the knee by eliminating axial rotation, varus, and hyperextension instability [9–11].

Classification of Posterolateral Instability of the Knee

Three types of posterolateral instability of the knee may be encountered: A, B, and C (4). These three types of posterolateral instability are determined by physical examination. Posterolateral instability includes at least 10 degrees of increased tibial external rotation compared to the normal knee at 30 degrees of knee flexion (positive dial test and external rotation thigh foot angle

G. C. Fanelli (✉)
Department of Medical Education, Geisinger Commonwealth School of Medicine, Scranton, PA, USA

Department of Orthopaedic Surgery and Sports Medicine, Danville, PA, USA

M. G. Fanelli · D. G. Fanelli
Department of Orthopaedic Surgery and Sports Medicine, Geisinger Medical Center, Danville, PA, USA

M. G. Doran
NYU Langone Department of Orthopedic Surgery, New York, NY, USA

M. J. Alaia, K. J. Jones (eds.), *Revision Anterior Cruciate Ligament Reconstruction*, https://doi.org/10.1007/978-3-030-96996-7_12

test) and variable degrees of varus instability depending upon the injured anatomic structures (3). Posterolateral instability (PLI) type A has increased external rotation only, resulting from attenuation of the popliteofibular ligament, popliteus tendon, and posterolateral capsule. PLI type B presents with increased external rotation and approximately 5–10 mm of increased lateral joint line opening with a soft end point to varus stress at 30-degree knee flexion compared to the normal knee. This occurs with attenuation or minor avulsion of the popliteofibular ligament, popliteus tendon, fibular collateral ligament, and midlateral and posterolateral capsule. Hyperextension compared to the normal knee may or may not be present. PLI type C presents with increased tibial external rotation, varus laxity with no discernible end point, and hyperextension compared to the normal knee. This occurs with major avulsion or disruption of the popliteofibular ligament, popliteus tendon, fibular collateral ligament, and midlateral and posterolateral capsule and often includes disruption of one or both cruciate ligaments.

The physical examination will vary depending on the type of posterolateral instability. All types of posterolateral instability will demonstrate increased external rotation compared to the patient's uninjured knee; however, the degree of varus laxity will vary depending upon the severity of injury to the involved structures. Multiple physical examination tests should be utilized to determine the classification of pathologic motion because this will determine the surgical treatment [4, 10–16].

Clinical Presentation

Patients with posterolateral instability will present with functional instability during pivoting, twisting, cutting, and ambulation on uneven surfaces. These patients may present with posterolateral knee pain, lateral or medial joint line pain, and peroneal nerve symptoms which may include sensory and/or motor disturbances. Posterolateral instability patients may display abnormal gait patterns including a varus thrust during the stance phase of gait and hyperextension instability with heel strike.

Physical examination will demonstrate axial rotation laxity demonstrated with a positive dial test. Variable amounts of varus laxity and hyperextension may be present and are demonstrated by varus stress testing, the heel lift off test, and the hyperextension external rotation recurvatum test [3, 12–15].

Plain radiographs are usually negative; however, they may demonstrate capsular avulsion fractures, fibular head avulsion fractures, and malalignment in chronic cases. MRI is helpful in the acute posterolateral instability in conjunction with a good clinical examination. Arthroscopic evaluation of posterolateral instability compliments the clinical examination and the MRI findings demonstrating a positive drive-through sign and the floating meniscus sign indicating the location of structural injuries (14).

Surgical Treatment Principles

The surgical treatment principles of posterolateral reconstruction are reproducible. Peroneal nerve decompression is performed in each case, and the peroneal nerve is protected throughout the procedure. It is essential to identify the abnormal planes of instability and to correct and eliminate abnormal tibial external rotation, varus laxity, and hyperextension external rotation recurvatum. The midlateral and posterolateral capsule must always be addressed by either primary repair, capsular shift, or a combination of the two [6–8, 17–26]. Primary repair of all injured structures when possible combined with posterolateral reconstruction is more successful than primary repair alone [27, 28].

Biomechanics of Surgical Reconstruction

The surgical reconstruction for posterolateral instability involves the creation of ligamentous substitutes positioned to resist varus rotation, posterolateral tibial rotation, and hyperextension external rotation recurvatum. These procedures all involve the creation of structural bands from either the fibular head or the posterolateral corner of the tibia to the region of the lateral femoral epicondyle. Structural bands are created from existing structures, autografts, or allografts. It is important when planning a surgical reconstruction to understand the ligament length relationships of the lateral knee so that tissues can be placed in near isometric positions and in positions of optimal mechanical advantage to resist varus rotation and posterolateral tibial rotation. Any injury to the midlateral and posterolateral capsule must also be addressed to ensure successful posterolateral reconstruction [5, 29].

A study of the isometry of the lateral side of the knee investigated length relationships between the fibular head and the lateral aspect of the femur (30). In particular, this study demonstrates that the entire fibular head is relatively isometric to the lateral femoral epicondyle throughout a functional range of knee motion and that there is slightly improved isometry from the posterior aspect of the fibular head to the anterior aspect of the epicondyle and from the anterior aspect of the fibular head to the posterior aspect of the epicondyle. It should be noted that the isometric region from the posterior aspect of the fibular head to the anterior aspect of the epicondyle represents the anatomic position of the popliteofibular ligament or the static portion of the popliteal tendon. The popliteofibular ligament is thus relatively isometric and can remain functional through a full range of knee motion. The area from the posterolateral corner of the tibia to the lateral femoral epicondyle is not isometric. This region of attachment for a "popliteus bypass procedure" if tensioned near full extension will be supportive in that range but will become somewhat less supportive as the knee passes into greater angles of flexion. In the normal situation, this portion of the popliteus tendon is tensioned by an intact popliteus muscle belly. Because of the near isometric behavior of the popliteofibular ligament, it is important when reconstructing for posterolateral instability to include tissue in the position of the popliteofibular ligament. The reconstruction of the popliteofibular ligament can be performed either with a free graft or by the technique of biceps tenodesis. Wascher et al. studied the effects of biceps tenodesis after a complete injury to the posterolateral corner (31). Under varus load and external tibial torque, tenodesis (using a fixation point located 1 cm anterior to the femoral insertion of LCL) restored varus laxity and external tibial rotation.

During posterolateral reconstruction, tissue attached at the fibular head or the posterolateral corner of the tibia and routed to the lateral femoral epicondyle will resist external tibia rotation as well as varus rotation. Tissue from the lateral femoral epicondyle to the posterior fibular head has a mechanical advantage over tissue from the epicondyle to the posterolateral corner of the tibia. If the axis of rotation of the tibia relative to the femur is considered to be near the PCL tibial attachment site, then the lever arm of graft attachment to the posterior fibular head is greater by approximately 50% than that of a graft attached to the posterolateral tibia. A graft attached to the posterior fibular head is proportionately more effective in resisting posterolateral rotations. It is therefore appropriate that a posterolateral reconstruction should in most instances include tissue from the posterior aspect of the fibular head to the lateral femoral epicondyle in the position of the popliteofibular ligament. In cases of acute tibiofibular joint disruption and cases with hyperextension external rotation recurvatum deformity, it is necessary to also include tissue from the lateral femoral epicondyle to the posterolateral corner of the tibia as well as reconstruct the proximal tibiofibular joint [5, 7, 8, 17–19, 30].

Surgical Timing and Decision-Making

Surgical timing in acute posterolateral instability of the knee is dependent upon the severity of the injury [3, 4, 6, 14–19, 32–39]. Posterolateral instability (PLI) type A presents with increased external rotation only, resulting from attenuation of the popliteofibular ligament, popliteus tendon, and posterolateral capsule. Surgical treatment of PLI type A can usually be performed within 3–4 weeks of the initial injury. PLI type B presents with increased external rotation and approximately 5–10 mm of increased lateral joint line opening with a soft end point to varus stress at 30-degree knee flexion compared to the normal knee, and the varus laxity decreases as one approaches full extension. This occurs with attenuation or minor avulsion of the popliteofibular ligament, popliteus tendon, fibular collateral ligament, and midlateral and posterolateral capsule. Hyperextension compared to the normal knee may or may not be present. Surgical treatment of PLI type B also can usually be performed within 3–4 weeks of the initial injury.

PLI type C presents with increased tibial external rotation, varus laxity with no discernible end point, and hyperextension compared to the normal knee. This occurs with major avulsion or disruption of the popliteofibular ligament, popliteus tendon, fibular collateral ligament, and midlateral and posterolateral capsule and often includes disruption of one or both cruciate ligaments. PLI type C, in our experience, is typically treated with a staged surgical procedure, however can also be performed in the same setting. Stage 1 is peroneal nerve decompression and neurolysis and posterolateral primary repair and capsular procedure combined with posterolateral reconstruction within the first 10 days of the injury. Stage 2 is cruciate ligament reconstruction approximately 4–6 weeks later.

The surgical timing scenario outlined here includes guidelines that may need to be altered based on the condition of the patient's skin, nerves, blood vessel meniscus, articular cartilage, fractures, remote orthopedic trauma, and other organ system trauma. The timing of the knee surgery is to be considered within the context of the patient's overall health and condition [16, 18, 19].

The surgical decision-making concerning the posterolateral corner is dependent on the pathology at the time and the planes of instability of the injured knee. In both acute and chronic cases, primary repair is performed when possible using suture anchors, sutures placed through bone tunnels, or screws and spiked washers. Primary repairs are then augmented with a posterolateral reconstruction procedure which has proven to be more effective than primary repair alone in posterolateral instability [27, 28].

Split biceps tendon transfer is most successful in types A and B posterolateral instability when local autogenous tissue is required [5, 7, 8, 32–36, 40–42]. This method of reconstruction is applicable in both the acute and chronic clinical scenario as long as the proximal tibiofibular joint is intact, the posterolateral capsular attachments to the common biceps tendon are intact, and the biceps femoris tendon insertion into the fibular head is intact.

Fibular head-based figure of eight posterolateral reconstruction using allograft or autograft tissue is applicable in the acute and chronic situation and with type A, type B, and some type C posterolateral instability patterns. In the case of type C posterolateral instability, there must be a functionally adequate midlateral and posterolateral capsule and the absence of hyperextension [5–8, 16–19, 32, 40, 43, 44].

Fibular head-based figure of eight posterolateral reconstruction combined with a proximal tibia-based popliteus tendon bypass posterolateral reconstruction is used in both the acute and chronic clinical scenarios. In addition, this combined posterolateral reconstruction surgical procedure is utilized when there is disruption of the proximal tibiofibular joint, in posterolateral instability type C when there is inadequate midlateral and posterolateral capsule, and when there is hyperextension compared to the normal knee demonstrated by the heel lift off test [5–8, 16–19, 32, 40, 43, 44].

Regardless of the posterolateral reconstruction surgical procedure chosen, the midlateral and posterolateral capsule are always addressed with primary repair of injured capsular tissues, a capsular shift procedure, or a combination of the two in both the acute and chronic situations. Failure to address the capsule will result in residual posterolateral laxity. Lower extremity alignment is important for successful posterolateral reconstruction, and osteotomy is utilized as necessary [5–8, 16–19, 32, 40, 41, 43, 44].

Primary Repair Surgical Technique

When reconstructing chronic lateral and posterolateral instabilities, it is important to perform primary repair when possible. Primary repair of acute posterolateral knee injuries is most easily accomplished within the first 2–3 weeks post-injury when possible; however, it is possible to repair these injured tissues in very chronic cases as well. Injuries to the lateral side structures can occur as avulsion of soft tissue from bone at the femoral, tibial, or fibular head attachments; mid-substance interstitial disruption leaving the injured structures in continuity but elongated; and displaced fibular head fractures. Our preferred surgical technique for soft tissue avulsion from bone is direct anatomic repair of the injured structures using suture anchors and permanent braided suture or screw and ligament washer fixation [12–15, 35, 36, 43, 44].

Displaced fibular head fractures cause posterolateral instability because most of the lateral side supporting structures attach to the fibular head, and these structures are no longer able to resist varus stress. Also, when the fibular head displaces in a proximal direction, the lateral, posterolateral capsule, and menisco-tibial ligaments are almost always avulsed from the tibia eliminating the ability of these structures to resist varus stress. Our preferred surgical technique for treating displaced fibular head fractures is direct anatomic repair of the injured lateral, posterolateral capsule, and menisco-tibial ligaments using suture anchors and permanent braided suture and anatomic open reduction and internal fixation with screw and washer of the displaced fibular head fracture. Additionally, suture fixation of a comminuted fracture can be performed using non-absorbable sutures via bone tunnels through the intact fibular head cortical bone.

Biceps Tendon Transfer Posterolateral Reconstruction

There are two types of biceps tendon transfer procedures described: the full biceps tendon transfer and the split biceps tendon transfer. Although the full biceps tendon transfer procedure is very effective, the split biceps tendon procedure is advantageous because it saves the dynamic stabilizing effect of the biceps femoris muscle tendon complex [5, 7, 8, 31–36, 40, 42].

The surgical technique for posterolateral reconstruction using the split biceps tendon transfer to the lateral femoral epicondyle recreates the function of the popliteofibular ligament and lateral collateral ligament, tightens the posterolateral capsule, and provides a post of strong autogenous tissue to reinforce the posterolateral corner. The requirements for this procedure include an intact proximal tibiofibular joint, the posterolateral capsular attachments to the common biceps tendon should be intact, and the biceps femoris tendon insertion into the fibular head must be intact [4, 5, 7–9, 14, 24, 31–36, 40, 42].

A lateral hockey stick incision is made. Peroneal nerve decompression and neurolysis are performed, and the peroneal nerve is protected throughout the procedure. The long head and common biceps femoris tendon is isolated, and the anterior 2/3 is separated from the short head muscle. The tendon is detached proximally and left attached distally to its anatomic insertion site on the fibular head. The strip of biceps tendon should be 12–14 cm long. The iliotibial band is incised in line with its fibers, and the fibular collateral ligament and popliteus tendon are exposed. A drill hole is made 1 cm anterior to the fibular collateral ligament femoral insertion.

A longitudinal incision is made in the lateral capsule just posterior to the fibular collateral ligament. The split biceps tendon is passed medial to the iliotibial band and secured to the lateral femoral epicondylar region with a screw and spiked ligament washer at the abovementioned point. The residual tail of the transferred split biceps tendon is passed medial to the iliotibial band and secured to the fibular head. The posterolateral capsule that had been previously incised is then shifted and sewn into the strut of transferred biceps tendon to eliminate posterolateral capsular redundancy, thus performing the posterolateral capsular shift procedure.

Biceps Tendon Procedure Results

Combined PCL Posterolateral Reconstructions

Fanelli and Edson, in 2004, published the 2–10-year (24–120-month) results of 41 chronic arthroscopically assisted combined PCL/posterolateral reconstructions evaluated pre- and postoperatively using the Lysholm, Tegner, and Hospital for Special Surgery knee ligament rating scales, KT 1000 arthrometer testing, stress radiography, and physical examination (36). Posterior cruciate ligament reconstructions were performed using the arthroscopically assisted single femoral tunnel-single bundle transtibial tunnel posterior cruciate ligament reconstruction technique using fresh frozen Achilles tendon allografts in all 41 cases. In all 41 cases, posterolateral instability reconstruction was performed with combined biceps femoris tendon tenodesis and posterolateral capsular shift procedures.

Postoperative physical exam revealed normal posterior drawer/tibial step off for the overall study group in 29/41 (70%) of knees. Normal posterior drawer and tibial step offs were achieved in 91.7% of the knees tensioned with the Biomet Sports Medicine mechanical graft tensioner. Posterolateral stability was restored to normal in 11/41 (27%) of knees and tighter than the normal knee in 29/41 (71%) of knees evaluated with the external rotation thigh foot angle test. Thirty-degree varus stress testing was normal in 40/41 (97%) of knees and grade I laxity in 1/41 (3%) of knees.

The authors concluded that chronic combined PCL/posterolateral instabilities can be successfully treated with arthroscopic posterior cruciate ligament reconstruction using fresh frozen Achilles tendon allograft combined with posterolateral corner reconstruction using biceps tendon tenodesis combined with posterolateral capsular shift procedure [7, 8, 36]. Statistically significant improvement is noted ($p = 0.001$) from the preoperative condition at 2–10-year follow-up using objective parameters of knee ligament rating scales, arthrometer testing, stress radiography, and physical examination.

Combined PCL ACL Reconstruction Without Mechanical Graft Tensioning

Fanelli and Edson, in 2002, published results of multiple ligament injured knee treatment without mechanical graft tensioning (35). This study presented the 2–10-year (24–120-month) results of 35 arthroscopically assisted combined ACL/PCL reconstructions evaluated pre- and postoperatively using the Lysholm, Tegner, and Hospital for Special Surgery knee ligament rating scales, KT 1000 arthrometer testing, stress radiography, and physical examination.

This study population included 26 males, 9 females, 19 acute knee injuries, and 16 chronic knee injuries. Ligament injuries included 19 ACL/PCL/posterolateral instabilities, 9 ACL/PCL/MCL instabilities, 6 ACL/PCL/posterolateral/MCL instabilities, and 1 ACL/PCL instability. All knees had grade III preoperative ACL/PCL laxity and were assessed pre- and postoperatively with arthrometer testing, three different knee ligament rating scales, stress radiography, and physical examination. Arthroscopically assisted combined ACL/PCL reconstructions were performed using the single incision endoscopic ACL technique and the single femoral tunnel-single bundle transtibial tunnel PCL technique. PCLs were reconstructed with allograft Achilles tendon (26 knees), autograft BTB (7 knees), and autograft semitendinosus/gracilis (2 knees). ACLs were reconstructed with autograft BTB (16 knees), allograft BTB (12 knees), Achilles tendon allograft (6 knees), and autograft semitendinosus/gracilis (1 knee). MCL injuries were treated with bracing or open reconstruction. Posterolateral instability was treated with biceps femoris tendon transfer, with or without primary repair, and posterolateral capsular shift procedures as indicated. A Biomet Sports Medicine graft tensioning boot was not utilized in this series of patients (Biomet Sports Medicine, Warsaw, Indiana).

Postoperative physical examination results revealed normal posterior drawer/tibial step off in 16/35 (46%) of knees, with normal Lachman and pivot shift tests in 33/35 (94%) of knees.

Posterolateral stability was restored to normal in 6/25 (24%) of knees and tighter than the normal knee in 19/25 (76%) of knees evaluated with the external rotation thigh foot angle test. 30° varus stress testing was normal in 22/25 (88%) of knees and grade I laxity in 3/25 (12%) of knees. 30° valgus stress testing was normal in 7/7 (100%) of surgically treated MCL tears and normal in 7/8 (87.5%) of brace-treated knees.

The conclusions of this study are that combined ACL/PCL instabilities can be successfully treated with arthroscopic reconstruction of the cruciate ligaments and the appropriate collateral ligament surgery [7, 8, 35]. Statistically significant improvement is noted from the preoperative condition at 2–10-year follow-up using objective parameters of knee ligament rating scales, arthrometer testing, stress radiography, and physical examination. Posterolateral stability was restored to normal in 6/25 (24%) knees and tighter than the normal knee in 19/25 (76%) knees evaluated with the external rotation thigh foot angle test (dial test). This indicated a 100% correction rate of pathologic external rotation. Thirty-degree varus stress testing was restored to normal in 22/25 (88%) knees and grade I laxity in 3/25 (12%) knees. This indicates an 88% correction rate of pathologic varus laxity in these multiple ligament injured knees utilizing primary posterolateral repair combined with biceps femoris tendon transfer and posterolateral capsular shift reconstruction. It was determined that biceps tendon transfer was not optimal for posterolateral instability type C.

Fibular Head-Based Figure of Eight Posterolateral Reconstruction

Our most commonly utilized surgical technique for posterolateral reconstruction is the fibular head-based figure of eight procedure utilizing semitendinosus allograft or other soft tissue allograft material. This is a biomechanically sound and effective surgical procedure (30). This procedure requires an intact proximal tibiofibular joint and the absence of a severe hyperextension external rotation recurvatum deformity. This technique combined with capsular repair and posterolateral capsular shift procedures mimics the function of the popliteus tendon-popliteofibular ligament and lateral collateral ligament, tightens the posterolateral capsule, and provides a post of strong allograft or autograft tissue to reinforce the posterolateral corner. When there is a disrupted proximal tibiofibular joint, or severe hyperextension external rotation recurvatum deformity (PLI type C), a two-tailed (fibular head, proximal tibia) posterolateral reconstruction is performed in addition to the posterolateral capsular shift procedure [5–8, 15, 17–30, 32, 43–45].

In acute cases, primary repair of all lateral side injured structures is performed with suture anchors, screws and washers, and permanent sutures through drill holes as indicated. The primary repair is then augmented with an allograft tissue reconstruction. Posterolateral reconstruction with the fibular head-based figure of eight posterolateral reconstruction surgical technique utilizes semitendinosus or other soft tissue allograft [17–19]. A curvilinear incision is made in the lateral aspect of the knee extending from the interval between Gerdy's tubercle and the fibular head to the lateral epicondyle and then proximal following the course of the iliotibial band. A peroneal nerve decompression and neurolysis are performed, and the peroneal nerve is protected throughout the procedure. The fibular head is identified, and a tunnel is created in an anterolateral to posteromedial direction at the area of maximal fibular head diameter.

The tunnel is created by passing a guide pin followed by a standard cannulated drill 7 mm in diameter. The peroneal nerve is protected during tunnel creation and throughout the procedure. The free tendon graft is passed through the fibular head drill hole. An incision is made in the iliotibial band in line with the fibers exposing the lateral femoral epicondyle area of the distal femur. The graft material is passed medial to the iliotibial band for the fibular collateral ligament limb and medial to the common biceps tendon and iliotibial band for the popliteus tendon popliteofibular ligament limb. The limbs of the graft are crossed to form a figure of eight with the fibular collateral ligament component being lateral to the popliteus tendon component.

A 3.2 mm drill hole is made to accommodate a 6.5-mm-diameter fully threaded cancellous screw that is approximately 35–40 mm in length. The drill hole is positioned in the lateral epicondylar region of the distal lateral femur so that after seating a 17–20 mm spiked ligament washer with the abovementioned screw, the washer will precisely secure the two limbs of the allograft tissue at the respective anatomic insertion sites of the fibular collateral ligament and popliteus tendon on the distal lateral femoral condyle. This drill hole is approximately 1 cm anterior to the fibular collateral ligament femoral insertion.

A longitudinal incision is made in the lateral capsule just posterior to the fibular collateral ligament, and the posterolateral capsular shift is performed. The graft material is tensioned at approximately 30–40 degrees of knee flexion, secured to the lateral femoral epicondylar region with a screw and spiked ligament washer at the abovementioned point. Fine-tuning of graft orientation is accomplished with multiple permanent braided sutures. The posterolateral capsule is then sewn into the strut of the figure of eight graft tissue material for additional reinforcement. The anterior and posterior limbs of the figure of eight graft material are sewn to each other to reinforce and tighten the construct.

The final graft tensioning position is approximately 30–40 degrees of knee flexion with a slight valgus force applied and slight internal tibial rotation. Number 2 non-absorbable suture is used to sew the tails of the graft together proximal to the washer to prevent slipping and also to sew the allograft to the deep capsular layers for additional reinforcement. The iliotibial band incision is closed. The procedures described are designed to eliminate posterolateral axial rotation and varus rotational instability.

When there is a disrupted proximal tibiofibular joint, or hyperextension external rotation recurvatum deformity (PLI type C), a two-tailed (fibular head, proximal tibia) posterolateral reconstruction is utilized combined with a posterolateral capsular shift [17–19]. A 7 or 8 mm drill hole is made over a guidewire approximately 2 cm below the lateral tibial plateau. Tibialis anterior or other soft tissue allograft is passed through this tibial drill hole and follows the course of the popliteus tendon to its anatomic insertion site on the lateral femoral epicondylar region. Nerves and blood vessels must be protected. The tibialis anterior or other soft tissue allograft is secured with a suture anchor and multiple number 2 braided non-absorbable sutures at the popliteus tendon anatomic femoral insertion site. The knee is cycled through multiple sets of full flexion and extension cycles, placed in 90 degrees of flexion, the tibia slightly internally rotated, slight valgus force applied to the knee, and the graft tensioned and secured in the tibial tunnel with a bioabsorbable interference screw and polyethylene ligament fixation button. The fibular head-based reconstruction and posterolateral capsular shift procedures are then carried out as described above. Number 2 permanent braided suture is used to sew the tails of the graft together proximal to the washer to prevent slipping and also to sew the allograft to the deep capsular layers for additional reinforcement.

Fibular Head-Based Figure of Eight Posterolateral Reconstruction Results

Isolated Posterolateral Reconstruction

Thirty-one knees with isolated type B chronic posterolateral instability were treated with a fibular head-based figure of eight posterolateral reconstruction using fresh frozen semitendinosus allograft combined with a posterolateral capsular shift [7, 8]. Mean postoperative follow-up was 2 years with a range of 1–6 years and a follow-up rate of 67.7% (21 of 31 knees available for follow-up evaluation). Postoperative evaluation was performed using physical examination and the Tegner, Lysholm, and Hospital for Special

Surgery Knee ligament rating scales. Physical examination compared the surgical knee to the normal knee using the dial test at 30° of knee flexion and the varus stress test at 30° and 0° of knee flexion and hyperextension.

Symmetrical varus stress tests were achieved in 95.2% of knees and grade I varus laxity in 4.8% of knees. The dial test was symmetrical to the normal knee in 95.2% and tighter (less external rotation) than the normal knee in 4.8% of knees. Range of motion was symmetrical to the normal knee in 85.7% of knees with loss of terminal flexion in 14.3% of the surgical knees compared to the normal knee. There were no flexion contractures in this series. The mean knee ligament rating scale scores were Lysholm 89.3/100 (range 67–100), Hospital for Special Surgery 82.2/100 (range 78–100), and Tegner 5.7/10 (range 3–9).

Combined ACL Posterolateral Reconstructions

Another study addressing combined anterior cruciate ligament and posterolateral reconstruction of the knee using allograft tissue in chronic knee injuries has been recently published (6). This study presents the results of 34 chronic combined anterior cruciate ligament with posterolateral reconstructions in 34 knees using allograft tissue and evaluating patient outcomes with KT 1000 knee ligament arthrometer and Lysholm, Tegner, and Hospital for Special Surgery knee ligament rating scales. Additionally, observations regarding patient demographics with combined ACL posterolateral instability, postoperative range of motion loss, post-injury degenerative joint disease, infection rate, return to function, and the use of radiated and non-irradiated allograft tissue were presented. Symmetrical physical examination of the surgical knee was achieved in 97% of Lachman, pivot shift tests, and varus stress tests. Ninety-four percent of dial tests are symmetrical, and 3% of dial tests are tighter than the normal side.

Combined PCL ACL Reconstruction with Mechanical Graft Tensioning

Results of multiple ligament injured knee treatment using mechanical graft tensioning are outlined below (43). This data presents the 2-year follow-up of 15 arthroscopically assisted ACL PCL reconstructions using the Biomet graft tensioning boot (Biomet Sports Medicine, Warsaw, Indiana). This study group consists of 11 chronic and 4 acute injuries. These injury patterns included six ACL PCL PLC injuries, four ACL PCL MCL injuries, and five ACL PCL PLC MCL injuries. The Biomet graft tensioning boot was used during the procedures as in the surgical technique described above. All knees had grade III preoperative ACL/PCL laxity and were assessed pre- and postoperatively using the Lysholm, Tegner, and Hospital for Special Surgery knee ligament rating scales, KT 1000 arthrometer testing, stress radiography, and physical examination.

Arthroscopically assisted combined ACL/PCL reconstructions were performed using the single incision endoscopic ACL technique and the single femoral tunnel-single bundle transtibial tunnel PCL technique. PCLs were reconstructed with allograft Achilles tendon in all 15 knees. ACLs were reconstructed with Achilles tendon allograft in all 15 knees. MCL injuries were treated surgically using primary repair, posteromedial capsular shift, and allograft augmentation as indicated. Posterolateral instability was treated with allograft semitendinosus free graft, with or without primary repair, and posterolateral capsular shift procedures as indicated. The Biomet graft tensioning boot was used in this series of patients.

Post-reconstruction physical examination results revealed normal posterior drawer/tibial step off in 13/15 (86.6%) of knees, normal Lachman test in 13/15 (86.6%) knees and normal pivot shift tests in 14/15 (93.3%) knees.

Posterolateral stability was restored to the level of the uninjured knee in all knees with posterolateral instability when evaluated with the external rotation thigh foot angle test also known as the dial test (nine knees equal to the normal knee and two knees tighter than the normal knee). Thirty-degree varus stress testing was restored to the level of the uninjured knee in all 11 knees with posterolateral lateral instability. Thirty- and zero-degree valgus stress testing were restored to the level of the uninjured knee normal in all nine knees with medial-sided laxity. This study demonstrates the effectiveness of posterolateral reconstruction using the fibular head-based figure of eight surgical technique combined with posterolateral capsular shift procedure in knee dislocations.

Multiple Ligament Reconstruction in Knees with Global Laxity with Long-Term Follow-Up

Two- to 18-year postsurgical results in combined PCL, ACL, medial, and lateral side knee injuries (global laxity) revealed the following information [44, 45]. Forty combined PCL-ACL-lateral-medial side (global laxity reconstructions) were performed by a single surgeon (GCF). Twenty-eight of 40 were available for 2- to 18-year follow-up (70% follow-up rate).

Varus and valgus stability were evaluated on physical examination at hyperextension and 0 and 30 degrees of knee flexion comparing the injured to the normal knee. Symmetrical varus stability was achieved in 93.3% of knees, and symmetrical valgus stability was achieved in 92.6% of knees. The dial test performed at 30 degrees of knee flexion to evaluate axial rotation posterolateral stability comparing the injured to the normal knee was symmetrical in 85.2%, tighter than the normal knee (less external rotation) in 11.1%, and more lax (greater external rotation) in 3.7% of knees. Thus, posterolateral axial rotation instability was corrected or overcorrected in 96.3% of knees.

Comparison of Surgical Techniques

A comparison of fibular head-based posterolateral reconstructions entitled "Surgical treatment of posterolateral instability of the knee with biceps tendon transfer procedures in posterolateral instability types A, B, and C" was presented at the Herodicus Society Annual Meeting [7, 8, 46]. The study compared the results of the full biceps tenodesis procedure, the split biceps tendon transfer procedure, and fibular head figure of eight posterolateral reconstruction procedure.

Conclusions from this study were that biceps femoris tendon transfer procedures provided excellent results for types A and B posterolateral instability of the knee when local autograft tissue is desired due to the inability to use allograft tissue. These results are applicable to both acute and chronic cases. Requirements for successful results with these biceps tendon transfer procedures include an intact proximal tibiofibular joint, intact posterolateral capsular attachments to the common biceps femoris tendon, and an intact common biceps femoris tendon insertion into the fibular head. Performing a concomitant posterolateral capsular shift procedure to reduce pathologic posterolateral and midlateral capsular laxity and capsular volume or reattaching avulsed midlateral and posterolateral capsule to bone is essential to the success of this surgical procedure. Biceps femoris tendon transfer procedures were not effective in restoring stability in cases of posterolateral instability type C.

Open Growth Plates

Posterolateral instability can occur in patients with open growth plates, and care must be taken during posterolateral reconstruction to preserve the physis. The fibular head-based figure of eight posterolateral reconstruction can be modified to protect the physis in patients with open growth plates. In acute cases, primary repair of all lateral side injured structures is performed with suture anchors and permanent sutures through drill holes as indicated. The primary repair is then augmented with an allograft tissue reconstruction. No fixation devices or bone plugs cross or violate the growth plates. Posterolateral reconstruction with the fibular head-based free graft figure of eight technique utilizes semitendinosus or other soft tissue allograft.

A lateral curvilinear incision is made. Dissection is carried down to the layer 1 fascia level. The peroneal nerve is identified, peroneal nerve neurolysis is performed, and the peroneal nerve is protected throughout the entire procedure. When the distal femoral growth plates are open, no hardware or drill holes are made on the lateral aspect of the knee. The common biceps tendon at its insertion into the fibular head is identified. A semitendinosus or other all soft tissue allograft is looped around the common biceps tendon insertion at the head of the fibula and sewn with number 2 permanent braided sutures where the common biceps tendon inserts into the fibular head. Care is taken to not damage the fibular physis.

The iliotibial band is incised in line with its fibers. Dissection is carried down to the anatomic insertion site of the fibular collateral ligament and the popliteus tendon. A longitudinal incision is made posterior and parallel to the fibular collateral ligament. This incision provides access to the posterolateral compartment of the knee to assess capsular insertion sites for primary repair and to enable the posterolateral capsular shift. Primary repair is performed as indicated. Posterolateral capsular shift is performed with permanent number 2 Ethibond suture.

The semitendinosus allograft limb positioned lateral to the common biceps femoris tendon is passed medial to the iliotibial band and parallel to the fibular collateral ligament. This represents the fibular collateral ligament arm of the fibular head-common biceps femoris tendon-based figure of eight posterolateral reconstruction. The semitendinosus allograft limb positioned medial to the common biceps femoris tendon is passed medial to the iliotibial band and medial to the fibular collateral ligament and parallel to the popliteus tendon. This limb represents the force vector of the popliteus tendon and popliteal fibular ligament. The two limbs of the semitendinosus allograft are sewn into the respective anatomic insertion sites of the fibular collateral ligament and popliteus tendon on the distal lateral aspect of the femur using number 2 permanent braided suture. The posterolateral capsule that had been previously incised is then shifted and sewn into the strut of figure of eight graft tissue material using number 2 permanent braided suture. The allograft tissue used for the posterolateral reconstruction is also sewn into the underlying fibular collateral ligament, popliteus tendon, and popliteofibular ligament also using number 2 permanent braided suture.

Throughout the procedure, there is protection of the fibula, tibia, and femoral physes and the peroneal nerve. At the completion of the lateral side procedure, the wound is thoroughly irrigated and closed in layers. Results evaluated with arthrometer measurements, stress radiography, and knee ligament rating scales demonstrate results similar to those achieved in adult patient populations with no incidence of growth arrest and resultant angular deformity about the knee after surgical intervention [8, 16, 47–50].

Postoperative Rehabilitation

The knee is maintained in full extension for 3–5 weeks non-weight bearing. This initial period of immobilization is followed by progressive range of motion and progressive weight bearing. Progressive closed kinetic chain strength training, proprioceptive training, and continued motion exercises are initiated very slowly beginning at postoperative week 11. The long leg range of motion brace is discontinued after the tenth week, and the patient may wear a global laxity functional brace for all activities for additional protection if necessary. Return to sports and heavy labor occur after the 12th postoperative month when sufficient strength, range of motion, and proprioceptive skills have returned [8, 51–54]. It is very important to carefully observe these complex knee ligament injury patients and get a feel for the "personality of the knee." The surgeon may need to make adjustments and individualize the postoperative rehabilitation program as necessary. Careful and gentle range of motion under general anesthesia is a very useful tool in the treatment of these complex cases and is utilized as necessary.

Case Presentation

The patient is a 39-year-old male who presents with right knee pain. The patient reports that his right knee buckled as he was getting off of a golf cart. This was followed by pain and swelling with difficulty ambulating long distances. He has a history of a right ACL reconstruction done 10 years prior with a BTB autograft and partial lateral meniscectomy.

On exam, he has healed prior surgical incisions with a moderate effusion. His range of motion was full extension to 130 degrees of flexion. A grade IIB Lachman was present, as well as 2+ opening to varus stress at 30 degrees and a 15–20-degree difference in external rotation at 30 degrees of knee flexion (Fig. 12.1). There was mild laxity on posterolateral drawer testing. There was no instability at full extension, nor was recurvatum present.

Alignment films and plane radiographs demonstrated neutral alignment with a vertical femoral tunnel position (Fig. 12.2). An MRI was obtained which showed rupture of the prior ACL graft with an intact LCL, biceps tendon, and popliteus (Fig. 12.3). The patient was indicated for revision ACL reconstruction with quadriceps autograft and posterolateral corner reconstruction.

Under anesthesia, the patient had a grade IIB Lachman and positive pivot shift. Again, he had increased laxity with posterolateral drawer and a 15-degree increase in external rotation at 30 degrees of flexion. A standard diagnostic arthroscopy was performed; there was noted to be complete rupture of the prior graft. Additionally, there was a drive-through sign in the lateral compartment. The prior graft was debrided, and tunnels were examined. Previous tunnels were deemed to without expansion, and new tunnels were reamed with 10 mm reamers. The graft was passed and secured with interference screws.

Attention was then turned to the posterolateral corner reconstruction which was performed through a separate incision. A 12 cm hockey stick incision was made from halfway between Gerdy's tubercle and the fibular head distally and extended proximally to the level of the lateral epicondyle. The peroneal nerve was located and found to be intact, and a 7 cm neurolysis was performed. The fibular head was then skeletonized, and a tunnel was drilled from anterior to posterior erring distal

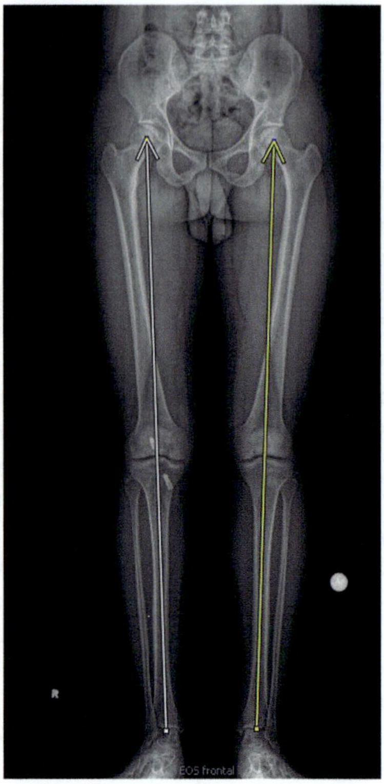

Fig. 12.2 Alignment films demonstrating neutral, bilateral alignment

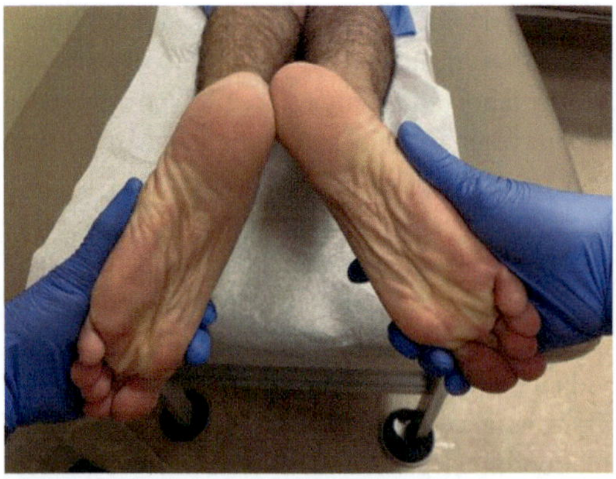

Fig. 12.1 Prone clinical image demonstrating significantly increased external rotation of the right limb at 30 degrees of knee flexion

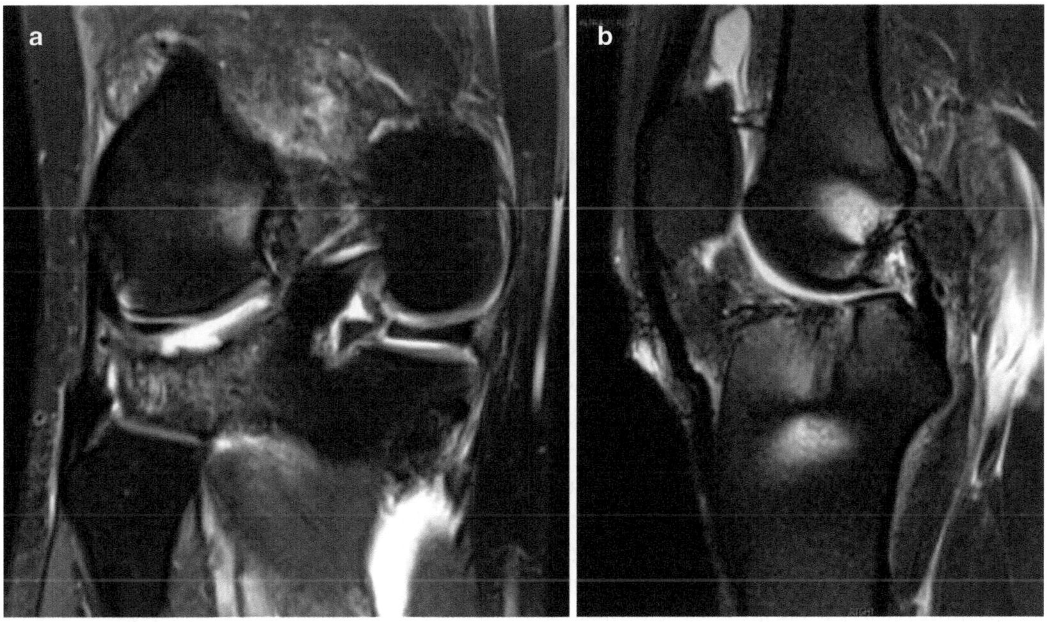

Fig. 12.3 (**a**) Coronal MRI demonstrating intact LCL and posterior horn medial meniscus tear. (**b**) Sagittal MRI demonstrating complete rupture of prior ACL graft

to proximal about 2 cm distal to the tip of the fibular head. A window was made in the IT band, and the lateral collateral ligament was found to be intact, but significantly attenuated. A horizontal arthrotomy was made over the epicondyle, and the popliteus tendon was visualized and found to be intact. Guidewires were then placed at the LCL origin. A hamstring allograft was prepared and was passed through the LCL tunnel with sutures out of the medial skin for tensions, and the graft was then passed through the fibula. The graft was fixed in the femur with an interference screw and then tensioned at 30 degrees of flexion with minimal internal rotation and valgus force applied and was then fixed to the fibula with an interference screw. Finally, a posterolateral capsular imbrication was performed to back up the reconstruction and provide more posterolateral stability. At this point, the knee was found to have a grade IA Lachman, was stable to posterolateral stress, and had equal external rotation at 30°.

Postoperatively, the patient did well and participated in standard postoperative therapy protocol. To date, the patient remains with a stable knee and is back to his preoperative activities.

Our treatment algorithm for PLC reconstruction is guided by physical exam and preoperative imaging. In this patient, examination revealed moderate rotational laxity without recurvatum which is why a fibular-based reconstruction was utilized with a capsular shift. In patients with more significant injury pattern, a two-tailed is certainly considered.

Summary

Accurate physical examination is essential for the diagnosis of posterolateral instability to identify the pathologic planes of instability, especially the type A posterolateral instability pattern. It is important to remember that MRI enhances the physical examination; however, the MRI may be "negative" in chronic situation even with an abnormal physical examination. Surgical timing in acute posterolateral instability is determined by the severity of the injury. Posterolateral instability types A and B are typically done as a single-stage operation within 3 to 4 weeks post-injury, and type C is typically done as a two-stage procedure. Specific patient considerations may affect surgical timing.

The surgical treatment goal is to correct pathologic external rotation, varus laxity, and hyperextension external rotation recurvatum. Posterolateral corner injuries treated with primary repair combined with reconstruction are more successful than primary repair alone. The fibular head-based figure of eight posterolateral reconstruction surgical technique combined with a posterolateral capsular shift is indicated when the heel lift test is symmetrical to the normal lower extremity and with varus laxity that diminishes from 30 degrees of knee flexion to hyperextension. A two-tailed posterolateral reconstruction, consisting of fibular head-based figure of eight posterolateral reconstruction combined with a popliteus bypass graft and posterolateral capsular shift, is indicated when the heel lift off test is positive, cases of revision posterolateral reconstruction, and proximal tibiofibular joint instability. It is essential to always address the midlateral and posterolateral capsule with either primary capsular repair, capsular shift, or a combination of the two.

Peroneal nerve decompression and neurolysis are always performed with posterolateral reconstruction surgical techniques. Screw and washer fixation of the graft allows adjustability of the tension of the reconstruction. No single surgical technique is best for every case of posterolateral instability, so the surgical procedure should be tailored to the specific case. Lower extremity alignment is very important for the success of posterolateral reconstruction surgical procedure, and osteotomies are to be performed as indicated. Recognition and correction of posterolateral instability and posteromedial instability is essential for successful posterior and anterior cruciate ligament surgery [8, 16].

References

1. Fanelli GC, Desai B, Cummings PD, Hanks G, Kalenak A. Divergent alignment of the femoral interference screw in single incision endoscopic reconstruction of the ACL. Contemp Orthop. 1994;28(1):21–5.
2. Fanelli GC, Edson CJ, Maish DR. Revision ACL reconstruction. Associated patholaxity, tibiofemoral malalignment, rehabilitation, and results. Am J Knee Surg. 2001;14(3):1–4.
3. Bleday RM, Fanelli GC, Giannotti BF, Edson CJ, Barrett TA. Instrumented measurement of the posterolateral corner. Arthroscopy. 1998;14(5):489–94.
4. Fanelli GC, Feldman DD. Management of combined anterior cruciate ligament/posterior cruciate ligament/posterolateral complex injuries of the knee. Oper Tech Sports Med. 1999;7(3):143–9.
5. Fanelli GC, Larson RV. Practical management of posterolateral instability of the knee. Arthroscopy. 2002;18(2) {February, Supplement 1}:1–8.
6. Fanelli GC, Fanelli DG, Edson CJ, Fanelli MG. Combined anterior cruciate ligament and posterolateral reconstruction of the knee using allograft tissue in chronic knee injuries. J Knee Surg. 2014;27(5):353–8.
7. Fanelli GC, Fanelli DG. Fibular head based posterolateral reconstruction of the knee combined with capsular shift procedure. Sports Med Arthrosc Rev. 2015;23(1):33–43.
8. Fanelli GC. Fibular head based posterolateral reconstruction of the knee: surgical technique and outcomes. J Knee Surg. 2015;28(6):455–63.
9. Muller W, editor. The knee: form, function, and ligamentous reconstruction. New York: Springer; 1983.
10. Skyhar MJ, Warren RF, Oritz GJ, et al. The effects of sectioning the posterior cruciate ligament and the posterolateral complex on the articular contact pressure within the knee. J Bone Joint Surg Am. 1993;75:694–9.
11. Veltri DM, Warren RF. Posterolateral instability of the knee. J Bone Joint Surg. 1994;76-A:460–72.
12. Fanelli GC. PCL injuries in trauma patients. Arthroscopy. 1993;9:291–4.
13. Fanelli GC, Edson CJ. PCL injuries in trauma patients: Part II. Arthroscopy. 1995;11(5):526–9.
14. Fanelli GC, Giannotti BF, Edson CJ. Current concepts review. The posterior cruciate ligament arthroscopic evaluation and treatment. Arthroscopy. 1994;10(6):673–88.
15. Fanelli GC, Orcutt DR, Edson CJ. Current concepts: the multiple ligament injured knee. Arthroscopy. 2005;21(4):471–86.
16. Fanelli GC. The multiple ligament injured knee: what I have learned. In: Fanelli GC, editor. The multiple ligament injured knee. A practical guide to management. Third ed. Springer Nature Switzerland AG. Cham: Switzerland; 2019. p. 3–21.
17. Fanelli GC. Rationale and surgical technique for PCL and multiple knee ligament reconstruction. Third ed. Warsaw: Biomet Sports Medicine; 2012.
18. Fanelli GC. Surgical treatment of combined PCL ACL medial and lateral side injuries (global laxity): acute and chronic. In: Fanelli GC, editor. The multiple ligament injured knee. A practical guide to management. Third ed. Springer Nature Switzerland AG. Cham: Switzerland; 2019. p. 295–316.
19. Fanelli GC. Combined PCL, ACL, posteromedial, and posterolateral reconstruction. In: Fanelli GC, editor.

Posterior cruciate ligament injuries. A practical guide to management. Second ed. New York: Springer; 2015. p. 173–88.
20. Arciero RA. Anatomic posterolateral corner knee reconstruction. Arthroscopy. 2005;21:1147.
21. Bicos J, Arciero RA. Novel approach for reconstruction of the posterolateral corner using a free tendon graft technique. Sports Med Arthrosc Rev. 2006;14:28–36.
22. Shi SY, Ying XZ, Zheng Q, Cao GP. Isometric reconstruction of the posterolateral corner of the knee. Acta Orthop Belg. 2009;75:504–11.
23. Niki Y, Matsumoto H, Otani T, Enomoto H, Toyama Y, Suda Y. A modified Larson's method of posterolateral corner reconstruction of the knee reproducing the physiological tensioning pattern of the lateral collateral and popliteofibular ligaments. Sports Med Arthrosc Rehabil Ther Technol. 2012;4:21.
24. Veltri DM, Warren RF. Operative treatment of posterolateral instability of the knee. Clin Sports Med. 1994;13(3):615–27.
25. Baker CL Jr, Norwood LA, Hughston JC. Acute combined posterior cruciate and posterolateral instability of the knee. Am J Sports Med. 1984;12(3):204–8.
26. Yoon KH, Bae DK, Ha JH, Park SW. Anatomic reconstructive surgery for posterolateral instability of the knee. Arthroscopy. 2006;22(2):159–65.
27. Stannard JP, Brown SL, Farris RC, McGwin G, Volgas DA. The posterolateral corner of the knee: repair versus reconstruction. Am J Sports Med. 2005;33:881–8.
28. Levy BA, Dajani KA, Morgan JA, Shah JP, Dahm DL, Stuart MJ. Repair versus reconstruction of the fibular collateral ligament and posterolateral corner in the multiligament-injured knee. Am J Sports Med. 2010;38:804–9.
29. Leiter JRS, Levy BA, Stannard JP, Fanelli GC, Whelan DB, Marx RG, Stuart MJ, Boyd JL, McDonald PB. Accuracy and reliability of determining the isometric point of the knee for multiligament knee reconstruction. Knee Surg Sports Traumatol Arthrosc. 2014;22:2187–93.
30. Sidles JA, Larson RV, Garbini JL, et al. Ligament length relationships in the moving knee. J Orthop Res. 1988;6:593–610.
31. Wascher DC, Grauer JD, Markoff KL. Biceps tendon tenodesis for posterolateral instability of the knee. An in vitro study. Am J Sports Med. 1993;21(3):400–6.
32. Fanelli GC. Surgical reconstruction for acute posterolateral injury of the knee. J Knee Surg. 2005;28(2):157–62.
33. Fanelli GC, Giannotti BF, Edson CJ. Arthroscopically assisted combined anterior and posterior cruciate ligament reconstruction. Arthroscopy. 1996;12(1):5–14.
34. Fanelli GC, Giannotti BF, Edson CJ. Arthroscopically assisted combined posterior cruciate ligament/posterior lateral complex reconstruction. Arthroscopy. 1996;12(5):521–30.
35. Fanelli GC, Edson CJ. Arthroscopically assisted combined ACL/PCL reconstruction. 2-10 year follow-up. Arthroscopy. 2002;18(7):703–14.
36. Fanelli GC, Edson CJ. Combined posterior cruciate ligament –posterolateral reconstruction with Achilles tendon allograft and biceps femoris tendon tenodesis: 2-10 year follow-up. Arthroscopy. 2004;20(4):339–45.
37. Levy B, Fanelli GC, Whalen D, Stannard J, MacDonald P, Boyd J, Marx R, Stuart M. Modern perspectives for the treatment of knee dislocations and multiligament reconstruction. J Am Acad Orthop Surg. 2009;17(4):197–206.
38. Levy B, Dajani KA, Whalen DB, Stannard JP, Fanelli GC, Stuart MJ, Boyd JL, MacDonald PA, Marx RG. Decision making in the multiple ligament injured knee: an evidence based systematic review. Arthroscopy. 2009;25(4):430–8.
39. Fanelli GC, Stannard JP, Stuart MJ, MacDonald PB, Marx RG, Whelan DB, Boyd JL, Levy BA. Management of complex knee ligament injuries. J Bone Joint Surg. 2010;92-A(12):2235–46.
40. Fanelli GC. Surgical treatment of lateral posterolateral instability of the knee using biceps femoris tendon procedures. Sports Med Arthrosc Rev. 2006;14(1):37–43.
41. Noyes FR, Barber-Westin SD, Hewett TE. High tibial osteotomy and ligament reconstruction for varus angulated anterior cruciate ligament-deficient knees. Am J Sports Med. 2000;28:282–96.
42. Clancy WG Jr. Repair and reconstruction of the posterior cruciate ligament. In: Chapman MW, editor. Operative orthopaedics. Philadelphia: JB Lippincott; 1998. p. 1651–65.
43. Fanelli GC, Edson CJ, Orcutt DR, Harris JD, Zijerdi D. Treatment of combined ACL-PCL-MCL-PLC injuries of the knee. J Knee Surg. 2005;18(3):240–8.
44. Fanelli GC, Edson CJ. Surgical treatment of combined PCL, ACL, medial, and lateral side injuries (global laxity): surgical technique and 2 to 18 year results. J Knee Surg. 2012;25(4):307–16.
45. Fanelli GC, Sousa P, Edson CJ. Long term followup of surgically treated knee dislocations: stability restored, but arthritis is common. Clin Orthop Relat Res. 2014;472(9):2712–7.
46. Fanelli GC. Surgical treatment of posterolateral instability of the knee with biceps tendon transfer procedures. In: 32nd Annual Herodicus Society Meeting, Hershey, 25–28 June 2006.
47. Fanelli GC, Fanelli DG. Multiple ligament injured knee in patients eighteen years of age and younger. In: Fanelli GC, editor. The multiple ligament injured knee. A practical guide to management. Third ed. Springer Nature Switzerland AG. Cham: Switzerland; 2019. p. 507–21.
48. Fanelli GC, Fanelli DG. Knee dislocations in patients 18 years of age and younger. Surgical technique and outcomes. J Knee Surg. 2016;29(4):269–77.
49. Fanelli GC, Fanelli DG. Multiple ligament knee injuries in the pediatric population. J Knee Surg. 2018;31(5):399–409.
50. Fanelli GC, Tomaschewski D. Allograft use in the treatment of the multiple ligament injured knee. Sports Med Arthrosc Rev. 2007;15(3):139–48.

51. Fanelli GC, Beck JD, Edson CJ. Postoperative rehabilitation of the posterior cruciate ligament. Sports Med Arthrosc Rev. 2010;18(4):275–9.
52. Edson CJ, Fanelli GC, Beck JD. Rehabilitation after multiple ligament reconstruction of the knee. Sports Med Arthrosc Rev. 2011;19(2):162–6.
53. Edson CJ. Rehabilitation following PCL reconstruction: scientific and theoretical basis. In: Fanelli GC, editor. Posterior cruciate ligament injuries. A practical guide to management. Second ed. New York: Springer; 2015. p. 311–20.
54. Edson CJ, Fanelli GC. Postoperative rehabilitation of the multiple ligament injured knee. In: Fanelli GC, editor. The multiple ligament injured knee. A practical guide to management. Third ed. Springer Nature Switzerland AG. Cham: Switzerland; 2019. p. 551–8.

13 Coronal Malalignment and Revision Anterior Cruciate Ligament Reconstruction

Paul M. Incan and Matthew J. Matava

Introduction

Reconstruction of the anterior cruciate ligament (ACL) is uniformly successful with long-term failure rates of approximately 10% (range, 2–26%) [1–3]. In general, the primary cause of failure can be due to either traumatic reinjury, biologic failure of graft incorporation, or surgical error. In some cases, a combination of these factors may be responsible. It has been widely assumed, based on expert opinion and case series, that the majority of failures can be attributed to either identifiable trauma or tunnel malposition [4, 5]. Osseous malalignment may also be a contributing cause of ACL reconstruction failure due to the tensile strain it places on the graft. This excessive tensile force may occur in the sagittal plane due to an elevated posterior tibial slope [6, 7]. As axial loading through the tibiofemoral joint occurs, vertical shear forces are converted to anteriorly directed tibial translation resulting in increased ACL strain.

Coronal plane malalignment is more commonly encountered in the revision setting and may be due to either congenital bilateral, or acquired unilateral, genu varum or valgum. This chapter will focus on coronal plane malalignment, which may be either a causative factor in primary ACL reconstruction failure or the end result of associated meniscal and/or chondral injury in these patients. In both cases, the unaddressed malalignment may compromise the revision reconstruction and exacerbate any preexisting cartilage damage. Surgical strategies must consider both the technical aspects of the revision reconstruction and the influence of a concurrent realignment procedure, which increases the complexity and risk for complications.

Individuals undergoing revision ACL reconstruction are significantly more likely to demonstrate varus malalignment than individuals undergoing primary reconstruction [8]. Noyes and Barber-Weston found that varus malalignment was a factor contributing to ACL reconstruction failure in 25% of their patients [9]. Varus malalignment has also been shown to predict the development of medial compartment osteoarthritis [10]. The status of the menisci and the alignment of the lower extremity are both likely to influence the prevalence of chondrosis in the medial and lateral tibiofemoral compartments at the time of revision reconstruction. Knees undergoing revision surgery have been shown to have more concomitant intra-articular injuries than knees undergoing primary reconstruction [11]. Ninety percent of knees undergoing revision ACL reconstruction have been found to have meniscal or chondral injury, and 57% had both [12]. Meniscal injury [13, 14] and the amount of

P. M. Incan · M. J. Matava (✉)
Department of Orthopaedic Surgery, Washington University School of Medicine, St. Louis, MO, USA

M. J. Alaia, K. J. Jones (eds.), *Revision Anterior Cruciate Ligament Reconstruction*,
https://doi.org/10.1007/978-3-030-96996-7_13

meniscus removed at the time of prior surgery [15] have been shown to be associated with the subsequent development of arthrosis. Partial meniscectomies occurring prior to revision ACL reconstruction are associated with a higher rate of chondrosis at the time of revision surgery compared with previous meniscal repair or no prior meniscal surgery [16]. Therefore, progressive coronal plane malalignment may arise from the associated meniscal and/or chondral damage from the prior injury and surgery.

Alternatively, tibiofemoral degeneration may be the result of an unaddressed coronal malalignment at the time of the primary reconstruction [4]. Irrespective of etiology, clinical and radiographic assessment of coronal plane alignment is a necessary component of the evaluation and management of patients requiring revision ACL reconstruction in order to prevent failure of the revision graft and to relieve symptoms resulting from tibiofemoral degeneration [17].

Coronal Plane Malalignment and Primary ACL Failure

The relationship between coronal malalignment and ACL graft failure must be understood from a biomechanical perspective. In the static knee, varus malalignment increases the tensile force on the ACL by up to 25% and is greatest with the knee in full extension [18]. This effect is exacerbated in patients with associated posterolateral ligamentous insufficiency [9]. Axial loading of the maligned knee during gait results in a dynamic varus force (increased adduction moment) [19], leading to cyclical lateral joint space diastasis [18]. This "varus thrust" results in increased tensile force transmitted to the ACL graft throughout the gait cycle, with ACL tension increasing linearly as the mechanical axis medializes [18, 20]. A pathologic condition is created that is functionally opposite of the mechanically neutral knee, which demonstrates joint space compression with axial load [18]. Furthermore, as the lateral soft tissues of the knee (i.e., the posterolateral corner [PLC], joint capsule, and iliotibial band) experience cyclical loading and resultant attenuation, lateral joint space separation may be accentuated resulting in even greater tension on the ACL throughout the gait cycle [21]. Therefore, varus malalignment results in both static and dynamic ACL graft strain, which may predispose the graft to either attritional or acute failure. Interestingly, the forces resulting from the elevated adduction moments associated with a varus thrust have not correlated with static alignment radiographs [19].

The spectrum between osseous malalignment and dynamic soft tissue attenuation is best conceptualized through the principle of the "primary," "double," and "triple varus" knee, as conceptualized by Noyes [21]. In the "primary varus" knee, the deformity is limited to the osseous alignment of the lower extremity [21]. Though such skeletal malalignment may be seen as an anatomic variant, the 30–40% rate of concurrent medial meniscal tears seen with ACL rupture [4, 22, 23] and resultant acceleration in chondral degeneration [24] may account for the relatively high rate of primary varus seen in patients undergoing revision ACL reconstruction [8]. With increasing osseous malalignment, the lateral soft tissues attenuate, as discussed above, allowing the lateral femoral condyle to separate ("lift-off") from the lateral tibial plateau during gait, resulting in the "double varus" knee. The quadriceps, biceps femoris, iliotibial band, and gastrocnemius muscles act dynamically to resist the adduction moment encountered during the gait cycle in an attempt to reduce the lateral condylar lift-off. If this dynamic restraint is insufficient, then lateral tibiofemoral separation ensues. Skeletal varus combined with insufficiency of the PLC [25] resulting in lateral tibiofemoral separation (dynamic varus) may be associated with recurvatum in extension resulting in the "triple varus" knee [21]. In these patients, varus recurvatum results in excessive external tibial rotation and hyperextension due to long-standing insufficiency of the PLC and often the ACL and/or posterior cruciate ligament (PCL). In these patients, both the ACL and PLC insufficiency must be corrected in addition to the osseous malalignment.

Clinical Evaluation

The physical examination for the patient being evaluated for a revision ACL reconstruction has been thoroughly outlined in prior chapters. The comprehensive assessment of a patient with a failed ACL reconstruction begins with an inspection of standing alignment and gait. It is imperative that the patient's lower extremities are exposed during the examination. Simple observation of the patient standing upright with the feet comfortably apart can provide information as to the presence of unilateral or bilateral coronal plane malalignment. Unilateral malalignment is usually an acquired deformity, whereas bilateral malalignment is more likely a normal anatomic variant. Bilateral malalignment results in either a "bow-legged" (genu varum) or a "knock-kneed" posture (genu valgum). An assessment of gait can be performed in any office setting and is most commonly accomplished while the patient simply walks down a hallway.

The most common gait abnormality in these patients is a varus thrust, described previously, which consists of a visible increase in tibiofemoral varus during the weight-bearing phase of the gait cycle with return to neutral alignment during the late stance phase [26]. Varus recurvatum may also be noted in the sagittal plane as an indicator of advanced insufficiency of the PLC resulting in hyperextension and external tibial rotation seen in the "triple varus" knee. A valgus thrust is less common and usually encountered with chronic attenuation of the superficial medial collateral ligament (sMCL). It is an exacerbation or abrupt onset of valgus malalignment during the stance phase, with a return to a more neutral alignment during lift-off and the swing phase of gait. In theory, a valgus thrust increases the compressive load transmitted to the lateral tibiofemoral compartment, potentially contributing to lateral compartment osteoarthritis. A formal gait analysis is typically reserved for those patients with significant gait alterations or for those in whom formal attempts at correction have been unsuccessful. Any preexisting gait abnormality should be corrected prior to the revision surgery with a 6-week program of gait training under the guidance of an experienced physical therapist. Correction of a varus thrust can be addressed with maintenance of a toe-out position during the gait cycle while maintaining a shortened stride length with the knee in 5° of flexion on initial heel strike. Failure to correct any preexisting gait abnormality will place the revision ACL graft and posterolateral structures at risk.

It is important to emphasize that the physical examination in these patients should be comprehensive in order to diagnose all clinically relevant conditions that may affect the final outcome (Table 13.1). The patellofemoral joint should be evaluated as a potential source of pain and instability due to the combined effects of increased external tibial rotation and varus recurvatum. Medial compartment pain and crepitus with varus malalignment may indicate articular cartilage and/or meniscal damage or insufficiency. Lateral compartment pain is more commonly due to soft tissue tensile overload but may also result from articular cartilage and meniscal damage with valgus malalignment.

Knee range of motion and instability testing should be compared with the contralateral knee. The Lachman test is performed at 30° of knee flexion and is the most sensitive test to detect ACL insufficiency. The pivot shift test is most specific for ACL insufficiency and is recorded on a scale of 0–3, with a grade of 0 indicating no pivot shift; grade 1 represents a pivot glide; grade 2 is defined as a distinct "clunk" indicative of subluxation of the posterior aspect of the lateral tibial plateau over the lateral femoral condyle; and grade 3 is represented as gross impingement of the lateral tibial plateau against the lateral femoral condyle. The anterior drawer is also assessed but is the least sensitive or specific test for ACL insufficiency.

The PCL is evaluated with direct observation of posterior tibial subluxation with the knee at 90° of flexion ("sag sign") compared to the contralateral knee. The medial tibiofemoral step-off is palpated with the knee at 90° with a 1 cm step-off considered normal and lesser amounts indicative of progressive posterior tibial subluxation. The posterior drawer test is also performed at 90° of flexion to confirm (1) the status of the PCL and

Table 13.1 Physical examination tests in the evaluation of patients with combined ACL insufficiency and coronal plane malalignment

Standing alignment
Gait assessment
Varus thrust
Varus recurvatum thrust
Active and passive range of motion
Patellofemoral examination
Alignment
Tracking
Compression pain
Crepitus
Anterior cruciate ligament
Lachman exam at 30°
Pivot shift
Anterior drawer
Posterior cruciate ligament
"Sag" sign
Tibiofemoral step-off
Posterior drawer
Quadriceps active test
Varus stress
Varus laxity at 30° *only* indicates isolated LCL injury
Varus laxity at 0° and 30° indicates both LCL and ACL injury
Dial test
>10° external rotation asymmetry at 30° only consistent with isolated PLC injury
>10° external rotation asymmetry at 30°and 90° consistent with PLC and PCL injury
External rotation recurvatum
Leg falls into external rotation and recurvatum when suspended by great toe in supine position
More common with chronic, multi-ligament injuries (i.e., ACL/PCL and PLC)
Posterolateral drawer test
Combined posterior drawer and external rotation force results in an increase in posterolateral tibial translation
Reverse pivot shift test
External rotation and valgus force applied to tibia as the knee is extended from 90° with a palpable clunk as the lateral tibial plateau reduces past the lateral femoral condyle at 20° of flexion to a reduced position in full extension

ACL anterior cruciate ligament, *LCL* lateral collateral ligament, *PLC* posterolateral corner

(2) that the tibia is not posteriorly subluxated indicating a partial or complete PCL tear which may give a false positive anterior drawer test. Posterior tibial translation is confirmed with the quadriceps active test in which the tibia translates anteriorly at 80° of flexion with active quadriceps.

Insufficiency of the lateral collateral ligament (LCL) is assessed by the application of varus stress at 0° and 30° of knee flexion. The quality of the endpoint and degree of lateral joint space opening (in millimeters) are compared to the contralateral normal knee. Patients with combined insufficiency of the ACL and LCL will have increased laxity at both 0° and 30° of knee flexion. It is important to distinguish true ligamentous laxity with varus stress from the false positive ("pseudolaxity") caused by loss of the lateral compartment articular cartilage. This can be avoided by initially applying a valgus and axial load. With pseudolaxity, the lateral joint opening noted with a varus stress returns the limb from a relative valgus alignment to a more neutral position and confirms the absence of true lateral ligamentous damage. The dial test is performed at both 30° and 90° of flexion with the patient prone or supine to indicate damage to the PLC. An asymmetric increase of 10° in the foot-thigh angle with the knee at 30° is indicative of isolated deficiency of the PLC, whereas a positive test at both 30° and 90° of flexion is indicative of combined injury to the PLC and PCL. The external rotation recurvatum test is positive for combined severe injury to the PLC and ACL when the knee falls into hyperextension and external tibial rotation while the lower limb is suspended from the great toe. The reverse pivot shift is indicated by a palpable reduction of the externally mal-rotated lateral tibial plateau across the lateral femoral condyle at 20° as the knee is extended from 90° to full extension.

An increase in medial joint space opening is also assessed at both 0° and 30° of flexion to identify associated damage to the sMCL in patients with valgus malalignment. The quality of the endpoint and degree of joint space opening (in millimeters) are determined and compared to the contralateral normal knee. Similar to assessing the lateral soft tissues, a false positive result may occur from "pseudolaxity" attributed to medial compartment narrowing associated with articular cartilage loss. This can be avoided by conducting the exam first with a varus and axial load applied. With pseudolaxity, the medial joint opening noted with a valgus stress returns the limb from a relative varus alignment to a more neutral position and confirms the absence of true medial ligamentous damage.

Radiographic Evaluation

Plain Radiographs

Initial radiographic evaluation of the knee should include an anteroposterior (AP), 30° lateral, patellofemoral (Merchant), and 45° flexion-weight-bearing posteroanterior (Rosenberg) [27] views. The lateral radiograph requires reasonable superimposition of the femoral condyles as alterations in patellar "height" may occur with high tibial osteotomy (HTO) [28]; therefore, presence of preexisting patella alta or baja must be appreciated. For this purpose, the Blackburn-Peel and Caton-Deschamps ratios produce the most reliable means of quantifying patellar height both preoperatively and following surgical intervention [29]. Additionally, elevated posterior tibial slope (>12°) should also be noted on the lateral radiograph because of the potentially deleterious effects it has on the ACL graft [30] discussed previously that may be corrected concurrently with coronal plane realignment [31]. An AP view with the knee in full extension may not show significant joint space narrowing since most condylar wear is present between 30° and 60° of knee flexion which is best identified with the 45° flexion, weight-bearing view (Fig. 13.1). Excessive medial or lateral compartment joint space narrowing greater than 50% of the articular cartilage thickness represents a relative contraindication to an osteotomy, as the articular degeneration is likely too great to be relieved solely by a realignment procedure [8].

Comprehensive radiographs can provide relevant information regarding the presence of hardware from prior surgery as well as femoral and tibial tunnel placement and their dimensions. Bone tunnel widening is theorized to be due to a complex interplay between biologic factors (i.e., synovial fluid-derived cytokines, inflammatory mediators, thermal necrosis) and mechanical stress (i.e., graft motion ["bungee cord" effect], non-aperture fixation, graft tension) [32–34]. Seen most commonly with the use of allograft tissues [34] and soft tissue grafts, tunnel expansion does not appear to be the cause of ACL graft failure but may affect the technical aspects of the revision reconstruction (Fig. 13.2).

Full-length standing AP radiographs from the hips to the ankles with the feet 10″ apart should also be performed on all patients considered for revision ACL reconstruction [17]. Though some surgeons may prefer standing single-leg or supine full-length radiographs [35], we prefer bilateral whole-limb radiographs for the evaluation of limb alignment (Fig. 13.3). Subtle positional changes of the extremity can significantly alter the mechanical axis measurements [36]. Therefore, reference foot templates on the radiograph platform and centering the patella over the femoral condyles may be necessary to ensure reproducible radiographs [8, 17].

The mechanical axis of the lower extremity is defined by a line connecting the center of the femoral head to the middle of the tibial plafond. In individuals with a neutral mechanical axis, this line should intersect the mid-line of the tibial plateau between the tibial spines [37]. Coronal plane deformity may be quantified as a percentage of tibial width where the mechanical axis intersects the tibia plateau. By convention, 0% indicates the medial tibial cortex, and 100% represents the lateral tibial cortex [38]. The mechanical axis of the femur is represented by a line connecting the center of the femoral head and the intercondylar notch. The mechanical axis of the tibia is represented by a line connecting the center of the tibial plafond and bisecting the tibial plateau (Fig. 13.4). These axis lines intersect to form the mechanical tibiofemoral angle, which normally forms essentially a straight line as the normal angle has been shown to be −0.7 ± 3° [37]. Increasing varus or valgus deformity, defined as the apex of the deformity at the tibiofemoral joint, results in an increase or decrease of this angle, respectively. As discussed below, the tibio-

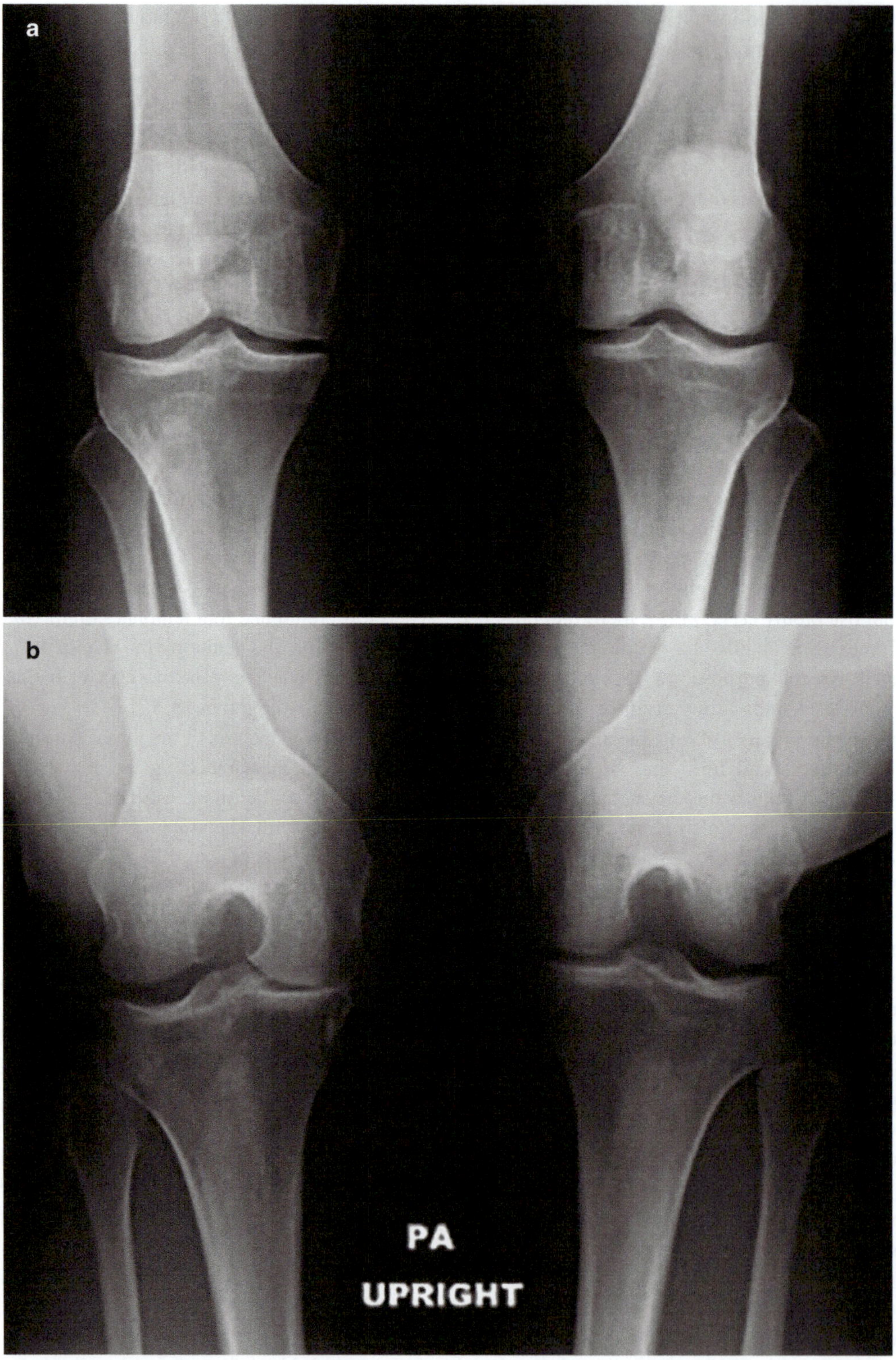

Fig. 13.1 Radiographs showing the importance of the flexion weight-bearing view in the same patient. (**a**) AP weight-bearing view showing maintenance of joint space. (**b**) 40° PA weight-bearing view illustrating loss of medial joint space of the right knee

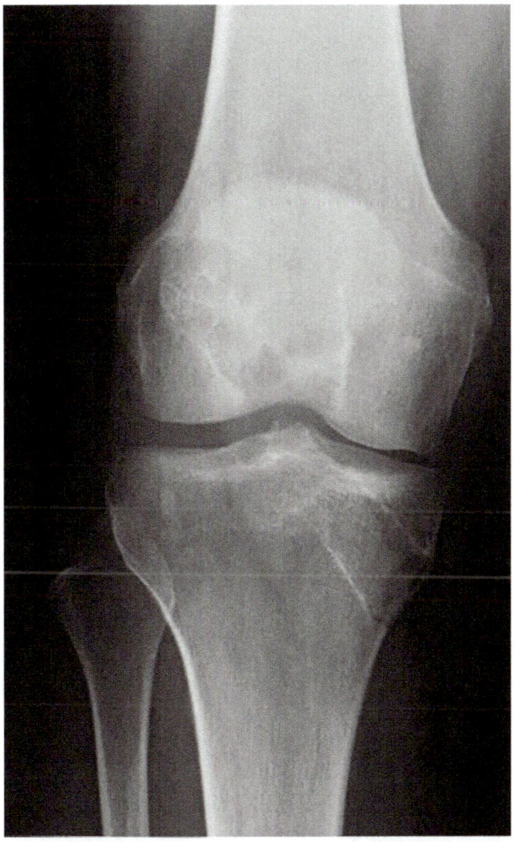

Fig. 13.2 AP radiograph showing femoral and tibial tunnel expansion often seen in patients undergoing revision ACL reconstruction

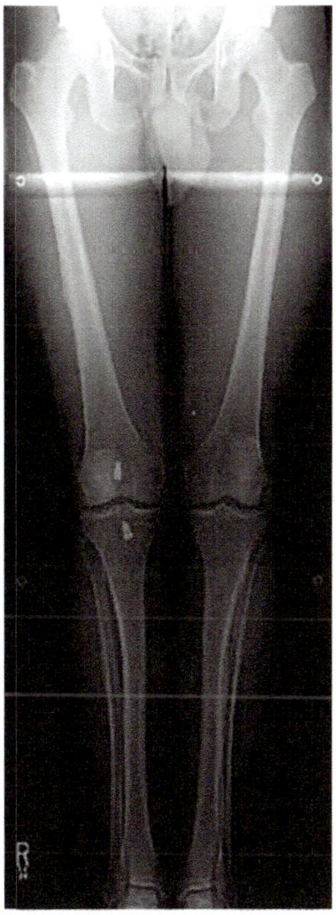

Fig. 13.3 Full-length standing AP radiographs from the hips to the ankles used to assess lower extremity alignment

femoral angle becomes vital for preoperative templating for deformity correction.

A joint convergence angle may be quantified by comparing a line across the femoral condyles and a line across the tibial plateau. In patients with a neutral mechanical axis, such lines should be grossly parallel, and 0–3° of medial convergence is considered normal [37]. In the "double" and "triple varus" knee, attenuation of the posterolateral soft tissues yields asymmetric lateral joint space diastasis increasing the medial convergence angle. As demonstrated in prior biomechanical studies [18, 19], this joint space diastasis is dynamic; thus, varus stress radiographs may be required to more accurately quantify the contribution of lateral condylar lift-off to a patient's varus deformity.

Magnetic Resonance Imaging

In addition to a complete radiographic assessment of the knee, magnetic resonance imaging (MRI) is obtained to provide relevant information regarding ACL status, associated ligamentous deficiencies, and meniscal and articular cartilage damage. Ferromagnetic implants will interfere with the quality and accuracy of MR images. To reduce MR artifact from metal instrumentation, use of a smaller field strength magnet (1.5T rather than 3.0T) is recommended as artifact is directly proportional to field strength. Inversion recovery/STIR (short tau inversion recovery) sequences are less prone to metal artifact, whereas normal frequency-selective fat suppression sequences and gradient echo sequences should be avoided as they are more prone to metal artifact.

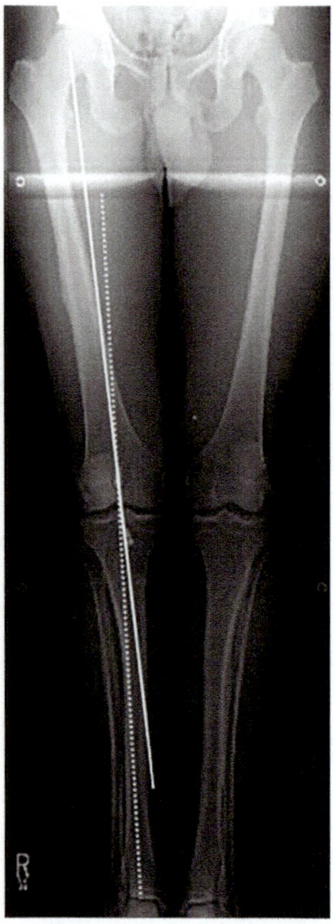

Fig. 13.4 The mechanical axis of the femur (solid white line) is represented by a line connecting the center of the femoral head and the intercondylar notch. The mechanical axis of the tibia (dashed white line) is represented by a line connecting the center of the tibial plafond and bisecting the tibial plateau

While some ACL grafts may be partially intact, they can be functionally incompetent if attenuated or misplaced. The location and diameter of prior bone tunnels in the sagittal and coronal planes must be considered prior to a revision reconstruction. For instance, a non-dilated tunnel placed too vertically in the intercondylar notch may lead to functional ACL instability despite the graft being intact on MRI (Fig. 13.5). In this case, the patient may demonstrate a positive pivot shift but have a normal Lachman examination. Alternatively, well-placed tibial and femoral tunnels created at the prior surgery may be excessively dilated (≥13 mm in diameter) necessitating a staged bone grafting prior to the revision surgery (Fig. 13.6).

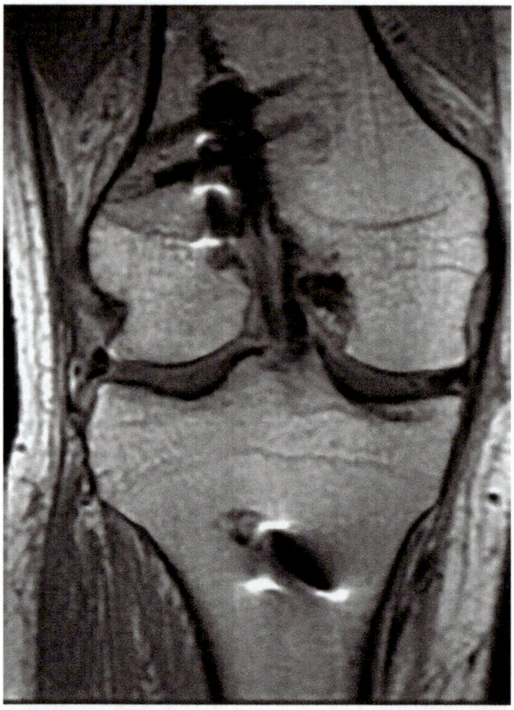

Fig. 13.5 Coronal T1-weighted MRI showing vertical femoral tunnel with hardware in place

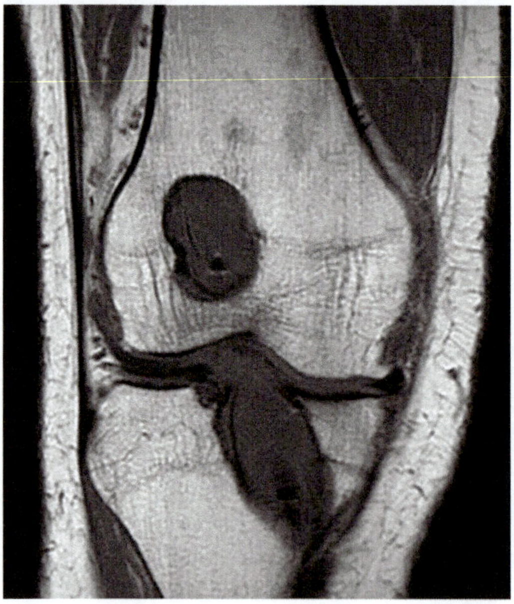

Fig. 13.6 Coronal T1-weighted MRI showing femoral and tibial tunnel expansion

Magnetic resonance imaging will detect both new and previously treated meniscal and articular cartilage pathology in the revision setting [4]. Advanced degenerative articular cartilage wear must be distinguished from contained focal defects. The former may be a contraindication to an osteotomy, while the latter may be corrected by an articular cartilage reconstructive procedure depending on the size, depth, and location of the defect. Meniscal irregularity from prior meniscectomy may be indistinguishable from a new tear on MRI. Significant meniscal resection that is symptomatic may indicate the need for concurrent meniscal allograft transplantation given the chondroprotective effect the meniscus has on the articular cartilage as well as its role as a secondary stabilizer to anterior tibial translation and rotational stability [39, 40]. A gadolinium-enhanced MRI arthrogram is reserved for those patients who have undergone a prior meniscal repair in which a recurrent tear cannot be distinguished from the scar tissue from a healed tear.

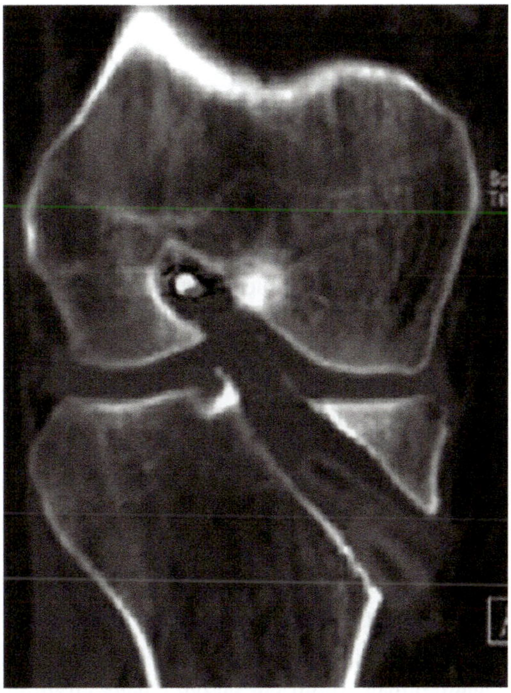

Fig. 13.7 Coronal CT image showing femoral and tibial tunnel expansion

Computerized Tomography

Computerized tomographic (CT) imaging has a limited role in the preoperative evaluation of patients being considered for a revision ACL reconstruction and realignment procedure given its limited utility and radiation exposure. However, in those patients with tunnel widening that requires more detailed three-dimensional imaging to quantify tunnel size, CT is the imaging modality of choice (Fig. 13.7). It is also useful in patients who undergo a staged bone grafting of a dilated tunnel, as it is more sensitive than plain radiographs or MRI to graft consolidation (Fig. 13.8). A CT arthrogram may also be useful in the rare patient in whom an MRI is precluded because of metallic implants elsewhere in the body that may be affected by the magnetic field. While its sensitivity is inferior to MRI, a CT arthrogram can provide general information about meniscal and articular cartilage status.

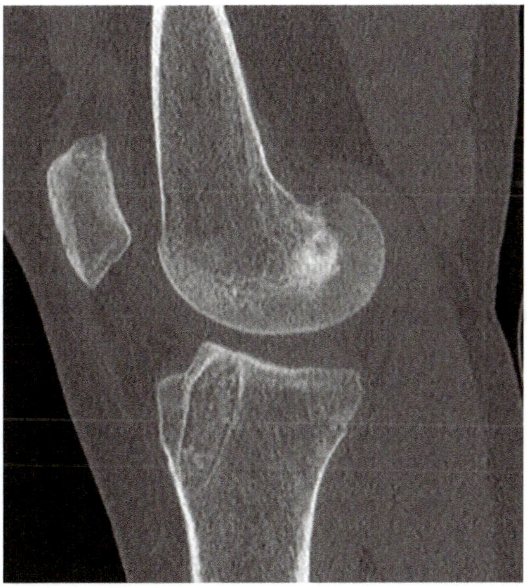

Fig. 13.8 Sagittal CT image showing consolidation of bone graft used to fill expanded tunnels prior to revision ACL reconstruction

Operative Indications and Contraindications

Indications

A combined revision ACL reconstruction and osteotomy is indicated for those younger (less than 60 years of age), active patients with instability symptoms coupled with coronal plane malalignment. Osteotomy initially gained wide acceptance for active patients with uni-compartmental osteoarthritis in whom a knee replacement (partial or total) is contraindicated because of their relatively young age.

Varus malalignment is corrected with a proximal ("high") tibial osteotomy (HTO); valgus malalignment is corrected with a distal femoral osteotomy (DFO). An HTO is also recommended for those patients with ACL insufficiency and associated physiologic genu varum in whom the malalignment would put undue tensile strain on the revision ACL graft. Patients considered for this combined procedure should have a history of functional instability with pivoting activities, a physical examination consistent with ACL insufficiency, and corresponding imaging studies confirming this diagnosis. The goal of the osteotomy in those patients with uni-compartmental osteoarthritis is to correct the mechanical abnormality by redistributing weight-bearing loads away from the involved arthritic compartment. Patients with varus malalignment are over-corrected into valgus. Patients with valgus malalignment are corrected only to a neutral mechanical axis as iatrogenic creation of genu varum would potentially strain the graft and increase compressive loads to the medial compartment. Patients undergoing revision ACL reconstruction who have the anatomic variant of bilateral varus or valgus alignment but no articular cartilage damage should also be corrected to neutral and not over-corrected to either compartment. Ideally, an osteotomy should only be performed in those patients with symptomatic mild-to-moderate osteoarthritis. Those with associated meniscal deficiency and/or focal uni-compartmental chondral defects can be treated either concurrently with the osteotomy and ACL reconstruction or in a staged fashion depending on the complexity of the procedure and comfort level of the surgeon.

Contraindications

The main contraindication to a combined revision ACL reconstruction and an HTO or DFO is advanced cartilage loss of the medial or lateral tibiofemoral compartments, respectively. In general, the majority of the compartment should have articular cartilage coverage. An uncorrected full-thickness cartilage defect of the tibia or femur greater than 15 mm ×15 mm is a contraindication to an osteotomy and is better addressed with a uni-compartmental arthroplasty and revision ACL reconstruction except in those patients too young (<50 years of age) or active for this procedure. Complete loss of medial or lateral joint space on 45° flexion, weight-bearing radiographs is also a contraindication. Other contraindications are cavitary defects of the medial or lateral tibial plateau, loss of flexion or extension >10°, tibial subluxation, and uncorrected complete or near-complete meniscectomy in the involved compartment.

Patients over the age of 60 who are candidates for a partial or total knee replacement are better served with this more definitive procedure. Patients with a body mass index (BMI) over 35 will likely not be symptomatically improved if they have arthritic symptoms in addition to instability. Concurrent patellofemoral arthritis is a relative contraindication to this procedure. Severe patellofemoral symptoms will not be improved following an HTO or DFO, while mild symptoms are not a contraindication to this procedure. Asymptomatic patellofemoral articular cartilage damage is not a contraindication despite the fact that these patients may develop patellofemoral symptoms over time. Medical contraindications to an osteotomy include inflammatory arthropathies that cause diffuse cartilage wear of all three knee compartments, diabetes mellitus, and malnutrition.

Non-compliance with rehabilitation restrictions and use of nicotine products are also contraindications. Nicotine use in the setting of an opening wedge tibial or femoral osteotomy (discussed below) is a significant risk factor for delayed union and nonunion because of the open void created that must fill with bone. An opening wedge HTO requires an incision on the medial aspect of the tibial plateau where there is limited subcutaneous soft tissue causing an elevated risk for wound healing complications in the setting of nicotine use or other factors that may interfere with wound healing. Cessation of smoking for at least 8 weeks is strongly recommended prior to an osteotomy and can be checked by serum or urine cotinine levels – a nicotine metabolite.

Correction of Varus Malalignment and ACL Insufficiency

Preoperative Considerations

Correction of varus malalignment is most readily accomplished with an HTO as most varus deformities are due to proximal tibia vara. This procedure has evolved over the past four decades, but at the present time, the two most common procedures involve either a medial opening wedge or a lateral closing wedge. Historically, the lateral closing wedge osteotomy was the predominant method despite the fact that it possesses several technical challenges that may compromise the final outcome. As a result, there has been increased interest in the medial opening wedge over the past several years for a variety of reasons independent of concurrent ACL revision surgery. Advantages of an opening wedge HTO include:

- Only a single bone cut is required.
- Less soft tissue disruption.
- No disruption of the proximal tibiofibular joint or fibular osteotomy is required.
- No risk to the peroneal nerve.
- The correction can be fine-tuned intraoperatively to achieve optimal alignment.
- Patellar height is maintained.
- Ideal if a PLC reconstruction is required by avoidance of fibular disruption.
- Preexisting patella alta may be corrected.

A medial opening wedge osteotomy is not without issues. Potential disadvantages of this technique in the setting of a revision ACL reconstruction include:

- Potential need for cortico-cancellous autograft or allograft
- Higher risk of delayed union/nonunion due to the need for increased bone consolidation
- Risk for fracture propagation with loss of the lateral cortical hinge or intra-articular extension into the lateral compartment
- Tendency to increase posterior tibial slope
- Exacerbation of preexisting patella baja
- Theoretical increased risk of wound complications in patients with compromised healing (i.e., smokers, diabetics)
- Delayed weight-bearing required during bone consolidation

Timing Issues

Consideration has to be given for patients with combined ligament deficiencies and malalignment such as the double varus and triple varus knee in which the HTO must be coupled with a revision ACL reconstruction and lateral ligamentous reconstructions. In patients with the double varus knee, the osteotomy and revision ACL reconstruction can be performed at one time depending on the experience and comfort level of the surgeon. Correction of the varus malalignment often causes a contracture of the lateral soft tissue structures once the weight-bearing tensile load is reduced by placing the mechanical axis in a position of relative valgus [21]. This would make reconstruction of the lateral ligamentous restraints unnecessary in patients with only moderate lateral ligamentous deficiencies (i.e., 6–8 mm of lateral joint space opening with varus stress). However, a lateral compartment gap greater than 10 mm with varus stress during arthroscopy would preclude a single-stage procedure as the residual lateral ligamentous deficiencies would place undue tensile strain on the ACL graft. Patients with the triple varus variant have a complex problem that is best treated in a staged fashion since a single-stage HTO and revision ACL and PLC reconstruction pose significant complications (i.e., arthrofibrosis, loss of fixation). In these patients, the HTO is performed first, and the revision ACL reconstruction and PLC can be addressed later once the osteotomy has healed.

Hardware and Tunnel Issues

As a general rule, preparation of the ACL revision graft should be deferred until after the removal of all potentially problematic hardware and it is confirmed that there is adequate bone stock available to drill the revision tunnels. It is imperative that all equipment needed for potential hardware removal is available prior to surgery. Most metallic interference screws can be removed with a large fragment (3.5 mm) screwdriver. Stripped screws may require reverse-threaded screw removal instrumentation for removal. Alternatively, these screws can be removed with a coring reamer 1–2 mm larger in diameter than the screw (Fig. 13.9). Bioabsorbable screws can potentially be left in place or drilled through during the revision procedure and the osteotomy. Non-aperture cortical fixation devices typically do not interfere with the revision graft or the osteotomy and can be left alone.

The index bone tunnels will be either anatomic and in the appropriate location, completely non-anatomic without contacting the new tunnel, or overlapping with the new tunnel potentially creating a "snowman" tunnel. Fixation hardware will likely require removal if located in an anatomic location or in an overlapping tunnel since it will interfere with drilling and placement of the revision hardware. Screws or other hardware located in femoral tunnels that are completely non-anatomic can be left in place in order to avoid a cavitary defect that may compromise fixation of the revision graft or require bone grafting (Fig. 13.10).

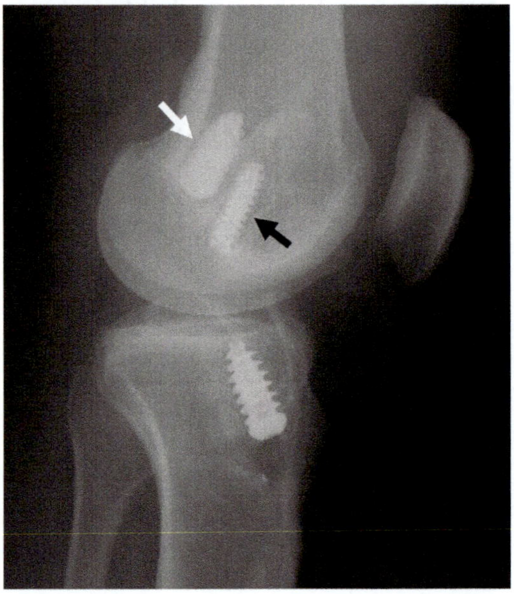

Fig. 13.10 Lateral x-ray showing misplaced femoral screw from primary reconstruction (black arrow) left in place as it did not interfere with placement of the revision screw (white arrow)

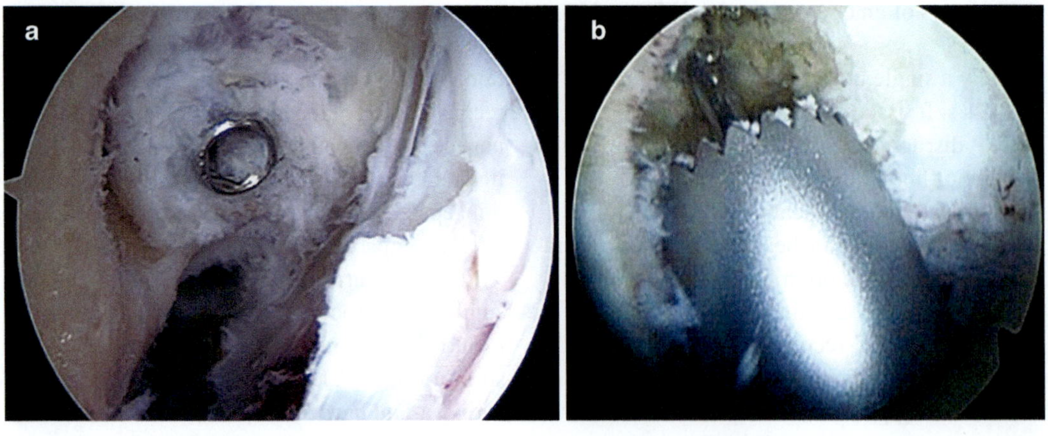

Fig. 13.9 (**a**) Retained femoral hardware. (**b**) Coring reamer used to remove stripped femoral screw

All metallic tibial hardware should be removed even if grossly non-anatomic as it will likely interfere with the tibial osteotomy or the revision graft and their associated fixation.

Once all hardware is removed, the index femoral and tibial tunnels should be assessed for their potential interference with the revision tunnels. A combination of shavers, burrs, curettes, and thermal ablation is used to remove all soft tissue remnants from the femoral notch and tibial plateau in order to adequately assess the quality of bone stock present. Tunnels that were anatomically appropriate without evidence of expansion on preoperative imaging can be reliably used for the revision tunnel. In general, our preference is to create a revision tunnel that is 1 mm in diameter larger than the prior tunnel in order to remove all sclerotic bone and achieve a viable cancellous surface (Fig. 13.11). Compaction drills can be useful to avoid bone loss and strengthen the surrounding bone to support interference fixation. Femoral tunnels that are ≤12 mm that result from overlapping tunnels can be filled with a larger bone plug from either a bone-patellar tendon-bone (B-PT-B) graft, quadriceps tendon-patellar bone (QT-B) graft, or Achilles allograft. Supplemental allograft chips or cortico-cancellous strips can also be placed adjacent to the bone plug, as can "stacked" interference screws to fill the bone void. Tibial tunnels that are ≤12 mm can also be bone grafted after the osteotomy is complete and before the ACL graft is secured. Interference screw fixation may be feasible in these cases depending on the type of HTO performed (opening wedge vs. closing wedge). However, an opening wedge HTO often requires suspensory cortical fixation with a screw and washer because of the presence of hardware from the HTO.

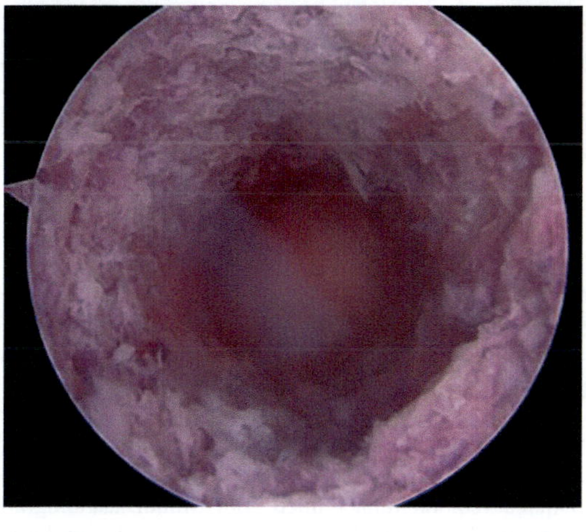

Fig. 13.11 Arthroscopic view of tibial tunnel showing circumferential cancellous bone

Tunnels that are ≥13 mm in diameter in any plane on preoperative imaging usually require a staged bone graft, especially if there is widening of the tunnel aperture (usually femoral) or "ballooning" of the tunnel. In these cases, reliable fixation cannot be achieved with either interference screws or suspensory cortical devices because of the potential "windshield wiper" effect of graft motion within the tunnel (Fig. 13.12). The tunnel surface is abraded back to bleeding bone and grafted with either allograft dowels, cancellous allograft chips, or iliac crest

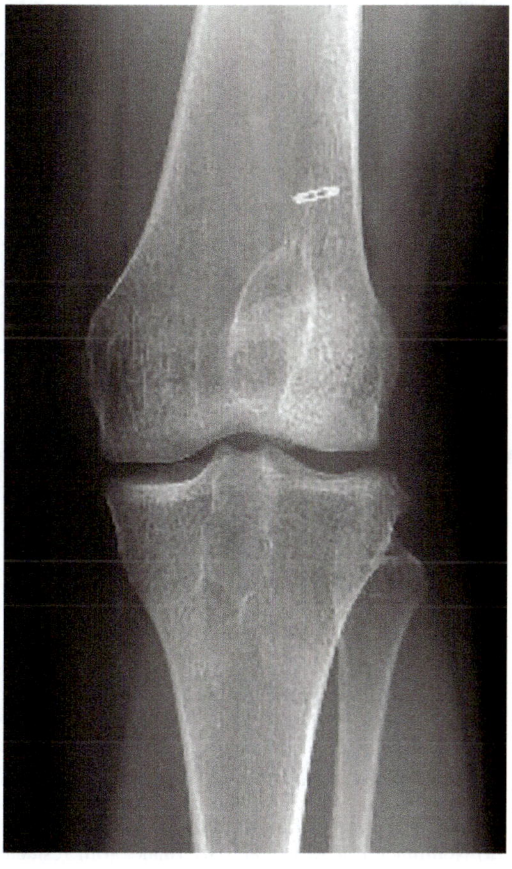

Fig. 13.12 Dilated, vertical femoral, and tibial tunnels greater than 13 mm in diameter may benefit from a staged bone graft prior to the revision ACL reconstruction

cortico-cancellous bone. An allograft dowel will provide structural support and can be inserted either through the anteromedial portal for the femoral side or directly through a metaphyseal window on the tibial side. Cancellous allograft chips can be inserted through a cut-off syringe or arthroscopy cannula with the graft impacted with a plunger or bone tamp. Demineralized bone matrix with reverse phase medium (StimuBlast®, Arthrex Inc., Naples, FL) can be added to the cancellous chips to resist fluid irrigation and displacement of the graft (Fig. 13.13). Tunnels that

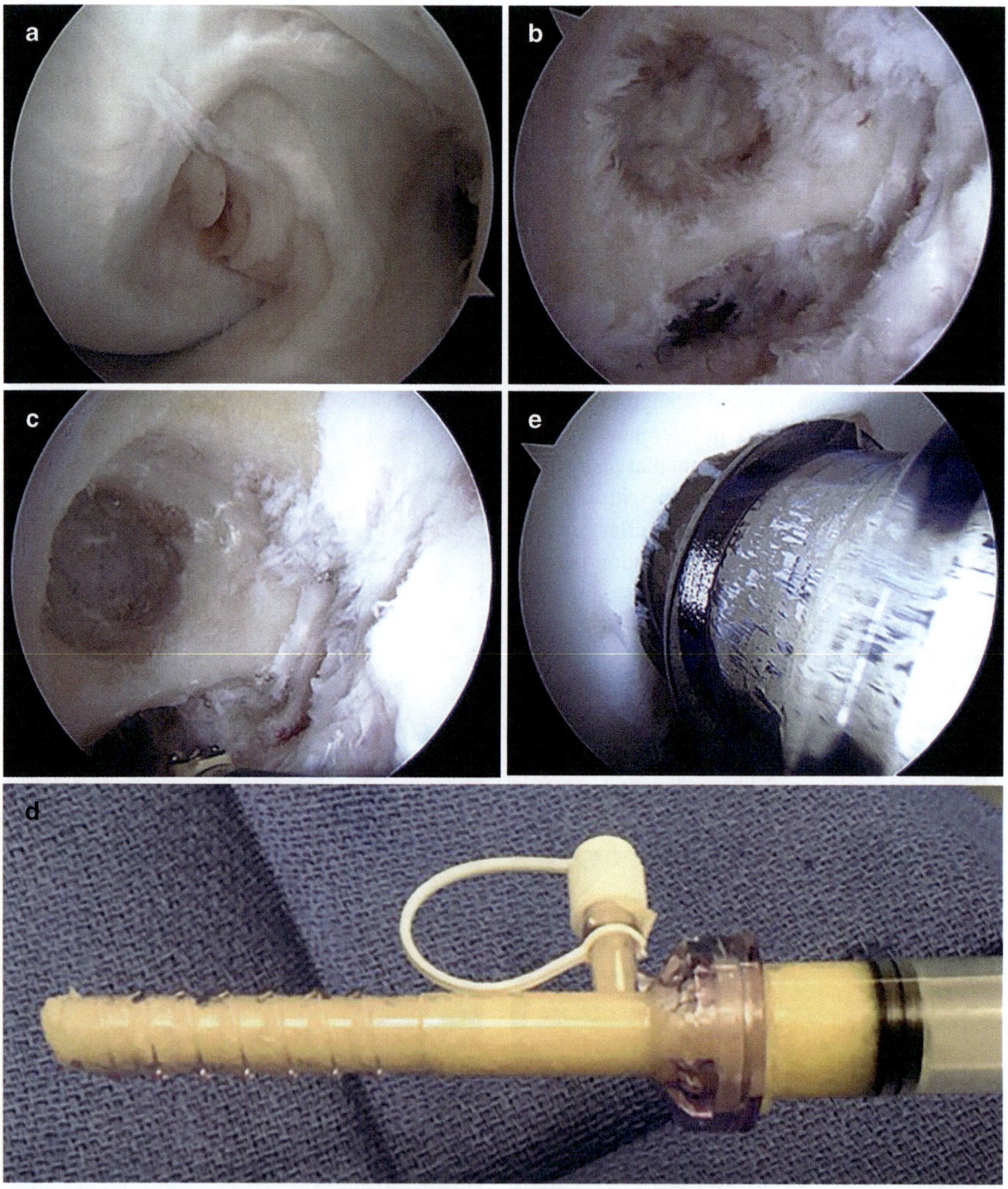

Fig. 13.13 Staged grafting of femoral and tibial tunnels. (**a**) Non-functional ACL graft. (**b**) Tunnel with residual graft and fibrous tissue debrided (**c**) Dilated femoral tunnel following complete graft removal. (**d**) Syringe with StimuBlast® demineralized bone matrix (Arthrex Inc., Naples, FL) and cancellous allograft chips placed inside arthroscopy cannula for ease of insertion. (**e**) Injection of StimuBlast and cancellous chips into femoral tunnel. (**f**) Dilated femoral tunnel filled with StimuBlast/allograft bone. (**g**) Tibial tunnel being filled similar to femoral tunnel. (**h**) Filled tibial tunnel. (**i**) Revision femoral tunnel drilled 5 months following grafting

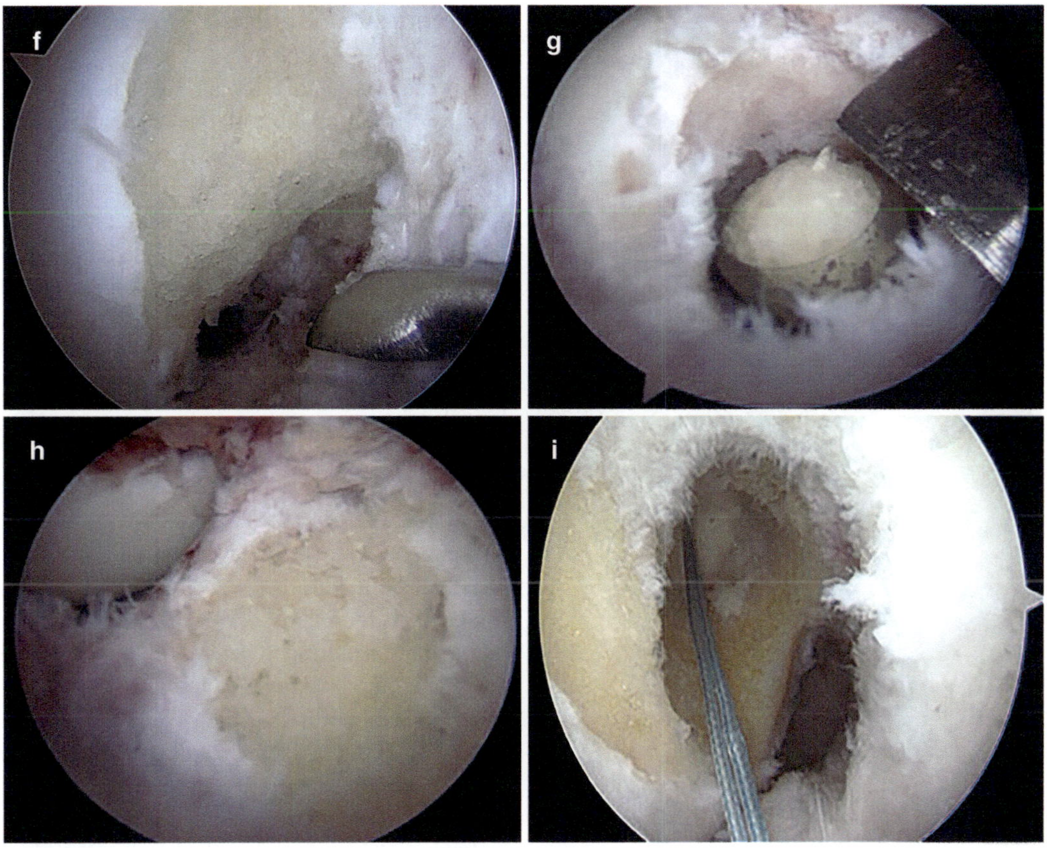

Fig. 13.13 (continued)

undergo a staged bone grafting are usually consolidated by 4–6 months as determined by plain radiographs or CT imaging (Fig. 13.14).

Graft Issues

It is imperative that the operative record from any prior ACL surgery is available since patients are often uncertain when asked about prior grafts. The choice of the revision graft is dependent on several factors. Prior graft harvest must be taken into consideration when choosing a revision graft in order to avoid wound healing complications associated with prior incisions that are closely parallel or that may cross any new incisions. Activity level is the most important factor when considering a primary ACL graft but may be less relevant in the setting of a concurrent osteotomy where decreased activity level is anticipated. Cosmesis, though a consideration, is the least important factor when choosing a revision graft.

Surgical options include the ipsilateral B-PT-B or quadriceps tendon autograft (with or without patellar bone plug) if the extensor mechanism is intact after the primary ACL reconstruction. A B-PT-B graft is not recommended if an HTO is also performed given the compromised tibial attachment of the remaining patellar tendon at the site of the osteotomy. If the B-PT-B or quadriceps tendon graft has already been harvested, re-harvest of these grafts is not recommended as they will be comprised predominantly of scar tissue rather than native tendon. An ipsilateral hamstring autograft, with or without a supplemental soft tissue allograft, can be considered in these patients and has the advantage of not being susceptible to graft-tunnel mismatch or requiring

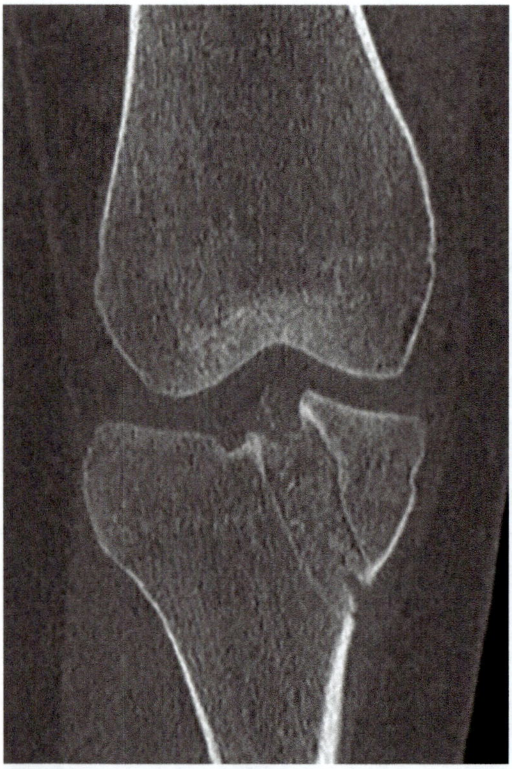

Fig. 13.14 Coronal CT scan showing consolidated tibial tunnel following bone grafting

interference fixation. Caution should be exercised in using a soft tissue graft if there is any evidence of tunnel widening since fixation and graft incorporation may be compromised. A contralateral B-PT-B or quadriceps tendon graft can also be used in the revision setting since prior skin incisions are not a factor and use of allograft tissues is avoided. Some patients are hesitant to consider surgery on the contralateral limb and would prefer to use an allograft. If an allograft is chosen, our preference is to use an Achilles tendon allograft since it is a robust graft that allows bone-to-bone healing and can accommodate a bone tunnel of any size. Patients who opt for an allograft should be apprised of the potential decreased success rate, risk for disease transmission, delayed incorporation, inflammatory immune response, and expense associated with allograft tissues [41].

Preoperative Planning

Preoperative planning for an HTO is achieved first by the calculation of the mechanical axis from full-length radiographs from the center of the femoral head to the center of the tibial plafond. In patients with varus malalignment, the mechanical axis passes medial to the medial tibial spine. The goal of an HTO is to move this weight-bearing line into the lateral compartment to unload the compromised medial compartment and to reduce tensile strain of the ACL graft and lateral soft tissues.

The Picture Archiving and Communication System (PACS) software can be very helpful in calculating the degree and amount of correction. A line is drawn across the widest portion of the proximal tibia with the medial cortex representing 0% and the lateral cortex 100% of this distance. The preferred location of the realigned mechanical axis is a point 62% of the width of the tibial plateau from medial to lateral, which equates to 3°–5° of mechanical valgus. This point, commonly referred to as the Fujisawa point [42], is half-way between a neutral mechanical axis (50%) and a point 75% across the tibial plateau in which nearly all weight-bearing forces are concentrated solely on the lateral compartment. One line representing the femoral weight-bearing line is drawn from the center of the femoral head to the 62% point, and a second line representing the tibial weight-bearing line is drawn from the center of the talus to this same point [43]. The angle formed by these two lines represents the angle of correction to achieve the desired mechanical axis (Fig. 13.15). If there is excessive lateral ligamentous laxity increasing the degree of varus alignment, the difference in the congruence angle formed by a line parallel to the tibial plateau and a second line along the condylar articular surface is subtracted from this correction angle.

The angle of correction is converted into millimeters of "opening" of the osteotomy by drawing a line across the tibia representing the anticipated site, angle, and length of the osteot-

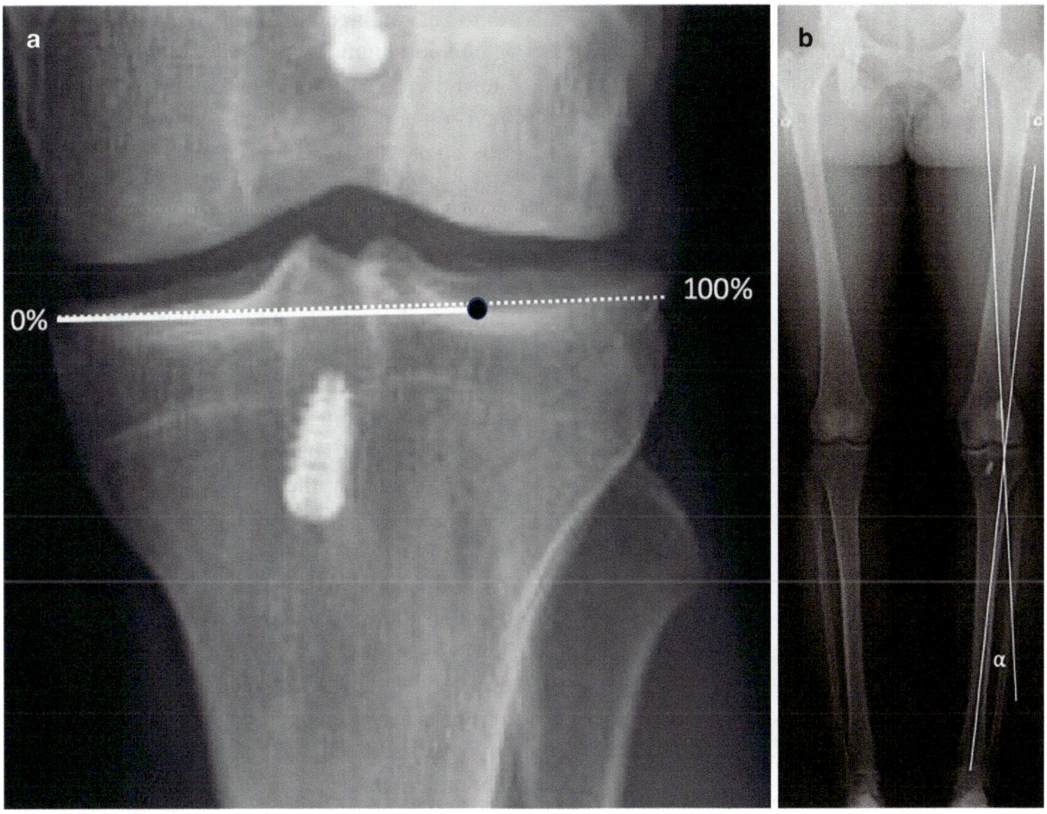

Fig. 13.15 Determination of desired mechanical axis following an HTO. (**a**) Calculation of the Fujisawa point which is 62% of the tibial plateau width from medial to lateral. This is the desired location for the realigned mechanical axis. (**b**) Full-length x-ray showing the calculated degree of correction for the amount of varus malalignment in order to put the realigned mechanical axis at the 62%ile of the tibial plateau width

omy. The length of this line is superimposed on the tibial weight-bearing line, and the distance at this location between the femoral and tibial weight-bearing lines is the amount of opening or closing of the osteotomy required to achieve the desired angular correction (Fig. 13.16).

Medial Opening Wedge High Tibial Osteotomy and Revision Anterior Cruciate Ligament Reconstruction: Surgical Technique

A combined opening wedge HTO and revision ACL reconstruction is a complicated procedure that is infrequently performed even by experienced knee surgeons. It is imperative that all equipment is available, including a fluoroscopic unit and a radiolucent table. Our preference is to use a large C-arm that is positioned on the opposite side of the patient. The patient is positioned supine with the operating room table flexed to 90° and a thigh holder placed on the proximal thigh to allow hyperflexion of the knee. Some surgeons prefer to perform all arthroscopic procedures with the knee in full extension. If a contralateral graft harvest is planned, then both lower extremities are prepped and draped free. If not, then sequential compression pumps are placed on the contralateral lower extremity for deep venous thrombosis prophylaxis. A tourniquet is used selectively, as necessary. Prophylactic antibiotics are given within 1 hour of the planned surgery in all patients.

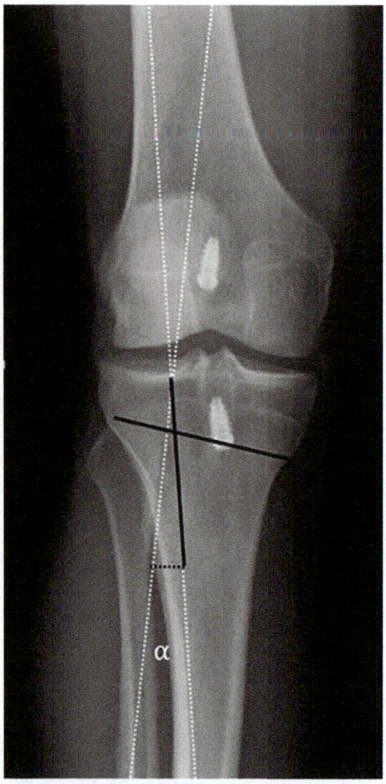

Fig. 13.16 The angle of desired correction (α) is converted into millimeters of “opening” of the osteotomy. A line across the tibia represents the anticipated site, angle, and length of the osteotomy (solid black line). The length of this line is superimposed on the tibial weight-bearing line, and the distance at this location between the femoral and tibial weight-bearing lines is the amount of opening, in millimeters, required to achieve the desired angular correction (dashed black line)

Surgical Technique

A routine knee arthroscopy is performed with standard portals to assess all compartments, debride or repair any meniscal pathology, address any chondral lesions, confirm the absence of a functional ACL, and assess the lateral compartment for any full-thickness cartilage lesions >15 mm that would preclude an HTO. If a cartilage restoration procedure is to be performed, it is typically done concurrently with the osteotomy.

The intercondylar notch is debrided of all nonviable ACL graft material to fully assess the femoral tunnel for expansion and to identify, and potentially remove, prior hardware. A notchplasty is often not necessary in a revision procedure but can be done to enhance visualization of the femoral tunnel site. At this stage, the surgeon must decide whether to proceed with the planned revision or perform a staged bone grafting, as discussed previously. If it is decided to proceed with the procedure, the revision ACL graft can be harvested from either the ipsilateral lower extremity or contralateral limb if an autograft is selected. Our goal is to harvest a revision graft that is 1 cm larger in diameter than the primary graft.

The revision femoral tunnel aperture is identified that would be in the center of the native ACL. This is sometimes difficult to identify in a revision setting. Therefore, a site is chosen that is at approximately the 1:30 or 10:30 position on the lateral wall of the intercondylar notch in a left or right knee, respectively. A guide pin is drilled with the assistance of a femoral offset guide through the anteromedial (AM) portal with the knee hyperflexed to 105° to prevent posterior wall “blowout” during tunnel drilling that may occur in lesser degrees of flexion. Alternatively, an outside-in technique can be used to create the femoral tunnel that is oriented away from the prior tunnel. A low-profile drill of appropriate diameter is used to create the femoral tunnel to a depth commensurate with the bone plug or the revision graft or at least 20 mm for a soft tissue graft. A Beath pin is used to pass a #2 shuttle suture out the lateral thigh that is left in the AM portal for later retrieval.

The operating table is fully extended if previously flexed and a new sterile drape applied under the knee, as is a foam knee wedge to elevate the operative limb above the contralateral lower extremity for fluoroscopic viewing. A 6–8 cm incision is made just distal to the medial joint line mid-way between the tibial tubercle and posterior edge of the proximal tibia. A needle tip electrocautery is used to carefully dissect the medial border of the patellar tendon to identify its insertion. Dissection is carried sharply down to the pes anserinus with identification and incision of the overlying sartorial fascia. In the setting of hamstring autograft, the underlying gracilis and semitendinosus can be identified and harvested to create a quadrupled graft [44]. The pes anserinus and sMCL are sharply dissected longitudinally and reflected posteriorly to the posterior tibial border. An elevator is used to release the sMCL to the flare of the medial tibial plateau. An osteotomy opening greater than 5 mm typically requires distal transection of the sMCL. A Z-retractor is placed behind the tibia to reflect the soft tissue envelope.

Our preferred technique is to use the opening wedge plate system (Arthrex Inc., Naples, FL). A perforated guide pin is drilled under fluoroscopic visualization starting 4 cm distal to the medial joint line at a 15° oblique angle across the proximal tibia at the predetermined location on the medial tibial metaphysis at which the radiographic corrections were calculated. The pin should be at or proximal to the tibial tubercle and directed at the proximal tibiofibular joint at least 1.5 cm distal to the lateral joint line. A second pin is drilled to an equal depth parallel to the first pin using the proprietary drill guide rotated posteriorly to match the slope of the tibial plateau. Lateral imaging is obtained to confirm adequate placement of both pins which should be parallel to the tibial plateau. The guide should be oriented to place the osteotomy just proximal to the patellar tendon insertion so that the osteotomy site is under compression with quadriceps contraction. A retractor is placed under the patellar tendon and the Z-retractor reoriented at the level of the osteotomy to protect the popliteal neurovascular bundle. An oscillating saw is used to begin the osteotomy under fluoroscopic visualization with care taken to make a precise single cut. The anterior and posterior tibial cortices are cut with a ¾-inch osteotome which is advanced medially under fluoroscopic guidance to a distance 1 cm from the lateral tibial cortex, which should correspond to the predetermined length of the osteotomy. Discontinuity of the anterior and posterior cortices is confirmed when there is slight separation of the proximal and distal bone fragments with gentle valgus force. Passage of a Kirschner wire across the lateral tibial cortex can be used to cause a "greenstick" effect which will allow opening of the osteotomy while maintaining continuity of the bone.

A calibrated wedge osteotome is inserted as far posterior as possible in the osteotomy in order to affect only coronal alignment (Fig. 13.17). More anterior placement would inadvertently increase the posterior tibial slope as a consequence of the medial tibial cortex being oriented at a 45° angle to the plane of the posterior tibial cortex that creates a triangular shape to the proximal tibia (Fig. 13.18) [38]. The osteotome is gen-

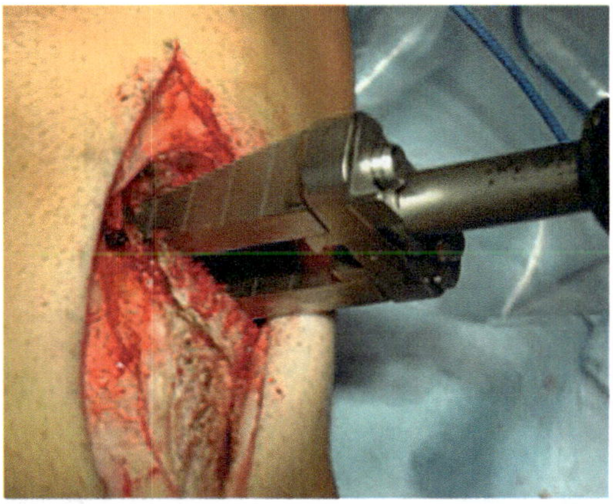

Fig. 13.17 Calibrated wedge osteotome used to open the osteotomy site the desired degree of correction in millimeters

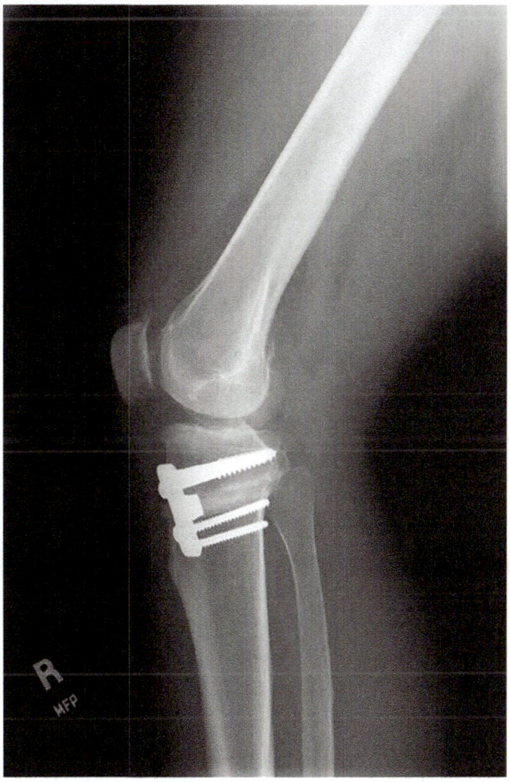

Fig. 13.18 Osteotomy plate placed too anteriorly which will inadvertently increase the tibial slope

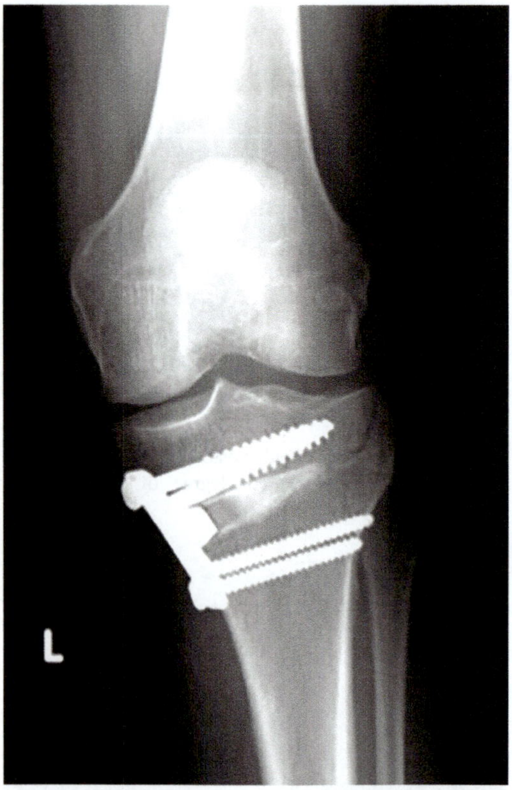

Fig. 13.19 Fracture of the lateral tibial cortex following an opening wedge HTO

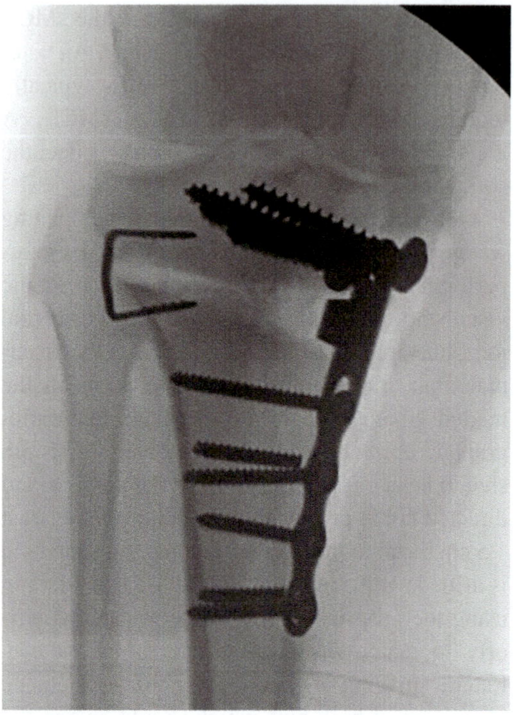

Fig. 13.20 Fracture of the lateral tibial cortex following an opening wedge HTO stabilized with a staple

tly advanced with a mallet laterally under fluoroscopic guidance to allow stress relaxation of the osteotomized tibial bone as it is opened. If the osteotome is advanced too forcefully, an iatrogenic fracture can occur through the lateral cortex or proximally into the lateral compartment (Fig. 13.19). If this occurs, a single staple or two-holed plate can provide stability to complete the osteotomy (Fig. 13.20).

Confirmation of appropriate realignment may be evaluated by placing a rigid guide rod from the center of the femoral head to the middle of the tibial plafond under fluoroscopic visualization. An axial load is applied to the foot, and the lower extremity is externally rotated 10° to provide a true assessment of lower limb alignment. Satisfactory realignment should result in the rod crossing the tibial plateau just lateral to the lateral tibial spine 62% of the distance across the tibial plateau. We have not found use of an electrocautery cord (as recommended by some authors) stretched from the center of the femoral head to the center of the tibial plafond to be particularly helpful due to its lack of rigidity [45].

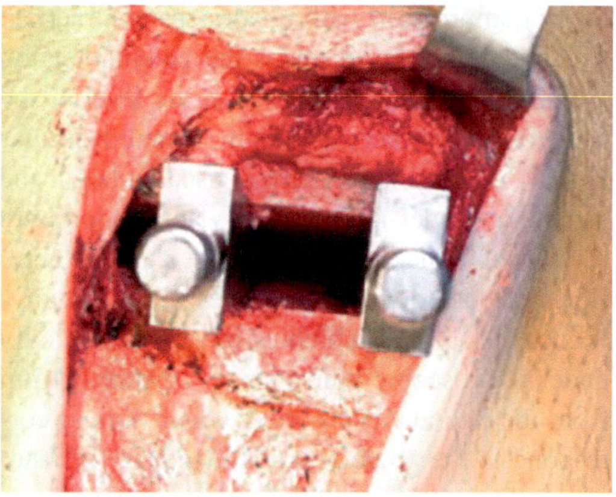

Fig. 13.21 Tines of the wedge osteotome left in place to allow for plate insertion

If the realignment is satisfactory, the handle of the osteotome is removed, while the two wedge tines remain in the tibia to preserve the opening wedge (Fig. 13.21). Based on preoperative mea-

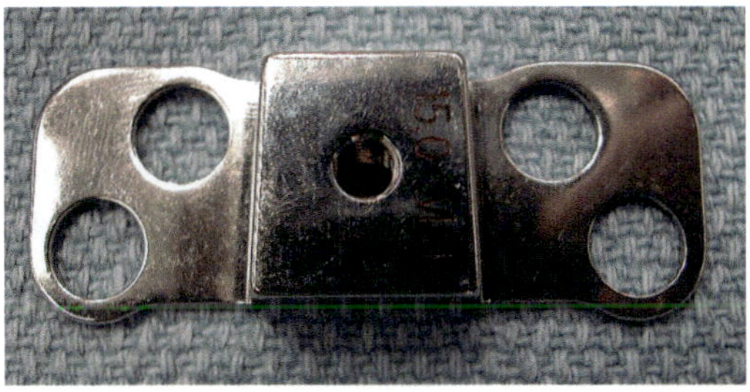

Fig. 13.22 Titanium Puddu plate (Arthrex Inc., Naples, FL) with sloped tooth to maintain opening of the osteotomy to the appropriate degree while preserving the tibial slope

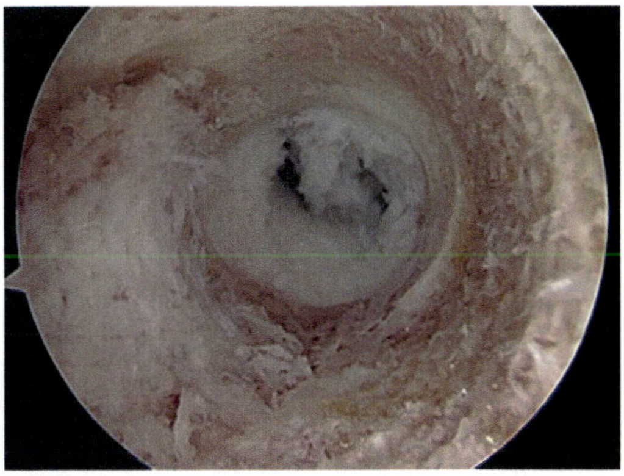

Fig. 13.23 Arthroscopic view within the ACL tibial tunnel following the HTO confirming absence of hardware that may interfere with graft passage

surements, a four-hole stainless plate with appropriate-sized tooth that will maintain the calculated degree of correction is inserted (Fig. 13.22). Multiple tooth thicknesses are available from 5 to 17.5 mm. The tooth can be either straight or sloped to maintain the slope of the tibial plateau. Alternatively, a titanium plate with locking screws can be used if bone density is in question. A single 6.5 mm cancellous screw is placed in the proximal posterior hole parallel to the osteotomy as far posterior as possible, and two 4.5 mm bi-cortical screws are directed distally through the distal holes. The proximal anterior screw is not inserted until the ACL tibial tunnel is drilled. Anteroposterior and lateral fluoroscopic images are obtained to confirm adequate placement of all hardware. If appropriately created, the osteotomy gap should be approximately twice as wide posterior to the plate as it is anterior in order to prevent an inadvertent increase of the tibial slope which would increase the strain transmitted to the revision ACL graft [46].

An alternative option for an opening wedge HTO consists of a nonabsorbable polyetheretherketone (PEEK) implant and screws (iBalance®, Arthrex, Inc., Naples, FL) that are buried within the tibial bone in order to prevent irritation of the overlying soft tissue envelope. A benefit of this system is that the proximal screws can be oriented in a more proximal direction to avoid the tibial ACL tunnel. The ACL graft can also be passed through and secured to the PEEK implant if desired.

Once fixation is complete, an arthroscopic tibial guide is placed at the center of the tibial ACL footprint, and a guide pin is inserted. If the prior bone tunnel is filled with soft tissue, pin purchase may be compromised. Advancing the guide pin into the room of the intercondylar notch will stabilize it for drilling. The guide pin should be anterior to the HTO plate and screws. The appropriately sized compaction drill is used to complete the tibial tunnel. An arthroscope can be inserted into the tunnel to confirm circumferential cancellous bone and the absence of the HTO hardware (Fig. 13.23). Shavers and thermal ablation devices should be used to debride all non-viable fibrous tissue which would affect graft-tunnel healing. The drill is left in place, and the knee is fully extended to confirm the absence of notch impingement. The final proximal cancellous screw is inserted into the plate with the drill still in the tunnel so that graft interference is avoided.

The shuttle suture is retrieved through the tibial tunnel and used to pull the revision ACL graft into the joint. Femoral fixation is accomplished with either interference screws or suspensory cortical fixation depending on graft type, surgeon preference, and femoral bone stock. Supplemental fixation may be required in certain situations. The knee is cycled from 0° to 90° to confirm isometricity, lack of impingement, and satisfactory fixation. Distal fixation is performed with the knee in 10° of flexion with 10 lbs. of traction to the distal graft sutures and a posterior drawer applied to the tibia. Interference screw fixation or cortical fixation is used depending on graft type, surgeon preference, and potential interference from the HTO screw(s).

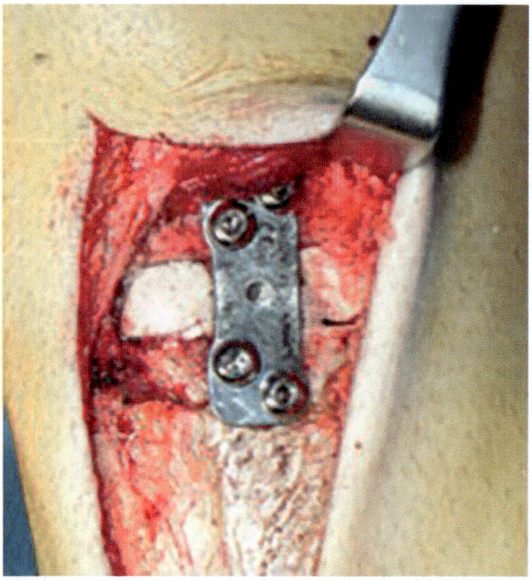

Fig. 13.24 Final HTO construct with plate in place and osteotomy site filled with a synthetic bone graft substitute

Once the plate and graft are secured, bone graft or a bone graft substitute can be placed anterior and posterior to the plate. Some surgeons do not use any bone graft material, except for larger defects. Our preference is to use morselized cancellous allograft chips to fill the defect and cortical allograft bone or synthetic osteoconductive bone graft substitute to provide cortical support (Fig. 13.24).

After copious irrigation, the deep soft tissue flap and overlying fascia are reapproximated to the sleeve of soft tissue remaining on the tibial cortex. Residual MCL laxity is not typically an issue even if it is released during the exposure. Following dermal and subcuticular closure, a soft dressing is placed, and the limb is wrapped with a compressive ACE bandage from the foot to the thigh. A long-leg hinged knee brace is used to protect the osteotomy and is locked in full extension.

Lateral Closing Wedge High Tibial Osteotomy and Revision Anterior Cruciate Ligament Reconstruction: Surgical Technique

Lateral closing wedge HTO was historically the most common method used for coronal plane realignment in the young, active patient. Despite the recent increased interest in the opening wedge technique, both lateral closing wedge and medial opening wedge osteotomies demonstrate similar clinical outcomes and complication profiles [47, 48]; therefore, the chosen technique is largely driven by surgeon preference.

Similar to the medial opening wedge osteotomy, the lateral closing wedge technique has several advantages and disadvantages in the setting of a revision ACL reconstruction. These advantages include:

- Cortical contact allowing for potentially earlier weight-bearing
- Faster healing
- Theoretically reduced risk of delayed union/nonunion
- More secure initial fixation
- Less interference with the ACL graft and hardware
- Tendency to decrease tibial slope

Unfortunately, there are several significant disadvantages of a closing wedge osteotomy that must be considered especially for surgeons unfamiliar with this technique. These include:

- Greater soft tissue dissection
- Converging dual osteotomies
- Difficulty achieving and changing the desired correction
- Risk for peroneal nerve injury
- Risk for fibular osteotomy nonunion
- Risk for proximal tibiofibular joint instability secondary to ligamentous disruption
- Potential increase in patellar height

Surgical Technique

In the setting of a combined closing wedge osteotomy and revision ACL reconstruction, the calculated correction of alignment, surgical set-up, and arthroscopic portion of the procedure are identical to the opening wedge technique. A reverse L-shaped incision is made from the fibular head to the tibial tubercle and curved distally to expose the fascia of the anterior compartment

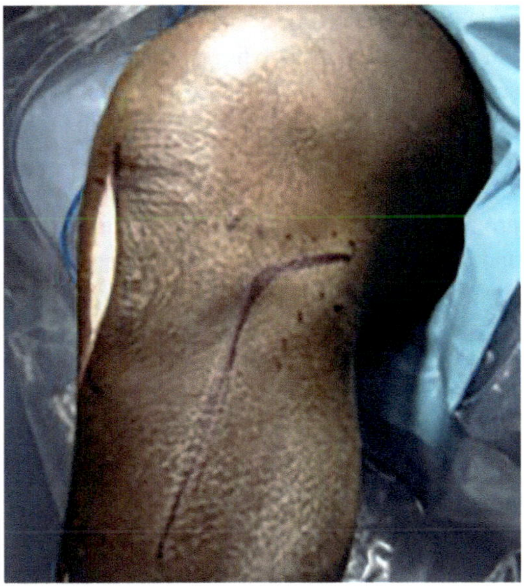

Fig. 13.25 L-shaped incision for closing wedge HTO

(Fig. 13.25). Though some authors advocate for alternative incisions and approaches, a parapatellar approach allows for easier exposure in the setting of an ACL reconstruction and for subsequent arthroplasty, if necessary [49]. Once the fascia is identified, the anterior compartment is incised parallel with the patellar tendon with electrocautery leaving a 1 cm strip of fascia to be used for later closure. The anterior compartment muscle is elevated off the tibia subperiosteally proximally to Gerdy's tubercle and laterally to the fibular head. Z-retractors are placed around the posterior aspect of the tibia to protect the popliteal neurovascular structures. The patellar tendon insertion is identified and protected.

There are three options to deal with the fibula when performing a closing wedge HTO. The proximal tibiofibular joint can be disrupted with a curved ½-inch osteotome to allow the fibula to slide proximally as the osteotomy is compressed. This is our choice for smaller corrections and in patients without PLC instability. A second alternative is an osteotomy of the fibular neck. This is especially useful for larger corrections but risks injury to the peroneal nerve and may compromise the fibular tunnel used for a lateral collateral ligament reconstruction. A third alternative is an oblique osteotomy of the fibula at the junction of the mid- and distal third. This option requires a secondary incision and is complicated by the potential risk for nonunion and injury to the superficial peroneal nerve [50].

Following division of the proximal tibiofibular joint, a guidewire is placed parallel to the joint line (approximately 2 cm distal to the articular surface) and advanced to the far medial cortex. A second guidewire is placed distal to the first wire, at a distance dictated by the preoperative planning, and drilled in a manner convergent with the first wire ending 1 cm from the medial tibial cortex. The second pin should be at or above the patellar tendon insertion. A commercially available guide can be used to ensure correct angulation of the second pin. The placement of these guidewires is confirmed with fluoroscopy, ensuring the planned osteotomy preserves a medial hinge. A cutting jig may be utilized to assist in the creation of the desired osteotomy to avoid complications while making two separate bone cuts [51]. With the knee in 30° of flexion to reduce tension on the popliteal neurovascular bundle and maximize distance between the bundle and the posterior tibia, the proximal osteotomy is made parallel to the tibial plateau 2 cm from the joint line. It is started with an oscillating saw with a posterior soft tissue protector in place. The second osteotomy is made parallel to the distal guide pin proximal to the patellar tendon insertion. Care is taken to maintain the medial tibial cortex which may be perforated with a Kirschner wire to allow closure without causing an acute fracture with loss of cortical contact. The bone wedge is removed as one triangular segment or in a piece-meal fashion (Fig. 13.26). Careful visualization of the posterior tibial cortex will help identify all remaining bone that may inhibit closure.

The osteotomy is closed either with a gentle valgus force or with a commercially available compression clamp. If a compression clamp is used, two proximal 6.5-mm-long (60 mm) cancellous screws are inserted through either an L- or T-shaped plate. Using shorter screws may cause them to cut out of the metaphyseal bone with compression. If the fibula was adequately released or osteotomized, there should be complete closure of the tibial osteotomy. Apposition of the bone fragments should be confirmed fluoroscopically and directly visualized. It is imperative that lateral closure does not result in medial cortical opening that may occur if the medial cortex cracks. If this occurs, a two-pronged staple or plate can be used to stabilize the medial cortex. Alignment is checked fluoroscopically to confirm that the desired mechanical axis was achieved.

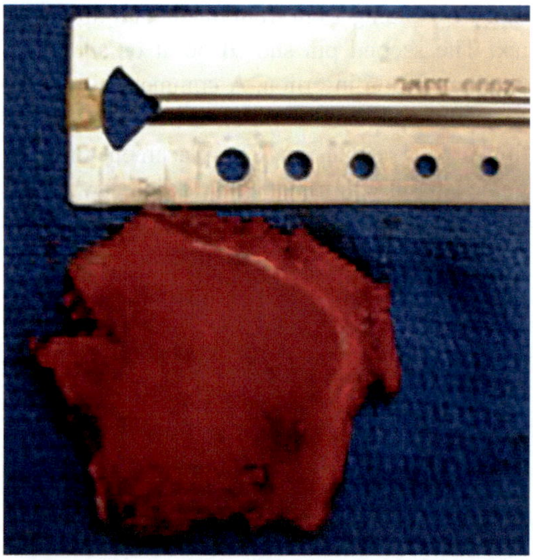

Fig. 13.26 Triangular wedge of bone removed during a closing wedge HTO

Distal plate fixation is achieved with 4.5 mm bi-cortical screws. The long proximal cancellous screws are removed, and shorter (approximately 35 mm) screws are inserted parallel to the tibial plateau to accommodate the ACL graft. The tibial ACL tunnel is drilled normally past the smaller proximal screws, and the revision graft is inserted and fixed in the usual fashion depending on graft type and surgeon preference (Fig. 13.27). The surgical site is thoroughly irrigated, and the anterior compartment fascia is reapproximated to the residual strip on the proximal tibia with absorbable suture. A prophylactic anterior compartment fasciotomy is routinely made to reduce the risk of a compartment syndrome. A layered closure is performed, and a soft dressing, compressive ACE bandage, and hinged knee brace locked in full extension are applied.

Outcomes Following Revision ACL Reconstruction and High Tibial Osteotomy

Little information is available regarding the outcomes of combined revision ACL reconstruction and coronal plane realignment, as the majority of studies evaluate outcome following HTO combined with primary ACL reconstruction [21, 31,

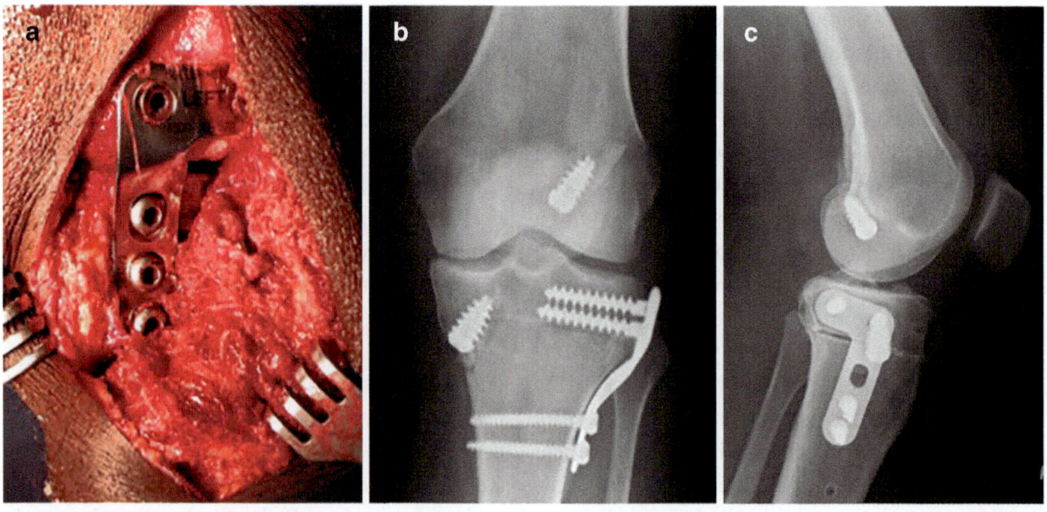

Fig. 13.27 Closing wedge HTO and revision ACL reconstruction. (**a**) Closing wedge HTO with L-shaped plate. (**b**) AP x-ray showing final construct with hardware in place. (**c**) Lateral x-ray

52–59]. Additionally, the literature also varies in terms of surgical technique (opening versus closing wedge), ACL graft source, and length of procedure (single- versus two-stage). In the primary setting, a combination HTO and ACL reconstruction typically results in a significant improvement in functional knee outcome scores [52]. Li et al. [53] conducted a systematic review of 11 studies that reported simultaneous ACL reconstruction and HTO. All cases of varus malalignment were corrected an average of 7.1°. Overall, 85.7% of patients had normal or nearly normal knee stability with a mean KT-1000 side-to-side difference of 2.4 mm. All subjective knee scores improved, and most patients returned to recreational sports activities. The most prevalent complication in this review was deep venous thrombosis (7.7%). Zaffagnini [59] reported only 2 failures at a mean follow-up of 6.5 years in 32 patients who underwent closing wedge HTO and primary or revision ACL reconstruction. Severe medial compartment osteoarthritis was noted in 22%. Arun et al. [54] retrospectively analyzed 30 patients who underwent a combined ACL reconstruction and medial opening wedge osteotomy. They found that decreasing the posterior tibial slope >5° resulted in better functional scores (International Knee Documentation Committee [IKDC] and Lysholm) compared to patients who had <5° decrease, thus emphasizing the importance of the tibial slope and its effect on ACL graft strain. Noyes et al. [21] treated 41 young patients with combined ACL insufficiency and varus malalignment with HTO followed by ACL reconstruction 8 months later. Eighteen patients required PLC reconstruction. After a mean follow-up of 4.5 years, pain was eliminated in 71%, and instability was improved in 66%. Thirty-seven percent rated their knee as normal or very good. Correction of varus malalignment was maintained in 80%, and the adduction moment documented with gait analysis was decreased to below normal values.

Lateral Opening Wedge Distal Femoral Osteotomy and Anterior Cruciate Ligament Reconstruction

Valgus malalignment is considerably less common than varus in the setting of a failed ACL reconstruction. In addition, fewer patients with uni-compartmental osteoarthritis have lateral compartment involvement than medial compartment involvement. Cooke et al. [60] reviewed the radiographs of 167 patients with osteoarthritis and noted valgus alignment in only 24% compared to 76% who were in varus. Normally, there is physiologic valgus of approximately 5°–7° due to 7°–9° of distal femoral valgus combined with 0°–3° of proximal tibial varus [61]. Despite this degree of physiologic valgus, the normal offset caused by the femoral neck results in the mechanical axis passing through the center of the knee. Pathologic valgus occurs when the distal femoral angle is elevated above normal causing the mechanical axis to pass through or lateral to the lateral compartment of the knee. This will lead to progressive wear of the lateral articular cartilage as well as contracture of the lateral capsule and ligamentous structures. Conversely, attenuation of the medial soft tissue restraints may develop over time.

The majority of patients with valgus malalignment have a deformity in the distal femur resulting in elevation in the distal femoral angle. Therefore, the correction of pathologic valgus is directed at realignment of the distal femur. Theoretically, correction of valgus malalignment could be accomplished at the proximal tibia, but this would likely cause joint line obliquity, increased sheer forces across the joint, and subsequent instability.

Surgical correction of valgus malalignment at the distal femur can be achieved with either a medial closing wedge or lateral opening wedge osteotomy similar to correction of varus malalignment at the tibia. Our preference, and that of most surgeons, is to perform a lateral opening wedge osteotomy due to the relative ease of exposure, need for a single osteotomy, ability to fine-tune the correction, and availability of less complicated fixation methods. However, many surgeons are still unfamiliar with this procedure because of its relative infrequency. Combining it with a revision ACL reconstruction increases the complexity and requires careful preoperative planning, accurate intraoperative imaging, and meticulous surgical technique to ensure a favorable outcome and avoid complications.

Preoperative Planning

Full-length, weight-bearing radiographs of both lower extremities are obtained in order to define the extent of the valgus malalignment and to calculate the required degree of correction similar to the preoperative assessment of patients with varus malalignment. However, unlike correction of a varus deformity in which the mechanical axis is shifted to the lateral compartment at the 62% point of the tibial plateau, over-correction of pathologic valgus is contraindicated in order to avoid compressive overload of the medial compartment. Rather, correction of valgus malalignment in patients with symptomatic lateral compartment cartilage wear should be no further medially than to the medial tibial spine. Patients with physiologic genu valgum without lateral compartment wear should only be corrected to neutral (50% of the tibial plateau width) (Fig. 13.28). The degree of correction calculated by the femoral and tibial weight-bearing lines is calculated similar to the planned correction of varus malalignment. In general, each degree of correction of coronal plane alignment is equal to the number of millimeters the osteotomy must be opened. However, this must be confirmed through preoperative calculation of the location, length, and obliquity of the osteotomy (Fig. 13.29).

Deciding which graft to use for the ACL revision in the setting of a combined DFO should follow the same thought process used when performing an HTO in combination with an ACL revision. The primary technical issue associated with the combined procedure is femoral fixation. It is imperative that the femoral tunnel is drilled through an anteromedial portal or via an outside-in approach rather than through a trans-tibial tunnel in order to prevent a relatively vertical femoral tunnel that may interfere with the DFO hardware. Outside-in drilling has the advantage in that it can be done through the same incision as that for the DFO in order to avoid the femoral hardware. Our preference is to drill the femoral tunnel prior to performing the DFO so the hyperflexion of the knee that is required to drill the femoral tunnel does not destabilize the osteotomy fixation.

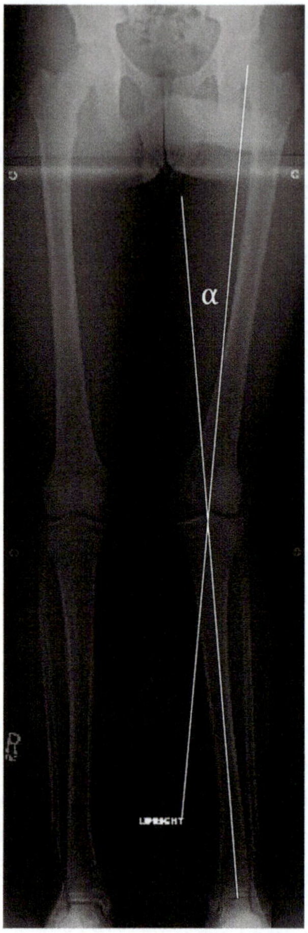

Fig. 13.28 Full-length x-ray showing the degree of correction calculated by the femoral and tibial weight mechanical axis lines needed to achieve a new mechanical axis that is at a point 50% of the width of the tibial plateau

Suspensory cortical fixation may not be feasible due to the presence of the lateral plate and screws, but interference fixation can usually be accomplished given the obliquity of the distal cancellous DFO screws and the location of a properly drilled femoral tunnel.

Surgical Technique

In the setting of a combined opening wedge DFO osteotomy and revision ACL reconstruction, patient positioning, arthroscopic meniscal/chondral procedures, and notch preparation are done

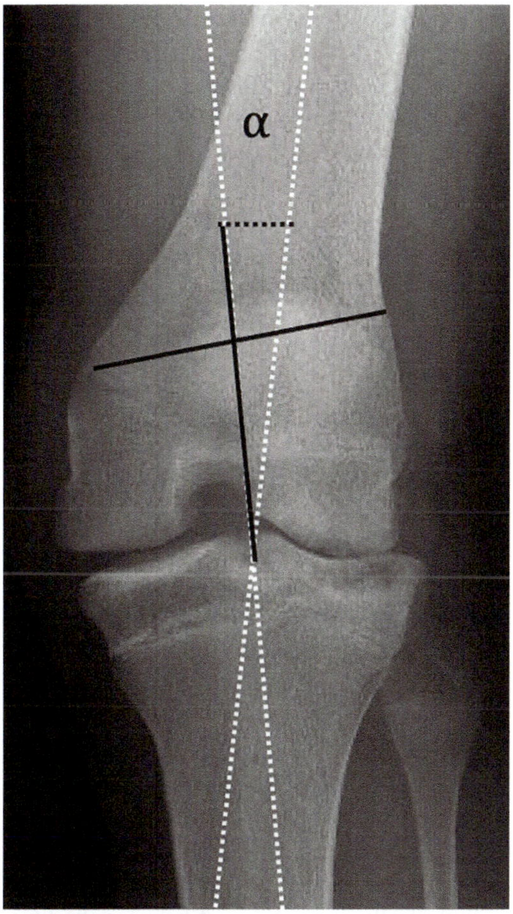

Fig. 13.29 The angle of desired correction (α) is converted into millimeters of "opening" of the osteotomy. A line across the distal femur represents the anticipated site, angle, and length of the osteotomy (solid black line). The length of this line is superimposed on the femoral weight-bearing line, and the distance at this location between the femoral and tibial weight-bearing lines is the amount of opening, in millimeters, required to achieve the desired angular correction (dashed black line)

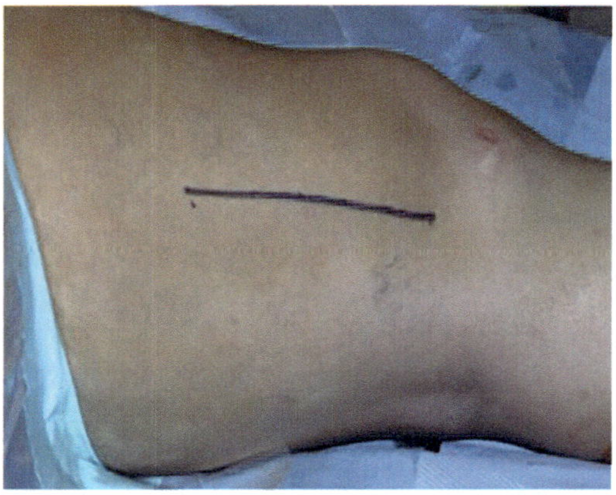

Fig. 13.30 Incision of the distal lateral thigh used for a DFO

as in the HTO. If it is decided to proceed with the combined procedure, the revision graft is harvested and is made 1 mm larger in diameter than the primary graft, if known. The femoral tunnel is drilled through the anteromedial portal or with a two-incision outside-in method using the appropriate over-the-top guide and a shuttle suture is passed for later use. The tibial tunnel is created using compression drills with care taken to achieve anatomic placement. Confirmation of circumferential cancellous in the tibial tunnel will aid graft fixation. This can be achieved with use of curettes and thermal ablation, while the tunnel is visualized from the intra-articular aperture with a 70° arthroscope.

A 10 cm incision is made along the lateral aspect of the distal thigh to 1 cm distal to the lateral epicondyle (Fig. 13.30). The iliotibial band is incised longitudinally, and the vastus lateralis is split in line with its fibers to the lateral intermuscular septum. A Cobb elevator is used to expose the anterior, lateral, and posterior surfaces of the distal femur. A Bennett retractor is used to facilitate exposure and protect the quadriceps muscle anteriorly (Fig. 13.31). A radiolucent or other curved retractor is used to protect the neurovascular structures posteriorly.

Under fluoroscopic visualization, a guide pin is drilled across the distal femur parallel to the joint line, and a second pin is drilled obliquely at a 15°–20° angle in the coronal plane to the level of the medial femoral cortex. It is imperative that the guide pin is placed *above* the level of the trochlear groove so that the patellofemoral joint is not breached with the osteotomy. A second guide pin is placed parallel with the first using a free-hand technique or the proprietary drill guide (Arthrex Inc., Naples, FL) (Fig. 13.32). Anteroposterior and lateral fluoroscopic images should confirm accurate pin placement to ensure a perpendicular osteotomy in relation to the femoral shaft in the sagittal plane. A flat cutting guide is inserted

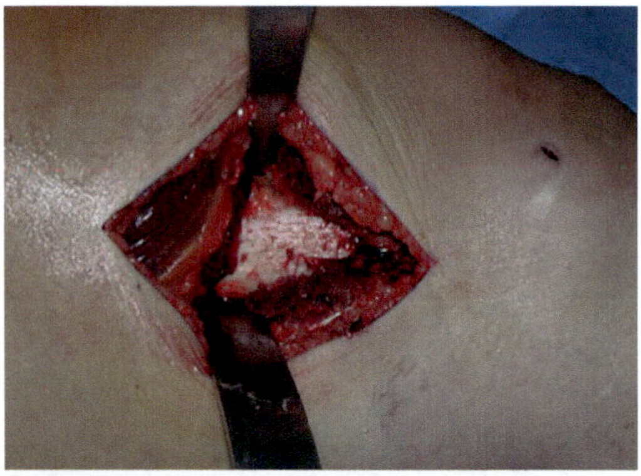

Fig. 13.31 Exposure of lateral femur following elevation of the vastus lateralis

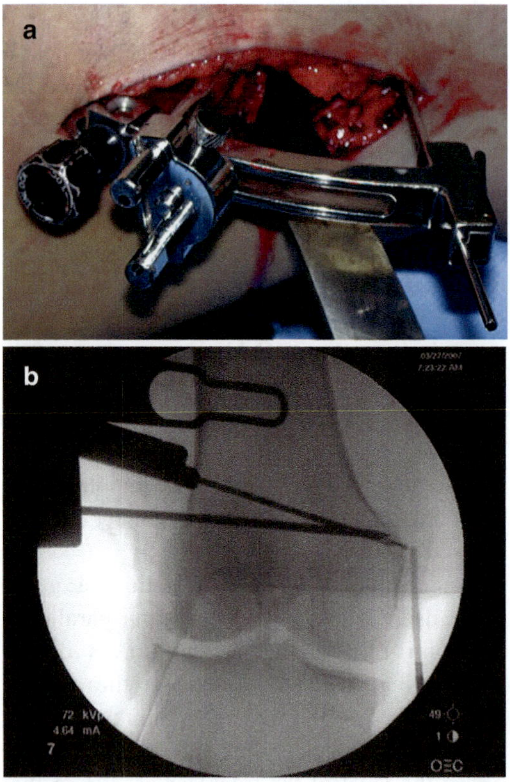

Fig. 13.32 Osteotomy of the distal femur. (**a**) Guide used to place two Kirschner wires at the correct location and angle for the cutting guide. (**b**) Fluoroscopic image of Kirschner wires in place showing the intended angle of the osteotomy

over the guide pins, and a 1″ oscillating saw is used to cut the lateral, anterior, and posterior femoral cortices under fluoroscopic guidance with soft tissue protectors in place at all times (Fig. 13.33). A straight osteotome is used to complete the osteotomy to a distance 1 cm from the medial femoral cortex (Fig. 13.34). A Kirschner wire can be used to perforate the medial cortex several times to cause a "green-stick" effect and allow the cortex to bend with a gentle varus force applied to the osteotome. It is imperative that the osteotomy is performed perpendicular to the femoral shaft in the sagittal plane in order to avoid flexion or extension of the femoral condyle as the osteotomy is opened.

Once the osteotomy is mobile, a wedged osteotome with removable handle is gently impacted with a mallet taking multiple pauses to allow for stress relaxation of the intact medial cortex. The osteotome is inserted with the distance calculated preoperatively (Fig. 13.35). If a fracture of the medial femoral cortex occurs, it should be stabilized with a two-hole plate and screws as the curvature of the medial femoral metaphysis precludes fixation with a staple. Loss of medial cortical fixation will cause loss of the realignment and risk malunion and nonunion of the osteotomy. Once the osteotomy is completed, adequate correction is confirmed with a rigid alignment rod as discussed previously. The rod should ideally cross the joint between the tibial spines and no further medial than the medial tibial spine. If the correction is adequate, the handle is removed from the wedge osteotome, and a T-shaped osteotomy plate (Arthrex Inc., Naples, FL) with appropriate-sized tooth corresponding to the degree of opening in millimeters is inserted between the tines of the osteotome (Fig. 13.36). Four 4.5 mm bi-cortical screws are used for proximal fixation, and three converging 6.5 mm cancellous screws inserted parallel to the obliquity of the osteotomy are used for distal fixation. Placement of an arthroscopic shaver or drill into the previously drilled femoral tunnel while the distal screws are inserted can ensure free passage of the ACL graft.

Once osteotomy fixation is complete, the bone defect is filled anterior and posterior to the plate with autograft or allograft bone or synthetic bone graft substitute to both fill the cancellous defect and provide structural support to the lateral cor-

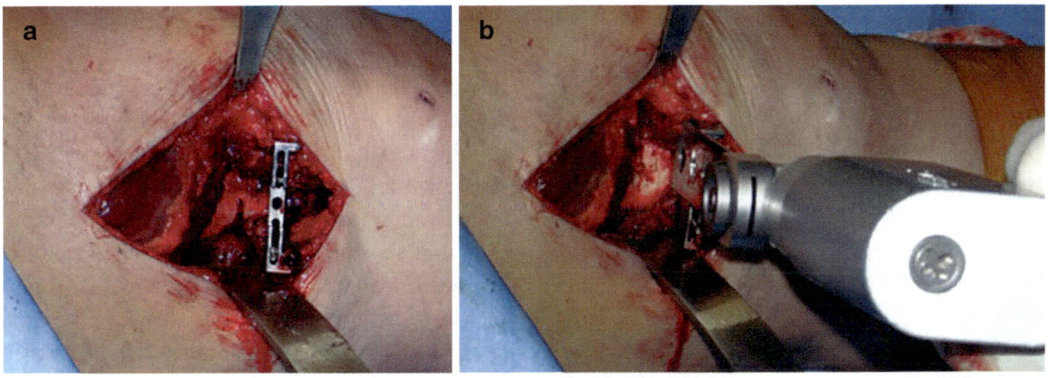

Fig. 13.33 (**a**) Cutting guide secured by the Kirschner wires. (**b**) Osteotomy performed with an oscillating saw with neurovascular structures protected by Z-retractors

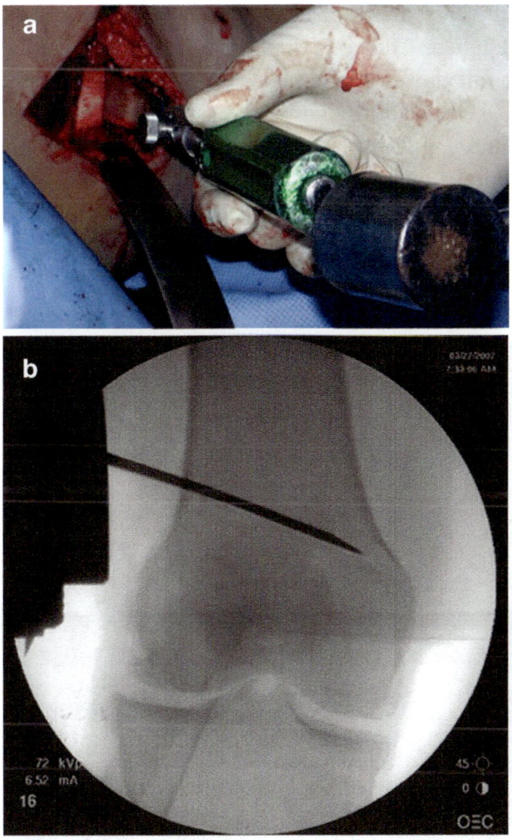

Fig. 13.34 (**a**) Osteotome used to complete the osteotomy. (**b**) AP fluoroscopic image showing osteotome at correct angle and depth

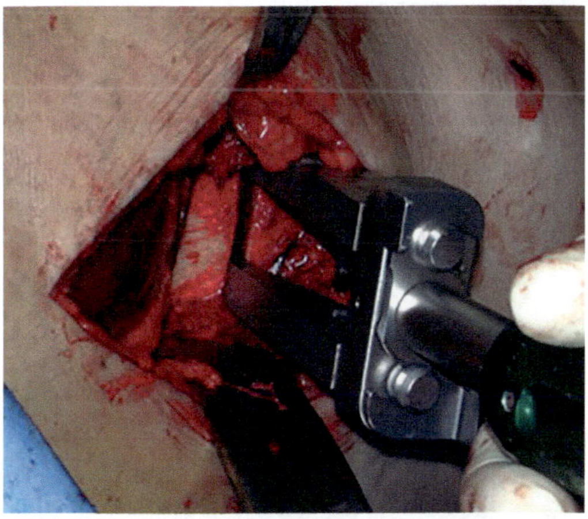

Fig. 13.35 Wedge osteotome used to progressively open the osteotomy to the desired degree in millimeters

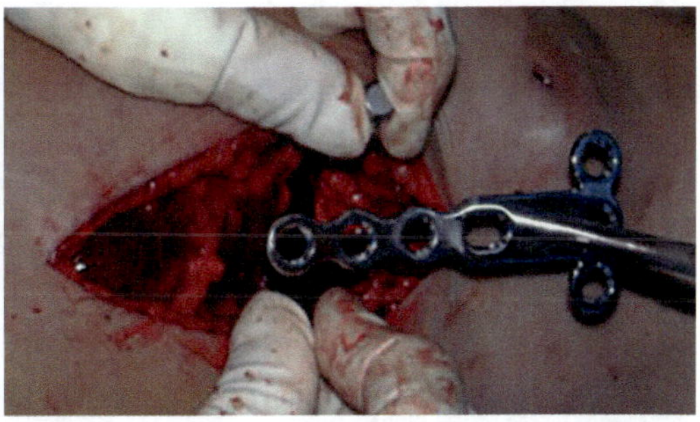

Fig. 13.36 T-shaped femoral Puddu plate (Arthrex Inc., Naples, FL) prior to insertion

tex (Fig. 13.37). The iliotibial band is closed with a running absorbable suture, and the skin is closed in layers.

The arthroscope is placed back in the joint, and the shuttle suture is used to pass the graft up the tibial tunnel and into the femoral tunnel. If a

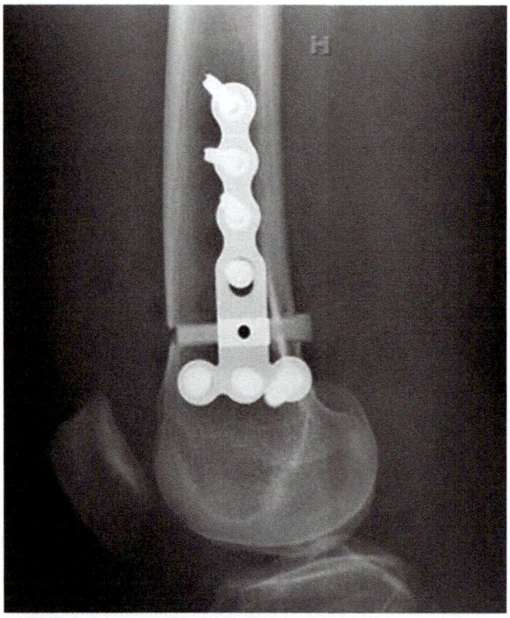

Fig. 13.37 Lateral x-ray showing femoral osteotomy plate in place with osteoinductive bone graft substitute filling the defect. Note the maintenance of normal femoral alignment

soft tissue graft is selected, suspensory cortical fixation may be feasible but must take the plate into consideration. The graft sutures may be tied around the distal cancellous screws to provide proximal fixation as an alternative option. If a graft with a femoral bone plug is used, interference fixation that is laterally oriented in the femoral tunnel should avoid the distal osteotomy screws. Adequate femoral fixation and graft isometricity are confirmed with 10 lbs. of tension applied to the distal graft sutures, while the knee is cycled multiple times from 0° to 90° of flexion. Two millimeters or less of graft migration within the tibial tunnel is acceptable with flexion and extension. Tibial fixation is accomplished with the knee in 10° of flexion and a posterior drawer applied. Choice of fixation is dependent on the graft chosen and surgeon preference (Fig. 13.38).

Once all wounds are closed, a well-padded dressing and an ACE wrap are applied to the entire lower extremity. A long-leg hinged knee brace is locked in full extension for 24 hours.

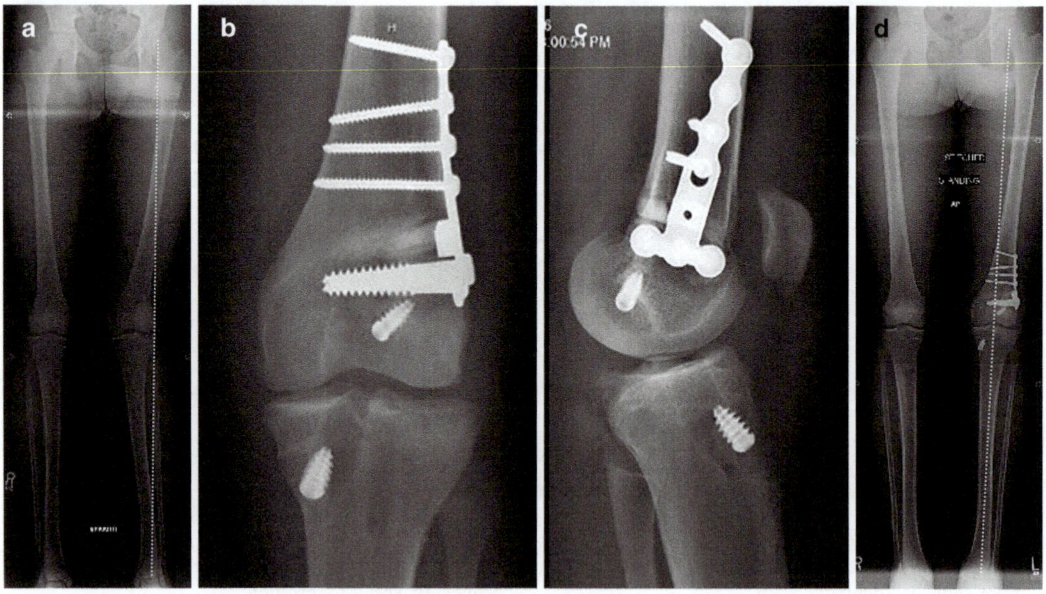

Fig. 13.38 A 17-year-old male who underwent ACL "repair" several years prior with pain and recurrent instability. (**a**) Full-length x-ray showing mechanical axis indicative of significant genu valgum (dashed white line). (**b**) AP x-ray following DFO and ACL reconstruction. (**c**) Lateral x-ray. (**d**) Postoperative full-length x-ray of lower extremities showing new mechanical axis at the 50th percentile of the joint line following realignment (dashed white line)

Postoperative Care Following Revision ACL Reconstruction and Osteotomy

The postoperative rehabilitation following an HTO or DFO combined with a revision ACL reconstruction is begun within the first week following surgery. Deep venous thrombosis (DVT) prophylaxis is recommended for 4 weeks given the magnitude of the procedure. Ankle pumps and elevation are helpful to facilitate venous blood flow. The rehabilitation regimen is generally less permissive than following an isolated ACL reconstruction due to the osteotomy that is solely dependent on the method of fixation for initial stability. Concurrent meniscal and/or cartilage restorative procedures may also necessitate limited weight-bearing. Patellar mobilization and isometric quadriceps contraction are performed as is aggressive use of cold therapy and compression to control swelling. Hamstring, gastrocnemius, and quadriceps stretching is performed throughout the rehabilitation period.

A long-leg hinged knee brace is worn for 8 weeks following surgery and is locked in full extension for the first 24 hours in order to reduce the risk of extension loss that may occur following a revision ACL reconstruction combined with an osteotomy. Range of motion is encouraged from 0° to 90° beginning on the day after surgery. Passive and active range of motion exercises are performed four times per day for 10 minutes per session with an emphasis on obtaining full, symmetrical extension. Patients should achieve 120° by 4 weeks and 135° by 8 weeks following surgery. Active range of motion is facilitated with a stationary cycle. Extension loss should be addressed immediately with an aggressive overpressure regimen, as necessary, to prevent arthrofibrosis.

The patient is allowed toe-touch weight-bearing for the first 4 weeks, after which plain radiographs are taken to assess healing and confirm satisfactory placement of all hardware. More permissive weight-bearing may be considered following a closing wedge HTO since there is immediate bone apposition. As healing progresses, patients are allowed to bear 25% of their body weight with emphasis on a normal heel-to-toe gait pattern. Full weight-bearing as tolerated is allowed when there is evidence of radiographic union and no tenderness at the osteotomy site, which usually occurs 8–10 weeks following surgery. Gait training is resumed with an emphasis on maintenance of a normalized gait pattern that was achieved preoperatively in those patients demonstrating pathologic gait patterns.

Quadriceps isometrics, straight leg raises, and ankle pumps are allowed within the first 2 weeks. Closed-chain exercises are started at 4 weeks. Hamstring curls and active open-chain knee extension from 90° to 30° are allowed at 8 weeks. Hip abduction, adduction, flexion, and extension are performed as tolerated. Balance and proprioceptive training are begun at 8 weeks if healing has occurred. Lower extremity conditioning, aquatherapy, treadmill ambulation, and walking for exercise are progressively allowed 3–4 months after surgery.

Patients who undergo an HTO or DFO are encouraged to return to low-impact, light activities (i.e., swimming, golf, cycling). Repetitive high-impact exercises such as running or jumping should be discouraged in those patients with meniscal or articular cartilage damage as they will potentially exacerbate preexisting cartilage damage. Sports that involve frequent cutting and pivoting should be avoided to reduce strain on the revision ACL graft. Light, recreational activity is typically allowed 6 months following surgery.

Complications

A combined revision ACL reconstruction and coronal plane osteotomy offers the advantage of correcting both knee instability and malalignment in a single stage, thus avoiding two separate procedures and a lengthier rehabilitation. Unfortunately, both procedures have significant potential complications common to more complex operations. General complications common to both an HTO and DFO include under-correction and over-correction of the realignment. This can be prevented with careful preoperative planning, accurate use of the saw and osteotome to the correct depth, and fluoroscopic confirmation. Delayed union, malunion, and nonunion may occur secondary to non-compliance with postoperative weight-bearing restrictions, loss of fixation, or nicotine use. Loss of fixation of the tibial or femoral cortical hinge may occur postoperatively because either it was not noticed by the surgeon intraoperatively, the patient was non-compliant with weight-bearing restrictions, or there was preexisting decreased bone density. Intra-articular extension of the osteotomy may occur for three reasons: (1) if, during a DFO, the guide pins are inserted too far distally below the proximal edge of the trochlear groove causing violation of the patellofemoral joint; (2) if the osteotomy is angulated toward the joint, a fracture can extend into the lateral or medial compartment during an HTO and DFO, respectively; and (3) if the cortical hinge has not been adequately cut and perforated causing a fracture to propagate once a valgus (HTO) or varus (DFO) force is applied.

Flexion or extension of the distal femoral condylar fragment may occur during a DFO if the osteotomy is not perpendicular to the femoral shaft. This is analogous to inadvertently increasing the posterior tibial slope during an HTO. Malalignment of the distal femur in the sagittal plane will result in loss of knee extension or flexion and is difficult to correct postoperatively. Iliotibial band irritation from the underlying DFO plate and screws may occur and is more common in thinner individuals. Similar irritation can occur at the medial tibial plateau following an HTO. The hardware can be removed once adequate healing has occurred but, in general, should be delayed for at least 12 months.

Complications following an isolated HTO are considerably more likely compared to a DFO due, in part, due to the relative frequency of the two procedures. Spahn [62] noted deep infection rates following an HTO of 4.7%. Hardware failure due to plate or screw fracture following opening wedge osteotomies has been described in 16.6% [62], and intra-articular fractures have been described in 14.6% of patients [62]. Warden et al. [63] reported delayed union rates of 6.6% with nonunion occurring in 1.6%. Fortunately, the patients considered for these complex combined procedures are relatively healthy. Despite this, patient compliance with weight-bearing and activity restrictions is crucial to the success of these complex procedures in order to avoid complications.

Complications following isolated revision ACL reconstruction are dependent on the presence of concurrent meniscal and/or chondral pathology, technical aspects to address prior tunnels and hardware, and choice of the revision graft. These variables limit the ability to generalize complication rates across all ACL revisions. In general, there is a three to four times higher failure rate following revision ACL reconstruction when compared to primary reconstructions [64]. Rates of deep infection [65] and DVT following ACL surgery are consistently less than 1% [66].

Prior literature has focused mainly on the surgical technique and complications of a *primary* ACL reconstruction combined with an osteotomy. There is no body of literature specifically evaluating the complication rates of *revision* ACL surgery combined with an osteotomy. Despite this, prior literature pertaining to complications is still informative. Willey et al. [67] found after a mean follow-up of 45 months, 37% of patients who underwent a primary ACL reconstruction, and either an HTO or DFO, experienced either a major (i.e., arthrofibrosis, over-correction, nonunion, infection, neurovascular injury) or minor (i.e., hardware pain, hematoma, delayed union, superficial infection) complication. A significant number of associated procedures were performed (i.e., chondral resurfacing, meniscal transplantation, extensor mechanism reconstruction) that may have contributed to the 20% rate of major complications and 25.7% incidence of minor complications. These authors concluded that a combined ACL reconstruction and coronal plane osteotomy was a relatively safe procedure with complication rates similar to an isolated osteotomy. Boss et al. [56] reported 5 patients who required arthroscopic debridement and manipulation for arthrofibrosis and 2 patients with sensory disturbances in 27 patients who underwent a combined ACL reconstruction and HTO. Dejour et al. [57] noted 3 major complications and 16 minor complications among 44 patients who underwent combined HTO and ACL reconstruction. As a result of the relatively low complication rates and favorable outcomes, these authors also favored a single-stage approach for this patient cohort. In contrast, Lattermann et al. [58] recommended a staged approach in patients under 40 with combined medial compartment osteoarthritis and ACL insufficiency. They recommended that the HTO be performed first followed by ACL reconstruction if instability persists. In their series of eight patients who underwent the combined procedure, six of eight sustained major complications including two ACL re-ruptures.

Conclusion

Assessment of coronal plane alignment is an essential element in the preoperative evaluation of patients considered for revision ACL reconstruction. Unaddressed malalignment places the revision ACL graft at risk and can lead to elevated compressive loads in the medial or lateral compartment for varus or valgus malalignment, respectively. A thorough physical examination is mandatory to diagnose all ligamentous insufficiencies and potential sources of pain. Graft options in the revision setting must take into consideration prior graft(s) and hardware used, hardware placement for the realignment procedure, concurrent pathology, and activity goals. Accurate preoperative calculation of the degree of coronal plane correction, anatomic placement of the revision graft, and treatment of all associated meniscal and chondral damage are imperative. The rehabilitation following these complex procedures is typically less permissive than following a primary ACL reconstruction as bone consolidation is the initial rate-limiting factor of the rehabilitation regimen. Low-impact activities should be emphasized to prevent further articular cartilage degeneration.

References

1. Maletis GB, et al. Comparison of community-based ACL reconstruction registries in the U.S. and Norway. J Bone Joint Surg Am. 2011;93 Suppl 3:31–6. ISSN 0021-9355.
2. Andernord D, et al. Patient predictors of early revision surgery after anterior cruciate ligament reconstruction: a cohort study of 16,930 patients with 2-year follow-up. Am J Sports Med. 2015;43(1):121–7. ISSN 0363-5465.
3. Crawford SN, Waterman BR, Lubowitz JH. Long-term failure of anterior cruciate ligament reconstruction. Arthroscopy. 2013;29(9):1566–71. ISSN 0749-8063.
4. Wright RW, et al. Descriptive epidemiology of the Multicenter ACL Revision Study (MARS) cohort. Am J Sports Med. 2010;38(10):1979–86. ISSN 0363-5465.
5. Morgan JA, et al. Femoral tunnel malposition in ACL revision reconstruction. J Knee Surg. 2012;25(5):361–8. ISSN 1538-8506 (Print) 1538-8506.
6. Zeng C, et al. Is posterior tibial slope associated with noncontact anterior cruciate ligament injury? Knee Surg Sports Traumatol Arthrosc. 2016;24(3):830–7. ISSN 0942-2056.
7. Giffin JR, et al. Effects of increasing tibial slope on the biomechanics of the knee. Am J Sports Med. 2004;32(2):376–82. ISSN 0363-5465 (Print) 0363-5465.
8. Won HH, et al. Coronal limb alignment and indications for high tibial osteotomy in patients undergoing revision ACL reconstruction. Clin Orthop Relat Res. 2013;471(11):3504–11. ISSN 0009-921x.
9. Noyes FR, Barber-Westin SD. Anterior cruciate ligament revision reconstruction: results using a quadriceps tendon-patellar bone autograft. Am J Sports Med. 2006;34(4):553–64. ISSN 0363-5465 (Print) 0363-5465.
10. Coventry MB. Osteotomy of the upper portion of the tibia for degenerative arthritis of the knee. A preliminary report. 1965. Clin Orthop Relat Res. 1989;(248):4–8. ISSN 0009-921X (Print) 0009-921x.
11. Borchers JR, et al. Intra-articular findings in primary and revision anterior cruciate ligament reconstruction surgery: a comparison of the MOON and MARS study groups. Am J Sports Med. 2011;39(9):1889–93. ISSN 0363-5465.
12. MARS Group. Radiographic findings in revision anterior cruciate ligament reconstructions from the Mars cohort. J Knee Surg. 2013;26(4):239–47.
13. Shelbourne KD, Gray T. Results of anterior cruciate ligament reconstruction based on meniscus and articular cartilage status at the time of surgery. Five- to fifteen-year evaluations. Am J Sports Med. 2000;28(4):446–52. ISSN 0363-5465 (Print) 0363-5465.

14. Wu WH, Hackett T, Richmond JC. Effects of meniscal and articular surface status on knee stability, function, and symptoms after anterior cruciate ligament reconstruction: a long-term prospective study. Am J Sports Med. 2002;30(6):845–50. ISSN 0363-5465 (Print) 0363-5465.
15. Fink C, et al. Long-term outcome of operative or nonoperative treatment of anterior cruciate ligament rupture – is sports activity a determining variable? Int J Sports Med. 2001;22(4):304–9. ISSN 0172-4622 (Print) 0172-4622.
16. Brophy RH, et al. Association between previous meniscal surgery and the incidence of chondral lesions at revision anterior cruciate ligament reconstruction. Am J Sports Med. 2012;40(4):808–14. ISSN 0363-5465.
17. Albright JP. Corr Insights (R): coronal limb alignment and indications for high tibial osteotomy in patients undergoing revision ACL reconstruction. Clin Orthop Relat Res. 2013;471(11):3512–3. ISSN 0009-921x.
18. Van De Pol GJ, et al. Varus alignment leads to increased forces in the anterior cruciate ligament. Am J Sports Med. 2009;37(3):481–7. ISSN 0363-5465.
19. Noyes FR, et al. The anterior cruciate ligament-deficient knee with varus alignment. An analysis of gait adaptations and dynamic joint loadings. Am J Sports Med. 1992;20(6):707–16. ISSN 0363-5465 (Print) 0363-5465.
20. Markolf KL, et al. Combined knee loading states that generate high anterior cruciate ligament forces. J Orthop Res. 1995;13(6):930–5. ISSN 0736-0266 (Print) 0736-0266.
21. Noyes FR, Barber-Westin SD, Hewett TE. High tibial osteotomy and ligament reconstruction for varus angulated anterior cruciate ligament-deficient knees. Am J Sports Med. 2000;28(3):282–96. ISSN 0363-5465 (Print) 0363-5465.
22. Brambilla L, et al. Prevalence of associated lesions in anterior cruciate ligament reconstruction: correlation with surgical timing and with patient age, sex, and body mass index. Am J Sports Med. 2015;43(12):2966–73. ISSN 0363-5465.
23. Mok YR, et al. Anterior cruciate ligament reconstruction performed within 12 months of the index injury is associated with a lower rate of medial meniscus tears. Knee Surg Sports Traumatol Arthrosc. 2019;27(1):117–23. ISSN 0942-2056.
24. Mcdermott ID, Amis AA. The consequences of meniscectomy. J Bone Joint Surg Br. 2006;88(12):1549–56. ISSN 0301-620X (Print) 0301-620x.
25. Nannaparaju M, et al. Posterolateral corner injuries: epidemiology, anatomy, biomechanics and diagnosis. Injury. 2018;49(6):1024–31. ISSN 0020-1383.
26. Wink AE, et al. Varus thrust during walking and the risk of incident and worsening medial tibiofemoral MRI lesions: the Multicenter Osteoarthritis Study. Osteoarthr Cartil. 2017;25(6):839–45. ISSN 1063-4584.
27. Rosenberg TD, et al. The forty-five-degree posteroanterior flexion weight-bearing radiograph of the knee. J Bone Joint Surg Am. 1988;70(10):1479–83. ISSN 0021-9355 (Print) 0021-9355.
28. Bin SI, et al. Changes in patellar height after opening wedge and closing wedge high tibial osteotomy: a meta-analysis. Arthroscopy. 2016;32(11):2393–400. ISSN 0749-8063.
29. Berg EE, Mason SL, Lucas MJ. Patellar height ratios: a comparison of four measurement methods. Am J Sports Med. 1996;24(2):218–21. ISSN 0363-5465. Disponível em: < 10.1177/036354659602400218 >. Acesso em: 2018/12/31.
30. Jaecker V, et al. Increased medial and lateral tibial posterior slopes are independent risk factors for graft failure following ACL reconstruction. Arch Orthop Trauma Surg. 2018;138(10):1423–31. ISSN 0936-8051.
31. Cantivalli A, et al. High tibial osteotomy and anterior cruciate ligament reconstruction/revision. Clin Sports Med. 2019;38(3):417–33. ISSN 0278-5919.
32. Hantes ME, et al. The effect of early motion on tibial tunnel widening after anterior cruciate ligament replacement using hamstring tendon grafts. Arthroscopy. 2004;20(6):572–80. ISSN 0749-8063.
33. Wilson TC, et al. Tunnel enlargement after anterior cruciate ligament surgery. Am J Sports Med. 2004;32(2):543–9. ISSN 0363-5465 (Print) 0363-5465.
34. Fahey M, Indelicato PA. Bone tunnel enlargement after anterior cruciate ligament replacement. Am J Sports Med. 1994;22(3):410–4. ISSN 0363-5465 (Print) 0363-5465.
35. Amendola A. Unicompartmental osteoarthritis in the active patient: the role of high tibial osteotomy. Arthroscopy. 2003;19 Suppl 1:109–16. ISSN 0749-8063.
36. Lee YS, et al. Effect of foot rotation on the mechanical axis and correlation between knee and whole leg radiographs. Knee Surg Sports Traumatol Arthrosc. 2013;21(11):2542–7. ISSN 0942-2056.
37. Paley D, et al. Deformity planning for frontal and sagittal plane corrective osteotomies. Orthop Clin North Am. 1994;25(3):425–65. ISSN 0030-5898 (Print) 0030-5898.
38. Noyes FR, Goebel SX, West J. Opening wedge tibial osteotomy: the 3-triangle method to correct axial alignment and tibial slope. Am J Sports Med. 2005;33(3):378–87. ISSN 0363-5465 (Print) 0363-5465.
39. Allen CR, et al. Importance of the medial meniscus in the anterior cruciate ligament-deficient knee. J Orthop Res. 2000;18(1):109–15. ISSN 0736-0266 (Print) 0736-0266.
40. Musahl V, et al. The effect of medial versus lateral meniscectomy on the stability of the anterior cruciate ligament-deficient knee. Am J Sports Med. 2010;38(8):1591–7. ISSN 0363-5465.
41. Young Sd TA. Complications of allograft use in anterior cruciate ligament reconstruction: a systematic review. Oper Tech Spots Med. 2012;14:20–6.

42. Fujisawa Y, Masuhara K, Shiomi S. The effect of high tibial osteotomy on osteoarthritis of the knee. An arthroscopic study of 54 knee joints. Orthop Clin North Am. 1979;10(3):585–608. ISSN 0030-5898 (Print) 0030-5898.
43. Dugdale TW, Noyes FR, Styer D. Preoperative planning for high tibial osteotomy. The effect of lateral tibiofemoral separation and tibiofemoral length. Clin Orthop Relat Res. 1992;(274):248–64. ISSN 0009-921X (Print) 0009-921x.
44. Frank RM, et al. ACL reconstruction basics: quadruple (4-Strand) hamstring autograft harvest. Arthrosc Tech. 2017;6(4):e1309–13. ISSN 2212-6287 (Print) 2212-6287.
45. Nha KW, et al. Navigated versus conventional technique in high tibial osteotomy: a meta-analysis focusing on weight bearing effect. Knee Surg Relat Res. 2019;31(2):81–102. ISSN 2234-0726 (Print) 2234-0726.
46. Bates NA, et al. External loads associated with anterior cruciate ligament injuries increase the correlation between tibial slope and ligament strain during in vitro simulations of in vivo landings. Clin Biomech (Bristol, Avon). 2019;61:84–94. ISSN 0268-0033.
47. Wang Z, et al. Is opening-wedge high tibial osteotomy superior to closing-wedge high tibial osteotomy in treatment of unicompartmental osteoarthritis? A meta-analysis of randomized controlled trials. Int J Surg. 2018;60:153–63. ISSN 1743-9159.
48. Smith TO, et al. Opening- or closing-wedged high tibial osteotomy: a meta-analysis of clinical and radiological outcomes. Knee. 2011;18(6):361–8. ISSN 0968-0160.
49. Marcheggiani Muccioli GM, et al. Lateral closing wedge high tibial osteotomy for medial compartment arthrosis or overload. Clin Sports Med. 2019;38(3):375–86. ISSN 0278-5919.
50. Barrett SL, et al. Superficial peroneal nerve (superficial fibularis nerve): the clinical implications of anatomic variability. J Foot Ankle Surg. 2006;45(3):174–6. ISSN 1067-2516 (Print)1067-2516.
51. Billings A, et al. High tibial osteotomy with a calibrated osteotomy guide, rigid internal fixation, and early motion. Long-term follow-up. J Bone Joint Surg Am. 2000;82(1):70–9. ISSN 0021-9355 (Print) 0021-9355.
52. Gupta A, et al. Surgical techniques, outcomes, indications, and complications of simultaneous high tibial osteotomy and anterior cruciate ligament revision surgery: a systematic review. HSS J. 2019;15(2):176–84. ISSN 1556-3316 (Print) 1556-3316.
53. Li Y, et al. Clinical outcome of simultaneous high tibial osteotomy and anterior cruciate ligament reconstruction for medial compartment osteoarthritis in young patients with anterior cruciate ligament-deficient knees: a systematic review. Arthroscopy. 2015;31(3):507–19. ISSN 0749-8063.
54. Arun GR, et al. Long-term follow up of single-stage anterior cruciate ligament reconstruction and high tibial osteotomy and its relation with posterior tibial slope. Arch Orthop Trauma Surg. 2016;136(4):505–11. ISSN 0936-8051.
55. Mehl J, et al. ACL deficiency and varus osteoarthritis: high tibial osteotomy alone or combined with ACL reconstruction? Arch Orthop Trauma Surg. 2017;137(2):233–40. ISSN 0936-8051.
56. Boss A, et al. Anterior cruciate ligament reconstruction combined with valgus tibial osteotomy (combined procedure). Knee Surg Sports Traumatol Arthrosc. 1995;3(3):187–91. ISSN 0942-2056 (Print) 0942-2056.
57. Dejour H, et al. Anterior cruciate reconstruction combined with valgus tibial osteotomy. Clin Orthop Relat Res. 1994;(299):220–8. ISSN 0009-921X (Print) 0009-921x.
58. Lattermann C, Jakob RP. High tibial osteotomy alone or combined with ligament reconstruction in anterior cruciate ligament-deficient knees. Knee Surg Sports Traumatol Arthrosc. 1996;4(1):32–8. ISSN 0942-2056 (Print) 0942-2056.
59. Zaffagnini S, et al. Combined ACL reconstruction and closing-wedge HTO for varus angulated ACL-deficient knees. Knee Surg Sports Traumatol Arthrosc. 2013;21(4):934–41. ISSN 0942-2056.
60. Cooke TD, Li J, Scudamore RA. Radiographic assessment of bony contributions to knee deformity. Orthop Clin North Am. 1994;25(3):387–93. ISSN 0030-5898 (Print) 0030-5898.
61. Luo CF. Reference axes for reconstruction of the knee. Knee. 2004;11(4):251–7. ISSN 0968-0160 (Print) 0968-0160.
62. Spahn G. Complications in high tibial (medial opening wedge) osteotomy. Arch Orthop Trauma Surg. 2004;124(10):649–53. ISSN 0936-8051 (Print) 0936-8051.
63. Warden SJ, et al. Delayed- and non-union following opening wedge high tibial osteotomy: surgeons' results from 182 completed cases. Knee Surg Sports Traumatol Arthrosc. 2005;13(1):34–7. ISSN 0942-2056 (Print) 0942-2056.
64. Wright RW, et al. Outcome of revision anterior cruciate ligament reconstruction: a systematic review. J Bone Joint Surg Am. 2012;94(6):531–6. ISSN 0021-9355.
65. Wang C, et al. Septic arthritis after arthroscopic anterior cruciate ligament reconstruction: a retrospective analysis of incidence, presentation, treatment, and cause. Arthroscopy. 2009;25(3):243–9. ISSN 0749-8063.
66. Williams JS Jr, et al. Incidence of deep vein thrombosis after arthroscopic knee surgery: a prospective study. Arthroscopy. 1995;11(6):701–5. ISSN 0749-8063 (Print) 0749-8063.
67. Willey M, et al. Complications associated with realignment osteotomy of the knee performed simultaneously with additional reconstructive procedures. Iowa Orthop J. 2010;30:55–60. ISSN 1541-5457.

Sagittal Plane Correction in Revision ACL Reconstruction

14

S. Mark Heard and Michaela Kopka

Introduction

Tibial osteotomy has been an accepted surgical technique for the treatment of knee osteoarthritis (OA) for over 50 years [1]. However, its utility in the setting of knee ligament insufficiency has only come to prominence in recent years. As soft tissue reconstructive techniques have evolved, the impact of bony morphology on knee stability has received increased attention. The importance of coronal alignment in anterior cruciate ligament (ACL)-deficient knees was addressed in detail in the previous chapter. This chapter will focus on the role of sagittal alignment and how osteotomy can be utilized to improve biomechanics and thereby optimize outcomes in revision ACL reconstruction.

Background

In the sagittal plane, posterior tibial slope (PTS) is best defined as the angle between a line perpendicular to the mid-diaphysis of the tibia and the posterior inclination of the tibial plateau. The normal values for the medial and lateral tibial plateau are 9–11° and 6–8°, respectively [2]. A number of biomechanical studies have demonstrated that increased PTS leads to increased anterior tibial translation and subsequently increased strain on the native ACL. Dejour and Bonnin [3] determined that every 10° increase in PTS resulted in a 6 mm increase in anterior tibial translation. McLean et al. [4] demonstrated that elevated PTS was significantly correlated with increased anterior tibial translation and acceleration, as well as peak anteromedial ACL bundle strain.

Clinical studies have corroborated these findings by revealing an increased risk of ACL injury among patients with elevated PTS. In a matched cohort study of 100 patients undergoing ACL reconstruction compared to 100 patients presenting with patellofemoral pain, Brandon et al. [5] demonstrated a statistically significant increase in PTS for the ACL-injured patients. A 15-year prospective longitudinal study of 200 patients following ACL reconstruction concluded that those who sustained further ACL injury (either ACL graft rupture or contralateral injury) had a mean PTS of 9.9° compared to 8.5° for those without further injury. The odds of sustaining a new injury increased fivefold when PTS ≥12° [6]. In adolescent ACL reconstruction patients, the hazard of increased PTS is even more profound with a 20-year ACL graft survival rate of only 22% in patients with PTS ≥12° [7].

Osteotomy aimed at decreasing PTS can effectively reduce the strain on the ACL graft and thereby decrease the risk of re-injury. In a

S. M. Heard (✉) · M. Kopka
Orthopaedic Surgery, Banff Sport Medicine, Banff, AB, Canada

M. J. Alaia, K. J. Jones (eds.), *Revision Anterior Cruciate Ligament Reconstruction*, https://doi.org/10.1007/978-3-030-96996-7_14

cadaveric study, Imhoff et al. [8] determined that tibial osteotomy significantly decreased anterior tibial translation in the ACL-deficient knee, as well as significantly decreased the force through the ACL graft in the reconstructed knee. Zaffagnini et al. [9] prospectively assessed a cohort of 32 patients following revision ACL reconstruction and concurrent lateral closing wedge osteotomy. At a mean follow-up of 6.5 years, the authors showed significant improvements in patient-reported outcomes with an overall failure rate of only 6%. Even in the re-revision scenario, combining ACL reconstruction with slope-reducing osteotomy has been proven to improve graft laxity and patient-reported outcomes [10, 11].

Indications

The decision to perform an osteotomy in the setting of revision ACL reconstruction depends on a range of factors including coronal and sagittal plane alignment, integrity of other ligamentous structures, associated meniscal and chondral pathology, as well as patient characteristics including age, comorbidities, and functional status. All of these factors must be considered when creating a preoperative plan.

The three most common types of osteotomies used to decrease tibial slope and, if necessary, correct coronal plane alignment are presented in Table 14.2. Careful patient evaluation and consideration of all contributing factors must be performed prior to determining which surgical approach is most appropriate.

In addition to the three osteotomies listed in Table 14.1, a medial closing wedge osteotomy can be utilized in a patient with failed ACL reconstruction, valgus alignment, *and* increased PTS. Although the distal femur is typically the site of correction in a valgus knee, if sagittal plane alignment needs to be addressed, then a tibial-based osteotomy may be necessary.

In selecting the most appropriate approach, it is also critical to consider the geometry of the proximal tibia and how different types of osteotomies will affect sagittal plane alignment. Based upon three-dimensional computed tomography modelling, Noyes et al. [12] described the proximal tibia as a triangle where the posterior cortex forms a 90° angle with the lateral cortex and a 45° angle with the medial cortex (Fig. 14.1). Due to this relationship, the "gap" angle of an anteromedial opening wedge osteotomy will influence not only coronal alignment but also tibial slope. These authors determined that in order to maintain tibial slope, the height of the anterior osteotomy gap must be half that of the posterior gap. Further, each 1 mm of gap error leads to a 2° increase in PTS. This relationship makes it challenging to maintain – and particularly difficult to *decrease* – PTS when performing a medial opening wedge osteotomy. In contrast, a lateral closing wedge osteotomy has been shown to be more likely to decrease PTS [13, 14]. Additional factors to consider when selecting between a medial and lateral osteotomy are outlined in Table 14.3.

Table 14.1 General indications and contraindications for performing a tibial osteotomy in the revision ACL setting

Indications	Contraindications
Correcting coronal alignment	Concurrent posterior cruciate ligament (PCL) deficiency
Decreasing PTS	Significant knee hyperextension (>10°)
Unloading the medial or lateral compartment (due to meniscal or chondral pathology or concurrent reconstructive procedure)	Grade 4 chondral injury in an isolated compartment
Decreasing stress on ligamentous structures (in the setting of bony malalignment)	Tricompartmental osteoarthritis
	Inflammatory arthritis
	Range of motion restrictions (>5° flexion contracture and/or < 120° of flexion)
	Older (>65 years) and lower demand patients
	Elevated body mass index (BMI >35)

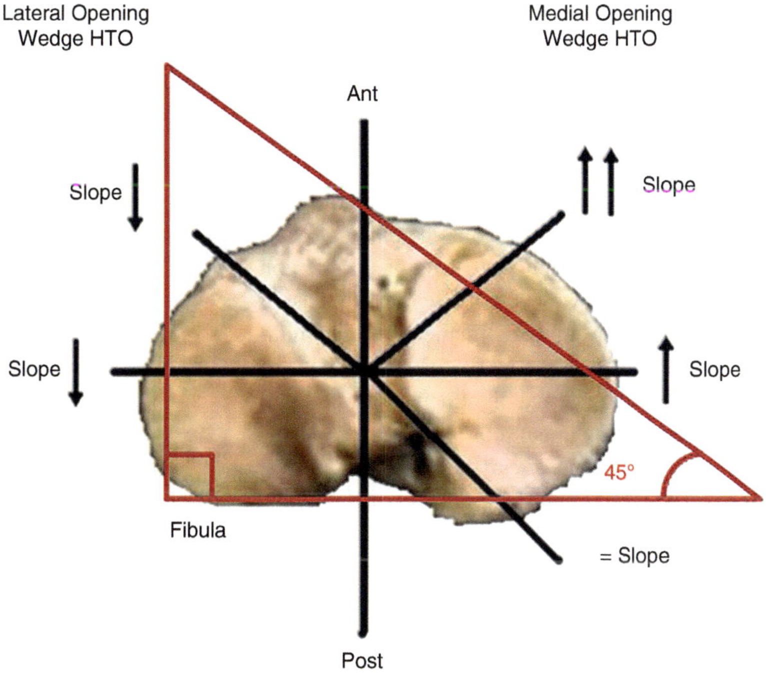

Fig. 14.1 The proximal tibia can be represented as a triangle with the medial and lateral cortices forming 45° and 90° angles with the posterior cortex, respectively. An anteromedial osteotomy is thus more likely to increase slope, while a lateral osteotomy will decrease it. (Modified from Noyes et al. [13])

Table 14.2 The three most common types of tibial osteotomies used to decrease tibial slope and correct coronal plane alignment as necessary

Type of osteotomy	Goal	Indications
Anterior closing wedge	Decrease PTS	Failed ACL reconstruction with PTS >12° and/or high-grade anterior instability
Medial opening wedge	Decrease PTS + correct varus alignment	Failed ACL reconstruction with PTS >12° and/or high-grade anterior instability *and* Early to moderate medial compartment degenerative changes Medial meniscus deficiency Concurrent osteochondral or meniscal transplant Lateral ligament insufficiency *with bony varus*
Lateral closing wedge	Decrease PTS + correct varus alignment	Same indications as for medial opening wedge

Table 14.3 Factors to consider when selecting between a medial opening and lateral closing wedge tibial osteotomy

Medial opening wedge osteotomy	Lateral closing wedge osteotomy
Difficult to decrease PTS	*Decreases PTS*
Ability to "fine-tune" correction intraoperatively	Immediate weightbearing possible
Need for bone graft	Decreased tension on lateral ligaments
Risk of non-union (i.e., smokers, large correction)	Risk of de-stabilizing the proximal tibia-fibula joint
Risk of patella baja	Risk of patella alta
Increases leg length	Decreases leg length

Preoperative Planning

Standard preoperative patient evaluation including a detailed history and thorough physical examination are essential when planning a revision ACL reconstruction. Specific to osteotomy, it is important to determine whether sagittal plane instability is the sole complaint or if there are other contributing factors such as pain or coronal plane instability. Physical examination begins with an inspection of alignment to assess for coronal and sagittal plane abnormalities such as varus and hyperextension. The patient's gait should be carefully evaluated for varus or hyperextension thrust. Leg length discrepancies should be measured as this may influence the type of osteotomy selected. Any asymmetries in range of motion (ROM) should also be documented, paying particular attention to restrictions of flexion and extension, as well as notable hyperextension deformities. A complete ligamentous examination should include a quantitative assessment of the ACL, PCL, medial ligament complex, and posterolateral ligament complex. Pseudolaxity due to meniscal and/or cartilage deficiency must be distinguished from true ligamentous laxity.

Radiographic (XR) evaluation begins with standard weightbearing anteroposterior (AP) and lateral views. A 45° flexion AP XR can be used to better assess the extent of degenerative change within the tibiofemoral joint. A skyline patellar view should also be included to determine if patellofemoral OA is present. A full-length standing XR is essential in order to evaluate for leg length discrepancy and accurately measure coronal alignment. A full-length lateral XR can also be considered to determine if any distal or proximal sagittal plane abnormalities exist. Computed tomography (CT) should be standard in all revision ACL cases to accurately assess tunnel position and the extent of tunnel enlargement. Magnetic resonance imaging (MRI) is helpful to identify other pathology, including chondral or meniscal injury, and to confirm the status of other ligamentous structures.

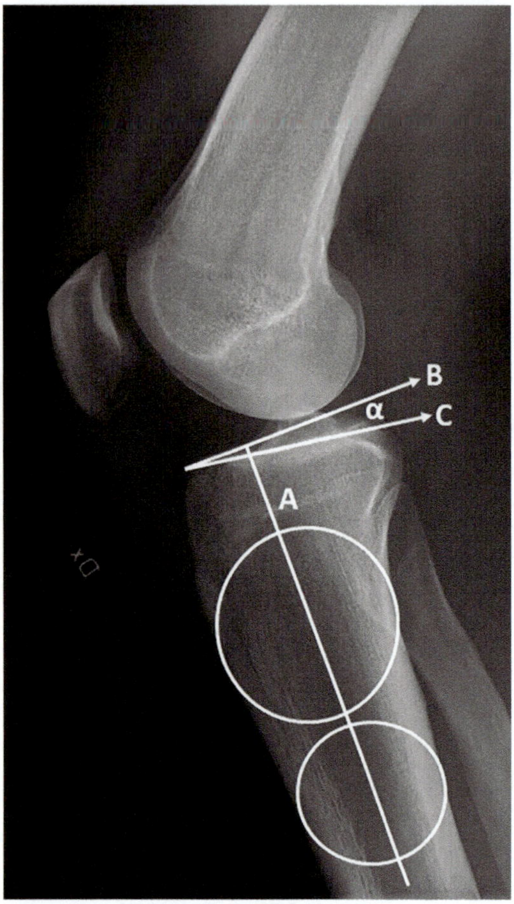

Fig. 14.2 The circle method for calculating posterior tibial slope (PTS). Two circles are drawn between the anterior and posterior cortex of the proximal tibia. The superior circle is in line with the tibial tubercle. The anatomic axis of the tibia is determined by connecting the midpoints of each circle (*A*). The PTS (α) is calculated as the angle between a line perpendicular to the anatomic axis (*B*) and the tibial plateau (*C*)

A number of methods have been described to measure the PTS. The authors' preferred technique is the circle method described by Hudek et al. [15]. This involves drawing two circles from the anterior to posterior cortex of the proximal tibia and connecting their midpoints to define the anatomic axis. The PTS is then calculated as the angle between a line perpendicular to the anatomic axis and the tibial plateau (Fig. 14.2). This technique can be employed with either a plain XR or cross-sectional imaging. It is important to obtain a true lateral XR to eliminate any joint obliquity. Cross-sectional imaging can permit the independent measurement of the lateral and medial tibial plateaus; however, there may not be sufficient proximal tibia included in the slices to fit the two measurement circles. A study comparing the circle method to three other methods of PTS measurement indicated that the circle method had the lowest inter- and intra-observer variability and was not dependent on the length of proximal tibia measured [16].

Another consideration of note in planning an osteotomy and revision ACL reconstruction is whether to proceed as a single or staged procedure. The first stage typically consists of osteotomy along with bone grafting of the ACL tunnels, if necessary. The second stage takes place once healing and bony consolidation have occurred and includes revision ACL reconstruction. The advantages of a staged approach include the following:

- The ability to address tunnel enlargement and/or malposition with bone grafting.
- Technically less challenging.
- Rehabilitation of the ACL reconstruction is not compromised.
- Decreased risk of arthrofibrosis.
- Some patients may not require later ligament reconstruction (i.e., a lower-demand patient with low-grade AP laxity and symptoms of OA).

The main benefits of a single-stage approach are a quicker return to function and decreased risk of anesthetic complications. These benefits must be balanced by the increased technical challenge of a combined procedure as well as the associated potential increase in surgical complications including thromboembolism, infection, and arthrofibrosis.

Cases

Case #1

A 29-year-old male presents with bilateral knee instability. He initially injured his left knee in 2015 while sliding into base during a baseball game. He underwent ACL reconstruction with hamstring autograft. No meniscal pathology was identified during the initial surgery. He suffered an atraumatic failure of his ACL within the first postoperative year and subsequently underwent revision reconstruction with soft tissue allograft. Unfortunately, this reconstruction also failed atraumatically, and he was advised to manage his symptoms conservatively with lifestyle modification and a stabilizing knee brace. Shortly thereafter, the patient tore his right ACL during a baseball game. He is employed in sales and hopes to return to baseball and volleyball at a recreational level.

On physical examination, he is 5 foot 11 inches and 250 pounds (he has gained 30 pounds since his initial injury), with a BMI of 34. He has neutral alignment and a normal gait with no thrust. ROM assessment reveals 5° of hyperextension and 140° of flexion, bilaterally. Ligamentous examination reveals a grade 3 Lachman and grade 3 pivot shift on the left and a grade 2 Lachman and grade 2 pivot shift on the right. No other ligamentous instability is evident with varus, valgus, posterior drawer, or Dial testing.

XR reveals interference screw fixation on both the femoral and tibial side from a previous left ACL reconstruction. There is no evidence of osteoarthritis or patella alta. The PTS is measured as 15° in both knees (Fig. 14.3). Full-length standing XR indicates neutral coronal alignment. Computed tomography confirms appropriate tunnel placement with no evidence of enlargement. An MRI is/was not performed.

This case highlights the importance of measuring PTS as part of the standard work-up in all ACL-deficient patients. This particular patient has an elevated PTS bilaterally. This bony morphology was not addressed at the initial and first revision surgeries and thus contributed to ACL graft failure. Accordingly, a slope-reducing osteotomy must be a component of the surgical plan for this revision ACL reconstruction scenario. This patient has neutral alignment in the coronal plane and no evidence of meniscal or chondral pathology; therefore, only sagittal plane correction is necessary.

Given that tunnel size and position were deemed appropriate, a revision ACL reconstruction was planned concurrent with the osteotomy. A patellar tendon autograft was selected for this patient. This is the authors' preferred graft in a revision scenario as it allows for early bone-to-bone healing and can fill large (up to 10 mm) tunnels. Additionally, the tibial bone plug can cross the osteotomy site, thus providing increased stability. In tunnels larger than 10 mm or if patellar tendon is not available, quadriceps tendon autograft (with or without a bone plug) may be utilized.

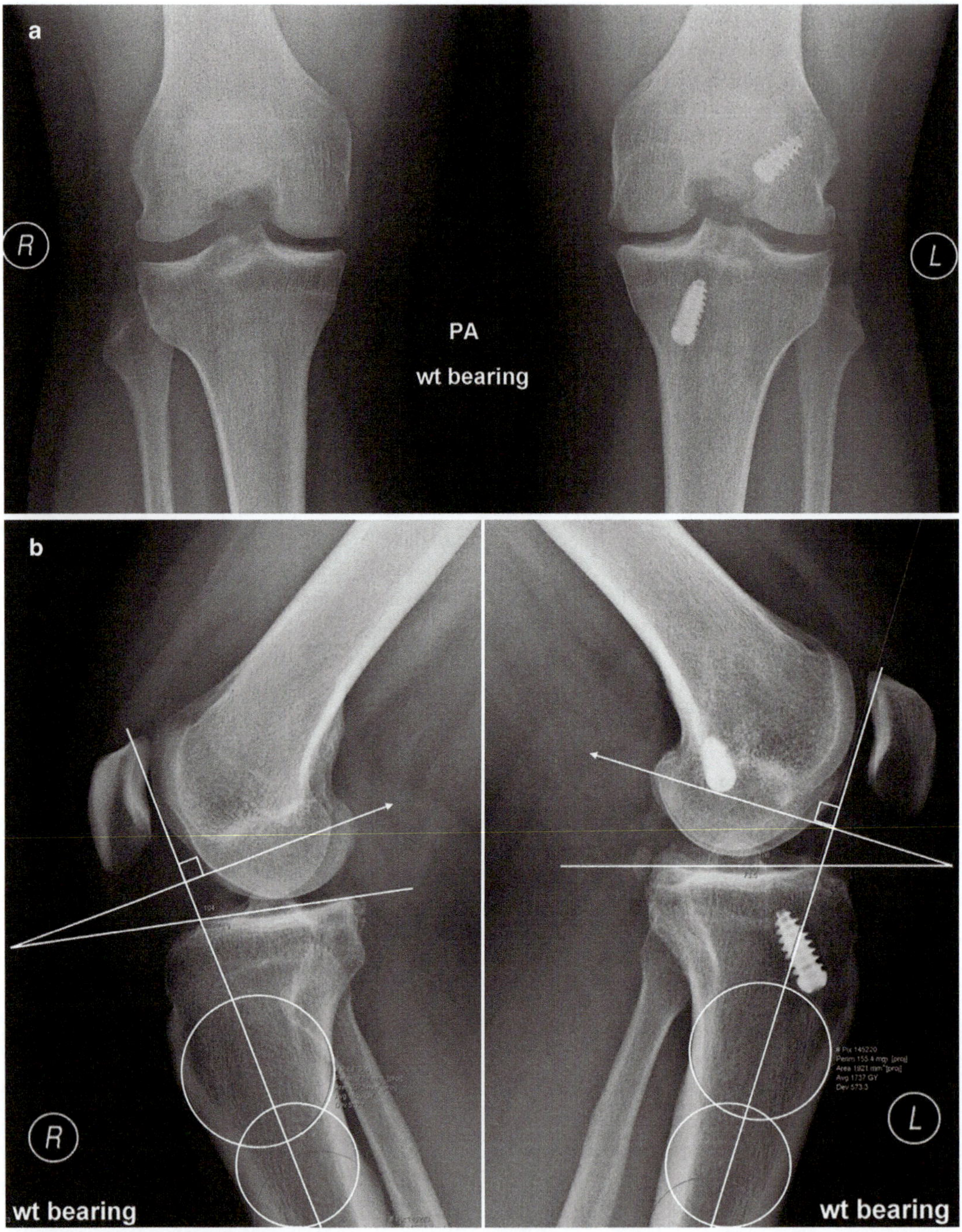

Fig. 14.3 (**a**) Preoperative, weightbearing AP XR, bilateral knees. Left knee shows a previous ACL reconstruction with interference screw fixation. (**b**) Preoperative, weightbearing lateral XR, bilateral knees. PTS is measured bilaterally as 15°

An anterior closing wedge osteotomy combined with revision ACL reconstruction was selected for this patient in order to address his elevated PTS without altering his coronal plane alignment. A tibial tubercle osteotomy was performed due to the large degree of correction necessary (8°) and so as to not alter the position of the patella. The ACL was reconstructed with patellar tendon allograft. This was performed as a single-stage procedure. The technical details are outlined below.

Four months postoperative from the above-mentioned left knee, a primary ACL reconstruction with patellar tendon autograft and concurrent anterior closing wedge osteotomy was performed on the contralateral (right) knee (Fig. 14.4). Although the use of osteotomy in the primary ACL reconstruction setting is controversial, the rationale in this case was the elevated PTS of 15°, as well as the patient's history of ACL graft failure on the contralateral (left) knee.

Case #2

A 48-year-old female presents with left knee pain and instability. She initially injured her left knee in 1991 in a twisting fall while skiing. She underwent ACL reconstruction with patellar tendon autograft and partial medial meniscectomy. She had two additional arthroscopic surgeries for recurrent meniscal tears. Two years ago, she reinjured her knee while playing soccer and sustained a rupture of her ACL graft. She is employed as a pharmaceutical representative and hopes to return to skiing and soccer at a recreational level.

On physical examination, the patient is 5 foot 9 inches and 185 pounds with a BMI of 28. She has neutral alignment and evidence of a slight

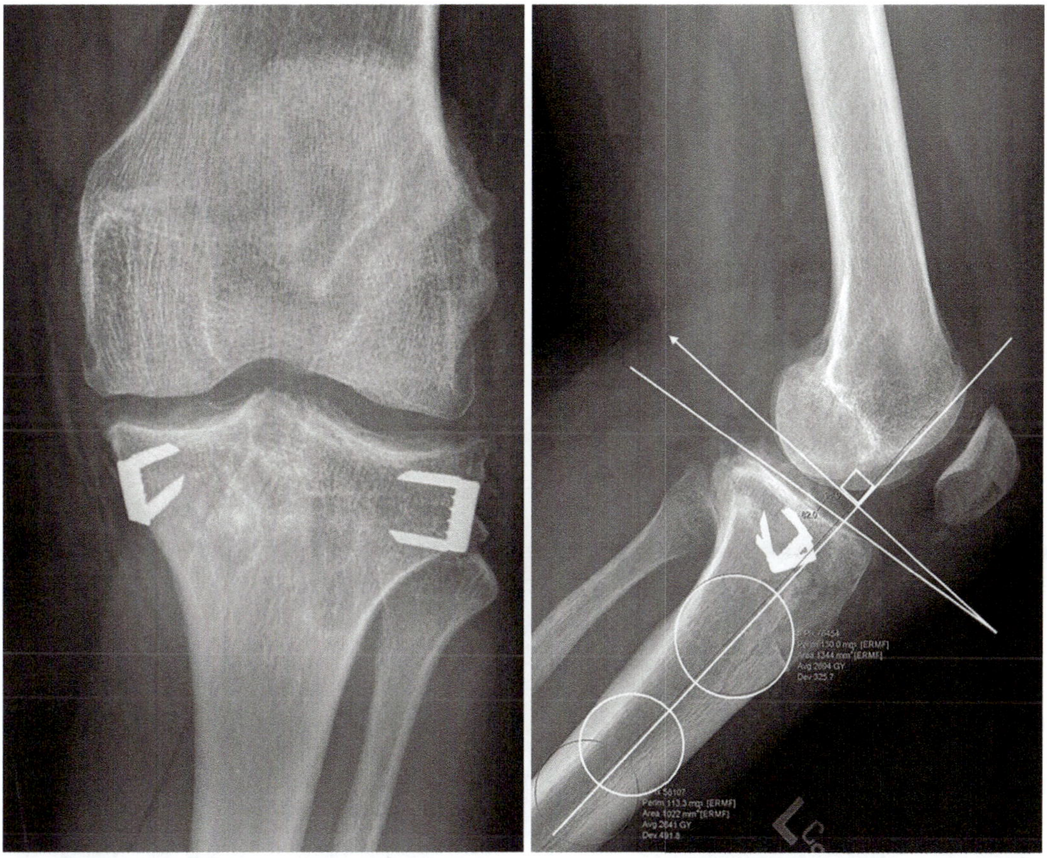

Fig. 14.4 Postoperative AP and lateral XR of the left knee. An anterior closing wedge HTO was performed and secured with two staples. The PTS was decreased to 6°. A concurrent ACL reconstruction with patellar tendon autograft was performed

varus thrust on gait assessment. Range of motion is 2–135° on the left and 0–140° on the right. Ligamentous examination of the left knee reveals a grade 2 Lachman and grade 1 pivot shift. There is some pseudolaxity to varus stress but no ligamentous instability to valgus, posterior drawer, or Dial testing.

X-rays reveal interference screw fixation on both the femoral and tibial side from a previous ACL reconstruction. Moderate OA is noted in the medial compartment, and PTS is measured as 12°. Full-length standing XR shows mild (<5°) varus alignment (Fig. 14.5). An MRI confirms complete rupture of the ACL graft, subtotal medial meniscectomy, and moderate chondral loss in the medial compartment. Articular surfaces in the lateral and patellofemoral compartments are preserved. Tunnel position is appropriate with no evidence of enlargement. A CT was not performed.

This case illustrates the not uncommon scenario of a patient with a failed ACL reconstruction and early medial compartment OA. Considering the increased PTS of 12° and mild varus deformity, this patient would benefit from a realignment osteotomy in both the sagittal and coronal planes. Accordingly, a lateral closing wedge osteotomy was selected due to its ability to decrease PTS and correct varus alignment. A revision ACL reconstruction was performed concurrently as there were no concerns regarding tunnel size or position. A patellar tendon allograft was used due to the patient's age (Fig. 14.6).

Surgical Technique for Anterior Closing Wedge Osteotomy and ACL Reconstruction

As with any complex procedure, the order of the surgical steps is of particular importance and should be clear to the entire operating room team. The authors recommend beginning with ACL graft harvest and preparation. The incision site should be carefully planned so as to incorporate the osteotomy whenever possible. A midline incision from the distal pole of the patella to the distal aspect of the tibial tubercle allows access to the patellar tendon for graft harvest and exposes the anterior tibia for optimal visualization of the osteotomy. Alternatively, a "lazy-S" incision can be utilized to expose the proximal medial tibia for visualization of the tibial tunnel and fixation of the osteotomy (Fig. 14.7).

An arthroscopic evaluation of the knee should be performed next. The chondral cartilage should

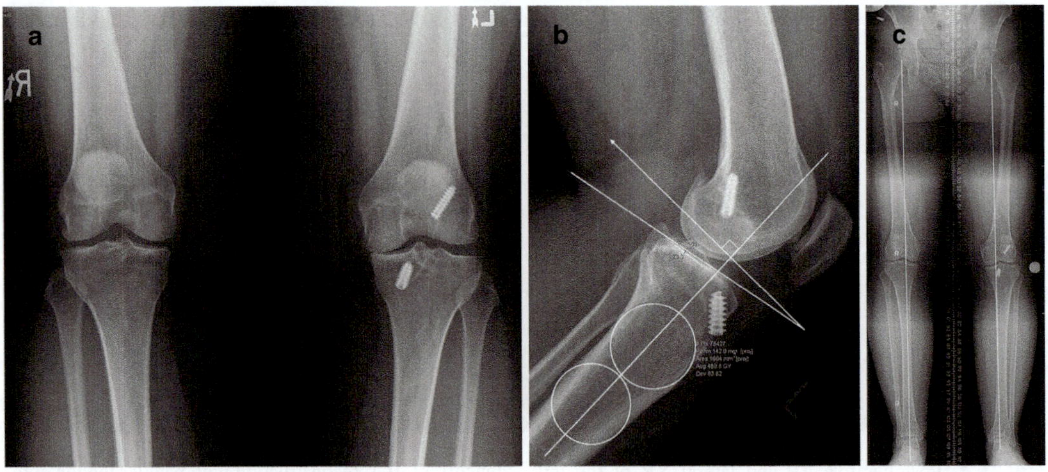

Fig. 14.5 (**a**) Preoperative, weightbearing AP XR, bilateral knees. Left knee shows a previous ACL reconstruction with interference screw fixation and medial compartment narrowing consistent with OA. (**b**) Preoperative, weightbearing lateral XR, left knee. PTS is measured as 12°. (**c**) Preoperative, full-length standing AP XR reveals slight varus alignment on the left

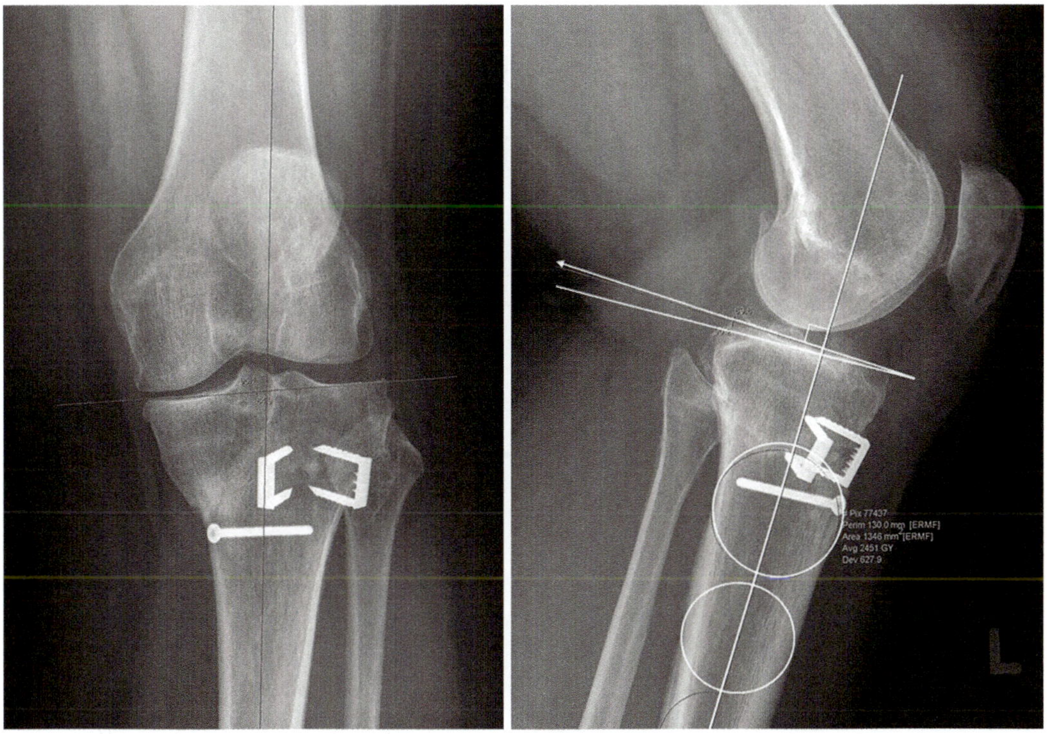

Fig. 14.6 Postoperative AP and lateral XR of the left knee. A lateral closing wedge HTO was performed and secured with two staples. The PTS was decreased to 5°. A concurrent ACL reconstruction with patellar tendon allograft was performed with secondary fixation of the tibia over a small-fragment screw

be carefully inspected, and any chondral or meniscal pathology can be addressed. The femoral tunnel of the ACL should be drilled in its anatomic location. The tibial tunnel is not drilled at this time but can be landmarked to facilitate drilling once the osteotomy is complete.

The tibial osteotomy should be performed as the next step. A tourniquet may be utilized as bleeding from the osteotomy site can obscure the surgical field. Although not always necessary in small corrections, the authors advocate for a tibial tubercle osteotomy concurrent with an anterior closing wedge osteotomy. The benefits of a tibial tubercle osteotomy are that it improves visualization of the anterior tibia, allows for greater correction of alignment if needed, and enables repositioning of the tubercle to prevent patella baja. The main disadvantage is delayed union. Note that a tibial tubercle osteotomy should not be performed with ipsilateral patellar tendon harvest. A long (6 cm) and thin (1–2 cm) tibial tubercle osteotomy is performed in a plane perpendicular to the anterior tibial cortex. The edges of the patellar tendon correspond to the medial and lateral borders of the osteotomy. Once the tubercle has been osteotomized, two Steinman pins can be placed in a converging fashion from anterior to posterior at the expected site of the anterior closing wedge osteotomy (Fig. 14.8). Fluoroscopy may be used to confirm the pin position and degree of correction. In general, removal of 1 millimeter of anterior tibial cortex corresponds to a 1 degree decrease in PTS. An oscillating saw should be used to initiate the cortical cuts, and osteotomes may be helpful to complete them as they provide more tactile and acoustic feedback and are less likely to cause neurovascular injury. The posterior cortex should not be disrupted in an anterior closing wedge osteotomy.

The osteotomized wedge of bone is removed, and curettes are used to extract cancellous bone until the posterior cortex of the tibia is exposed.

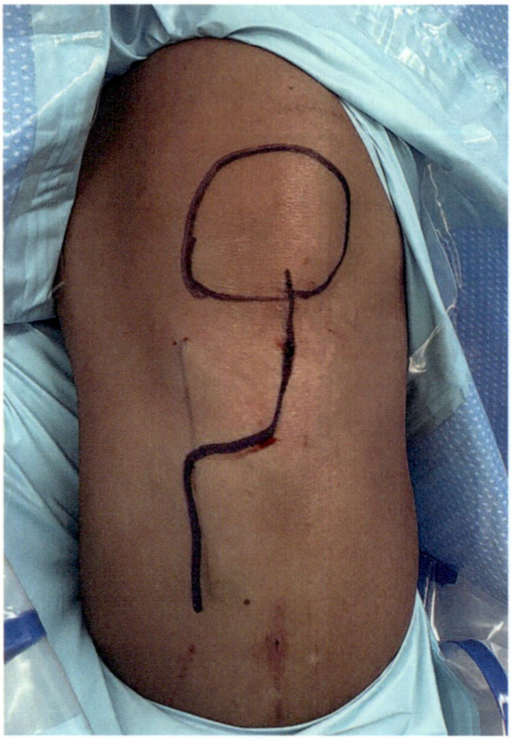

Fig. 14.7 A “lazy-S” incision can be used to expose the patellar tendon for graft harvest and the proximal medial tibia for visualization of the ACL tibial tunnel and anterior osteotomy site.

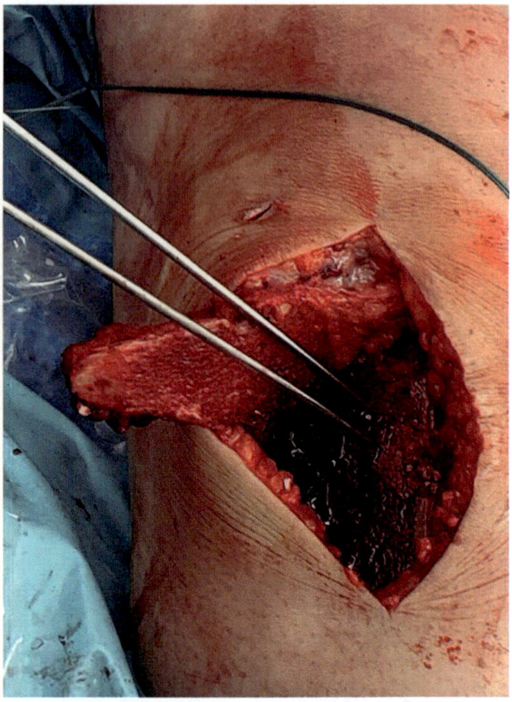

Fig. 14.8 Intraoperative photo showing a TTO exposing the anterior tibia with two converging Steinman pins indicating the planned osteotomy site and orientation

This can be used for bone graft along the osteotomy site once complete. The knee is then placed into hyperextension to close the osteotomy gap. In large corrections, the proximal tibia-fibula joint will need to be released to ensure complete closure of the osteotomy laterally. This is typically performed from the medial aspect of the joint so as to not injure the common peroneal nerve. Complete closure of the osteotomy and the degree of correction are confirmed clinically and fluoroscopically. The osteotomy is fixated with two crossing 3.5 mm screws directed from anteromedial/lateral to posterolateral/medial or two large staples. Fixation of the tibial tubercle is performed with two 3.5 mm screws in an anterior to posterior fashion ensuring bicortical fixation and adequate compression to minimize the risk of delayed union. When placing the osteotomy hardware, consideration should be given to the position of the ACL tibial tunnel.

The tibial tunnel of the ACL should be drilled next. The arthroscope is re-introduced into the knee and the tunnel landmarked in the anatomic footprint on the tibia. It is preferable that the tunnel crosses the osteotomy site to improve fixation. Finally, the ACL graft should be passed and secured in the standard fashion.

The incision should be closed in layers, using interrupted sutures or staples for the skin to facilitate drainage of the wound and decrease the risk of hematoma and compartment syndrome. Thromboembolic prophylaxis is recommended for 2 weeks postoperative. A stabilizing brace is typically not needed, and early range of motion is encouraged. Isometric strengthening exercises are initiated as tolerated. The patient can begin partial weightbearing with the use of crutches immediately postoperative, and full weightbearing is permitted at 6 weeks. Plyometric exercises begin around 4 months. Return to sport is delayed for at least 1 year and until the patient has passed appropriate clinical and functional assessments.

Discussion

Assessment of alignment in the sagittal plane is a critical step in preoperative planning for revision ACL reconstruction. In general, a slope-reducing osteotomy should be considered if PTS is measured as ≥12°. In Case #1, an inherently elevated PTS was not recognized and thereby contributed to ACL graft failure. An anterior closing wedge osteotomy is most effective at reducing PTS without affecting coronal plane alignment. When coronal plane correction is desired, as in Case #2, a lateral or medial osteotomy should be considered. The advantages and disadvantages of a medial opening or lateral closing wedge osteotomy to correct varus alignment and address tibial slope were previously reviewed. Of particular importance in the setting of ACL deficiency are the geometry of the proximal tibia and the effect of the osteotomy "gap" on tibial slope [12]. Due to this relationship, a lateral closing wedge osteotomy is much more likely to decrease PTS, while a medial opening wedge osteotomy is more likely to increase it (Fig. 14.9). In light of these findings, the authors' preferred approach to correct varus alignment and decrease PTS in an ACL-deficient knee is a lateral closing wedge osteotomy.

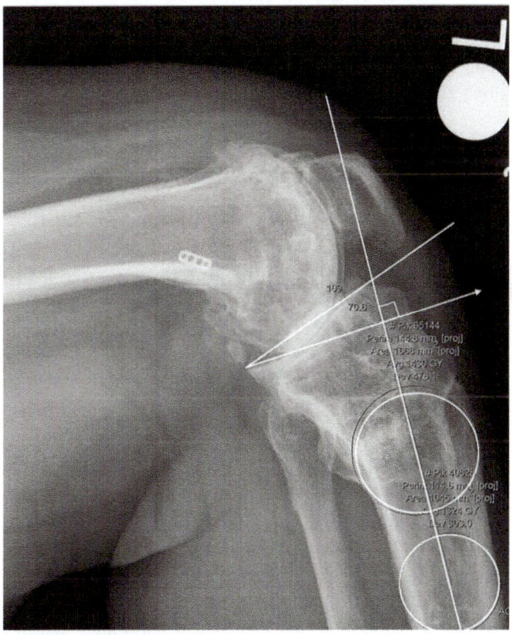

Fig. 14.9 Lateral XR of a patient whose PTS was inadvertently increased in performing a MOW-HTO for early medial compartment OA. They subsequently developed sagittal plane instability, and osteoarthritis continued to progress

Another important consideration in osteotomy planning is the position of the patella. In general, closing osteotomies tend to increase patellar height (alta), while opening osteotomies tend to decrease it (baja). A tibial tubercle osteotomy to shift the patella proximally or distally should be considered if there is concern about patellar malposition following a planned osteotomy. A distalizing tibial tubercle osteotomy was performed in Case #1 due to the need for a large sagittal plane correction that could have resulted in a patella alta. When needed, the tubercle will be translated distally to equal the correction from the sagittal plane osteotomy. We also find it optimal to have the tubercle positioned on both sides of the osteotomy, and, if possible, to have screw purchase on both sides of the osteotomy cut.

Leg length should also be taken into account in planning for either an opening or closing osteotomy. Many individuals have some degree of congenital leg length discrepancy, and, in general, up to 10 mm is reasonably well tolerated. However, it is important to be mindful of not over-lengthening the limb with an opening osteotomy or substantially shortening it with a closing wedge osteotomy. Importantly, limb length is affected by both coronal and sagittal plane corrections. For example, a medial opening wedge osteotomy will increase leg length both due to the osteotomy gap and by the degree of coronal realignment. Similarly, a lateral closing wedge osteotomy will decrease leg length due to the osteotomy gap and *increase* it by the degree of coronal plane correction. It is critical to consider these relationships in preoperative planning and surgical decision-making.

Finally, the complete ligamentous status of the knee must be carefully evaluated in any revision ACL scenario. Collateral ligament instability in the setting of coronal plane malalignment will benefit from osteotomy, and this should be incorporated into the surgical plan. In some cases, osteotomy can correct both the sagittal and coronal plane instability without the need for subsequent ligament reconstruction. Conversely,

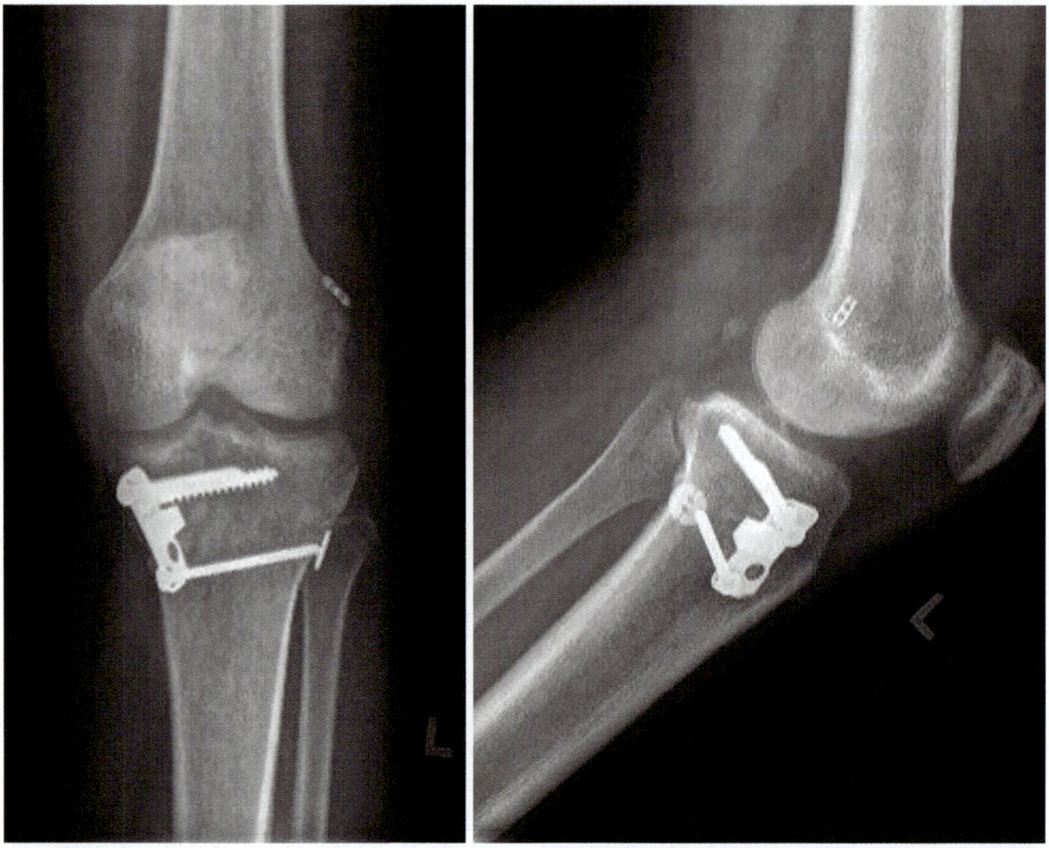

Fig. 14.10 XR of a patient who underwent concurrent ACL and posterolateral corner (PLC) reconstruction combined with MOW-HTO. A medial approach was selected in this case so as not to compromise the PLC reconstruction, and careful attention was paid to maintain tibial slope as it was not elevated

an osteotomy can be combined with ligamentous reconstruction in order to restore sagittal and coronal plane stability (Fig. 14.10).

Conclusion

Failed ACL reconstruction is a frustrating situation for both the patient and surgeon. It is essential that all modifiable factors predisposing to graft failure are eliminated prior, or concurrent to, proceeding with revision reconstruction. Increased posterior slope of the proximal tibia has been well documented to contribute to ACL rupture and should thus be addressed with a slope-reducing osteotomy. The best approach is dependent on a variety of factors, and each patient should be evaluated independently. The addition of tibial osteotomy to a surgeon's toolbox can greatly enhance the management of complex knee instability cases and thereby contribute to reduced ACL graft failure and improved patient outcomes.

References

1. Coventry MB. Osteotomy of the upper portion of the tibia for degenerative arthritis of the knee. A preliminary report. J Bone Joint Surg Am. 1965;47:984–90.
2. Genin P, Weill G, Julliard R. The tibial slope. Proposal for a measurement method. J Radiol. 1993;74(1):27–33.
3. Dejour H, Bonnin M. Tibial translation after anterior cruciate ligament rupture. Two radiological tests compared. J Bone Joint Surg Br. 1994;76(5):745–9.
4. McLean SG, Oh YK, Palmer ML, Lucey SM, Lucarelli DG, Ashton-Miller JA, et al. The relation-

ship between anterior tibial acceleration, tibial slope, and ACL strain during a simulated jump landing task. J Bone Joint Surg Am. 2011;93(14):1310–7.
5. Brandon ML, Haynes PT, Bonamo JR, Flynn MI, Barrett GR, Sherman MF. The association between posterior-inferior tibial slope and anterior cruciate ligament insufficiency. Arthroscopy. 2006;22(8):894–9.
6. Webb JM, Salmon LJ, Leclerc E, Pinczewski LA, Roe JP. Posterior tibial slope and further anterior cruciate ligament injuries in the anterior cruciate ligament-reconstructed patient. Am J Sports Med. 2013;41(12):2800–4.
7. Salmon LJ, Heath E, Akrawi H, Roe JP, Linklater J, Pinczewski LA. 20-year outcomes of anterior cruciate ligament reconstruction with hamstring tendon autograft: the catastrophic effect of age and posterior tibial slope. Am J Sports Med. 2018;46(3):531–43.
8. Imhoff FB, Mehl J, Comer BJ, Obopilwe E, Cote MP, Feucht MJ, et al. Slope-reducing tibial osteotomy decreases ACL-graft forces and anterior tibial translation under axial load. Knee Surg Sports Traumatol Arthrosc. 2019;27(10):3381–9.
9. Zaffagnini S, Bonanzinga T, Grassi A, Marcheggiani Muccioli GM, Musiani C, Raggi F, et al. Combined ACL reconstruction and closing-wedge HTO for varus angulated ACL-deficient knees. Knee Surg Sports Traumatol Arthrosc. 2013;21(4):934–41.
10. Dejour D, Saffarini M, Demey G, Baverel L. Tibial slope correction combined with second revision ACL produces good knee stability and prevents graft rupture. Knee Surg Sports Traumatol Arthrosc. 2015;23(10):2846–52.
11. Sonnery-Cottet B, Mogos S, Thaunat M, Archbold P, Fayard JM, Freychet B, et al. Proximal tibial anterior closing wedge osteotomy in repeat revision of anterior cruciate ligament reconstruction. Am J Sports Med. 2014;42(8):1873–80.
12. Noyes FR, Goebel SX, West J. Opening wedge tibial osteotomy: the 3-triangle method to correct axial alignment and tibial slope. Am J Sports Med. 2005;33(3):378–87.
13. Hohmann E, Bryant A, Imhoff AB. The effect of closed wedge high tibial osteotomy on tibial slope: a radiographic study. Knee Surg Sports Traumatol Arthrosc. 2006;14(5):454–9.
14. Ranawat AS, Nwachukwu BU, Pearle AD, Zuiderbaan HA, Weeks KD, Khamaisy S. Comparison of lateral closing-wedge versus medial opening-wedge high tibial osteotomy on knee joint alignment and kinematics in the ACL-deficient knee. Am J Sports Med. 2016;44(12):3103–10.
15. Hudek R, Schmutz S, Regenfelder F, Fuchs B, Koch PP. Novel measurement technique of the tibial slope on conventional MRI. Clin Orthop Relat Res. 2009;467(8):2066–72.
16. Lipps DB, Wilson AM, Ashton-Miller JA, Wojtys EM. Evaluation of different methods for measuring lateral tibial slope using magnetic resonance imaging. Am J Sports Med. 2012;40(12):2731–6.

15 Lateral Extra-articular Tenodesis in Revision Anterior Cruciate Ligament Reconstruction

Michelle E. Arakgi, Lachlan M. Batty, and Alan M. J. Getgood

Case 1

A 21-year-old female soccer player initially suffered a non-contact knee injury resulting in an ACL tear. She underwent a successful ACL reconstruction with hamstring autograft, had an uneventful recovery and returned to sport at 8 months post-op. At 10 months post-op, she suffered a repeat non-contact injury with graft failure. Clinical examination demonstrated full range of motion with a grade 2 Lachman, grade 2 pivot shift, intact PCL and collateral ligament exams. No significant recurvatum was seen on the examination. Radiographs demonstrated appropriate tunnel placement with no widening. Given the patient's young age, activity level and role as an elite soccer player, the decision was made to augment the revision with an extra-articular tenodesis. She underwent a single-stage revision ACL reconstruction with BTB autograft and LET (Fig. 15.1). Her recovery was uneventful, and full return to sport was accomplished.

M. E. Arakgi · A. M. J. Getgood (✉)
Fowler Kennedy Sport Medicine Clinic, University of Western Ontario, London, ON, Canada

L. M. Batty
Fowler Kennedy Sport Medicine Clinic, University of Western Ontario, London, ON, Canada

St Vincent's Hospital Melbourne, Fitzroy, VIC, Australia

Case 2

A 24-year-old male football player suffered a non-contact football injury, resulting in an ACL rupture and an irreparable medial meniscus tear. He underwent ACL reconstruction with hamstring autograft and a very small partial medial meniscectomy, removing less than 10% of the meniscal tissue and leaving a sufficient rim of more than 5 mm. The patient then suffered a second deceleration injury 6 months post-op, resulting in graft failure without a change in the status of the meniscus. He underwent revision ACL with BTB autograft. At 10 months post-revision ACL reconstruction, he was playing baseball and suffered another twisting injury resulting in a second re-tear.

Clinical examination at the time demonstrated neutral limb alignment, excellent muscle tone, grade 3 Lachman, grade 3 pivot shift, no external rotation laxity and intact collaterals. Lateral radiographs demonstrated an increased posterior slope of 14 degrees without significant recurvatum on exam (Fig. 15.2a). Given the multiple graft failures, the decision was made to address slope and ACL deficiency concurrently. The patient underwent anterior closing wedge high tibial osteotomy with revision ACL reconstruction with quadriceps tendon autograft and LET (Fig. 15.2b, c). LET in this case was especially helpful, given the potential for hyper-extension after anterior closing wedge high tibial osteot-

M. J. Alaia, K. J. Jones (eds.), *Revision Anterior Cruciate Ligament Reconstruction*,
https://doi.org/10.1007/978-3-030-96996-7_15

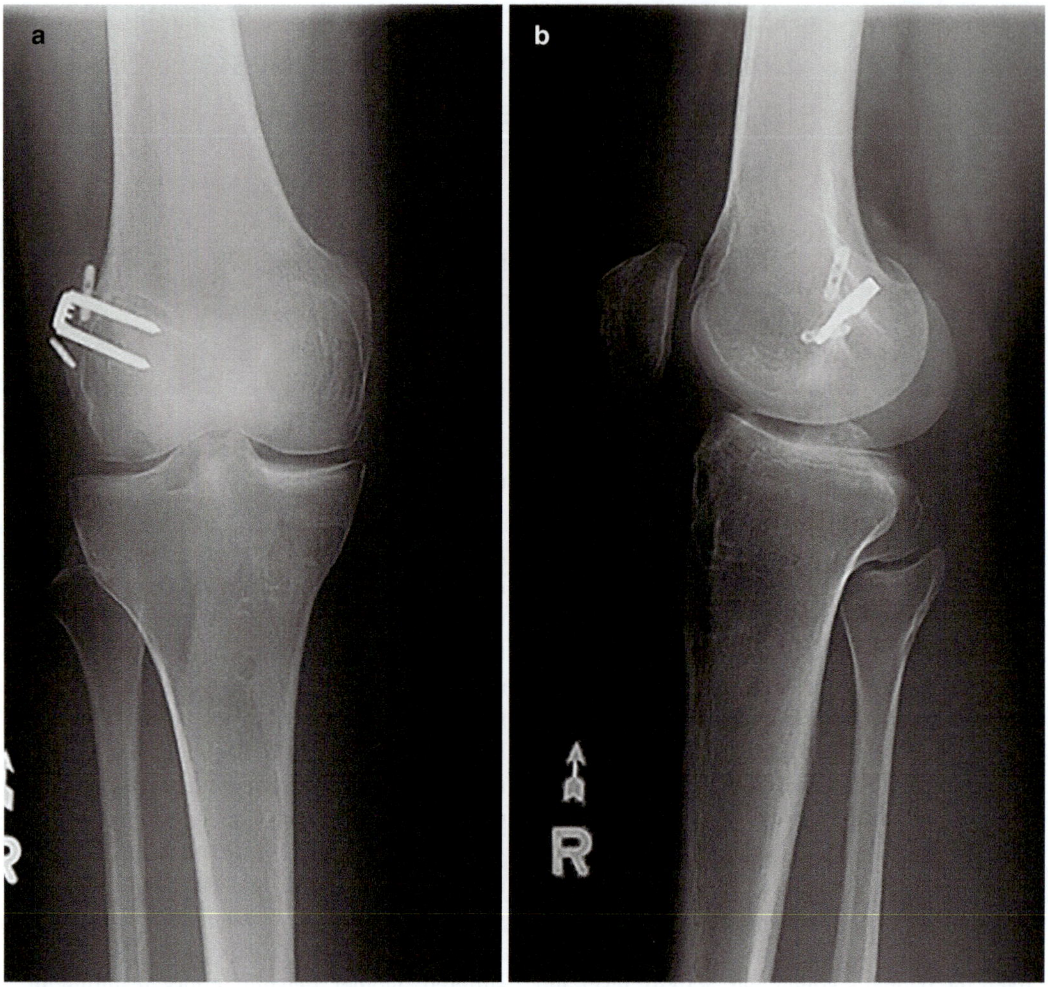

Fig. 15.1 Case 1. Post-operative radiograph demonstrating the position of the staple on both (**a**) anteroposterior and (**b**) lateral radiographs

omy. As the meniscal deficiency was minute, we did not indicate the patient for medial meniscus allograft transplantation. He has subsequently returned to athletics with no residual instability.

Introduction

Anterior cruciate ligament (ACL) reconstruction (ACLR) has generally favourable outcomes. However, there remains a subset of patients who go on to fail [1, 2]. Graft failure can occur as a result of traumatic rupture, biologic factors (failure of graft to incorporate), technical errors of tunnel placement or unrecognized concomitant laxity [3]. Clinical failure may present with residual rotatory laxity resulting in instability, unacceptable stiffness or pain. A systematic review in 2011 suggested a 19% incidence of increased anterolateral rotatory laxity (pivot shift grade 2 and higher) after ACL reconstruction [4].

Undiagnosed concomitant injury to the anterolateral complex (ALC), which includes the iliotibial band (ITB) and anterolateral ligament (ALL), has been proposed to cause anterolateral rotatory instability (ALRI) that leads to increased failure of ACLR. ALRI is accentuated by other ligamentous deficiencies, particularly the ACL

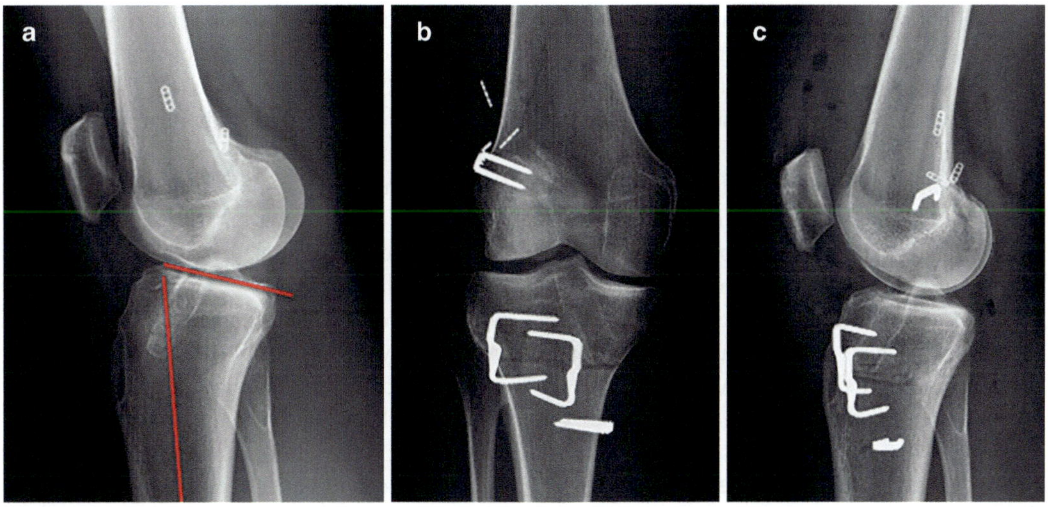

Fig. 15.2 Case 2. Radiographs demonstrate (**a**) pre-operative increased tibial slope of 14 degrees. Post-operative radiographs demonstrating reduced posterior slope and revision ACL reconstruction with LET (**b**, **c**)

[5]. The role of the ALC, and the ALL in particular, has been an area of intense controversy and recent study in regard to knee stability in recent years [6, 7].

Lateral extra-articular tenodesis (LET) procedures are a diverse group of nonanatomic operations that have been described to help control ALRI. Additionally, LET has been proposed to protect the ACL graft from strain during the initial healing period [5, 8]. Definitive evidence supporting the indications for LET procedures and long-term outcomes in revision ACLR are still emerging. The ALC Consensus Group, however, met in 2018 to discuss the available literature regarding the ALC and LET procedures. Based on the current evidence, they concluded that they were unable to make definitive recommendations on when to add LET to ACLR. The group suggested that LET procedures may be indicated in the context of revision ACLR and in primary ACLR in patients who present with a high-grade pivot shift and generalized ligamentous laxity and in young patients wishing to return to pivot sports [9]. Recent studies support these indications in the primary ACLR setting [10, 11]. The aim of the current chapter is to examine the relevant anatomy and biomechanics in ALRI and the role of LET in revision ACL reconstruction.

Relevant Anatomy

The ALC is comprised of the superficial iliotibial band (ITB), the deep ITB and its capsulo-osseous layer attachments from the distal femur to the proximal tibia and the ALL, a ligamentous structure within the anterolateral capsule [7, 9].

The anterolateral ligament (ALL) was first described by Segond in 1879 [12]. The ALL is a ligamentous structure within the anterolateral capsule of the knee. The ALL is best visualized with the knee flexed at 60 degrees and the tibia maximally internally rotated after sectioning the ACL [6]. In this position, the firm fibres can be seen running from the lateral epicondyle to the femur to the anterolateral portion of the tibia.

Differing dissection techniques and difficulty distinguishing the ALL from the anterolateral capsule can make the ALL challenging to identify [7, 9, 13]. Therefore, the prevalence of the ALL in the knee in cadaveric studies has ranged from 45% to 100% [13–16]. Additionally, authors have also described the ALL as being under the ITB and within the anterolateral capsule [17].

Histologically, there again is controversy observed in the literature. A 2020 cadaveric study in paediatric knees demonstrated that there was no discernible ligamentous tissue found within the ALC with histological, immunohistochemical or molecular analyses [18]. In adult cadaveric studies, however, others have found the ALL to be differentiated from the capsular tissue as it is comprised of dense connective tissue collagen bundles which are more consistent with ligamentous tissue [7, 19]. This band of connective tissues is often surrounded by loose synovial tissue [20]. Anti-human neurofilament protein stains have also revealed a large amount of peripheral nerves and mechanoreceptors suggesting a potential proprioceptive role of the ALL [21].

Biomechanical Rationale for Lateral Augmentation

Multiple cadaveric studies have investigated the role of the ALC on knee stability [22–26]. The anterolateral structures have been demonstrated to act as secondary stabilizers to anterolateral rotation in the knee. The ALL begins to load share beyond the physiological limits of the ACL [25, 26]. This indicates that the ALL has little role in controlling internal rotation in the ACL intact knee. A 2015 study demonstrated that sectioning of the ALL was observed to result in a statistically significant increase in anterior translation and internal rotation after the ACL was sectioned during an early-phase pivot shift [22].

In knees with combined ALL and ACL injury, ACL reconstruction alone has been shown to be inadequate at restoring anterolateral stability, resulting in significant residual rotational laxity [23, 27]. A 2016 in vitro robotic study examined the biomechanical effect of reconstruction of the ALL on rotatory stability when performed in combination with ACLR [23]. Kinematic differences between ACLR with an intact ALL, ACLR with ALL reconstruction using semitendinosus allograft and ACLR with a deficient ALL were compared with the intact state. In this study, combined anatomic ALL reconstruction and ACLR significantly improved the rotatory stability of the knee compared with isolated ACLR in the face of a concurrent ALL deficiency. Additionally, during pivot shift testing, ALL reconstruction significantly reduced internal rotation and axial plane tibial translation when compared with ACLR alone with an ALL deficiency [23].

When examining the effects of LET on in vitro knee kinematics, a 2016 study demonstrated that both the modified Lemaire procedure and modified MacIntosh procedure restored rotational kinematics to the intact knee state [27]. Similar results were demonstrated in a 2019 study that examined multiple types of lateral augmentation procedures on the ACL- and ALC-deficient knee. In this study, the ACL and ALC (including ALL, capsule, and Kaplan fibres) were sectioned. After ACLR, the knees underwent five different lateral augmentation procedures. It was again noted that ACLR alone could not restore normal knee kinematics. The study found that ALL reconstruction and Ellison procedures were able to restore physiologic knee kinematics. Lemaire and MacIntosh procedures resulted in supra-physiologic constraint in this study [28].

Types of LET Procedures

Multiple different LET procedures have been described in the literature. Many were initially proposed for the treatment of ACL-deficient knees in isolation, without concomitant intra-articular ACLR [29–35]. Many of these techniques have also undergone modifications over the years. The original Lemaire technique forms the basis for many LET procedures [5]. The original Lemaire technique described using a 1.5 × 18 cm strip of ITB autograft [29]. This graft was left attached distally at Gerdy's tubercle and passed under the fibular collateral ligament (FCL) and through a femoral bone tunnel back under the FCL and anchored in a tibial bone tunnel at Gerdy's tubercle (Fig. 15.3a). The current modified Lemaire technique uses a single 7–8 cm strip of ITB left attached to Gerdy's tubercle, passed under the FCL and secured to the femur within a bone tunnel or via a staple/suture anchor (see author's technique and Fig. 15.4a–g) [30, 31].

The Ellison procedure uses an ITB graft that is detached distally from its insertion with the use of a bone block [32]. The graft is passed deep to

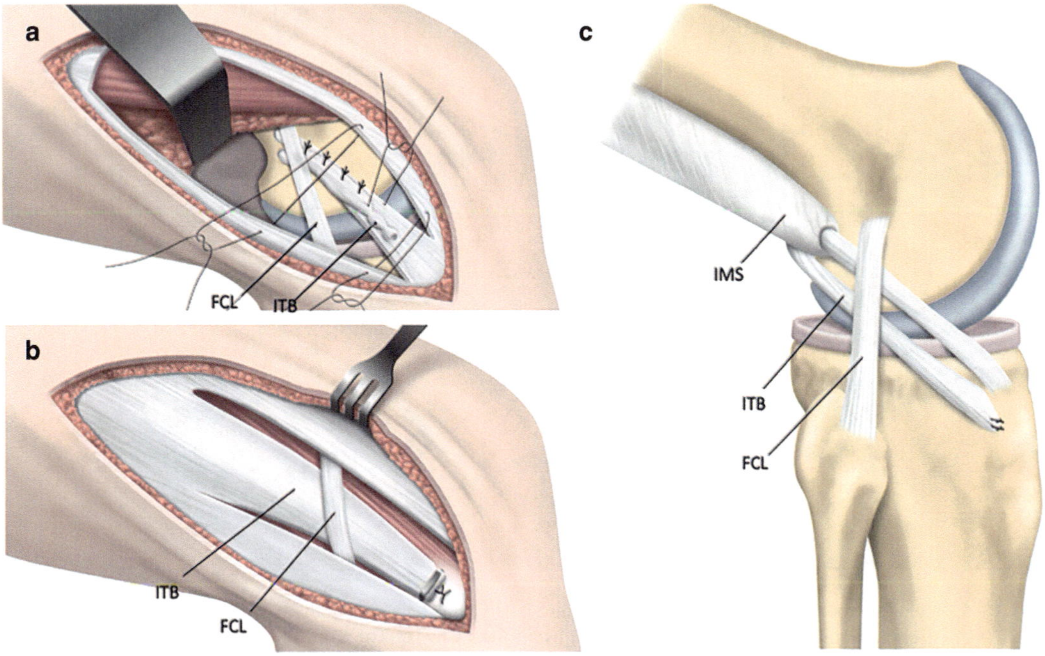

Fig. 15.3 LET procedures. (**a**) Lemaire technique; (**b**) Ellison technique; (**c**) MacIntosh technique (*FCL* fibular collateral ligament, *ITB* iliotibial band, *IMS* intermuscular septum)

the FCL and anchored just anterior to Gerdy's tubercle with a staple (Fig. 15.3b). A capsular plication is also performed in conjunction to the tenodesis deep to the FCL.

The original MacIntosh procedure is similar to the Lemaire in that it uses an ITB autograft left attached distally to Gerdy's tubercle [35]. The 20 × 2 cm graft is passed deep to the FCL, through a subperiosteal tunnel behind the FCL, then through a proximal tunnel in the intermuscular septum. The graft is then sutured back onto itself (Fig. 15.3c). A modification of this procedure has been described where a 2 cm strip of ITB is passed deep to the proximal FCL where it is sutured. It is then passed over top of itself and secured at Gerdy's tubercle with the use of a staple [33]. The MacIntosh technique has also been described as a combined intra- and extra-articular technique [34]. In this "over-the-top" procedure, a 25 × 4 cm strip of ITB is left attached distally to Gerdy's tubercle. It is passed deep to the FCL. It is then passed subperiosteally anterior to the intermuscular septum and then over the femoral condyle and into the knee to be used for ACLR.

Patient Assessment and Indications for LET in Revision ACLR

LET procedures should be considered in the revision setting when other factors predisposing a patient to graft failure have been excluded. Patients with primary graft failure should be investigated with complete history, physical examination and appropriate imaging.

History should include details of primary surgery including arthroscopic findings, postoperative rehabilitation course, time to return to sport and onset of recurrent instability (insidious versus acute traumatic rupture). Additionally, delineating the patients sporting and activity aspirations can help guide treatment.

Physical examination begins with assessment of weight-bearing alignment and gait abnormalities. In-depth assessment of collateral and cruciate ligaments including posterolateral, posteromedial, anterolateral and anteromedial corners should be completed to assess overall soft tissue integrity. When considering LET, particular attention should be paid to residual

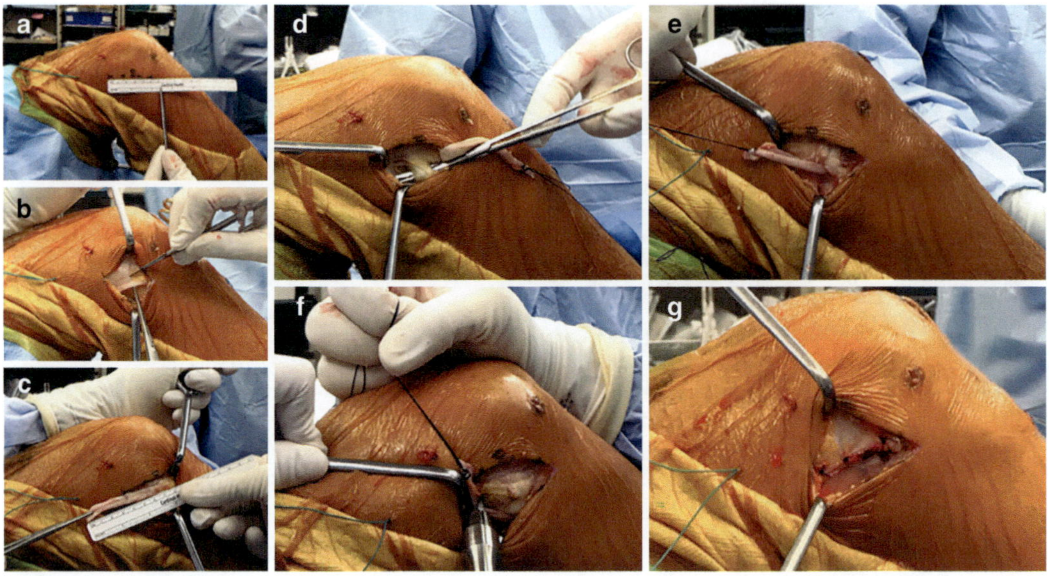

Fig. 15.4 Senior author's technique of modified Lemaire LET. (**a**) A 6 cm longitudinal skin incision is made just posterior to the lateral epicondyle, stopping 2 cm from Gerdy's tubercle. (**b**) The subcutaneous tissue is dissected down to the ITB. (**c**) A 1-cm-wide by 8-cm-long strip of the posterior half of the ITB is harvested, leaving intact the distal attachment at Gerdy's tubercle as well as the Kaplan fibre complex. (**d**) The fibular collateral ligament (FCL) is located and dissected. A Kelly is passed beneath the FCL. (**e**) The graft is tunnelled deep to the FCL. (**f**) Fixation of the tenodesis is performed with a staple, with the graft tensioned to no more than 20 N with the knee held at 60° of flexion and neutral rotation of the tibia. (**g**) The ITB is tacked closed with number 1 Vicryl suture. (Ethicon Inc., Somerville, NJ)

ALRI. Evidence of high-grade pivot shift test is indicative of ALRI [36, 37].

Appropriate imaging should include plain radiographs (weight-bearing films including hip-to-ankle alignment films), MRI and CT scan. Plain radiographs provisionally assess tunnel position and size and existing hardware. Alignment radiographs can also identify bony malalignment that can contribute to graft failure such as increased tibial slope or coronal malalignment with particular attention paid to asymmetry [38]. MRI can further reveal ligamentous or meniscal deficiency that contributes to residual instability. CT is regarded as the gold standard to evaluate tunnel widening and tunnel position [39]. Stress radiographs can augment clinical examination in the assessment of concomitant ligamentous injury such as the posterolateral corner.

Once other factors contributing to the index ACL failure have been identified and addressed, the authors suggest the following possible clinical scenarios where addition of LET would be appropriate:

1. Traumatic graft rupture in a young patient with previously well-functioning graft and well-positioned tunnels where the patient has a desire to return to multidirectional sports
2. Clinical graft failure with non-modifiable risk factors including meniscal deficiency, unresponsive to appropriate rehabilitation program, generalized ligamentous laxity or high-grade pivot shift
3. Graft failure with no clear cause for failure
4. Residual ALRI with intact graft

Outcomes of LET in Revision Surgery

Initial studies examining LET procedures in isolation showed variable outcomes and failed to definitively demonstrate the efficacy of the procedure [40, 41]. With the renewed interest in the ALL and its modern use in combination with ACLR and revision ACLR, the outcomes have been more promising. Recent studies have demonstrated improved patient-reported outcomes and decreased rates of failure with combined ACLR and LET compared to ACLR alone in both the primary and revision setting [42–47].

A study in 2006 evaluated revision ACLR with hamstring autograft combined with modified MacIntosh LET [43]. Thirty patients were evaluated at a mean 5 years post-operatively. A graft was considered to have failed when a revision was done or when the side-to-side difference on KT-1000 arthrometer testing was >5 mm and/or the pivot shift test grade was greater than a trace. At the time of final follow-up, one patient had undergone repeat revision for graft failure at 3 years post-operatively. Pivot shift was normal in 15 patients (50%), slightly positive in 11 patients (37%) and positive in 2 patients. Overall rate of failure was 10%. There were no degenerative changes noted on radiographs.

Similarly, a 2019 study examined the functional results of combined LET and ACLR in professional soccer players. In the retrospective review, 24 professional soccer players were analysed at a mean of 42 months post-operatively [42]. ACLR revision was performed with an autologous bone–patellar tendon–bone autograft or a hamstring graft. LET was performed using a MacIntosh procedure. At the time of final follow-up, AP laxity was significantly reduced ($p < 0.0001$). Twenty-two patients (92%) had a negative pivot shift, and two had a residual glide (8%). The mean subjective IKDC and Lysholm score improved from 69.5 ± 11.1 (range: 56–90) to 88.4 ± 8.9 (range: 62.1–100) and from 58.1 ± 11.7 (range: 33–72) to 97.4 ± 3.2 (range: 88–100), respectively, with significant improvement ($p < 0.0001$) over pre-operative values. There was a 92% return to sport at the same level. Failure rate was reported as 8% [42].

A 2012 study directly compared revision ACL alone to revision ACL with the addition of LET [47]. The retrospective multicentre study included patients operated on from 1994 to 2003 at ten different centres with a minimum of 2 years follow-up. There were 163 patients included in the study. An associated LET was performed in 84 patients (51%). Type of LET performed and specific indications for the procedure were not disclosed by the authors. Failure was defined as grade 2 or 3 pivot shift or KT-1000 test showing a difference of greater than 5 mm. Failure rate was 15% in the revision ACLR group and 7% in the revision ACLR with LET group. At final follow-up, 63% of patients in the revision ACLR alone group had a negative pivot shift compared to 80% in the revision ACLR with LET ($p = 0.03$). There was, however, no statistical difference between groups with respect to IKDC scores.

A 2018 study investigated radiographic changes in patients who underwent ACLR with semitendinosus autograft combined with LET. Patients were evaluated at a mean of 10 years follow-up. There was a 7.6% failure rate based on side-to-side KT-1000 evaluation, >2 or higher pivot shift or patient-reported instability. Severe degenerative changes were seen in 25% of patients. The only risk factor that correlated with degenerative changes was previous meniscectomy [48].

The French Society of Arthroscopy investigated the rate of complications associated with combined primary ACLR and LET [46]. Thirteen surgical centres prospectively studied 392 cases of ACLR with LET with a minimum of 1-year follow-up. Multiple techniques for LET were used including both single continuous grafts and separate grafts for each procedure. Outcome measures included range of motion, time to return to normal gait, Lachman testing, adverse events and re-tear. Two patients (0.5%) required manipulation under anaesthesia for flexion deficit, and four patients (1%) underwent arthroscopic lysis of adhesions for extension deficit. At the time of arthroscopy, this was found to be related to cyclops lesion and not the LET. During the first year, there was 1.7% rate of revision surgery specific to LET (three tibial screw and three femoral screw removal). Overall re-tear rate was 2.8% at 2 years follow-up. This study indicates the low morbidity associated with the lateral extra-articular procedures and highlights the increased post-operative stability and reduced failure rate.

Senior Author's Preferred Surgical Technique

The modified Lemaire technique is used by the senior author (AG) [30]. The leg is positioned in 80 degrees of flexion. A 6 cm longitudinal skin incision is made just posterior to the lateral epicondyle, stopping 2 cm from Gerdy's tubercle (Fig. 15.4a). The subcutaneous tissue is dissected down to the iliotibial band (Fig. 15.4b). A 1-cm-wide by 8-cm-long strip of the posterior half of the ITB is harvested, leaving intact the distal attachment at Gerdy's tubercle as well as the Kaplan fibre complex (Fig. 15.4c). The free end of the tendon is whipstitched with a number 1 Vicryl suture (Ethicon Inc., Somerville, NJ). The fibular collateral ligament (FCL) is located and dissected. A Kelly is passed beneath the FCL (Fig. 15.4d). The graft is tunnelled deep to the fibular collateral ligament (FCL) (Fig. 15.4e). The graft is then attached to the femur just proximal to the metaphyseal flare of the lateral femoral condyle, proximal and posterior to the FCL femoral attachment and just anterior to the insertion of the distal Kaplan fibres of the ITB. Care must be taken during dissection at this point to avoid compromise of the ACL femoral fixation which is in the vicinity of this area. Fixation of the tenodesis is performed with a staple (Fig. 15.4f), with the graft tensioned to no more than 20 N with the knee held at 60° of flexion and neutral rotation of the tibia. The graft is then sutured back onto itself over the staple using the remainder of the whipstitched number 1 Vicryl suture [30]. The ITB is tacked closed with number 1 Vicryl suture (Fig. 15.4g). There is no change in the post-operative rehabilitation protocol with the addition of the LET. Generally, LET is completed at the end of the case (i.e. after ACL reconstruction is completed).

Conclusion

Though ACLR has generally favourable outcomes, there remains a subset of patients who go on to clinical graft failure or re-rupture. Multiple factors can lead to ACLR failure. ALRI or excessive residual laxity can contribute to ACLR failure. Modern LET procedures add minimal morbidity and have been shown to be effective in addressing ALRI in revision ACLR and decreasing graft failure rates.

References

1. Tashman S, Collon D, Anderson K, Kolowich P, Anderst W. Abnormal rotational knee motion during running after anterior cruciate ligament reconstruction. Am J Sports Med. 2004;32(4):975–83.
2. Ristanis S, Stergio N, Patras K. Excessive tibial rotation during high demand activities is not restored by anterior cruciate ligament reconstruction. Arthroscopy. 2005;21.1323–9.
3. Wright RW, Huston LJ, Spindler KP, Dunn WR, Haas AK, Allen CR, et al. Descriptive epidemiology of the Multicenter ACL Revision Study (MARS) cohort. Am J Sports Med. 2010;38(10):1979–86.
4. Mohtadi NG, Chan DS, Dainty KN, Whelan DB. Patellar tendon versus hamstring tendon autograft for anterior cruciate ligament rupture in adults. Cochrane Database Syst Rev. 2011;(9):CD005960.
5. Batty L, Lording T. Clinical results of lateral extra-articular tenodesis. Tech Orthop. 2018;33(4): 232–8.
6. Ahn JH, Patel NA, Lin CC, Lee TQ. The anterolateral ligament of the knee joint: a review of the anatomy, biomechanics, and anterolateral ligament surgery. Knee Surg Relat Res. 2019;31(1):12.
7. Roessler PP, Schüttler KF, Heyse TJ, Wirtz DC, Efe T. The anterolateral ligament (ALL) and its role in rotational extra-articular stability of the knee joint: a review of anatomy and surgical concepts. Arch Orthop Trauma Surg. 2016;136(3):305–13.
8. Engebretsen L, Lew WD, Lewis JL and Hunter RE. The effect of an iliotibial tenodesis on intraarticular graft forces and knee joint motion. Am J Sports Med. 1990;18(2):169–76.
9. Getgood A, Brown C, Lording T, Amis A, Claes S, Geeslin A, et al. The anterolateral complex of the knee: results from the International ALC Consensus Group Meeting. Knee Surg Sports Traumatol Arthrosc. 2019;27(1):166–76.
10. Getgood AMJ, Bryant DM, Litchfield R, Heard M, McCormack RG, Rezansoff A, et al. Lateral extra-articular tenodesis reduces failure of hamstring tendon autograft anterior cruciate ligament reconstruction: 2-year outcomes from the STABILITY study randomized clinical trial. Am J Sports Med. 2020;48(2):285–97.
11. Sonnery-Cottet B, Saithna A, Cavalier M, Kajetanek C, Temponi EF, Daggett M, et al. Anterolateral ligament reconstruction is associated with significantly reduced ACL graft rupture rates at a minimum follow-up of 2 years: a prospective comparative study of 502

patients from the SANTI study group. Am J Sports Med. 2017;45(7):1547–57.
12. Segond P. Recherches cliniques et experimentales sur les epanchements sanguins du genou par entorse. Prog Med. 1879;7:297–341.
13. Roessler P, Schuttler K, Stein T, Gravius S, Heyse T, Prescher A. Anatomic dissection of the anterolateral ligament (ALL) in paired fresh-frozen cadaveric knee joints. Arch Orthop Trauma Surg. 2017;137(2):249–55.
14. Daggett M, Ockuly AC, Cullen M, Busch K, Lutz C, Imbert P, et al. Femoral origin of the anterolateral ligament: an anatomic analysis. Arthroscopy. 2016;32(5):835–41.
15. Runer A, Birkmaier S, Pamminger M, Reider S, Herbst E, Künzel KH, et al. The anterolateral ligament of the knee: a dissection study. Knee. 2016;23(1):8–12.
16. Stijak L, Bumbaširević M, Radonjić V, Kadija M, Puškaš L, Milovanović D, et al. Anatomic description of the anterolateral ligament of the knee. Knee Surg Sports Traumatol Arthrosc. 2016;24(7):2083–8.
17. Helito CP, do Amaral C, Nakamichi YD, Gobbi RG, Bonadio MB, Natalino RJ, et al. Why do authors differ with regard to the femoral and meniscal anatomic parameters of the knee anterolateral ligament?: Dissection by layers and a description of its superficial and deep layers. Orthop J Sports Med. 2016;4(12):2325967116675604.
18. Iseki T, Rothrauff B, Kihara S, Novaretti J, Shea K, Tuan R, et al. Paediatric knee anterolateral capsule does not contain a distinct ligament: analysis of histology, immunohistochemistry and gene expression. J ISAKOS. 2020;0:1–6.
19. Helito CP, Demange MK, Bonadio MB, Tírico LE, Gobbi RG, Pécora JR, et al. Anatomy and histology of the knee anterolateral ligament. Orthop J Sports Med. 2013;1(7):2325967113513546.
20. Vincent JP, Magnussen RA, Gezmez F, Uguen A, Jacobi M, Weppe F, et al. The anterolateral ligament of the human knee: an anatomic and histologic study. Knee Surg Sports Traumatol Arthrosc. 2012;20(1):147–52.
21. Caterine S, Litchfield R, Johnson M, Chronik B, Getgood A. A cadaveric study of the anterolateral ligament: re-introducing the lateral capsular ligament. Knee Surg Sports Traumatol Arthrosc. 2015;23(11):3186–95.
22. Spencer L, Burkhart TA, Tran MN, Rezansoff AJ, Deo S, Caterine S, et al. Biomechanical analysis of simulated clinical testing and reconstruction of the anterolateral ligament of the knee. Am J Sports Med. 2015;43(9):2189–97.
23. Nitri M, Rasmussen MT, Williams BT, Moulton SG, Cruz RS, Dornan GJ, et al. An in vitro robotic assessment of the anterolateral ligament, part 2: anterolateral ligament reconstruction combined with anterior cruciate ligament reconstruction. Am J Sports Med. 2016;44(3):593–601.
24. Rasmussen MT, Nitri M, Williams BT, Moulton SG, Cruz RS, Dornan GJ, et al. An in vitro robotic assessment of the anterolateral ligament, part 1: secondary role of the anterolateral ligament in the setting of an anterior cruciate ligament injury. Am J Sports Med. 2016;44(3):585–92.
25. Huser LE, Noyes FR, Jurgensmeier D, Levy MS. Anterolateral ligament and iliotibial band control of rotational stability in the anterior cruciate ligament-intact knee: defined by tibiofemoral compartment translations and rotations. Arthroscopy. 2017;33(3):595–604.
26. Thein R, Boorman-Padgett J, Stone K, Wickiewicz TL, Imhauser CW, Pearle AD. Biomechanical assessment of the anterolateral ligament of the knee: a secondary restraint in simulated tests of the pivot shift and of anterior stability. J Bone Joint Surg Am. 2016;98(11):937–43.
27. Inderhaug E, Stephen J, Williams A, Amis A. Anterolateral tenodesis or anterolateral ligament complex reconstruction: effect of flexion angle at graft fixation when combined with ACL reconstruction. Am J Sports Med. 2017;45:3089–97.
28. Neri T, Dabirrahmani D, Beach A, Putnis S, Oshima T, Cadman J, et al. A biomechanical comparison of the main anterolateral procedures used in combination with anterior cruciate ligament reconstruction. Orthop J Sports Med. 2020;8:2.
29. Lemaire M. Chronic knee instability. Technics and results of ligament plasty in sports injuries. J Chir (Paris). 1975;110(4):281–94.
30. Jesani S, Getgood A. Modified Lemaire lateral extra-articular tenodesis augmentation of anterior cruciate ligament reconstruction. JBJS Essent Surg Tech. 2019;9(4).
31. Christel P, Djian P. Anterio-lateral extra-articular tenodesis of the knee using a short strip of fascia lata. Rev Chir Orthop Reparatrice Appar Mot. 2002;88(5):508–13.
32. Ellison AE. Distal iliotibial-band transfer for anterolateral rotatory instability of the knee. J Bone Joint Surg Am. 1979;61(3):330–7.
33. Arnold JA, Coker TP, Heaton LM, Park JP, Harris WD. Natural history of anterior cruciate tears. Am J Sports Med. 1979;7(6):305–13.
34. Bertoia JT, Urovitz EP, Richards RR, Gross AE. Anterior cruciate reconstruction using the MacIntosh lateral-substitution over-the-top repair. J Bone Joint Surg Am. 1985;67(8):1183–8.
35. Macintosh D. Lateral substitution reconstruction. In proceedings of the Canadian Orthopaedic Association. J Bone Joint Surg. 1976;58.
36. Larson RL. Physical examination in the diagnosis of rotatory instability. Clin Orthop Relat Res. 1983;172:38–44.
37. Hughes JD, Rauer T, Gibbs CM, Musahl V. Diagnosis and treatment of rotatory knee instability. J Exp Orthop. 2019;6(1):48.
38. Giffin JR, Vogrin TM, Zantop T, Woo SL, Harner CD. Effects of increasing tibial slope on the

biomechanics of the knee. Am J Sports Med. 2004;32(2):376–82.
39. de Beus A, Koch JE, Hirschmann A, Hirschmann MT. How to evaluate bone tunnel widening after ACL reconstruction – a critical review. Muscles Ligaments Tendons J. 2017;7(2):230–9.
40. Neyret P, Palomo JR, Donell ST, Dejour H. Extra-articular tenodesis for anterior cruciate ligament rupture in amateur skiers. Br J Sports Med. 1994;28(1):31–4.
41. Ireland J, Trickey EL. Macintosh tenodesis for anterolateral instability of the knee. J Bone Joint Surg Br. 1980;62(3):340–5.
42. Alessio-Mazzola M, Formica M, Russo A, Sanguineti F, Capello AG, Lovisolo S, et al. Outcome after combined lateral extra-articular tenodesis and anterior cruciate ligament revision in professional soccer players. J Knee Surg. 2019;32(9):906–10.
43. Ferretti A, Conteduca F, Monaco E, De Carli A, D'Arrigo C. Revision anterior cruciate ligament reconstruction with doubled semitendinosus and gracilis tendons and lateral extra-articular reconstruction. J Bone Joint Surg Am. 2006;88(11):2373–9.
44. Grassi A, Zicaro JP, Costa-Paz M, Samuelsson K, Wilson A, Zaffagnini S, et al. Good mid-term outcomes and low rates of residual rotatory laxity, complications and failures after revision anterior cruciate ligament reconstruction (ACL) and lateral extra-articular tenodesis (LET). Knee Surg Sports Traumatol Arthrosc. 2020;28(2):418–31.
45. Marcacci M, Zaffagnini S, Giordano G, Iacono F, Preti M. Anterior cruciate ligament reconstruction associated with extraarticular tenodesis: a prospective clinical and radiographic evaluation with 10- to 13- year follow-up. Am J Sports Med. 2009;37(4):707–14.
46. Panisset JC, Pailhé R, Schlatterer B, Sigwalt L, Sonnery-Cottet B, Lutz C, et al. Short-term complications in intra- and extra-articular anterior cruciate ligament reconstruction. Comparison with the literature on isolated intra-articular reconstruction. A multicenter study by the French Arthroscopy Society. Orthop Traumatol Surg Res. 2017;103(8S):S231–S6.
47. Trojani C, Beaufils P, Burdin G, Bussière C, Chassaing V, Djian P, et al. Revision ACL reconstruction: influence of a lateral tenodesis. Knee Surg Sports Traumatol Arthrosc. 2012;20(8):1565–70.
48. Redler A, Iorio R, Monaco E, Puglia F, Wolf MR, Mazza D, et al. Revision anterior cruciate ligament reconstruction with hamstrings and extra-articular tenodesis: a mid- to long-term clinical and radiological study. Arthroscopy. 2018;34(12):3204–13.

The Role of Anterolateral Procedures: Anterolateral Ligament Reconstruction

16

Daniel J. Kaplan, Brian J. Mannino, Guillem Gonzalez-Lomas, and Laith M. Jazrawi

Background

Despite the overall success of anterior cruciate ligament reconstruction (ACLR procedure), failure rates remain unacceptably high, ranging from 1.1% to 14% [1, 2]. Despite anatomically placed femoral and tibial tunnels, 1.7–7.7% of ACLR patients are thought to fail due to persistent rotational instability [3–5]. This realization has led researchers to investigate the concept of tibial rotational restraint. This includes the role of the anterior cruciate ligament (ACL) as a primary stabilizer, along with several lateral-sided structures serving as important secondary stabilizers. Interest in anterolateral rotatory instability (ALRI) of the knee, and its possible responsibility for a percentage of ACLR failures, was further heighted following renewed interest in the anterolateral complex (ALC), specifically the anterolateral ligament (ALL).

Credit for the original description of what is now considered the ALL (or mid-third capsular ligament) belongs to Paul Segond, who described an avulsion fracture (now referred to as the eponymous "Segond fracture") in 1879, along the anterolateral aspect of the tibia [6]. At the location of the fracture, Segond noted the presence of a "pearly, resistant, fibrous band, which invariably showed extreme amounts of tension during forced internal rotation." [6] Despite occasional reference to an anterolaterally based knee structure in the literature, it was not named until 2012, when Vincent et al. published their anatomical work [7]. However, popularization of the ALL, and the ensuing controversy around its function (and existence), is often credited to Claes et al., who published a detailed anatomic description of the ALL based on a series of cadaveric dissections [8]. Since the "rediscovery" of the ALL, significant research has been done on its structure, function, and potential implications in ALRI, specifically as it relates to ACLR and ACLR failures. This chapter will provide an overview of the ALL, including relevant anatomy and the biomechanical role of the ALL with knee stabilization. It will explore the indications for ALL reconstruction (ALLR), particularly in the setting of revision ACLR, delineate patient workup after an ACL injury (or failed ACLR), and describe the surgical techniques for ALLR. It will conclude with outcomes and complications of the procedure based on a review of the literature and considerations regarding the choice between an ALLR and a lateral extra-articular tenodesis (LET).

D. J. Kaplan (✉) · B. J. Mannino
G. Gonzalez-Lomas · L. M. Jazrawi
Orthopaedic Department, Sports Medicine Division, New York University Langone Health, New York City, NY, USA

M. J. Alaia, K. J. Jones (eds.), *Revision Anterior Cruciate Ligament Reconstruction*, https://doi.org/10.1007/978-3-030-96996-7_16

Anatomy of the Anterolateral Complex of the Knee

The complexity of the lateral knee anatomy has led to challenges regarding structure identification and contributed to the opacity around the ALL definition. While controversy still exists, a layer-by-layer approach to the anterolateral knee helps elucidate its various components, including the layers of the iliotibial band (ITB), ALL, and anterolateral joint capsule (Table 16.1).

Iliotibial Band

The ITB is a thickening of deep fascia, intimately connected with the tensor fasciae latae (TFL) anteriorly and the gluteus maximus posteriorly. It extends laterally from the iliac crest to the tibia, with connecting fibers to the femur along its length. The complexity of lateral and anterolateral knee anatomy is due to the various layers of the ITB and the difficulty in distinguishing them from the other components of the ALC. The ITB is made up of the superficial ITB (sITB), Kaplan fibers, and deep ITB (dITB).

The sITB originates, as a continuation of the TFL and gluteus maximum fascia, with attachments along the intermuscular septum to the linea aspera of the femur [9]. It then courses laterally, with its posterior fibers reinforcing the fascia of the anterior aspect of the biceps femoris. Anteriorly, it curves obliquely, merging with the fascia of the vastus lateralis and partially inserting on the lateral aspect of the patella (forming the iliopatellar band fascia) [10]. Distally, the sITB inserts at Gerdy's tubercle. An important component of the sITB is the Kaplan fibers, which connect the sITB to the distal femoral metaphysis, primarily at the lateral femoral supraepicondylar region [11].

The dITB originates posterior and medial (deep) to the sITB along the lateral intermuscular septum, in the vicinity of the Kaplan fibers. It courses anteromedially, to combine with the sITB distal to the lateral femoral epicondyle, ultimately inserting on Gerdy's tubercle [12].

The capsulo-osseous layer represents the deepest (most medial) layer of the ITB. The layer begins proximally, contiguous with the fascia of the plantaris and lateral gastrocnemius muscle. It then runs deep and slightly posterior to the sITB, merging with the sITB and dITB distally at Gerdy's tubercle [12].

Table 16.1 Components of the anterolateral complex of the knee

Iliotibial band (from superficial to deep)	sITB
	Kaplan fibers
	dITB
	Capsulo-osseous layer
Anterolateral ligament	
Anterolateral capsule (from posterior to anterior)	Posterior division (superficial and deep layers to the LCL)
	Mid-third capsular ligament
	Anterior division

sITB superficial iliotibial band, *dITB* deep ITB, *LCL* lateral collateral ligament

Anterolateral Ligament and Anterolateral Capsule

The anterolateral joint capsule, as described by Hughston et al., consists of a superficial and deep layer, relative to the LCL [13]. The layers then become confluent anterior to the LCL [14]. The capsule can be further separated into anterior, mid-third, and posterior divisions [13]. The anterior division is thin without a femoral attachment; however, the mid-third capsular ligament is a discrete thickening, with femoral and tibial bony insertions which inserts on the lateral meniscus, forming the meniscofemoral and meniscotibial ligaments (coronary ligament) [15].

While it remains controversial, the evidence is increasingly pointing to the ALL as a ligamentous structure, separate from the capsule. However, there is considerable definitional overlap with the mid-third capsular ligament, and the question of whether these are two distinct structures is not yet settled [16]. A cadaver study by Getgood et al. found the ALL to be a ligamentous structure, which differentiated it from the surrounding capsule. It was not however a completely discrete ligament, the way the LCL is, however [17].

Accordingly, the ALL has been likened to the glenohumeral ligaments (GHL) of the shoulder, which are dense condensations of tissue that provide static joint stability [16]. Recent evidence points toward the ALL as a ligamentous structure embedded within capsular tissue.

The femoral origin of the ALL is perhaps one of the most controversial elements to its anatomic characterization and is largely responsible for the continued difficulty in identification. The femoral origin has variably been reported as anterior, directly on, or posterior and proximal to the lateral epicondyle [8, 18, 19]. Further research has led to an increasing consensus that the ligament primarily originates proximal and posterior to the lateral epicondyle [20]. This origin is most commonly posterior and proximal to the attachment site of the LCL, but it has been reported as anterior and distal as well [21, 22]. It has a large, fan-like footprint, which overlaps the LCL origin [23]. The diameter of the ALL at its femoral origin is 11.85 mm [24].

The ALL then courses anterolaterally, inserting onto the lateral aspect of the lateral meniscus, roughly at the junction between the anterior horn and body, for a mean length of 5.6 mm [25]. It then inserts onto the tibia, roughly halfway between Gerdy's tubercle and the anterior aspect of the fibular head [8]. Cadaver dissection has found the insertion to be on average 24.7 mm posterior to the center of Gerdy's tubercle and 26.1 mm anterior to the anterior margin of the fibular head [22]. The ALL has been found to be on average 9.5 mm distal to the joint line, just proximal to the insertion of the biceps femoris (Fig. 16.1) [22, 23].

The ALL is not an isometric ligament. Rather, the length of the ALL increases with progressive knee flexion (loosens). The critical clinical importance of this fact will be explored further in the surgical technique section [26].

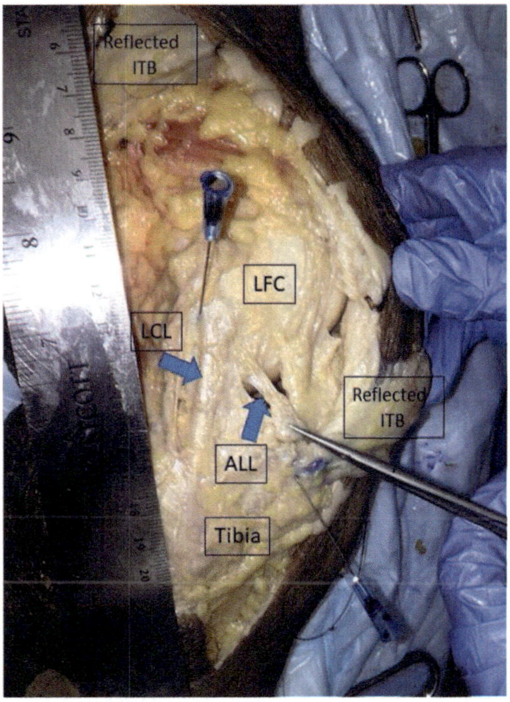

Fig. 16.1 Dissection of right knee cadaveric specimen. The anterolateral ligament (ALL) can be appreciated coursing from its origin just proximal and posterior to the LCL origin to its insertion between Gerdy's tubercle and the fibular head. *LCL* lateral collateral ligament, *ITB* iliotibial band

Primary and Secondary Stabilizers of Tibial Rotation

To understand the concept behind, and potential value of, ALLR, one must understand the synergistic relationship between the ACL and the ALC in limiting tibial rotation (Table 16.2). Butler and colleagues introduced the concept of primary restraint. [27] This was further expanded upon, and defined by Andersen as, "cutting a primary restraint results in an increase in joint motion, whereas cutting a secondary restraint will result in an increase of joint motion only in the absence of the primary restraint." [28] This notion was used as the foundation for future biomechanical studies establishing the significance of various restraints [29].

The Primary Stabilizer of Tibial Rotation: The Anterior Cruciate Ligament

Based on available evidence, the ACL is likely the primary stabilizer of tibial IR, particularly from 0 to 30° of flexion [30]. At flexion >30°, the ACL is likely still the chief restraint to tibial IR,

Table 16.2 Stabilizers of tibial rotation

	Structure	Function (knee position with highest contribution to stability)
Primary stabilizer	ACL	Low flexion angles (at or near full extension)
Secondary stabilizers	ITB—superficial	High flexion angles
	ITB—deep	Low flexion angles (at or near full extension)
	ALL	Likely contributes at all flexion angles (more evidence required)
	Lateral meniscus	Contributes at all flexion angles

ACL anterior cruciate ligament, *ALL* anterolateral ligament

but with a greater relative contribution of the ALC [28, 32–35]. Biomechanically, the mechanism of restraint is believed to be winding of the ACL bundles around each other, which loads the ligament and resists rotation [31].

Secondary Stabilizers

Evidence suggests the ITB is an important secondary stabilizer of tibial IR, particularly at higher flexion angles [36, 37]. The sITB provides more restraint at higher flexion angles, while the dITB contributes more at lower flexion angles [9, 36, 37]. Because the ACL resists more IR at extension, the dITB likely works synergistically at low flexion angles to assist the ACL in resisting rotation here. As the knee flexes, the sITB then takes over to help resist IR.

Additionally, based on available evidence, the ALL is an important secondary stabilizer to tibial IR, particularly in the ACL-deficient state. The ITB however may be a more important contributor to IR restraint, specifically the dITB at lower flexion angles and the sITB at higher flexion angles [1, 29, 35, 38–44]. Given this role, one can see how neglecting an anterolateral injury in the setting of an ACL rupture (or ACLR failure) could lead to increased stress on the ACL graft and risk future failure. With this in mind, the concept of a lateral-based extra-articular procedure has been re-visited, in the forms of lateral extra-articular tenodesis (LET) and anterolateral ligament reconstruction (ALLR).

Unlike the medial meniscus, the lateral meniscus does not contribute much to resisting anterior translation. It has, however, been shown both biomechanically and clinically to be an important secondary stabilizer to tibial IR [44–47].

Biomechanical Evidence for Anterolateral Ligament Reconstruction

Efficacy of ALLR

As ALLR is still a relatively nascent procedure, the majority of evidence of its efficacy comes from biomechanical studies [48–52]. These studies have attempted to evaluate the value of reconstructing the ALLR in the setting of ACLR, particularly in terms of additional IR restraint provided (Table 16.3). Conversely, several studies have demonstrated conflicting results, casting doubt on the ability of the ALLR to provide clinically relevant rotational stability. These studies reported not only a lack of overconstraint but a lack of restoration of native stability [1, 51–53].

Due to the mixed biomechanical and clinical results, a consensus has not yet been reached on the efficacy of ALLR. While most studies find it improves rotational stability, enough well-performed biomechanical investigations have found evidence to the contrary. Additionally, some studies that did find improved rotational control with ALLR found it only did so by simultaneously overconstraining the knee. For these reasons, a systematic review of biomechanical outcomes by DePhillipo et al. concluded only, "there is inconsistency in terms of femoral origin, flexion angle, and performance of the ALLR at this time" [53].

Femoral Origin for Graft Placement

There is also lack of agreement regarding the native femoral origin of the ALL, and it is of little surprise that various locations have been used for

Table 16.3 Selected biomechanical studies investigating the ALL

Key biomechanical studies evaluating the efficacy of ALLR in restoring knee kinematics			
Reference information			
Lead author, year	Journal	Methods	Main findings
Nitri, 2016	*AJSM*	6DFR, 10 cadaveric knees	Isolated ACLR did not restore rotation
		Compared various states of ACL deficiency and anterolateral deficiency, with ACLR and ALLR permutations	ACLR with ALLR SS↑ IR stability
Geeslin, 2018	*AJSM*	6DFR, 10 cadaveric knees	Isolated ACLR did not restore rotation
		Compared ALLR to LET in various states of ACL and anterolateral deficiency	Both ALLR and LET with ACLR resulted in overconstraint
		Fixed LET or ALLR at either 30° or 70° kf and at 20 or 40 N of tension	KF and graft tension did not significantly affect results
Jette, 2019	*Knee*	6DFR, 12 cadaveric knees	Both ALLR and LET with ACLR resulted in overconstraint
		Compared ALLR to LET in various states of ACL and anterolateral deficiency	KF and graft tension did not significantly affect results
Spencer, 2015	*AJSM*	6DFR, 12 cadaveric knees	ALLR did not reduce IR after ACLR
		Compared ALLR to LET in various states of ACL and anterolateral deficiency	LET did restore IR stability after ACLR
			Neither procedure resulted in overconstraint
Noyes, 2017	*AJSM*	6DFR, 7 cadaveric knees	ALLR produced only corrected modest amount of IR and only at high kf
		Evaluated effects of concomitant ALLR with ACLR in various states of ACL and anterolateral deficiency	ALLR only reduced a very modest amount of ACL graft stress
Inderhaug, 2017	*AJSM*	6DFR, 12 cadaveric knees	Isolated ACLR did not restore rotational stability
		Compared ALLR to LET in various states of ACL and anterolateral deficiency	ALLR did not provide sufficient additional stability
			LET at 20 N of tensioning restored kinematics

6DFR 6-degree-of-freedom robot, *SS* statistically significant, *LET* lateral extra-articular tenodesis, *kf* knee flexion

reconstruction. The 2017 DePhillipo systematic review found the six surgical technique articles, with the most common femoral origin site described being the posterior and proximal to the LCL origin (four studies) [54–57] vs two studies using a point anterior and distal to the LCL origin [58, 59].

Interestingly, in a comparison of four biomechanical outcome studies, two studies that did not find any overconstraint used the anterior and distal origin point [1, 48, 60, 61]. These studies also did not find any significant increase in rotational control following ALLR when using the anterior and distal origin. This indicates the anterior point likely cannot adequately tension the graft. Additional studies have demonstrated length changes depending on the location of the femoral origin, and accordingly the posterior and proximal position has been recommended for reconstruction [18, 26, 35, 62].

Knee Flexion Angle

The degree the graft is fixed may potentially affect efficacy of the procedure and may alter knee kinematics. While the optimal fixation angle has not yet been determined, the available evidence supports placing the graft with the knee in full extension (and with the leg in neutral rotation) is likely safest to prevent overconstraint [20, 49, 52, 60].

Graft Isometry

Unlike other ligament reconstructions where isometry is key, the ALL has surprisingly been found to be non-isometric [26, 63]. This lack of isometry should be considered when fixing the graft. During assessment, the graft should be slightly looser in flexion (because the native ligament lengthens with flexion) than in extension. If the graft is found to tighten with knee flexion, the femoral origin point may be too anterior and distal and should be revised to a more posterior and proximal position [20].

Indications

Currently, there are no consensus indications for an ALLR in the setting of an ACLR. This is due to the lack of sufficient clinical data with adequate follow-up to determine which patients benefit most from the procedure. However, several indications have been cited in the literature repeatedly (Table 16.4).

Irrespective of if it is a revision scenario or not, indications revolve around signs, or likely signs, of concomitant anterolateral injury. For instance, a high-grade pivot shift (defined as either 2+ or more typically 3+) is an indication for many authors. The higher pivot shift, however, is taken as a sign that secondary stabilizers must also be injured [16, 20, 56, 64]. Similarly, chronic ACL injuries are often considered for ALLR, as the chronic instability may weaken the secondary stabilizers [65]. Evidence of a Segond fracture has also been cited as an indication, as it represents an avulsion of the ALL off of the tibia [19, 56, 66]. Other indications include patients returning to high-risk sports/activities, such as those that require pivoting [20, 64], though this is more controversial than the other indications listed. Generalized hyperlaxity (measured via Beighton score) [67] should also prompt consideration for an ALLR, as the excess stress may be put on the graft without additional constraint [64].

Table 16.4 Indications and contraindications for ALLR

Potential indications and contraindications for concomitant ALLR	
Indications	High-grade pivot shift (2+ or 3+) [16, 20, 56, 64]
	Chronic ACL injuries [65]
	Evidence of Segond fracture [19, 56, 66]
	Participates in high-risk sports [20, 64]
	Generalized hyperlaxity [64]
	Revision ACLR [16]
Contraindications	Multi-ligament knee injuries [64]

Another factor is if a soft tissue or allograft is selected for ACLR, one may give stronger consideration to performing the ALLR, as it may help protect a potentially weaker graft (one that takes longer to incorporate without bone-to-bone healing). This concept is anecdotal and has not yet been studied.

In the revision setting, specifically, there is debate if ALLR should be performed in all (or the majority) of cases or if it should be more limited to revisions that also meet the above criteria [16]. More evidence is required before any definitive statements can be made.

Contraindications are also still being developed, but strong consideration should be given to not performing an ALLR in the setting of a multi-ligament knee injury (MLKI). Given that stiffness is one of the most common complications following MLKI reconstruction, avoiding a procedure that may lead to overconstraint is advisable. Additionally, by addressing the additional soft tissue injuries, the instability may improve, obviating the potential benefits of ALLR [64].

The authors' definitive indications for ALLR in the setting of a revision ACL include a pivot shift of 2+ or greater, knee recurvatum (as an indication of laxity), and a young or contact/collision athlete. Other causes of laxity or risk increases, addressed at length in other chapters, must be remedied as well.

Patient Evaluation

History

While a thorough history should be taken for all patients, when considering an ALLR, several key points should be highlighted. In regard to the ALLR, the physician should try to understand the status of the patient's anterolateral knee structures, their prior injury history, and their future risk.

The patient's injury history/mechanism of injury should be determined, with specific attention to rotational mechanisms. Surgical history is crucial, including prior ACLR in the setting of revisions, including type of grafts, implants, and if any concomitant procedures were performed. The patient should be asked if their knee ever felt stable after the primary surgery. In regard to risk, the patient's functional goals, occupation, and athletic activity should all be discussed.

Physical Examination

A standard knee and ligamentous exam should be performed. Special attention should again be paid to the lateral side of the knee for any signs of specific instability. For instance, a varus gait or thrust may suggest damaged lateral structures [64]. Additionally, a good pivot shift exam is essential to help assess the amount of ALRI; however, this typically can only be done properly under anesthesia. Finally, inspection of any prior surgical incisions should be performed to assist in surgical planning.

General laxity testing should also be performed to calculate a Beighton score [67]. Patients with elevated Beighton scores should be considered for ALLR.

Imaging

Standard knee x-rays, including an AP, lateral, and merchant/sunrise view, should be obtained at baseline. In addition to identifying other injuries, their main use in consideration of ALLR is to look for the presence of a Segond fracture, indicating ALL injury [66]. These can also be used to assess prior tunnel placement, tunnel lysis, and prior fixation. Additional radiographs that should be considered are full-length AP and lateral weightbearing views to assess for coronal and sagittal alignment. CT scans should also be obtained in the revision setting to help further assess tunnel lysis and tunnel placement.

Because the ALL is extra-articular, ultrasonography (US) has been proposed as a means of radiologic assessment. Furthermore, because the ligament tightens with internal rotation, it has been posited that ultrasound, which can dynamically evaluate structures, could be a cheap, effective method of investigating potential ALL injury [68]. Based on these principles, Cavaignac et al. conducted an anatomic dissection study using US to identify the ALL and reported excellent interrater agreement (Cohen *k*, 0.88–0.94) [68]. However, a similar study by Capo et al. using ten fresh-frozen cadaver knees and ultrasound found ultrasound to be unreliable and did not recommend its use in routine work-up [69]. More evidence is required at this time before a determination on the utility of US can be made in diagnosing ALL injuries.

Studies attempting to use magnetic resonance imaging (MRI) to identify the ALL, and characterize ALL injuries, have also had mixed results. Visualization of the ALL has been reported at 11–100% of patients (including cadaveric specimens) [70–72]. Though some studies have reported high sensitivities, most appear to be plagued by low-to-moderate inter- and intra-rater reliability. For example, a study by Hartigan et al. had two musculoskeletal radiologists visualize the ALL on 1.5 Tesla MRI [71]. Though they reported the ability to visualize the ALL in 100% of cases, one reviewer found the ALL to be torn in 26% of patients, while the second reviewer found the ALL to be torn in 62% of patients [71]. Of note, the tibia portion has been demonstrated to be the most consistently seen on MRI [73]. MRI appears to be a more promising modality to detect ALL injuries, though more research needs to be done, and protocols need to be improved before it can be considered a reliable diagnostic tool.

Surgical Procedure

Native ALL Properties and Graft Selection

An ideal graft choice would be one that mimics the properties of the native ALL as close as possible. Several studies have attempted to quantify the biomechanical properties of the native ALL in order to improve graft selection. The range of load to failure in these studies was 49.9 ± 14.62 N to 319.7 ±212.6 N [74, 75]. The stiffness of the ALL has been reported at 21 ± 8.2 N to 41.9 ± 25.7 N [74, 76, 77]. A consensus group led by Sonnery-Cottet reported the mean load to failure as "around 180 N" and the mean stiffness as 31 N/mm [20].

ALL Compared to Possible Grafts

The ideal graft for ALLR has not yet been determined, and multiple options have been described [23]. Kernkamp et al. described using an ITB-based autograft, by taking a free slip of it (similar to performing a modified Lemaire, but transecting the distal attachment) [78]. The most common graft used in the literature for both biomechanical and surgical technique articles is a gracilis graft (auto- and allo- have both been described) [54, 56, 59]. A tripled semitendinosus graft and a doubled gracilis graft have also been described [54]. Sonnery-Cottet et al. prefer a doubled gracilis tendon, but place the graft in an inverted Y formation, with two distal points of fixation in the tibia [55].

While limited comparative data exists regarding graft properties, Wytrykowski et al. compared the properties of the native ALL with the ITB and a two-strand gracilis graft in cadaveric knees. They found the ITB to be most consistent with the ALL; however, they did not describe their tissue harvesting technique [77]. Additionally, there is some concern about harvesting a portion of the ITB, which is a known important stabilizer to tibial IR, to reconstruct the ALL, with the goal of improving tibial IR (i.e., "robbing Peter to pay Paul") [79–81].

Set-Up

The patient is placed supine on a standard operating table with the feet brought to the edge of the bed. An exam under anesthesia is performed to confirm the diagnosis. If work-up regarding ALRI was equivocal up to this point, results of the pivot test exam can be critical in deciding whether an ALLR is indicated. Following the exam, a tourniquet is placed high on the thigh. The operative extremity is secured with a leg holder, high on the thigh to allow lateral access. We prefer to use a semitendinosus allograft for reconstruction, sized to a 4 mm diameter. This is prepared on the back table while the diagnostic arthroscopy is performed.

Procedure

After the leg is prepped and draped in the usual sterile fashion, landmarks are marked on the skin. These include the lateral epicondyle, Gerdy's tubercle, and the fibular head (Fig. 16.2). The ACLR (or revision ACLR) is performed first, up to and including drilling the femoral and tibial tunnels. Pearls and pitfalls of dealing with specific challenges of revision ACLR cases, such as

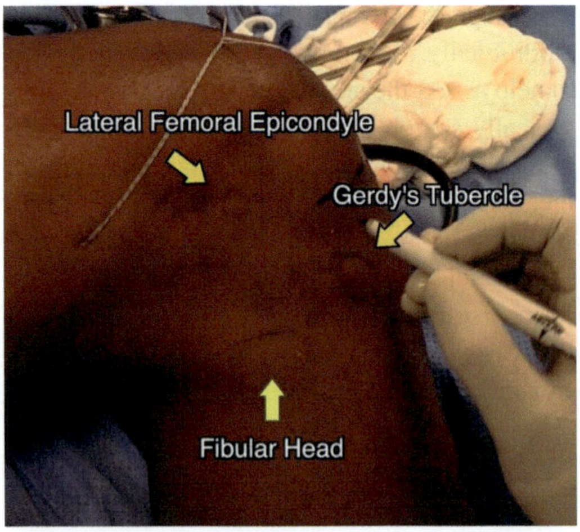

Fig. 16.2 Relevant landmarks for the anterolateral ligament reconstruction. The femora origin will be proximal and posterior to the lateral femoral epicondyle. The tibial insertion will be approximately halfway between Gerdy's tubercle and the fibular head

graft choice, osteolysis, tunnel widening, prior implant management, etc., are covered in prior chapters. The reason for drilling the femoral and tibial tunnels (particularly the femoral tunnel) prior to the ALLR is so that the femoral tunnel can be visualized through the anteromedial portal while drilling the ALL femoral tunnel. However, with experience and proper positioning and angling of the tunnels, this becomes less necessary.

Following ACL tunnel drilling, we proceed with the ALLR portion. A guide pin is placed at the femoral origin of the ALL, approximately 8 mm proximal and 4 mm posterior to the lateral epicondyle at the anatomic origin (Fig. 16.3). This guide pin is directed anteriorly and proximally to avoid tunnel convergence as well as the femoral trochlea. As the guide pin is placed, the femoral tunnel for the ACLR is visualized for any signs of convergence from the guide pin. If the pin is seen on arthroscopy, it is redirected. Once the guide pin is in place, the ACL graft is fixed in the femoral tunnel.

For the ALLR, one can do either a percutaneous approach, which has the advantages of improved cosmesis and limited soft tissue insult, or a larger incision from just proximal to the lateral epicondyle to about the midway point between Gerdy's and the anterior fibular head (tibial insertion point). The advantage of doing the open rather than percutaneous approach is it permits landmark palpation and direct visualization, which may better assist tunnel placement. The percutaneous approach is described below.

Following ACL graft fixation, a small skin incision is made over the femoral guidewire, and blunt dissection is carried out until bone is reached. A 4.5 mm reamer is used to overdrill the guidewire to a depth of 25 mm in preparation for a SwiveLock anchor (Arthrex, Naples, FL). The one limb of the graft is then inserted into the femoral tunnel and secured with the screw (Fig. 16.4). Sutures are tied over the anchor as back-up fixation. Other options for femoral fixation may include interference screw fixation [57].

Landmarks, including Gerdy's tubercle and the fibular head, are again palpated for confirma-

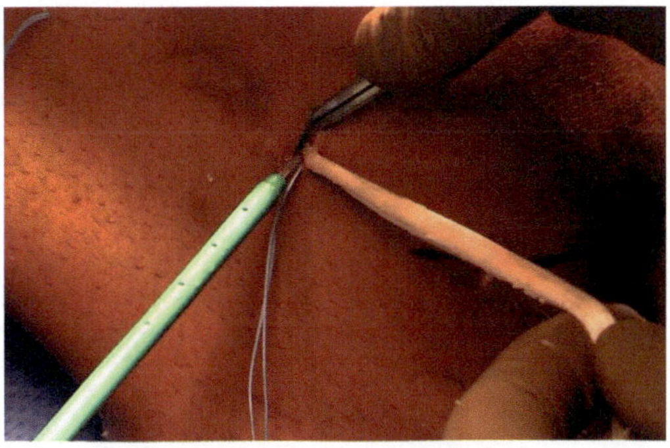

Fig. 16.4 Fixation of the femoral side of the ALLR graft

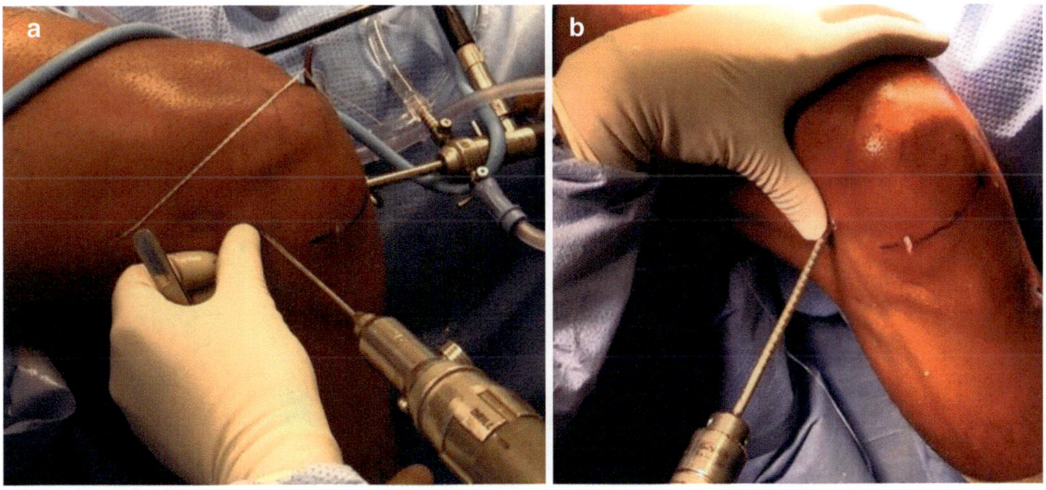

Fig. 16.3 (**a**, **b**) Femoral tunnel guidewire placement. This is followed by reaming to a depth of 25 mm

tion. A skin incision midway between the two and about 1 cm distal to the joint line is then made. Blunt dissection is performed until bone is reached. A guidewire is then passed from the anatomic ALL insertion in a slight superomedial orientation (Fig. 16.5). A 7.5 mm reamer is then used to overdrill the guidewire, again to a depth of 25 mm.

A clamp is passed from distal to proximal subcutaneously, and the suture on the distal limb of the grasp is fed to the clamp. The graft is then tunneled under the IT band and then subcutaneously (Fig. 16.6). At this point, the graft is provisionally fixed, and the knee is taken through a range of motion to assess graft isometry. Our preference is for the graft either to be isometric or to slightly loosen with flexion and tighten with extension (similar to the native ALL). If the graft position is felt to be adequate, a fork-tipped PEEK tenodesis screw (Arthrex, Naples, FL) is used to fix the graft to the tibia (Fig. 16.7). Anatomic ALLR tunnel position is critical for appropriate graft tension and function through knee range of motion (Fig. 16.8).

It is important to avoid overtension on the graft at any flexion angle. The ALL acts as a

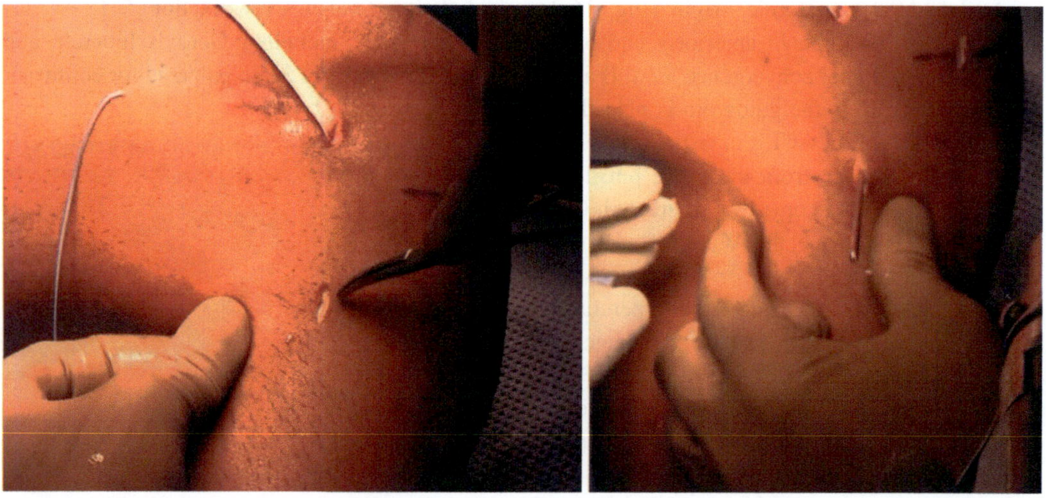

Fig. 16.5 Identification and guidewire placement into the tibial insertion site for ALLR

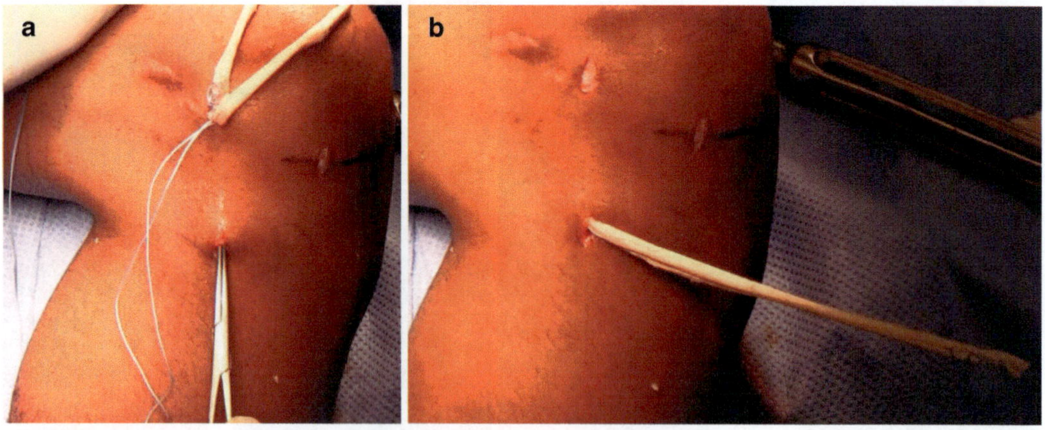

Fig. 16.6 (**a**, **b**) Percutaneous passage of the ALLR graft. A clamp is tunneled from distal to proximal and used to shuttle the graft distally to its tibial insertion site

checkrein, and overtightening can lead to overconstraint. As the primary concern following this procedure is stiffness, we typically fix our grafts in 0–30 degrees of flexion and neutral rotation. It is critical to assess isometry prior to ultimate fixation; the graft should become looser in flexion. Pearls and pitfalls can be seen in Table 16.5.

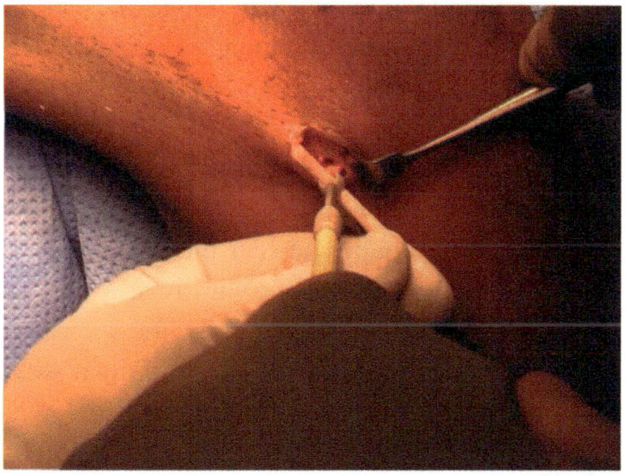

Fig. 16.7 Fixation of the tibial portion of the graft

Postoperative Protocol

As stiffness is one of the primary concerns with the addition of a lateral extra-articular procedure, we utilize a standard ACLR protocol. This includes weightbearing as tolerated with crutches and early range of motion as tolerated on postoperative day 1 while in the hinged knee brace (locked in extension for ambulation during the first week). Physical therapy focuses on quadri-

Table 16.5 Pearls and pitfalls of anterolateral ligament reconstruction

Pearls	Pitfalls
Confirm exam and ALRI under anesthesia	
Drill ACL femoral tunnel prior to ALLR femoral tunnel	Avoid ALLR femoral tunnel convergence with ACLR femoral tunnel
Look through ACL femoral tunnel to monitor for break from ALLR tunnel	Do not fix graft in external rotation, as this will lead to overconstraint
Drill ALLR femoral tunnel angled superomedially	

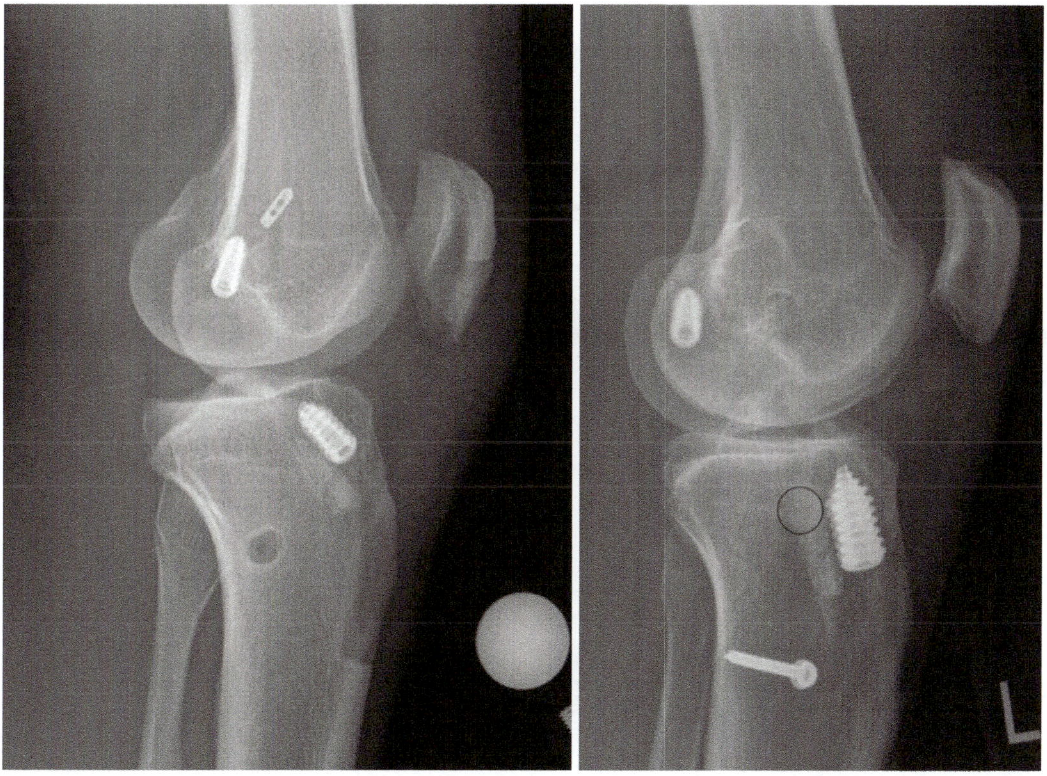

Fig. 16.8 Tibial tunnel malposition (posterior and distal) on the left. Appropriate tibial tunnel position on the right

ceps and hamstring strengthening and regaining range of motion, particularly extension.

After 2 weeks, crutches are weaned, and the brace can be discontinued once full extension without evidence of an extensor lag is reached, typically by 3–4 weeks post-op. The patient also begins closed-chain extension exercises and hamstring curls and use of a stationary bike.

At 3 months, the patient should achieve full, painless ROM. They can begin straight ahead running at this point. By 8 months, the patient may begin gradual return to athletic activity as tolerated with the goal of competitive play by 10 months.

Additional Case Examples

Case 1

A 44-year-old male had previously undergone an ACLR at an outside institution 11 years prior to presentation. He had been doing well until about 2 years prior to presentation (9 years status-post index ACLR) when he had a rotational injury associated with hemarthrosis. Since this incident, he has had recurrent swelling, pain, and recurrent instability. He also reported mechanical symptoms (clicking and catching).

On exam, the patient was noted to have a mild effusion, standing grossly physiologic valgus standing alignment, with range of motion of 0–135 degrees. For ligamentous assessment, he was found to have a 2B Lachman and a positive pivot shift. He otherwise was stable to posterior, varus, and valgus stress testing, as well as posterolateral corner testing. Dial test was also negative. Additionally, he had medial joint line tenderness and a positive McMurray test.

Imaging was notable primarily for a vertical femoral tunnel (Fig. 16.9). MRI confirmed ACL re-rupture, as well as a medial meniscal tear (Fig. 16.10). Given the patient's symptoms, he was indicated for ACLR.

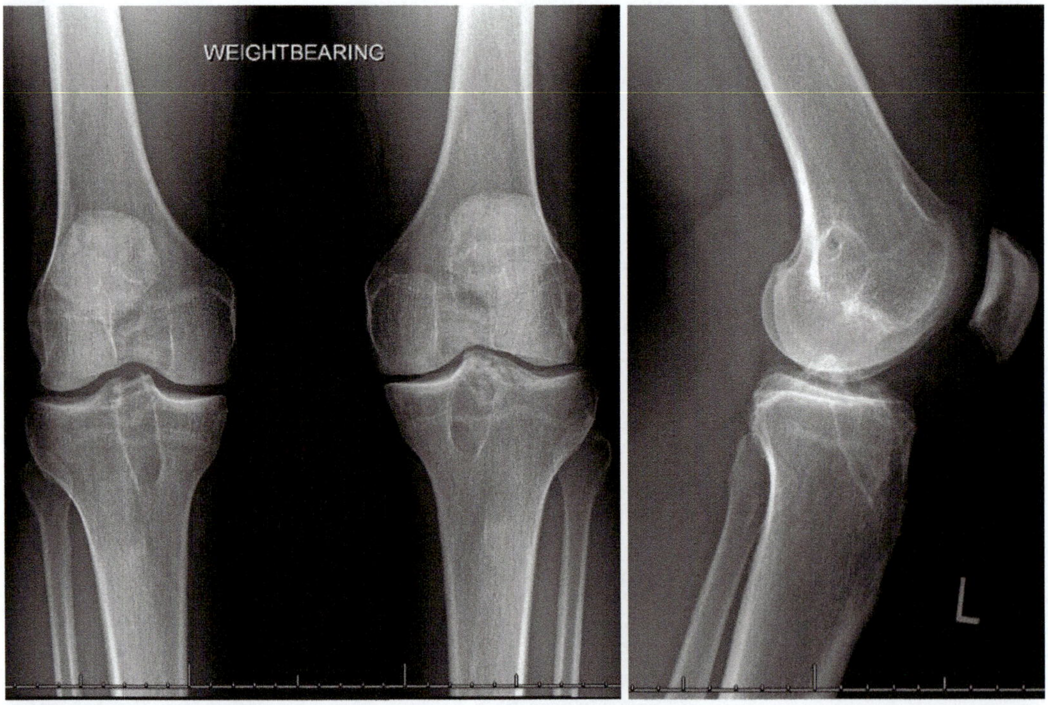

Fig. 16.9 Preoperative x-rays of a 44-year-old male with left knee recurrent pain and instability 11 years after ACLR at outside institution. Vertical femoral tunnel position can be appreciated

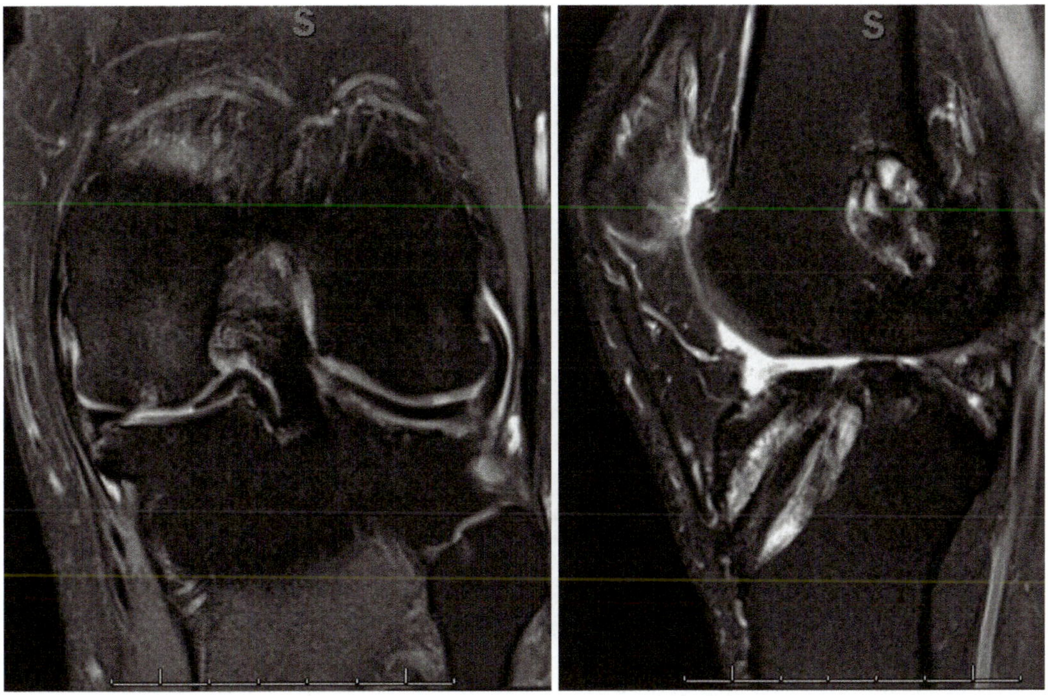

Fig. 16.10 MRI of the left knee demonstrating rupture of prior ACLR graft, including empty notch sign

Case 1 Considerations

The femoral tunnel in this case is positioned anterior. This likely was ultimately responsible for the graft failure, given the poor rotational control associated with vertical tunnel placement. In terms of other possible failure etiologies, the patient did not have any unidentified concomitant ligamentous injuries or pathologic coronal or sagittal alignment. There was also a small meniscal tear, but one that appeared stable, without root compromise.

In this scenario, it was felt that in addition to creating a separate femoral tunnel in a more anatomic position, performing an ALLR would help provide further rotational control, improving stability and taking stress off the new graft.

For the ACL, a new femoral tunnel was drilled, and a large bone-patellar-bone allograft was used to address the tibial tunnel widening. The femoral and tibial sides were fixed with interference screws. The tibial fixation was backed up with a screw and washer (Fig. 16.11). For the ALLR, a semitendinosus allograft with suture anchor fixation was used following the ACLR.

At 5 years follow-up, the patient has not had any recurrent instability and returned to his prior level of activity (recreational basketball).

Case 2

A 23-year-old male presented with recurrent right knee pain and instability 6 months after a revision ACLR with BTB allograft at an outside institution (first failure was BTB autograft). He reports he began feeling unstable during a recent physical therapy session and had not yet returned to any sports.

On exam, he had a large effusion, and range of motion of 0–135°. For ligamentous testing, he had a 2B Lachman and positive pivot shift test. He otherwise did not have any instability to posterior, varus, or valgus stress or posterolateral corner testing. Dial test was also negative. He did not have any medial or lateral joint line tenderness.

Imaging revealed physiologic coronal alignment and tunnel widening of the femoral and tibial tunnels (Figs. 16.12, 16.13, and 16.14a, b).

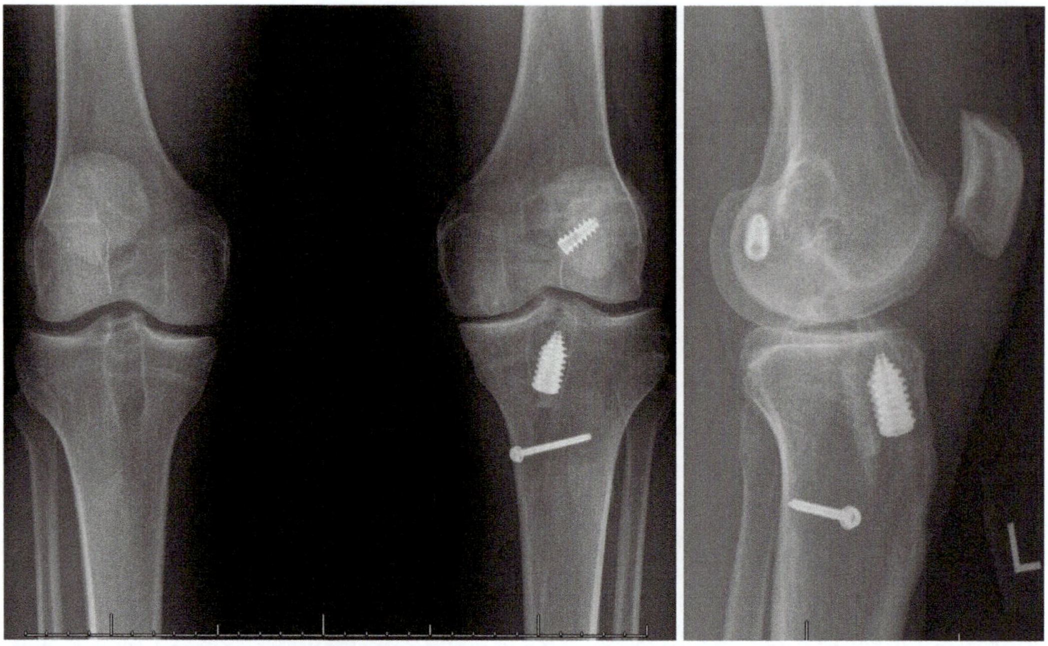

Fig. 16.11 Postoperative images demonstrating revision ACLR, with bone-patellar-bone allograft, fixed with interference screws on the femoral and tibial sides, with additional screw and washer back-up fixation. Visualization of the ALLR tunnels can be appreciated

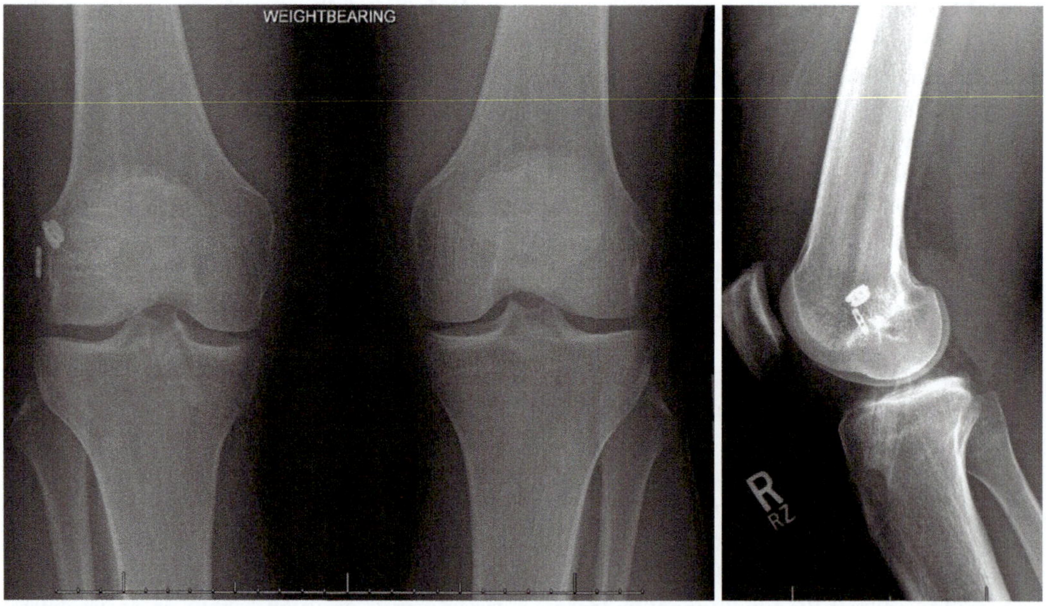

Fig. 16.12 AP and lateral x-rays of the right knee, demonstrating prior ACLR in a 23-year-old male. The patient had undergone two prior ACLR before presenting with recurrent instability

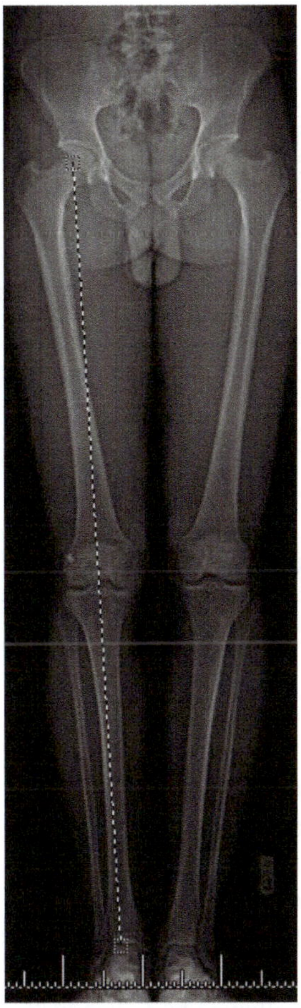

Fig. 16.13 Full-length weightbearing films of the patient's lower extremities, demonstrating neutral alignment in the coronal plane

MRI demonstrated ACL graft rupture (Fig. 16.15). Due to recurrent instability symptoms in the setting of ACLR failure, the patient was indicated for revision surgery.

Case 2 Considerations

Similar to case 1, there were no other anatomic factors contributing to the patient's ACLR failure. The patient's coronal and sagittal alignments were within normal range, there were no missed concomitant injuries, and tunnel positions seemed appropriate. One possible source of failure in this patient is the use of an allograft in a patient under 30 years old.

With this in mind, it was decided to treat this patient in a staged fashion, due to the tunnel widening. The first stage included bone grafting of the femoral and tibial tunnels. Following confirmation of graft incorporation (Fig. 16.14c, d), the patient was taken for re-revision ACLR.

Given the lack of any other failure sources, it was felt the patient would benefit from a lateral extra-articular procedure to help improve rotational control. The patient was therefore indicated for an ALLR, in addition to the revision ACLR. A contralateral BTB autograft was utilized for the ACL. A semitendinosus allograft was utilized for the ALLR, which was secured with a knotless anchor device in the femur and a metal screw in the tibia.

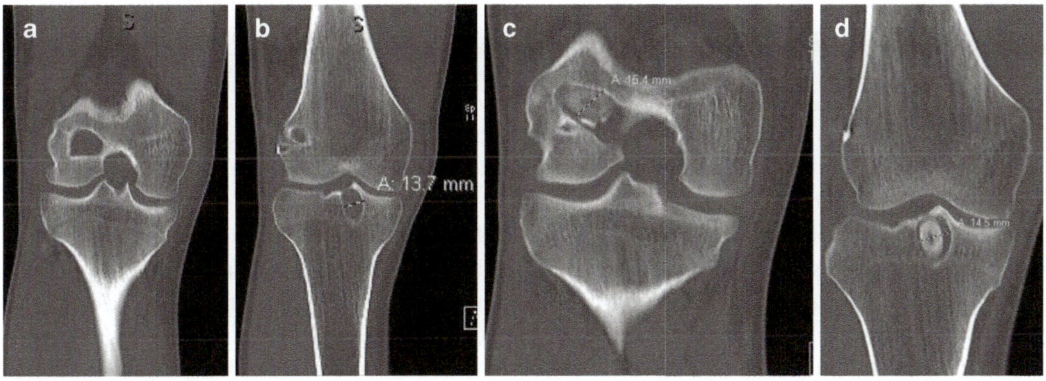

Fig. 16.14 Panels (**a**, **b**) demonstrate preoperative tunnel widening. Panels (**c**, **d**) represent a follow-up CT scan after the patient underwent a tunnel bone grafting procedure, demonstrating incorporation of the graft

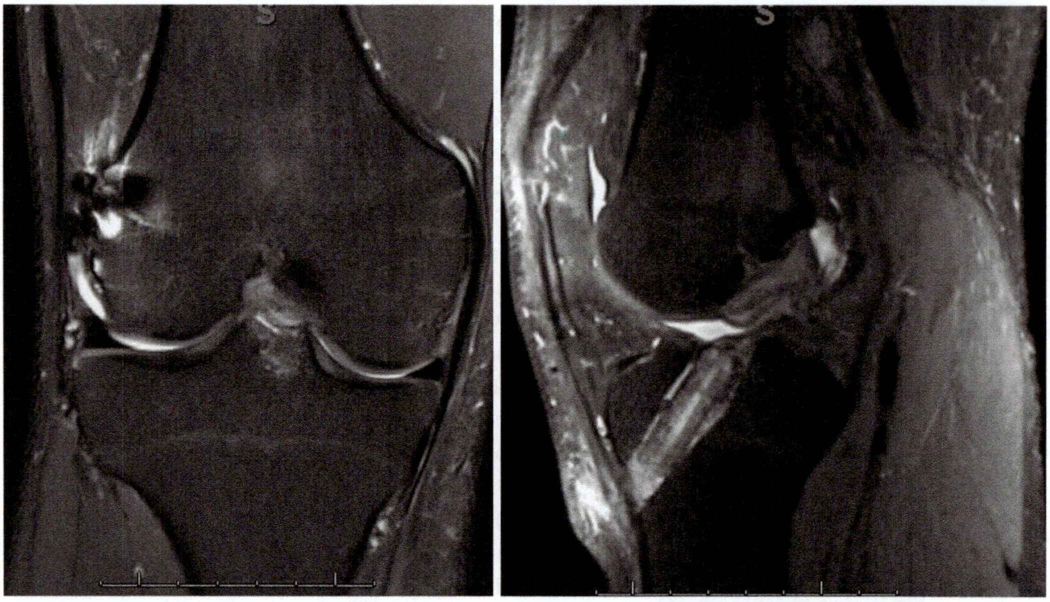

Fig. 16.15 Right knee MRI of a 23-year-old patient, demonstrating failure of prior ACLR

At 6 years follow-up, the patient has returned to his prior level of activity, without any recurrent instability events or pain.

Case 3

A 20-year-old female collegiate basketball player that had undergone an L knee ACLR with hamstring autograft 14 months presented with recurrent instability after a non-contact pivoting injury during practice.

On exam, she had a small effusion and range of motion of 0–130°. For ligamentous testing, she had a 1B Lachman with significant guarding. It was not possible to perform a pivot shift due to this guarding. Otherwise, no instability was noted to posterior, varus, or valgus stress or posterolateral corner testing. Dial test was also negative. She also was noted to have lateral joint line tenderness and a positive lateral McMurray sign.

Imaging demonstrated a likely ACL re-tear on MRI (Fig. 16.16), though this was not definitive. Alignment films demonstrated a slight 2–3 valgus malalignment (Fig. 16.17).

Case 3 Considerations

The patient's recurrent instability was strongly suggestive of re-tear; however, given the patients guarding on multiple exam attempts, and somewhat equivocal MRI, it was felt that diagnosis would be confirmed with an exam under anesthesia (EUA), followed by a diagnostic arthroscopy if the EUA was felt to be suggestive of a tear.

Under anesthesia, the patient was found to have a positive pivot shift and 2B Lachman, so the decision was made to proceed with diagnostic arthroscopy and tunnel bone grafting. Follow-up x-ray 3 months later confirmed graft consolidation (Fig. 16.18). The patient was indicated for revision ACLR 4 months after the bone grafting procedure. A partial lateral meniscectomy was also performed at this time.

In terms of options for this patient, while she did have some valgus malalignment, this was felt to be minimal (only 2–3°) and likely not contributory. She did not have any increased posterior tibial slope necessitating a closing wedge osteotomy. No other concomitant injuries were appreciated. Given she had already failed a prior soft tissue autograft, the patient was indicated for a BTB autograft ACLR. Similar to the cases above,

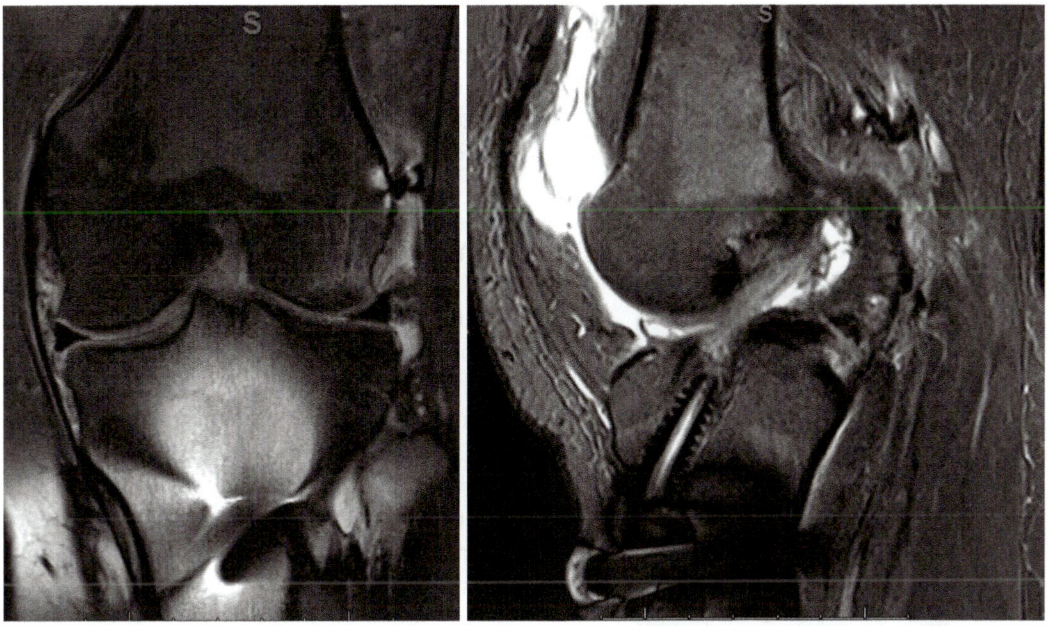

Fig. 16.16 Left knee MRI of a 20-year-old female with likely recurrent ACL tear. Because the imaging here was somewhat equivocal, final diagnosis was made at th time of the bone grafting procedure through a combination of EUA and diagnostic arthroscopy

given the lack of other etiologies for her failure, it was felt that this patient likely would benefit from additional rotational control in the form of a lateral extra-articular procedure. She was therefore indicated for an ALLR, in addition to ACLR.

One thing to always be cognizant of is the danger of overconstraint. It is important to avoid overtension on the graft at any flexion angle. Because the ALL only acts as a checkrein, overtightening it can lead to overconstraint. This can both limit ROM and increase contact pressures in the lateral compartment, leading to premature osteoarthritis. To avoid this, one should try to always fix the graft with the leg in neutral rotation, as opposed to external rotation, which may lead to overtightening. Additionally, the leg should be kept in 0–30°, which has been shown to result in the least overconstraint. Most importantly, it is critical to assess isometry prior to ultimate fixation; the graft should become looser in flexion.

At 5 years follow-up, the patient was able to return to sport and has not had any instability symptoms since her revision surgery.

All three cases above serve to illustrate the same principles. It is imperative to always evaluate any patient with an ACL tear, particularly in the revision setting, for sources of failure etiology. This may include alignment, concurrent injuries, tunnel position, graft choice, and graft fixation. Performing an anterolateral extra-articular tenodesis procedure, such as an ALLR, can help provide additional rotational stability, limiting the stress on ACL grafts. In a revision setting, when there is not another cause for failure, this can be a particularly useful tool to help minimize failure rate.

Clinical Outcomes

At the time of this writing, the only study evaluating outcomes in patients undergoing revision ACLR (and thus most relevant to this textbook chapter) is a 2019 paper by Lee et al. In a retrospective study of revision ACLR patients that underwent either isolated revision ACLR or combined revision ACLR with ALLR, the group

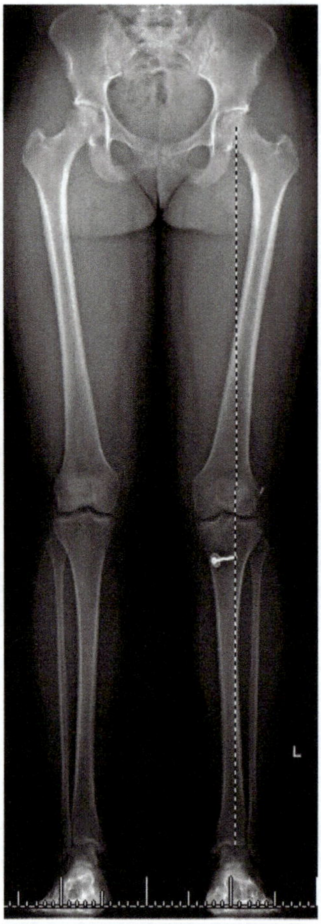

Fig. 16.17 Full-length alignment films demonstrating slight valgus malalignment of 2–3 degrees

found the combined ACLR ALLR group had significantly less patients with postoperative pivot shifts, significantly more patients returning to sport at the same level of activity pre-injury, and significantly higher IKDC [85]. The group theorized that the extra-articular procedures participate in a load-sharing effect with the ACLR, limiting stress on the ACLR and preventing delayed healing and ultimately failure [85].

Given the relative paucity of available evidence, particularly mid- and long-term studies, ALLR cannot be unequivocally recommended. In clinical studies, it does appear to improve stability and outcome scores and possibly reduce rerupture rates [82–84]. However, no information exists regarding the effect on lateral compartment cartilage following combined ALLR. Until long-term studies on combined ACLR and ALLR patients can be reported, some question about the clinical effects of potential overconstraint will remain. A summary table of clinical outcome studies can be found in Table 16.6.

Complications

While no specific clinical complications have been reported in the literature, as discussed in the biomechanics section above, several studies have found evidence of overconstraint with both ALLR and LET procedures [49, 50, 52, 60]. Conversely, well-performed studies, like that by Noyes et al., have found ALLR to not even improve rotational laxity, let alone result in overconstraint [51]. Importantly, no clinical data about overconstraint exists. If ALLR does result in slight overconstraint, there is no information regarding the clinical effects of this.

There are two primary concerns with overconstraint from lateral extra-articular procedures. Overconstraint generally refers to reduced tibial internal rotation and anterior translation as compared to the intact state [49]. The first is that the constraint may limit knee range of motion. This is particularly evident, as the studies that did find evidence of overconstraint found it primarily at higher knee flexion angles [49, 50]. This could lead to knee stiffness. The other concern is the effect of constraint on the lateral compartment of the knee. With increased constraint, compartment pressures may increase, which could lead to accelerated degeneration. This has not been demonstrated yet in the literature, but is a very real theoretical concern. Until long-term clinical research can be performed, the value of increased stability with extra-articular procedures must be balanced against the risk of overconstraint.

If one elects to proceed with ALLR, steps should be taken to avoid the risk of overconstraint. This includes fixing the graft at a lower degree of knee flexion (either full extension or at most 30 degrees based on surgeon preference/patient laxity). It is also important to have the leg in neutral rotation (avoiding external rotation), which can also possibly lead to overconstraint

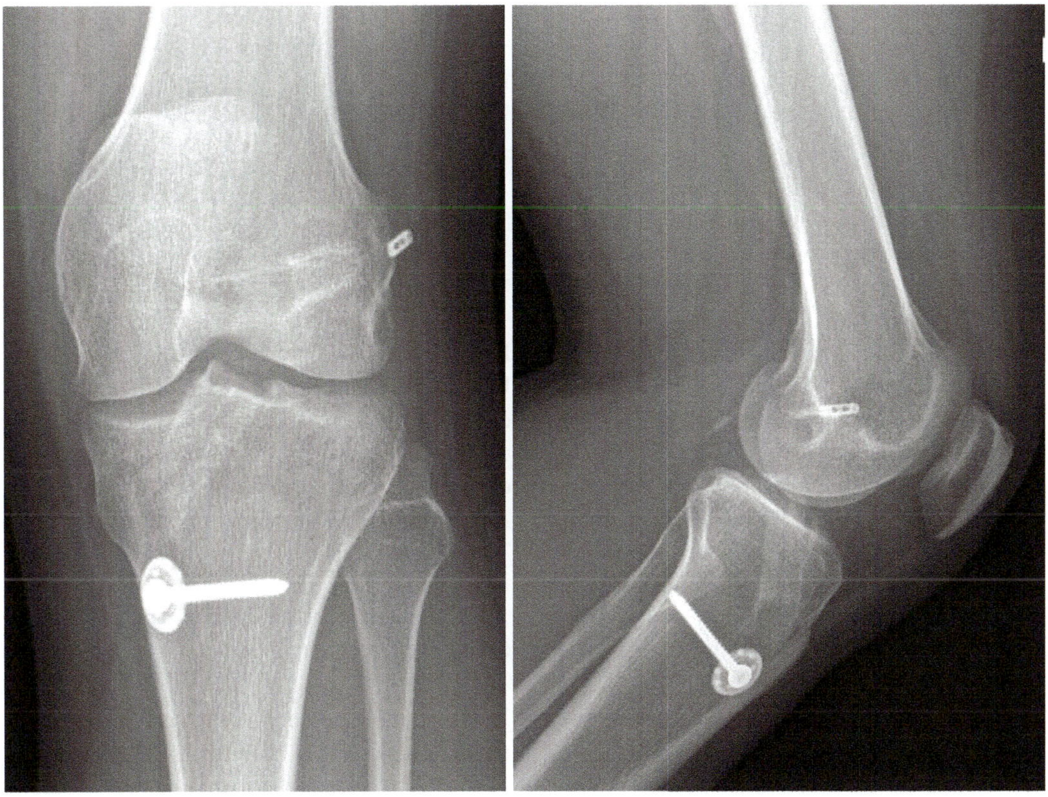

Fig. 16.18 Left knee AP and lateral x-rays taken 3 months after bone grafting procedure, demonstrating graft consolidation

Table 16.6 Selected clinical studies investigating ALLR

Key clinical studies evaluating the efficacy of ALLR in restoring knee kinematics			
Reference information			
Lead author, year	Journal	Methods	Main findings
Sonnery-Cottet, 2015	*AJSM*	Retrospective case series, of patients that underwent ACLR with ALLR for primary ACL rupture	SS↑ functional scores
		Minimum 2-year follow-up	6.6% contralateral ACL rupture rate, 1.1% ipsilateral re-rupture rate
Rosensteil, 2019	*Arthroscopy*	Retrospective case series of professional athletes that underwent ACLR with ALLR for primary ACL rupture	SS↑ functional scores
		Minimum 2-year follow-up	85.7% return to sport
			5.7% revision ACLR
Ibrahim, 2017	*AJSM*	Prospective RCT	No SS differences in functional scores
		Randomization to isolated ACLR or ACLR with ALLR	Slight SS↑ in stability with ALLR
Lee, 2019	*AJSM*	Retrospective review of revision ACL patients	SS↓ pivot shifts in ALLR group
		Treated with isolated revision ACLR or ACLR with ALLR	SS↑ patients returning to sport at the same level
			SS↑ IKDC score

[64, 65, 86]. After demonstrating restoration of knee kinematics with the ALLR in a cadaveric study, Smith et al. noted the importance of placing the femoral origin of the tunnel posterior and proximal to the LCL origin, and having the graft tighten in extension, while remaining slightly lax with flexion. They noted using this position, and fixing the graft in extension, ensures that the graft is tightest in extension where the pivot shift mechanism comes into play. Conversely, having the graft be tighter in flexion was shown to lead to overconstraint while simultaneously being less effective at resisting the pivot shift [86].

Other complications are related to the surgical technique itself. Femoral tunnel convergence can occur if the ALLR tunnel is not directed anterior and proximal. The surgeon may also use the arthroscope to view the ACL femoral tunnel while the femoral ALL tunnel is drilled. If any breach is noted, ALLR tunnel drilling should be stopped and redirected [55, 57]. Though relatively far from the zone of surgery, one must always be cognizant of the common peroneal nerve, initially deep and then posterior to the biceps femoris, until it wraps around the fibular neck. There are also the extra-surgical scar and potential hematoma from the lateral genicular artery.

Considerations for ALLR vs Modified Lemaire

When considering which lateral extra-articular procedure to use, it is important to note that the current state of literature is, at best, equivocal. While some advantages and disadvantages of each procedure have been offered, very little of how these biomechanical or theoretical concerns will clinical affect patients is actually known at this time.

Which procedure is biomechanically, or, more importantly, clinically, more effective is unknown at this time. ALLR may be more anatomic and may require less surgical insult [12, 20, 55, 86]. It also may be less prone to overconstraint [52]. However, it does not address a potentially injured ITB, does not benefit from the pulley effect of the LCL, and may be more expensive [29, 35, 64]. Ultimately, when directly compared, neither procedure has proven superior [49, 53]. The decision on which to use (if any at all) should be up to the discretion of the operating surgeon. A list of ALLR and LET considerations can be found in Table 16.7.

Table 16.7 ALLR vs LET considerations

ALLR advantages	ALLR disadvantages
Smaller surgical insult	LET may better limit IR
Avoids further trauma to ITB and LCL	LET addresses ITB injury/ weakness
More anatomic procedure	ALLR is more expensive (if allograft used)
May lead to less overconstraint than LET	

Conclusion

The ACL is the primary restraint to tibial internal rotation. Secondary stabilizers, including the ITB, ALL, anterolateral capsule, and lateral meniscus, provide additional restraint. When the ACL is injured, these secondary stabilizers may also be injured, particularly in patients with large pivot shifts. Biomechanical studies have demonstrated that ACLR alone may not restore knee IR kinematics. When combined with ACLR, ALLR has been shown in some studies to restore stability, though there is a risk of overconstraint. Multiple techniques for ALLR exist, but the most important keys are to avoid femoral tunnel convergence and fixing the graft in external rotation or significant knee flexion, which may lead to overtightening. Clinical outcome studies appear promising, but only short- to mid-term data exists.

References

1. Spencer L, Burkhart TA, Tran MN, et al. Biomechanical analysis of simulated clinical testing and reconstruction of the anterolateral ligament of the knee. Am J Sports Med. 2015;43(9):2189–97.
2. Tanaka M, Vyas D, Moloney G, Bedi A, Pearle AD, Musahl V. What does it take to have a high-grade

pivot shift? Knee Surg Sports Traumatol Arthrosc. 2012;20(4):737–42.
3. Hettrich CM, Dunn WR, Reinke EK, Group M, Spindler KP. The rate of subsequent surgery and predictors after anterior cruciate ligament reconstruction: two- and 6-year follow-up results from a multicenter cohort. Am J Sports Med. 2013;41(7):1534–40.
4. Hussein M, van Eck CF, Cretnik A, Dinevski D, Fu FH. Individualized anterior cruciate ligament surgery: a prospective study comparing anatomic single- and double-bundle reconstruction. Am J Sports Med. 2012;40(8):1781–8.
5. Lind M, Menhert F, Pedersen AB. Incidence and outcome after revision anterior cruciate ligament reconstruction: results from the Danish registry for knee ligament reconstructions. Am J Sports Med. 2012;40(7):1551–7.
6. Segond P-F. Recherches cliniques et expérimentales sur les épanchements sanguins du genou par entorse. Paris: Hachette Livre; 2017. p. 1879.
7. Vincent JP, Magnussen RA, Gezmez F, et al. The anterolateral ligament of the human knee: an anatomic and histologic study. Knee Surg Sports Traumatol Arthrosc. 2012;20(1):147–52.
8. Claes S, Vereecke E, Maes M, Victor J, Verdonk P, Bellemans J. Anatomy of the anterolateral ligament of the knee. J Anat. 2013;223(4):321–8.
9. Kaplan EB. The iliotibial tract; clinical and morphological significance. J Bone Joint Surg Am. 1958;40-A(4):817–32.
10. Terry GC, LaPrade RF. The biceps femoris muscle complex at the knee. Its anatomy and injury patterns associated with acute anterolateral-anteromedial rotatory instability. Am J Sports Med. 1996;24(1):2–8.
11. Lobenhoffer P, Posel P, Witt S, Piehler J, Wirth CJ. Distal femoral fixation of the iliotibial tract. Arch Orthop Trauma Surg. 1987;106(5):285–90.
12. Musahl V, Herbst E, Burnham JM, Fu FH. The anterolateral complex and anterolateral ligament of the knee. J Am Acad Orthop Surg. 2018;26(8):261–7.
13. Hughston JC, Andrews JR, Cross MJ, Moschi A. Classification of knee ligament instabilities. Part II. The lateral compartment. J Bone Joint Surg Am. 1976;58(2):173–9.
14. Seebacher JR, Inglis AE, Marshall JL, Warren RF. The structure of the posterolateral aspect of the knee. J Bone Joint Surg Am. 1982;64(4):536–41.
15. Herbst E, Albers M, Burnham JM, et al. The anterolateral complex of the knee: a pictorial essay. Knee Surg Sports Traumatol Arthrosc. 2017;25(4):1009–14.
16. Musahl V, Getgood A, Neyret P, et al. Contributions of the anterolateral complex and the anterolateral ligament to rotatory knee stability in the setting of ACL injury: a roundtable discussion. Knee Surg Sports Traumatol Arthrosc. 2017;25(4):997–1008.
17. Caterine S, Litchfield R, Johnson M, Chronik B, Getgood A. A cadaveric study of the anterolateral ligament: re-introducing the lateral capsular ligament. Knee Surg Sports Traumatol Arthrosc. 2015;23(11):3186–95.
18. Dodds AL, Halewood C, Gupte CM, Williams A, Amis AA. The anterolateral ligament: anatomy, length changes and association with the Segond fracture. Bone Joint J. 2014;96-B(3):325–31.
19. Zhang H, Qiu M, Zhou A, Zhang J, Jiang D. Anatomic anterolateral ligament reconstruction improves postoperative clinical outcomes combined with anatomic anterior cruciate ligament reconstruction. J Sports Sci Med. 2016;15(4):688–96.
20. Sonnery-Cottet B, Daggett M, Fayard JM, et al. Anterolateral Ligament Expert Group consensus paper on the management of internal rotation and instability of the anterior cruciate ligament – deficient knee. J Orthop Traumatol. 2017;18(2):91–106.
21. Helito CP, Demange MK, Bonadio MB, et al. Anatomy and histology of the knee anterolateral ligament. Orthop J Sports Med. 2013;1(7):2325967113513546.
22. Kennedy MI, Claes S, Fuso FA, et al. The anterolateral ligament: an anatomic, radiographic, and biomechanical analysis. Am J Sports Med. 2015;43(7):1606–15.
23. Kraeutler MJ, Welton KL, Chahla J, LaPrade RF, McCarty EC. Current concepts of the anterolateral ligament of the knee: anatomy, biomechanics, and reconstruction. Am J Sports Med. 2018;46(5):1235–42.
24. Daggett M, Ockuly AC, Cullen M, et al. Femoral origin of the anterolateral ligament: an anatomic analysis. Arthroscopy. 2016;32(5):835–41.
25. Helito CP, Bonadio MB, Soares TQ, et al. The meniscal insertion of the knee anterolateral ligament. Surg Radiol Anat. 2016;38(2):223–8.
26. Helito CP, Helito PV, Bonadio MB, et al. Evaluation of the length and isometric pattern of the anterolateral ligament with serial computer tomography. Orthop J Sports Med. 2014;2(12):2325967114562205.
27. Butler DL, Noyes FR, Grood ES. Ligamentous restraints to anterior-posterior drawer in the human knee. A biomechanical study. J Bone Joint Surg Am. 1980;62(2):259–70.
28. Andersen HN, Dyhre-Poulsen P. The anterior cruciate ligament does play a role in controlling axial rotation in the knee. Knee Surg Sports Traumatol Arthrosc. 1997;5(3):145–9.
29. Kaplan DJ, Jazrawi LM. Secondary stabilizers of tibial rotation in the intact and anterior cruciate ligament deficient knee. Clin Sports Med. 2018;37(1):49–59.
30. Lorbach O, Pape D, Maas S, et al. Influence of the anteromedial and posterolateral bundles of the anterior cruciate ligament on external and internal tibiofemoral rotation. Am J Sports Med. 2010;38(4):721–7.
31. Markolf KL, Park S, Jackson SR, McAllister DR. Anterior-posterior and rotatory stability of single and double-bundle anterior cruciate ligament reconstructions. J Bone Joint Surg Am. 2009;91(1):107–18.
32. Lipke JM, Janecki CJ, Nelson CL, et al. The role of incompetence of the anterior cruciate and lateral ligaments in anterolateral and anteromedial instability. A biomechanical study of cadaver knees. J Bone Joint Surg Am. 1981;63(6):954–60.
33. Engebretsen L, Wijdicks CA, Anderson CJ, Westerhaus B, LaPrade RF. Evaluation of a simulated

pivot shift test: a biomechanical study. Knee Surg Sports Traumatol Arthrosc. 2012;20(4):698–702.
34. Amis AA, Scammell BE. Biomechanics of intra-articular and extra-articular reconstruction of the anterior cruciate ligament. J Bone Joint Surg Br. 1993;75(5):812–7.
35. Kittl C, El-Daou H, Athwal KK, et al. The role of the anterolateral structures and the ACL in controlling laxity of the intact and ACL-deficient knee. Am J Sports Med. 2016;44(2):345–54.
36. Huser LE, Noyes FR, Jurgensmeier D, Levy MS. Anterolateral ligament and iliotibial band control of rotational stability in the anterior cruciate ligament-intact knee: defined by tibiofemoral compartment translations and rotations. Arthroscopy. 2017;33(3):595–604.
37. Terry GC, Norwood LA, Hughston JC, Caldwell KM. How iliotibial tract injuries of the knee combine with acute anterior cruciate ligament tears to influence abnormal anterior tibial displacement. Am J Sports Med. 1993;21(1):55–60.
38. Rasmussen MT, Nitri M, Williams BT, et al. An in vitro robotic assessment of the anterolateral ligament, part 1: secondary role of the anterolateral ligament in the setting of an anterior cruciate ligament injury. Am J Sports Med. 2016;44(3):585–92.
39. Sonnery-Cottet B, Lutz C, Daggett M, et al. The involvement of the anterolateral ligament in rotational control of the knee. Am J Sports Med. 2016;44(5):1209–14.
40. Bonanzinga T, Signorelli C, Grassi A, et al. Kinematics of ACL and anterolateral ligament. Part I: combined lesion. Knee Surg Sports Traumatol Arthrosc. 2017;25(4):1055–61.
41. Monaco E, Ferretti A, Labianca L, et al. Navigated knee kinematics after cutting of the ACL and its secondary restraint. Knee Surg Sports Traumatol Arthrosc. 2012;20(5):870–7.
42. Ruiz N, Filippi GJ, Gagniere B, Bowen M, Robert HE. The comparative role of the anterior cruciate ligament and anterolateral structures in controlling passive internal rotation of the knee: a biomechanical study. Arthroscopy. 2016;32(6):1053–62.
43. Thein R, Boorman-Padgett J, Stone K, Wickiewicz TL, Imhauser CW, Pearle AD. Biomechanical assessment of the anterolateral ligament of the knee: a secondary restraint in simulated tests of the pivot shift and of anterior stability. J Bone Joint Surg Am. 2016;98(11):937–43.
44. Guenther D, Rahnemai-Azar AA, Bell KM, et al. The anterolateral capsule of the knee behaves like a sheet of fibrous tissue. Am J Sports Med. 2017;45(4):849–55.
45. Musahl V, Citak M, O'Loughlin PF, Choi D, Bedi A, Pearle AD. The effect of medial versus lateral meniscectomy on the stability of the anterior cruciate ligament-deficient knee. Am J Sports Med. 2010;38(8):1591–7.
46. Musahl V, Rahnemai-Azar AA, Costello J, et al. The influence of meniscal and anterolateral capsular injury on knee laxity in patients with anterior cruciate ligament injuries. Am J Sports Med. 2016;44(12):3126–31.
47. Hosseini A, Li JS, Gill TJt, Li G. Meniscus injuries alter the kinematics of knees with anterior cruciate ligament deficiency. Orthop J Sports Med. 2014;2(8):2325967114547346.
48. Nitri M, Rasmussen MT, Williams BT, et al. An in vitro robotic assessment of the anterolateral ligament, part 2: anterolateral ligament reconstruction combined with anterior cruciate ligament reconstruction. Am J Sports Med. 2016;44(3):593–601.
49. Geeslin AG, Moatshe G, Chahla J, et al. Anterolateral knee extra-articular stabilizers: a robotic study comparing anterolateral ligament reconstruction and modified Lemaire lateral extra-articular tenodesis. Am J Sports Med. 2018;46(3):607–16.
50. Jette C, Gutierrez D, Sastre S, Llusa M, Combalia A. Biomechanical comparison of anterolateral ligament anatomical reconstruction with a semi-anatomical lateral extra-articular tenodesis. A cadaveric study. Knee. 2019;26(5):1003–9.
51. Noyes FR, Huser LE, Jurgensmeier D, Walsh J, Levy MS. Is an anterolateral ligament reconstruction required in ACL-reconstructed knees with associated injury to the anterolateral structures? A robotic analysis of rotational knee stability. Am J Sports Med. 2017;45(5):1018–27.
52. Inderhaug E, Stephen JM, Williams A, Amis AA. Biomechanical comparison of anterolateral procedures combined with anterior cruciate ligament reconstruction. Am J Sports Med. 2017;45(2):347–54.
53. DePhillipo NN, Cinque ME, Chahla J, Geeslin AG, LaPrade RF. Anterolateral ligament reconstruction techniques, biomechanics, and clinical outcomes: a systematic review. Arthroscopy. 2017;33(8):1575–83.
54. Ferreira Mde C, Zidan FF, Miduati FB, Fortuna CC, Mizutani BM, Abdalla RJ. Reconstruction of anterior cruciate ligament and anterolateral ligament using interlinked hamstrings – technical note. Rev Bras Ortop. 2016;51(4):466–70.
55. Sonnery-Cottet B, Barbosa NC, Tuteja S, Daggett M, Kajetanek C, Thaunat M. Minimally invasive anterolateral ligament reconstruction in the setting of anterior cruciate ligament injury. Arthrosc Tech. 2016;5(1):e211–5.
56. Helito CP, Bonadio MB, Gobbi RG, et al. Combined intra- and extra-articular reconstruction of the anterior cruciate ligament: the reconstruction of the knee anterolateral ligament. Arthrosc Tech. 2015;4(3):e239–44.
57. Chahla J, Menge TJ, Mitchell JJ, Dean CS, LaPrade RF. Anterolateral ligament reconstruction technique: an anatomic-based approach. Arthrosc Tech. 2016;5(3):e453–7.
58. Wagih AM, Elguindy AM. Percutaneous reconstruction of the anterolateral ligament of the knee with a polyester tape. Arthrosc Tech. 2016;5(4):e691–7.
59. Smith JO, Yasen SK, Lord B, Wilson AJ. Combined anterolateral ligament and anatomic anterior cruciate ligament reconstruction of the knee. Knee Surg Sports Traumatol Arthrosc. 2015;23(11):3151–6.
60. Schon JM, Moatshe G, Brady AW, et al. Anatomic anterolateral ligament reconstruction of the knee

leads to overconstraint at any fixation angle. Am J Sports Med. 2016;44(10):2546–56.
61. Tavlo M, Eljaja S, Jensen JT, Siersma VD, Krogsgaard MR. The role of the anterolateral ligament in ACL insufficient and reconstructed knees on rotatory stability: a biomechanical study on human cadavers. Scand J Med Sci Sports. 2016;26(8):960–6.
62. Katakura M, Koga H, Nakamura K, Sekiya I, Muneta T. Effects of different femoral tunnel positions on tension changes in anterolateral ligament reconstruction. Knee Surg Sports Traumatol Arthrosc. 2017;25(4):1272–8.
63. Kernkamp WA, Van de Velde SK, Hosseini A, et al. In vivo anterolateral ligament length change in the healthy knee during functional activities-a combined magnetic resonance and dual fluoroscopic imaging analysis. Arthroscopy. 2017;33(1):133–9.
64. Lau BC, Rames J, Belay E, Riboh JC, Amendola A, Lassiter T. Anterolateral complex reconstruction augmentation of anterior cruciate ligament reconstruction: biomechanics, indications, techniques, and clinical outcomes. JBJS Rev. 2019;7(11):e5.
65. Weber AE, Zuke W, Mayer EN, et al. Lateral augmentation procedures in anterior cruciate ligament reconstruction: anatomic, biomechanical, imaging, and clinical evidence. Am J Sports Med. 2019;47(3):740–52.
66. Vundelinckx B, Herman B, Getgood A, Litchfield R. Surgical indications and technique for anterior cruciate ligament reconstruction combined with lateral extra-articular tenodesis or anterolateral ligament reconstruction. Clin Sports Med. 2017;36(1):135–53.
67. Naal FD, Hatzung G, Muller A, Impellizzeri F, Leunig M. Validation of a self-reported Beighton score to assess hypermobility in patients with femoroacetabular impingement. Int Orthop. 2014;38(11):2245–50.
68. Cavaignac E, Wytrykowski K, Reina N, et al. Ultrasonographic identification of the anterolateral ligament of the knee. Arthroscopy. 2016;32(1):120–6.
69. Capo J, Kaplan DJ, Fralinger DJ, et al. Ultrasonographic visualization and assessment of the anterolateral ligament. Knee Surg Sports Traumatol Arthrosc. 2017;25(10):3134–9.
70. Taneja AK, Miranda FC, Braga CA, et al. MRI features of the anterolateral ligament of the knee. Skelet Radiol. 2015;44(3):403–10.
71. Hartigan DE, Carroll KW, Kosarek FJ, Piasecki DP, Fleischli JF, D'Alessandro DF. Visibility of anterolateral ligament tears in anterior cruciate ligament-deficient knees with standard 1.5-tesla magnetic resonance imaging. Arthroscopy. 2016;32(10):2061–5.
72. Porrino J Jr, Maloney E, Richardson M, Mulcahy H, Ha A, Chew FS. The anterolateral ligament of the knee: MRI appearance, association with the Segond fracture, and historical perspective. AJR Am J Roentgenol. 2015;204(2):367–73.
73. Helito CP, Helito PV, Costa HP, et al. MRI evaluation of the anterolateral ligament of the knee: assessment in routine 1.5-T scans. Skelet Radiol. 2014;43(10):1421–7.
74. Rahnemai-Azar AA, Miller RM, Guenther D, et al. Structural properties of the anterolateral capsule and iliotibial band of the knee. Am J Sports Med. 2016;44(4):892–7.
75. Zens M, Feucht MJ, Ruhhammer J, et al. Mechanical tensile properties of the anterolateral ligament. J Exp Orthop. 2015;2(1):7.
76. Helito CP, Bonadio MB, Rozas JS, et al. Biomechanical study of strength and stiffness of the knee anterolateral ligament. BMC Musculoskelet Disord. 2016;17:193.
77. Wytrykowski K, Swider P, Reina N, et al. Cadaveric study comparing the biomechanical properties of grafts used for knee anterolateral ligament reconstruction. Arthroscopy. 2016;32(11):2288–94.
78. Kernkamp WA, van de Velde SK, Bakker EW, van Arkel ER. Anterolateral extra-articular soft tissue reconstruction in anterolateral rotatory instability of the knee. Arthrosc Tech. 2015;4(6):e863–7.
79. Fetto JF, Marshall JL. The natural history and diagnosis of anterior cruciate ligament insufficiency. Clin Orthop Relat Res. 1980;147:29–38.
80. Fox JM, Blazina ME, Del Pizzo W, Ivey FM, Broukhim B. Extra-articular stabilization of the knee joint for anterior instability. Clin Orthop Relat Res. 1980;147:56–61.
81. Ellison AE. Distal iliotibial-band transfer for anterolateral rotatory instability of the knee. J Bone Joint Surg Am. 1979;61(3):330–7.
82. Sonnery-Cottet B, Thaunat M, Freychet B, Pupim BH, Murphy CG, Claes S. Outcome of a combined anterior cruciate ligament and anterolateral ligament reconstruction technique with a minimum 2-year follow-up. Am J Sports Med. 2015;43(7):1598–605.
83. Rosenstiel N, Praz C, Ouanezar H, et al. Combined anterior cruciate and anterolateral ligament reconstruction in the professional athlete: clinical outcomes from the scientific anterior cruciate ligament network international study group in a series of 70 patients with a minimum follow-up of 2 years. Arthroscopy. 2019;35(3):885–92.
84. Ibrahim SA, Shohdy EM, Marwan Y, et al. Anatomic reconstruction of the anterior cruciate ligament of the knee with or without reconstruction of the anterolateral ligament: a randomized clinical trial. Am J Sports Med. 2017;45(7):1558–66.
85. Lee DW, Kim JG, Cho SI, Kim DH. Clinical outcomes of isolated revision anterior cruciate ligament reconstruction or in combination with anatomic anterolateral ligament reconstruction. Am J Sports Med. 2019;47(2):324–33.
86. Smith PA, Thomas DM, Pomajzl RJ, Bley JA, Pfeiffer FM, Cook JL. A biomechanical study of the role of the anterolateral ligament and the deep iliotibial band for control of a simulated pivot shift with comparison of minimally invasive extra-articular anterolateral tendon graft reconstruction versus modified Lemaire reconstruction after anterior cruciate ligament reconstruction. Arthroscopy. 2019;35(5):1473–83.

17 Management of the Medial Meniscus-Deficient Knee with Revision Anterior Cruciate Ligament Reconstruction

Bogdan A. Matache, Eoghan T. Hurley, Amit K. Manjunath, and Eric J. Strauss

Introduction

The medial meniscus and meniscotibial ligaments provide both static and dynamic stabilizations to the medial side of the knee. Medial meniscal deficiency can be a source of pain and can contribute to rotational instability of the knee, as well as increase the amount of anterior tibial translation [1–3]. In the setting of a revision anterior cruciate ligament reconstruction (ACLR), meniscal deficiency may predispose the patient to an increased risk of failure. Musahl et al. [2] found, in a cadaveric study, that resection of the medial meniscus in ACL-deficient knees produced increased anterior tibial translation on Lachman testing as compared to the meniscus-intact state. Additionally, there is a linear relationship between the volume of meniscus removed and the tibiofemoral contact stresses, with total meniscectomy having been shown to increase peak contact stresses by 235% [4–8]. As a result, patients who undergo isolated ACLR in the setting of medial meniscal deficiency have been shown to exhibit poor long-term outcomes and an increased risk of osteoarthritis [9, 10]. Thus, the medial meniscal deficiency is often addressed with either a meniscal allograft transplantation (MAT) or high tibial osteotomy (HTO), depending on the status of the articular cartilage and overall mechanical alignment.

This chapter will review the decision-making process involved in the management of failed ACL reconstruction with medial meniscal deficiency, as well the surgical techniques for revision surgery and clinical outcomes.

B. A. Matache · E. T. Hurley (✉) · A. K. Manjunath
E. J. Strauss
New York University Langone Health, Department of Orthopedic Surgery, New York, NY, USA

Indications and Contraindications

Indications

In general, medial MAT is performed in the setting of revision ACLR in young patients with symptomatic medial meniscal deficiency (instability, pain, swelling or a combination) and minimal medial compartment arthritic changes (Outerbridge Grade 0–2) [11]. Deficiencies in these patients are typically the result of recurrent meniscal tear, failed repair, or a previous subtotal or total meniscectomy. In this patient population, MAT is indicated to both improve symptoms related to the meniscal deficiency and reduce the risk of graft re-rupture after revision ACL reconstruction by restoring more normal knee biomechanics.

An HTO is performed in the setting of revision ACLR in patients with varus malalignment, excessive posterior tibial slope, and/or significant medial compartment osteoarthritic changes (Outerbridge grade ≥3 or Fairbank's changes on

M. J. Alaia, K. J. Jones (eds.), *Revision Anterior Cruciate Ligament Reconstruction*,
https://doi.org/10.1007/978-3-030-96996-7_17

plain radiographs) [12]. Varus malalignment increases the forces across the ACL, thereby placing patients at risk for re-tear, while excessive posterior tibial slope, often defined as being greater than 12°, causes excessive anterior tibial translation and supraphysiologic stresses on the reconstructed ACL. Both of these factors constitute an increased risk of re-rupture after revision ACL reconstruction [13].

Contraindications

Contraindications for medial MAT in the setting of revision ACL reconstruction include age greater than 50 years, advanced medial compartment chondral osteoarthritis, uncorrectable varus malalignment, knee ROM ≤5–120°, inflammatory arthritis, synovial disease, and obesity [11]. Focal chondral lesions and malalignment that can be concomitantly corrected are not considered contraindications.

Contraindications for an HTO in the setting of revision ACL reconstruction include age greater than 65 years, neutral or valgus alignment, open physes, significant lateral compartment or patellofemoral osteoarthritis, knee ROM ≤5–120°, poor soft tissue envelope, and heavy smoking [12]. Additionally, if the location of the planned osteotomy is at risk of breaching into the ACL tibial tunnel, the patient should be treated in two stages, with bone grafting of the tunnels performed during the first stage.

Patient Evaluation

Patient History and Clinical Evaluation

The evaluation and management of patients presenting with a failed ACLR begin with obtaining a thorough history and performing a comprehensive physical examination of the knee. A complete history includes a description of the mechanism and timeline of the injury, as well as details surrounding the prior interventions, including previous graft selection and status of the menisci and articular cartilage, while often non-specific, symptom quality and severity should be assessed to rule out possible concomitant pathologies such as meniscal and chondral injuries. These may present predominantly with symptoms of pain, catching or locking, and articular effusions rather than giving way of the knee. The patient's regular activities and goals should be discussed and understood in order to set appropriate physician and patient expectations prior to proposing further treatment.

Physical examination begins with an assessment of gait, with a particular focus on whether any varus thrust is present. Varus thrust in the setting of failed ACL reconstruction is suggestive of an associated injury to the lateral collateral ligament and posterolateral corner (especially in the context of a varus knee), which is an independent risk factor for re-rupture if left unaddressed at the time of revision surgery. While standing, a patient's overall lower extremity alignment and patellar position can be assessed. Next, with the patient supine on the examination table, the knee is inspected for previous incisions, which may provide insight on the procedures the patient previously underwent, and quadriceps atrophy. The knee is then assessed for the presence of intra-articular effusion, and the joint lines are palpated to elicit point tenderness suggestive of meniscal pathology. Knee range of motion (ROM) with observation of patellar tracking is then assessed, and special tests including the varus and valgus stress, Lachman, anterior and posterior drawer, pivot shift, dial, and McMurray tests are performed. Any abnormalities detected on any of these maneuvers should alert the clinician to perform additional complementary special testing as indicated.

Imaging Studies

Imaging modalities used in the work-up of a patient with a failed ACL reconstruction includes plain radiographs of the knee, lower extremity coronal and sagittal plane alignment films (Fig. 17.1), magnetic resonance imaging (MRI), and potentially computed tomography (CT). A

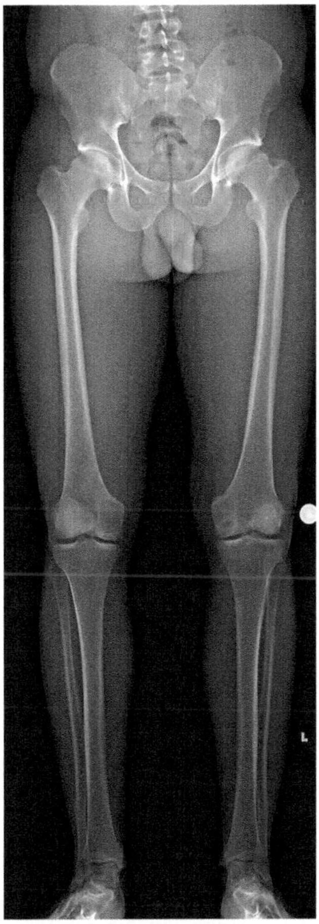

Fig. 17.1 Leg length alignment films

full set of weight-bearing radiographs (anterior-posterior [AP] view, lateral view, Merchant view, full-length weight-bearing AP and lateral, and Rosenberg view) is used for gross assessment of osteoarthritis and localization of previous bone tunnels. Full-length radiographs are useful in identifying any malalignment that may require a corrective osteotomy at the time of revision surgery. If injury to the posterior cruciate ligament (PCL) or collateral ligaments is suspected, stress views specific to each of these can be obtained. MRI is used to assess soft tissue structures, including the menisci, cruciates, collaterals, articular cartilage, and status of the subchondral bone. MRI can also be used to assess tunnel position and measure tunnel width in patients whom CT may be contraindicated. Prior bone tunnels are best assessed using CT, but these benefits must be weighed against the risks associated with radiation exposure secondary to its usage.

Surgical Technique

Medial MAT and Revision ACL Reconstruction

Graft Selection

The most commonly utilized type of meniscus graft for allograft transplantation is non-irradiated, fresh frozen allograft. This method of graft preparation allows for a more prolonged surgical window as compared to fresh grafts while reducing the risk of disease transmission. After harvesting, these grafts are stored at −80 °C for up to 5 years [14]. Sizing is a critical aspect of MAT, as oversizing results in increased tibio-femoral contact stresses, while under-sizing increases the forces borne by the meniscal graft and subjects the graft to a risk of tearing and failure.

The most commonly utilized method for medial meniscal graft sizing is the Pollard method, which utilizes the AP radiograph to determine medial meniscus width by measuring the distance between two parallel vertical lines extending from the medial proximal tibial metaphysis and the medial tibial eminence [15]. Medial meniscal length is then obtained by measuring the distance between two parallel vertical lines extending from the anterior proximal tibial metaphysis and the posterior tibia at the level of the joint line on the lateral X-ray. Each of these measurements is then multiplied by a correction factor of 80% [15]. Additionally, newer three-dimensional sizing methods utilizing MRI are often preferred by tissue banks, as these may improve the accuracy of graft sizing as compared to conventional radiography [16].

The choice of graft used in revision ACL reconstruction is individualized for each patient based on their age, prior graft usage, and patient preference [17]. Generally speaking, autograft is preferred in the setting of a failed previous ACL reconstruction due to its reduced risk of re-rupture as compared to allograft [17–19].

Alternatively, allograft is a reasonable choice if the patient is older and lower demand and has few remaining autograft options or if a concomitant extra-articular augmentation procedure is planned. In addition, allograft is the preferred graft source when tunnel widening is present and the revision procedure is to be performed as a single stage. Graft selection in revision ACL reconstruction is discussed in greater detail in Chap. 5.

Graft Preparation

Historically, the meniscal allograft was stabilized using a soft tissue fixation technique after introduction into the joint. However, this is no longer recommended as studies have demonstrated that without any form of bony fixation, the load transmission profile of the knee after MAT approximates that of the meniscus-deficient knee, thereby eliminating the biomechanical advantage conferred to the knee after transplantation [20]. Therefore, current techniques rely on bony fixation of the anterior and posterior horns, which can be achieved either using the bone plug or bridge-in-slot technique.

The double bone plug technique (Fig. 17.2) is the most commonly utilized technique for medial MAT and will be the focus of this technical description. While the bridge-in-slot technique (Fig. 17.3) has been shown to yield similar biomechanical results as the bone plug technique, it requires partial resection of the ACL tibial footprint when used for medial MAT and is therefore mostly indicated for lateral MAT [21]. The double bone plug technique involves reverse-reaming two sockets into the medial tibial plateau at the locations of the anterior and posterior horns of the medial meniscus and in setting the graft bone plugs into these tunnels.

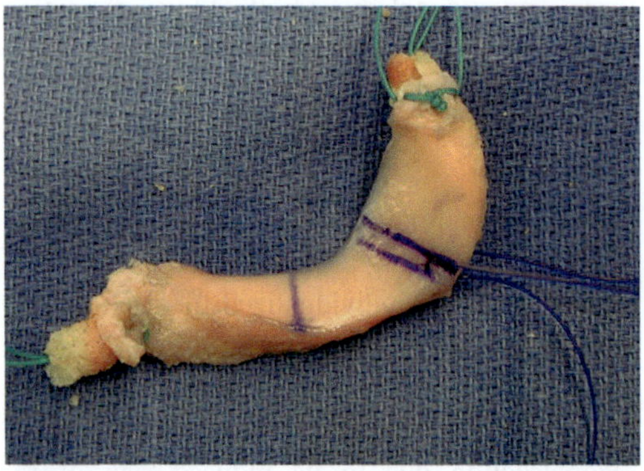

Fig. 17.2 Bone plug MAT

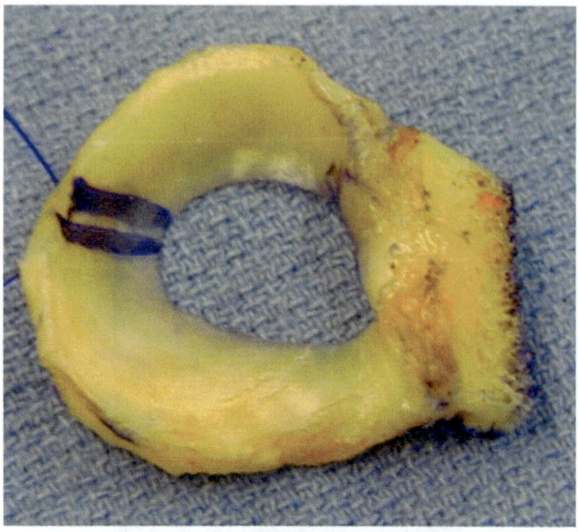

Fig. 17.3 Bridge-in-slot MAT

Preparation of the medial meniscus allograft for the bone plug technique of medial MAT begins with first excising any synovial attachments to the meniscus, followed by identifying the posterior root attachment and marking its center with a marking pen. Next, a 1.1 mm K-wire is drilled through the mark and out the inferior aspect of the graft at an angle that approximates the socket to be reamed into the tibia. A 2.4 mm cannulated drill is then loaded over the wire and drilled in a retrograde fashion toward the posterior root attachment, with care taken to exit the meniscus by hand so as to avoid wrapping and damaging the tissue. Next, a 9 mm coring reamer is loaded over the cannulated drill and also reamed in a retrograde manner, once again finishing the process by hand. A 15-blade scalpel is then used to cut around the coring reamer and remove any excess tissue while preserving the posterior root attachment to the tibial bone plug. The posterior bone plug is then freed from the reamer, the cannulated drill is removed, and the bone plug is cut to the depth of 8 mm with a small microsagittal saw. Finally, a No. 2 FiberLoop suture (Arthrex, Naples, FL) is looped around the posterior root and passed through the drill hole in the bone plug in an antegrade fashion. The same process is then repeated for preparation of the anterior root bone plug. The junction of the posterior horn and meniscal body is then marked with a marking pen, and a No. 2 PDS suture is passed through the meniscus at this location in a vertical mattress configuration. This suture will aid with reduction of the meniscus allograft. After preparation, the allograft is wrapped in wet gauze and placed in a basin until it is ready for implantation.

Patient Positioning

With the patient supine on the table, a tourniquet is applied high on the thigh, and the operative leg is placed in a circumferential leg holder. The distal bracket of the bed is lowered, allowing for easy maneuverability of the leg during surgery and unobstructed access to the posteromedial aspect of the knee for inside-out allograft repair. A folded blanket is placed under the proximal thigh of the contralateral leg to bring the hip into slight flexion and prevent any tension on the femoral nerve. The operative leg is then prepped and draped in the usual sterile fashion, and appropriate anatomic landmarks are marked, including the site of the posteromedial incision.

Diagnostic Arthroscopy and Meniscal Debridement

Using standard anterolateral and anteromedial portal sites, a diagnostic arthroscopy is performed. A spinal needle is used for creation of a low and lateral anteromedial portal that is 1–2 mm inferior and lateral to a standard anteromedial portal. Positioning the anteromedial portal as such allows for improved access to the medial compartment. The meniscal deficiency is confirmed (Fig. 17.4), and the condition of the articular cartilage is assessed before proceeding. In cases where a subtotal meniscectomy was previously performed, an arthroscopic biter and 4.5 mm shaver are used to debride the native meniscus, aiming to preserve a 1–2 mm peripheral rim to provide enhanced stability for allograft fixation. In cases where a total meniscectomy

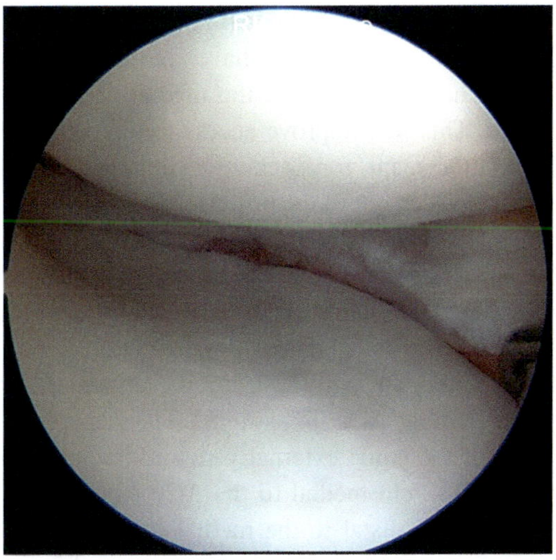

Fig. 17.4 Medial meniscus insufficiency

was previously performed, an arthroscopic rasp is used to abrade the capsule until a bleeding bed is created to encourage healing of the allograft to the capsule. We routinely release the MCL at the level of the proximal tibia, joint line, or distal femur using a pie-crusting technique, as this allows for excellent access and minimizes risk of iatrogenic chondral injury with no morbidity to the patient.

ACL Tunnel Preparation

The prior ACL graft and tunnels are debrided, and the revision femoral tunnel is drilled over a Beath pin through the standard anteromedial portal. A high-strength suture is then looped and passed into the femoral tunnel using the Beath pin. The loop is then retrieved out the anterolateral portal and clamped to its tails that are exiting percutaneously out the lateral thigh. This avoids suture crowding on the medial side of the knee. The tibial tunnel is then exposed with a 4–5-cm-long anteromedial incision and drilled. The incision should be long enough to allow for easy retraction of the medial soft tissue flap for creation of the two tibial sockets for allograft implantation. An appropriately sized portal plug is then inserted into the external aperture of the tibial ACL tunnel to maintain intra-articular fluid pressure.

Tibial Socket Preparation

A 5.5 mm bone cutting shaver is then used to resect the medial half of the medial tibial eminence. This will improve access to the posterior root attachment for socket drilling and avoid medial placement of the posterior socket. A tibial PCL FlipCutter guide (Arthrex, Naples, FL) is then inserted through the anteromedial portal and positioned internally on the location of the posterior root attachment and externally on the anteromedial tibia through the same incision used for creation of the ACL tibial tunnel. The ideal placement of the guide externally should be approximately 1–2 cm medial to the ACL tibial tunnel and 5–6 cm distal to the medial joint line. The posterior socket is then created using an 8.5 mm FlipCutter (Arthrex, Naples, FL) to a depth of 12–15 mm. A FiberStick (Arthrex, Naples, FL) is inserted into the posterior socket, and the suture loop is retrieved out the anteromedial portal.

The anterior tibial socket can then either be created in a similar fashion or under direct visualization using an outside-in technique, through the arthrotomy. If a retrograde tunnel technique is used, one must ensure that the two drill tunnels don't converge and that there is a sufficient bone bridge between it and the ACL tibial tunnel. This is made possible by placing the tibial guide 2 cm proximal and 1 cm medial to the location of the posterior socket drill tunnel on the anteromedial tibia. A crab claw instrument is then passed over both suture loops into the medial compartment through the anteromedial portal they are both exiting, ensuring absence of a suture bridge, and the sutures are clamped externally. If an outside-in technique is utilized, the anterior tibial socket is created after securing the posterior meniscal plug attachment.

Posteromedial Approach

A standard limited posteromedial approach to the knee is utilized for safe passage of inside-out sutures for repair of the MAT. The medial epicondyle is palpated, and the course of the medial collateral ligament (MCL) is drawn. The incision extends from 1–2 cm proximal to the medial tibiofemoral joint line to 2–3 cm distal to it, placed 0.5–1 cm posterior to the MCL. Sharp dissection is carried down to fascia, at which point the interval between the medial head of gastrocnemius and semimembranosus is exploited to the level of the posterior capsule of the knee. Flexion and extension of the foot can assist with identification of the medial head of gastrocnemius. The exposure is adequate when a sterile spoon can easily be inserted in the interval.

Meniscal Allograft Introduction and Repair

Before introducing the graft into the knee, the anteromedial portal is extended into a mini-open arthrotomy large enough to permit passage of the graft. A zone-specific cannula is then placed into the anteromedial portal, and a meniscal repair needle is passed through the meniscal remnant at the junction of the body and posterior horn. The needle is then retrieved through the posteromedial incision under direct visualization. The prevailing needle is removed, and the suture is tied into a loop and used to shuttle the graft passage sutures from the allograft through the posteromedial incision. The FiberLoop suture around the posterior bone plug is then passed into the suture loop exiting the posterior tibial socket and shuttled out the corresponding tibial tunnel.

Gentle traction is first maintained on posterior bone plug sutures, while the allograft is passed through the arthrotomy and then on the graft passage sutures until it is docked into the recipient socket. Once seated posteriorly, this process is repeated for the anterior bone plug. The knee can be cycled to aid with proper seating of the meniscus in the knee.

With the allograft in position, the meniscus is secured peripherally with 2–0 nonabsorbable sutures using an inside-out vertical mattress repair technique. Suture placement alternates between the superior and inferior aspects of the meniscal body for a balanced repair. The repair progresses anteriorly from the level of the graft passage sutures, and the sutures are retrieved through the posteromedial incision. All corresponding sutures are clamped but not tied with each successive pass. This protects the meniscal allograft by allowing for greater mobility to translate with femoral rollback during the ACL

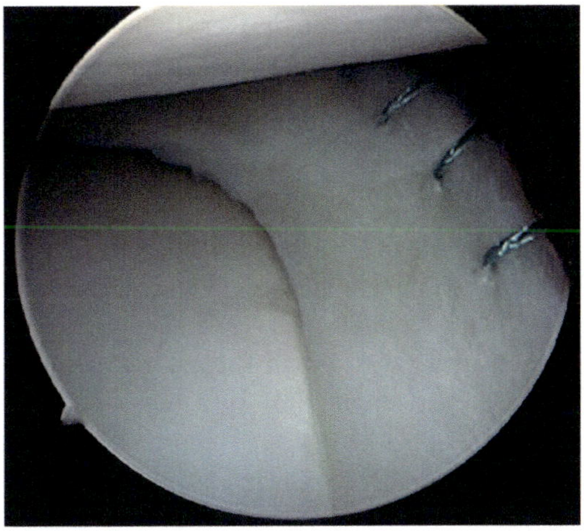

Fig. 17.5 MAT after implantation

reconstruction portion of the procedure. An all-inside technique is then used for fixation of the posterior horn (Fig. 17.5).

ACL Graft Passage and Fixation

Once the medial meniscal allograft is properly situated and all repair sutures are passed, the ACL graft can be introduced into the knee and fixated.

Meniscal Allograft Fixation

The final step of the procedure consists of securely fixating the meniscal allograft. The knee is placed in full extension, and all corresponding meniscal repair sutures from the previous step are tied under direct visualization with the arthroscope in the anterolateral portal. Once this is done, fixation of the anterior and posterior bone plugs is achieved by loading their corresponding sutures into a knotless anchor that is drilled and inserted into the anterior tibia distal to the bone tunnels. Alternatively, a suture button technique also provides secure fixation. The graft is then probed to confirm adequate stabilization.

Key Steps

1. ACL femoral tunnel preparation (anteromedial portal drilling technique)
2. ACL tibial tunnel preparation (outside-in drilling technique)
3. Posterior meniscus root tunnel preparation (retrograde drilling technique)
4. Posteromedial approach
5. Graft passage and docking (not yet fixed)
6. Meniscal repair (inside-out technique with sutures left untied)
7. ACL graft passage and fixation
8. Meniscal fixation

Closure

The posteromedial approach and anteromedial arthrotomy are irrigated and closed in layers. The portals are closed in a subcuticular manner, skin adhesive is applied to the incisions, and sterile dressings are applied. A hinged knee brace is then locked in extension and applied.

HTO and Revision ACL Reconstruction

When correction of varus malalignment is required in the setting of revision ACL reconstruction, there are a number of important technical factors to consider. The location of the previous tibial tunnel requires careful assessment to determine whether the revision procedure is conducive to a single stage or not. For example, a long, vertical tunnel will likely be in the way of the location of the tibial osteotomy. If a new, more horizontal, independent revision tibial tunnel can be drilled proximal to the location of the planned osteotomy, then it may be feasible to proceed in a single stage. Similarly, if the previous tibial tunnel is very horizontal, then it may be possible to avoid it altogether and perform the osteotomy distal to it. However, a properly placed and widened tibial tunnel will likely be in the way of the site of the planned osteotomy. It also carries a high risk of fracture propagation into the tibial plateau during opening of the medial wedge if the decision is made to traverse it with the osteotomy. Such cases may require a two-staged procedure, with preparation and bone grafting of the tunnels during the first stage, followed by HTO and revision ACL reconstruction during the second.

A detailed technical description of coronal plane correction in the setting of revision ACL reconstruction can be found in Chap. 15.

Postoperative Rehabilitation

To date, there is no well-established postoperative rehabilitation protocol that has been shown to provide superior outcomes compared to other protocols, with wide variation reported between studies [22].

Weight-Bearing

Both MAT and HTO resulted in prolonged rehabilitation following revision ACL. The patients are initially kept partially weight-bearing for 2 weeks, followed by 2–4 weeks of progressive weight-bearing to allow full weight-bearing with crutches at 4–6 weeks, after which full weight-bearing without crutches is allowed, pending normal gait cycle.

Bracing

Following MAT and HTO, patients are kept in a knee brace locked in extension for the first 2 weeks at all times, followed by locking in extension for 2 weeks for ambulation. Then at 4 weeks, the brace is opened to 90 for a further 2 weeks for ambulation, after which the brace is discontinued if the patient is capable of performing a straight leg raise without extensor lag.

Range of Motion

The goal is to achieve 90 deg by 4 weeks, and 120 deg by 6 weeks, and full range of motion by 8 weeks.

Return to Activity

Jogging and sport-specific exercises are allowed at 6 months, followed by running and agility exercises.

Outcomes

High Tibial Osteotomy

There is currently limited literature on the outcomes following concomitant revision ACLR and HTO. Gupta et al. [12] performed a systematic review on combined revision ACLR and HTO, with 7 studies and 77 patients included. Overall, there was a high success rate with no failures reported, and 88% of patients exhibit a negative pivot-shift test postoperatively. Additionally, there was a significant reduction in the posterior tibial slope – mean reduction of 7° among patients with a preoperative slope of greater than 12° – thus reducing the strain placed on the reconstructed ACL graft. The only revision reported in the included studies was a patient with stiffness requiring arthrolysis. There was a paucity of data on return to play, with 6/7 athletes playing sports pre-injury being able to return to play. This review found radiographic signs of osteoarthritis preoperatively in 51.6% and postoperatively in 58.3% of the 60 patients examined for osteoarthritis, which is lower than the mean rate of osteoarthritis following revision ACLR reported in literature (80.7%) [23]. However, surgeons should consider the possible associated difficulties with performing a future total knee replacement in patients who have an HTO implant in place when weighing the risks and benefits of the initial procedure [24, 25].

Meniscal Allograft Transplantation

Similar to performing a concomitant HTO in the setting of revision ACL reconstruction, there is limited literature on the outcomes following concomitant revision ACLR and MAT. Zaffagnini et al. [26] evaluated 18 patients undergoing combined revision ACL reconstruction and MAT, at a mean of 4 years follow-up. They found a significant reduction in pain, improvement in functional outcome scores, and a high satisfaction rate. Overall, 13 patients were able to return to play, with only 1 of those unable to return to play being due to residual symptoms. However, four patients required further surgery, including two graft failures and two with persistent pain, one of whom required an HTO.

Case Study

A 33-year-old male presented complaining of right knee instability and pain. He had a history of ACL reconstruction using allograft back 3 years prior. He noted he has had multiple buckling episodes with lateral movement, with the first one being a noticeable trauma while dancing 3 months after his initial procedure. He reports intermittent swelling in his knee with buckling episodes, and he denies mechanical symptoms. On examination, he had full range of motion with mild symmetric varus and 2B Lachman with a positive pivot shift. He was non-tender at the joint lines and had a negative McMurray test. An X-ray with alignment films, a CT, and an MRI were performed. Firstly, the X-ray showed minimal arthritic change, and alignment films showed minimal bilateral symmetrical varus deformity with the weight-bearing line falling just medial to the medial spine (Fig. 17.6). The CT scan showed acceptable prior tunnel position, without significant bone tunnel widening. The MRI demonstrated a full-thickness ACL tear and a deficient medial meniscus with some joint space narrowing in the medial compartment, without gross osteochondral lesions (Fig. 17.7).

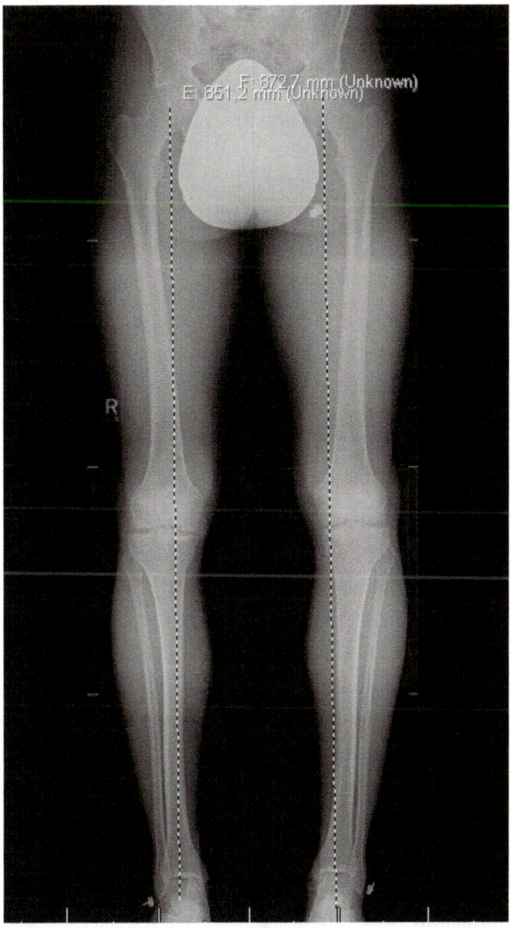

Fig. 17.6 Case study alignment films

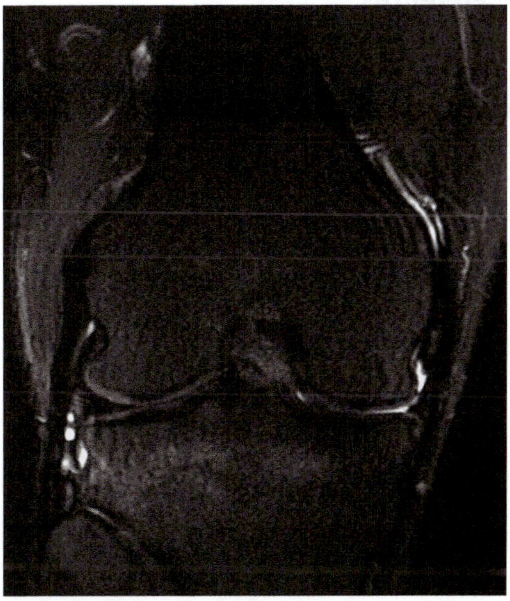

Fig. 17.7 Case study MRI

As this patient had a failed ACL reconstruction in slight varus with good bone tunnels and medial meniscal deficiency, a long discussion was about risks, benefits, and alternatives of revising the ACL ± MAT or HTO. We agreed that although he may have a slightly higher failure rate and without an osteotomy his varus is relatively symmetric, a MAT may be a better alternative as it addresses his medial meniscal deficiency, and he would likely have a successful outcome given the minimal arthritic change in the joint. Additionally, it was determined that a bone-patellar tendon-bone autograft for the ACL reconstruction revision should be utilized due to his relatively young age and having failed a prior autograft. His MRI was sent for matching with the tissue bank, and he ultimately underwent surgery 6 weeks later. At final follow-up, the patient is doing well and has resumed all of his activities of daily living.

Conclusion

Revision anterior cruciate ligament reconstruction in the setting of medial meniscal deficiency is a challenging problem for the practicing sports medicine surgeon. Options to manage this include medial meniscal allograft transplantation or valgus-producing high tibial osteotomy, depending on the patient's age, activities, overall kinematic alignment, and status of the articular surfaces. In general, meniscal allograft transplantation is performed in the setting of revision anterior cruciate ligament reconstruction in patients with symptomatic medial meniscal deficiency, neutral or correctable alignment, and intact articular surfaces. In contrast, valgus-producing high tibial osteotomy is performed in patients with varus malalignment, medial compartment osteoarthritis, or excessive posterior tibial slope to reduce the risk of re-rupture and improve symptoms and function.

References

1. Nishida K, Matsushita T, Hoshino Y, Araki D, Matsumoto T, Niikura T, et al. The influences of chronicity and meniscal injuries on pivot shift in anterior cruciate ligament-deficient knees: quantitative evaluation using an electromagnetic measurement system. Arthroscopy. 2020;36(5):1398–406. Epub 2020/02/01.
2. Musahl V, Rahnemai-Azar AA, Costello J, Arner JW, Fu FH, Hoshino Y, et al. The influence of meniscal and anterolateral capsular injury on knee laxity in patients with anterior cruciate ligament injuries. Am J Sports Med. 2016;44(12):3126–31. Epub 2016/08/11.
3. Arner JW, Irvine JN, Zheng L, Gale T, Thorhauer E, Hankins M, et al. The effects of anterior cruciate ligament deficiency on the meniscus and articular cartilage: a novel dynamic in vitro pilot study. Orthop J Sports Med. 2016;4(4):2325967116639895. Epub 2016/04/23.
4. Lee SJ, Aadalen KJ, Malaviya P, Lorenz EP, Hayden JK, Farr J, et al. Tibiofemoral contact mechanics after serial medial meniscectomies in the human cadaveric knee. Am J Sports Med. 2006;34(8):1334–44. Epub 2006/04/26.
5. Verma NN, Kolb E, Cole BJ, Berkson MB, Garretson R, Farr J, et al. The effects of medial meniscal transplantation techniques on intra-articular contact pressures. J Knee Surg. 2008;21(1):20–6. Epub 2008/02/28.
6. McDermott ID, Amis AA. The consequences of meniscectomy. J Bone Joint Surg. 2006;88(12):1549–56. Epub 2006/12/13.
7. Bai B, Shun H, Yin ZX, Liao ZW, Chen N. Changes of contact pressure and area in patellofemoral joint after different meniscectomies. Int Orthop. 2012;36(5):987–91. Epub 2012/01/05.
8. Baratz ME, Fu FH, Mengato R. Meniscal tears: the effect of meniscectomy and of repair on intraarticular contact areas and stress in the human knee. A preliminary report. Am J Sports Med. 1986;14(4):270–5. Epub 1986/07/01.
9. Oiestad BE, Holm I, Aune AK, Gunderson R, Myklebust G, Engebretsen L, et al. Knee function and prevalence of knee osteoarthritis after anterior cruciate ligament reconstruction: a prospective study with 10 to 15 years of follow-up. Am J Sports Med. 2010;38(11):2201–10. Epub 2010/08/18.
10. Costa-Paz M, Garcia-Mansilla I, Marciano S, Ayerza MA, Muscolo DL. Knee-related quality of life, functional results and osteoarthritis at a minimum of 20years' follow-up after anterior cruciate ligament reconstruction. Knee. 2019;26(3):666–72. Epub 2019/05/20.
11. Gilat R, Cole BJ. Meniscal allograft transplantation: indications, techniques, outcomes. Arthroscopy. 2020;36(4):938–9. Epub 2020/02/02
12. Gupta A, Tejpal T, Shanmugaraj A, Horner NS, Simunovic N, Duong A, et al. Surgical techniques, outcomes, indications, and complications of simultaneous high tibial osteotomy and anterior cruciate ligament revision surgery: a systematic review. HSS J. 2019;15(2):176–84. Epub 2019/07/23.
13. van de Pol GJ, Arnold MP, Verdonschot N, van Kampen A. Varus alignment leads to increased forces in the anterior cruciate ligament. Am J Sports Med. 2009;37(3):481–7. Epub 2008/12/18.
14. Mickiewicz P, Binkowski M, Bursig H, Wróbel Z. Preservation and sterilization methods of the meniscal allografts: literature review. Cell Tissue Bank. 2014;15(3):307–17. Epub 2013/09/04.
15. Pollard ME, Kang Q, Berg EE. Radiographic sizing for meniscal transplantation. Arthroscopy. 1995;11(6):684–7. Epub 1995/12/01.
16. Beeler S, Jud L, von Atzigen M, Sutter R, Fürnstahl P, Fucentese SF, et al. Three-dimensional meniscus allograft sizing-a study of 280 healthy menisci. J Orthop Surg Res. 2020;15(1):74. Epub 2020/02/26.
17. Rahardja R, Zhu M, Love H, Clatworthy MG, Monk AP, Young SW. Factors associated with revision

following anterior cruciate ligament reconstruction: a systematic review of registry data. Knee. 2020;27(2):287–99. Epub 2020/02/06.
18. Wang S, Zhang C, Cai Y, Lin X. Autograft or allograft? Irradiated or not? A contrast between autograft and allograft in anterior cruciate ligament reconstruction: a meta-analysis. Arthroscopy. 2018;34(12):3258–65. Epub 2018/11/07.
19. Mohan R, Webster KE, Johnson NR, Stuart MJ, Hewett TE, Krych AJ. Clinical outcomes in revision anterior cruciate ligament reconstruction: a meta-analysis. Arthroscopy. 2018;34(1):289–300. Epub 2017/09/04.
20. Ambra LF, Mestriner AB, Ackermann J, Phan AT, Farr J, Gomoll AH. Bone-plug versus soft tissue fixation of medial meniscal allograft transplants: a biomechanical study. Am J Sports Med. 2019;47(12):2960–5. Epub 2019/08/28.
21. Brial C, McCarthy M, Adebayo O, Wang H, Chen T, Warren R, et al. Lateral meniscal graft transplantation: effect of fixation method on joint contact mechanics during simulated gait. Am J Sports Med. 2019;47(10):2437–43. Epub 2019/07/18.
22. Hurley ET, Davey MS, Jamal MS, Manjunath AK, Kingery MT, Alaia MJ, et al. High rate of return-to-play following meniscal allograft transplantation. Knee Surg Sports Traumatol Arthrosc. 2020. Epub 2020/04/10.
23. Diamantopoulos AP, Lorbach O, Paessler HH. Anterior cruciate ligament revision reconstruction: results in 107 patients. Am J Sports Med. 2008;36(5):851–60. Epub 2008/02/15.
24. Parvizi J, Hanssen AD, Spangehl MJ. Total knee arthroplasty following proximal tibial osteotomy: risk factors for failure. J Bone Joint Surg Am. 2004;86(3):474–9. Epub 2004/03/05.
25. Haslam P, Armstrong M, Geutjens G, Wilton TJ. Total knee arthroplasty after failed high tibial osteotomy long-term follow-up of matched groups. J Arthroplast. 2007;22(2):245–50. Epub 2007/02/06.
26. Zaffagnini S, Grassi A, Romandini I, Marcacci M, Filardo G. Meniscal allograft transplantation combined with anterior cruciate ligament reconstruction provides good mid-term clinical outcome. Knee Surg Sports Traumatol Arthrosc. 2019;27(6):1914–23. Epub 2018/08/08.

Management of Lateral Meniscus Deficiency in Revision ACL Reconstruction

18

Trevor Gulbrandsen, Olivia O'Reilly, Ian Gao, and Seth L. Sherman

Introduction

Menisci in the tibiofemoral joint are essential, providing pivotal roles in knee stability and joint health including load transmission, stabilization, shock absorption, joint lubrication, and articular cartilage nutrition [1–3]. The two tibiofemoral menisci are biomechanically and anatomically unique with specific functions. While the medial tibial plateau is concave, the lateral tibial plateau is convex with the meniscus covering 80–85% of the surface and bearing up to 70% of the compartment axial load [1, 4, 5]. Complete meniscal deficiency in the form of total meniscectomy significantly decreases tibiofemoral contact area leading to 2–3× the contact force transmitted [4, 6]. The femur is also convex, creating complex kinematics and driving the unique "posterior roll-back" motion on the lateral side [7] (Fig. 18.1). These dynamic biomechanics lead to greater risk of chondral degeneration and collapse with earlier clinical symptoms when compared to medial compartment [8]. Therefore, lateral meniscus tears should be repaired when indicated, especially in young athletic patients. Lateral meniscus deficiency is often poorly tolerated with a higher prevalence of post-meniscectomy syndrome.

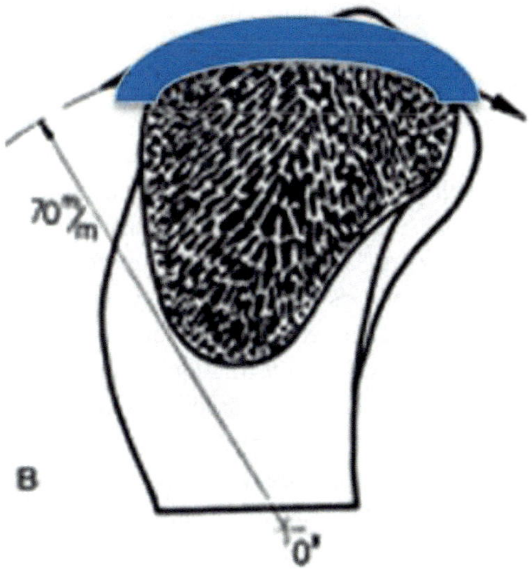

Fig. 18.1 The lateral tibial plateau is convex with the meniscus covering 80–85% of the surface and bearing up to 70% of the lateral compartment axial load

It is well known that the medial meniscus has a role in stability of the knee and acts as a secondary stabilizer to anterior-posterior displacement [9]. However, while previously believed to provide no secondary restraint, the lateral meniscus has recently been found to play a crucial role in the axial and rotatory stability of the knee [8, 10, 11]. It has been demonstrated that patients who

T. Gulbrandsen · O. O'Reilly
University of Iowa Hospitals and Clinics, Iowa City, IA, USA

I. Gao · S. L. Sherman (✉)
Department of Orthopaedic Surgery, Stanford University, Stanford, CA, USA

M. J. Alaia, K. J. Jones (eds.), *Revision Anterior Cruciate Ligament Reconstruction*,
https://doi.org/10.1007/978-3-030-96996-7_18

have undergone lateral meniscectomy experience decreased rotatory stability along with increased functional deterioration [12–14]. Lateral meniscal injuries including tears and posterior root avulsions are a common associated injury with anterior cruciate ligament (ACL) tears, occurring in up to 12–14% of cases [15–21]. This combined injury is more common with acute ACL tears and in active males who sustain a contact injury [11, 21, 22].

Although the meniscus should be preserved and repaired whenever possible, functional or subtotal meniscectomy is sometimes unavoidable. While providing symptomatic relief, lateral meniscal deficiency places the knee at greater risk for post-operative instability and is a significant risk factor for graft failure in ACL reconstruction [23–26]. Parkinson et al. reported meniscal deficiency as the most significant risk factor associated with graft failure after ACL reconstruction [24]. Robb et al. demonstrated similar results in 123 primary ACL reconstructions, reporting a 3.5 times increased risk of ACL graft failure in the presence of lateral meniscal deficiency [25]. In the setting of ACL reconstruction, meniscectomy (medial or lateral) is also associated with lower subjective outcome scores, significant activity limitations, and progressive radiographic abnormalities [26, 27]. Lateral meniscus deficiency contributes to the accelerated deterioration of the lateral compartment chondral surfaces, particularly in patients with valgus malalignment and/or ACL deficiency [8].

MAT has been demonstrated to be one of the few treatment options for meniscal deficient knees in young patients. There have been considerable advancements since the first meniscal transplantation in 1984 [28], with expansion of evidence-based indications and techniques contributing to improved long-term outcomes. The fundamental goal of the MAT procedure is to attempt to re-establish the biomechanical properties of the native meniscus in an attempt to reduce pain, restore knee function, improve patient quality of life, and possibly delay osteoarthritis [29–31].

Given the detrimental effect of lateral meniscal deficiency on knee stability, ACL reconstruction graft failure rates, patient-reported outcomes, and radiographic degeneration, we consider performing lateral meniscal allograft transplantation (MAT) (Fig. 18.2) in select patients with lateral meniscal deficiency undergoing revision ACL reconstruction [8, 29–31]. Patient education is critical to successful revision surgery. Careful preoperative planning, meticulous surgical technique, and a stepwise and progressive rehabilitation plan are required to increase the chance of a successful outcome.

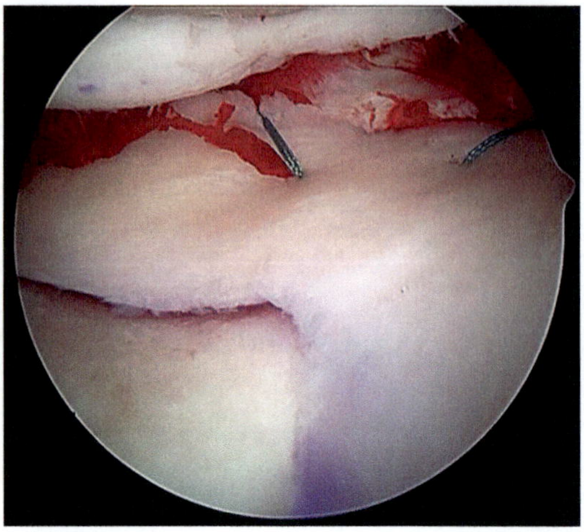

Fig. 18.2 Intraoperative photograph depicting a lateral meniscus allograft transplant (MAT)

Revision ACL Reconstruction: Preoperative Workup

The surgeon must perform a thorough and comprehensive evaluation including history, physical examination, and imaging studies. History should elucidate the reason for primary ACL graft failure. Lateral meniscus deficiency can be suspected from information found in previous operative report(s) or surgical pictures including prior meniscectomy or attempted lateral meniscus repair. This will be confirmed by imaging studies (i.e., MRI) and/or staging arthroscopy. Other causes of ACL failure must be systematically categorized (i.e., patient demographics, activity level, traumatic vs. insidious failure, suspicion for infection, prior graft choice, tunnel position, bony alignment, missed posterolateral or posteromedial corner injury). Localizing lateral pain, swelling, or mechanical symptoms may provide clues toward symptomatic lateral meniscal deficiency. Patient goals and expectations must be determined (i.e., occupation, recreation, level of competition).

Physical exam in patients with failed ACL and lateral meniscus deficiency may demonstrate an explosive grade III pivot shift. While the medial meniscus functions as a critical secondary stabilizer to anterior translation of the tibia during a Lachman maneuver, the lateral meniscus has been shown to be an important restraint to anterior tibial translation during combined valgus and rotatory loads applied during the pivot shift [8, 26, 32]. Multiple cadaveric studies have shown increased anterior tibial translation and tibial internal rotation with deficiency of the lateral meniscal root and meniscofemoral ligaments [33, 34]. Lateral joint line tenderness and effusion may also be present in patients with lateral meniscus deficiency and lateral chondral defects.

Standard imaging for revision ACL surgery includes comparison weightbearing AP, PA flexion, lateral, Merchant, mechanical axis radiographs as well as magnetic resonance imaging (MRI). Additionally, computed tomography (CT) imaging with 2D and 3D reconstructions allows the surgeon to precisely evaluate ACL tunnel position and tunnel widening and to measure tibial slope.

The above information is utilized to create a problem list for revision ACL surgery. If this list includes tunnel widening requiring bone grafting, malalignment requiring osteotomy, suspicion for meniscus deficiency, and/or focal chondral defect requiring cartilage restoration, a two-stage approach is reasonable. The first stage includes examination under anesthesia with direct comparison to the non-operative limb. Arthroscopy will confirm meniscus deficiency and will determine the exact size, depth, and location of any concomitant cartilage lesions. The surgeon may consider cartilage biopsy for future autologous-cultured chondrocytes (MACI®) or measure any defects for future osteochondral allograft. Unstable flaps of meniscus or cartilage are debrided, synovectomy performed, tunnels are inspected and bone grafted as needed, and realignment osteotomy performed if indicated. Second stage should include all definitive intra-articular procedures including revision ACL reconstruction, lateral meniscus transplantation, and cartilage restoration as indicated (Fig. 18.3).

Autograft ACL graft should be utilized when available. In 2014, a Multicenter ACL Revision Study (MARS) compared the outcomes of ACL graft choice at 2 years following revision ACL reconstruction [35]. This large cohort study demonstrated increased sports function and Patient Reported Outcomes (PRO) as well as decreased incidence of graft re-rupture when an autograft is

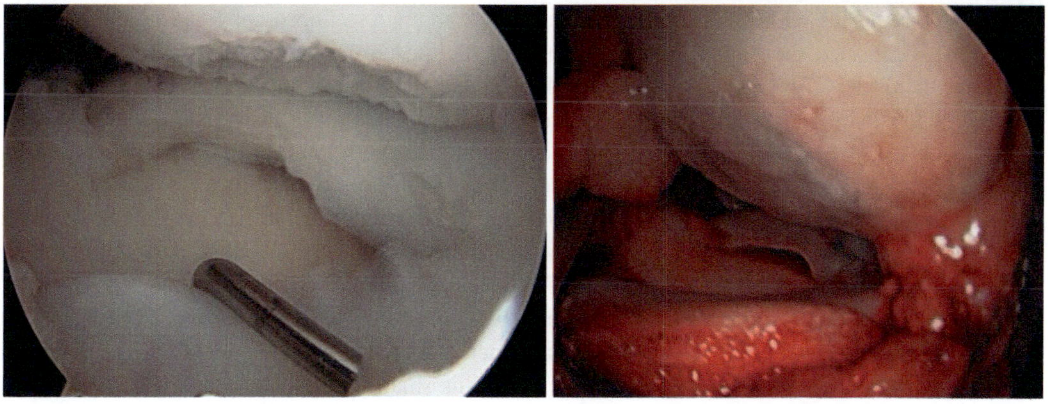

Fig. 18.3 Arthroscopic photograph of lateral MAT with concomitant cartilage repair procedure

utilized. Any osteotomy hardware may be removed at second stage if the bone has previously healed.

In the setting of a failed ACL reconstruction, indications for lateral MAT include painful effusions and/or functional instability (i.e., explosive pivot shift) associated with lateral meniscus deficiency. Patient alignment should be neutral or corrected to between the tibial spines. Tibial slope should be normal or corrected at the first stage. Chondral defects ICRS grade III-IV should be addressed concomitantly with MAT in the lateral compartment. Other secondary stabilizers should be addressed at the time of revision ACL reconstruction (i.e., posteromedial and posterolateral reconstruction). Standard contraindications for MAT should apply including elevated BMI, smokers, non-compliant patients, inflammatory disorders, and active infection. Care should be taken when considering concomitant MAT in contact/collision athletes. Alternative strategies for knee joint stabilization (i.e., lateral tenodesis and osteotomy) may be better suited to this very challenging high-demand population. Prolonged conservative rehabilitation and risk of graft breakdown with high-impact load limit the utility of MAT in this specific population [36].

MAT Sizing

Proper preoperative sizing of the allograft is an important aspect of meniscal transplantation. Inadequate sizing of the graft can lead to improper biomechanics, meniscus extrusion, and transplant failure requiring additional surgical procedures [37]. Graft size should be within 10% of the native meniscus [22]. Oversized grafts result in increased risk of graft extrusion, which can cause increased compressive forces across the articular cartilage and ultimately graft failure [23]. However, an undersized allograft experiences increased biomechanical load across the graft, which can result in graft disruption [37, 38]. Therefore, correct preoperative measurements along with the availability of a reliable tissue bank is necessary.

Several different methods have been recommended for meniscus sizing by utilizing radiographs, computed tomography (CT), magnetic resonance imaging (MRI), and arthropometric data [38]. The Yoon equation for length and arthropometric method for width are often preferred when planning for preoperative lateral MAT procedure. It is important to consider that the mediolateral sizing is more important than anteroposterior sizing [39]. Lee and colleagues recommend that when both dimensions cannot be matched, the graft size should be determined by the width [40]. Obtaining an MRI of the contralateral knee may be beneficial [41]; however, this should be used for select cases only. Shaffer et al. reported data that suggests that compared to radiographs, the use of MRI is only moderately more accurate in determining the correct size of the meniscus [42]. Additionally, MRI has the associated burden of increased cost [26].

Surgical Technique for Revision ACL Reconstruction and Lateral MAT

For revision ACL and lateral MAT, order of operations should be systematic and stepwise. Patient is taken to the operating room after regional anesthesia is administered in the holding area. In general, a motor-sparing adductor canal catheter are utilized but a femoral block may be considered. Following induction of general anesthesia, an examination under anesthesia is performed for both limbs. Comparison of joint ROM (i.e., hyperlaxity), as well as ligamentous laxity (Lachman, pivot shift), should be performed. Note that stress fluoroscopy to rule out posteromedial/posterolateral injuries is performed as indicated during the initial staging arthroscopy in the majority of these cases. Tourniquet is placed but not inflated. We typically begin with ipsilateral ACL graft harvest. In most revision cases, quadriceps autograft is harvested without bone and prepared as an all-inside construct using suspensory cortical fixation. Graft has a diameter of 9–10 mm and a length of 70 mm. The extensor is meticulously repaired. A damp sponge is placed in this small wound which is closed toward the end of the case. The graft is prepared and pretensioned on the back table.

Standard arthroscopy is performed. Synovectomy and scar lysis of adhesion are performed as indicated. ACL tunnels have been previously evaluated, debrided, and/or bone grafted. The lateral meniscus is prepared to leave a 2–3 mm rim of healthy tissue. A shaver and/or biter are utilized for this step. The meniscal rasp is used to create bleeding rim and fresh synovium/capsule.

The lateral meniscus is oval shaped, vertically oriented in the axial plane with less distance between the anterior and posterior roots than on the medial side of the joint (Fig. 18.4). For this reason, lateral MAT has classically been performed with bone bridge techniques [43–45]. Advantages include strong time-zero root fixation and maintained relationship between the anterior and posterior horns attached to the same bone block. There are limitations including technical difficulty flipping the meniscus into the joint, loss of bone stock, inability to handle graft mismatch, among others. Classic bone plug technique has advantages including easier passage into the joint, ability to accommodate for graft mismatch, and no associated risk of any ACL disruption and tissue loss for either medial or lateral MAT (Fig. 18.5) [11, 15, 21]. Known disadvantages include challenges seating an 8–10 mm deep plug into the tibial sockets and lower time-zero root fixation strength. There is also concern regarding tunnel convergence laterally with standard drilling techniques, given the close proximity of the roots. Soft tissue–only MAT is technically easiest and often performed around the globe. Concerns include decreased root fixation strength with classic suturing techniques and the increased risk of MAT extrusion when compared to bony techniques.

We have developed a hybrid technique that harnesses the advantages of all techniques (soft tissue, bone plug, and bone-bridge MAT) while limiting several of the disadvantages. Our techniques described fulfills several important criteria: (1) anatomic footprint restoration, (2) minimally invasive (all-arthroscopic), (3) technically straightforward passing the MAT into the joint (4), strong time-zero fixation allowing for early ROM, (5) ability to handle graft mismatch in real time, (6) attempt to handle extrusion with capsular fixation to the tibia (capsulodesis), and (7) maintenance of bone stock in the event a revision is required in the future.

The lateral MAT is prepared on the back table. Each lateral root has small bone plugs of 9 mm width and 3 mm depth. The posterior bone plug and adjacent root soft tissue are prepared similar

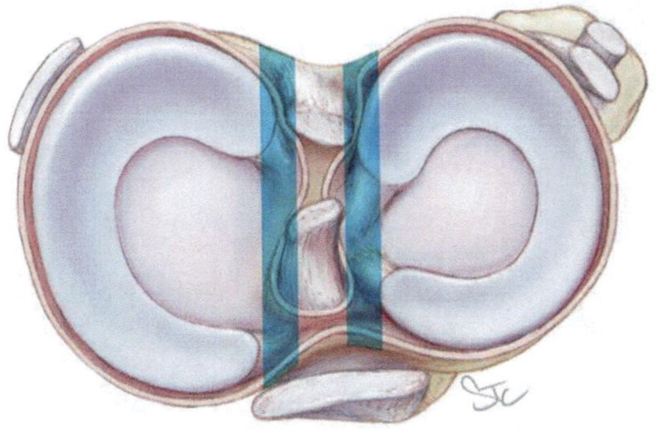

Fig. 18.4 Axial view illustration depicting medial and lateral meniscus anatomy and lines depicting the location for meniscal transplant trough placement both medially and laterally in relation to the cruciate ligaments

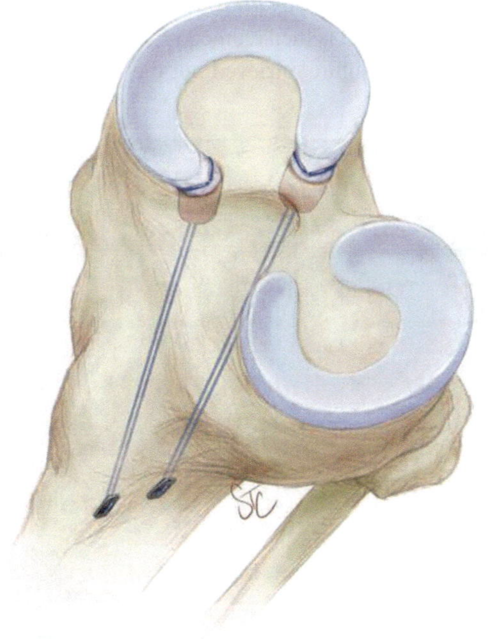

Fig. 18.5 Illustration depicting the bone plug meniscus allograft transplant (MAT) technique

to a QuadLink® Tightrope ABS suspensory fixation (Arthrex, Naples, Florida). This will allow modulation of the posterior root depth to accommodate either graft mismatch or time-zero graft extrusion during the case. The anterior root is prepared with FiberLoop suture tape (Arthrex, Naples, Florida) that is whip-stitched to include both soft tissue and bone. A labral tape is placed in horizontal mattress fashion at the junction of the mid-meniscus with the posterior horn of the MAT. This can be utilized as a shuttle stitch to deliver the MAT into the joint. The femoral surface of the MAT is marked with an "A" for anterior and "P" for posterior for orientation purposes.

In the Fig. 18.4 position, a retrocutter is utilized through the medial portal directed at the posterior root insertion of the lateral meniscus (Fig. 18.6). Incision is made longitudinal on the tibial cortex midway between anterior crest and posterior border. This incision can be utilized for ACL and lateral MAT cortical fixation. A 9 mm wide by 10 mm deep socket is reamed and a shuttle suture is passed and retrieved out the lateral portal. The socket is reamed deeper than the size of the posterior root bone plug (9 mm × 3 mm) to accommodate for any graft mismatch. The femoral ACL tunnel is then reamed in standard fashion and shuttle suture retrieved out the lateral portal. The tibial ACL socket is reamed and shuttle retrieved medially. Finally, a retrocutter is utilized through medial portal (visualizing high and lateral) to create the anatomic socket for the anterior root of the lateral meniscus. The ACL tibial socket is typically more vertical and exits the tibia just medial to the tibial tubercle. The lateral MAT socket is adjacent but not overlapping the ACL footprint and reamed to a 3–5 mm depth. The shuttle suture exits the tibial cortex posterior and medial in relation to the ACL socket.

The lateral meniscus is more mobile than the medial meniscus, with no additional attachments to the LCL or the popliteal hiatus. There is concern regarding limiting lateral MAT mobility if meniscotibial fixation is performed. However, there is also concern regarding lateral MAT extrusion if there is weak capsule or minimal native remnant for fixation. For these reasons, we utilize a lateral capsulodesis to try and reduce the risk of lateral MAT extrusion but minimize overconstraint [46, 47]. A spinal needle is utilized to pierce the lateral capsule just above the meniscus remnant at the junction of the mid-meniscus with the anterior and posterior horns respectively (Fig. 18.7). Two pairs of horizontal mattress labral tape sutures are shuttled into the capsule using the spinal needles and a plastic cannula in the lateral portal. These sutures are anchored

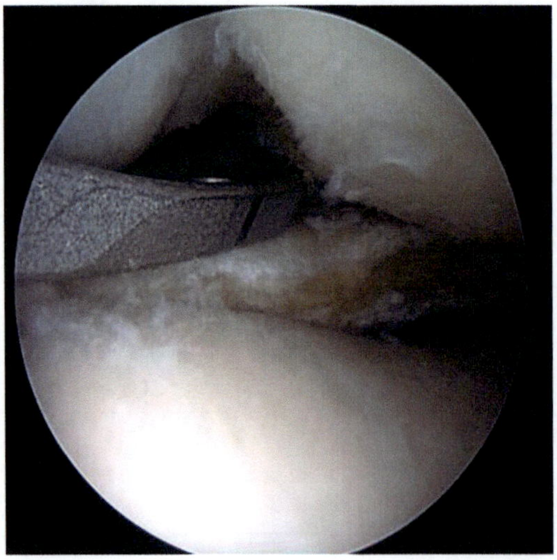

Fig. 18.6 Arthroscopic photograph of the retrocutter positioned on the posterior root of the lateral meniscus

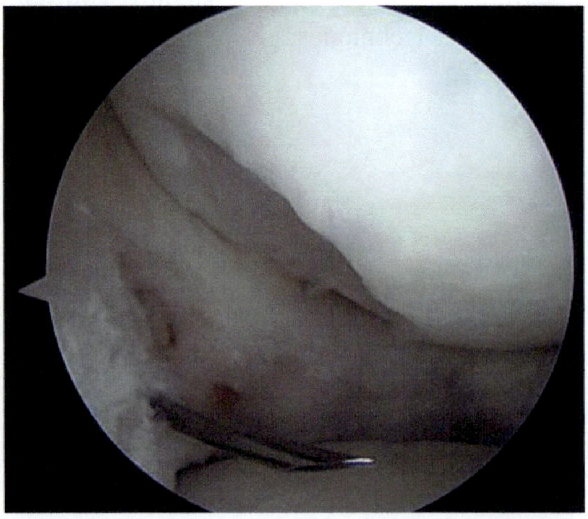

Fig. 18.7 Spinal needle at the lateral capsule. Surgeon should place the needle above the meniscus remnant at the junction of the mid-meniscus with the anterior and posterior horns to complete the lateral capsulodesis

(Pushlock Anchors® Arthrex, Naples, Florida) to the lateral tibia just below the meniscus remnant through small central open lateral incision. This brings the capsule to the tibia prior to shuttling the MAT into the joint. An inside-out device is utilized to pass a shuttle stitch at the junction of the native mid-meniscus with the posterior horn. This is retrieved out the lateral portal.

After a cannula is placed, the sutures for the anterior and posterior root sockets and posterolateral shuttle stitch are retrieved. The cannula is then removed. The posterior root and posterolateral shuttle stitch are utilized to shuttle the respective aspects of the lateral MAT into the joint through lateral portal under direct arthroscopic visualization. The anterior horn/root is then shuttled into the anterior socket. The attachable button is applied, and provisional fixation is performed for the posterior root. The anterior root is seated and firmly fixed with knotless anchor (SwiveLock Anchor® Arthrex, Naples, Florida) (Fig. 18.8). At this point, graft mismatch is assessed. If the graft is too large, the suspensory cortical mechanism may be shortened to bring some of the posterior horn/root deeper into the posterior socket. Usually, no more than 3–5 mm of mismatch is initially present. Hybrid fixation is then performed including all-inside posterior, inside-out for mid-meniscus, and outside-in as needed. In total, 6–8 points of fixation are typically utilized. The MAT is probed carefully and taken through ROM arc after final fixation.

At this point, attention is turned to completion of the ACL reconstruction in standard fashion. If concomitant cartilage restoration is to be performed, the ACL graft may be passed but not fixated on the tibial side. A limited lateral arthrotomy can be performed for cartilage restoration. Once complete, final ACL tensioning can be performed along with direct repair of the anterior horn of the MAT to the native meniscus rim and capsule. Final fluoroscopic images are taken. Examination under anesthesia is again performed. Wound is closed and dressing applied in standard fashion.

Below is a list of the steps:

1. *MAT prepared (bone plugs: 9 mm × 3 mm)*
2. *Posterior root drilled (*Fig. 18.4 *position; retrocutter through medial portal; 9 mm × 10 mm socket)*
3. *Femoral ACL tunnel reamed (shuttle retrieved laterally)*
4. *ACL socket reamed (shuttle retrieved medially)*
5. *Retrocutter utilized to create anterior root socket (3–5 mm depth)*
6. *Lateral capsulodesis*

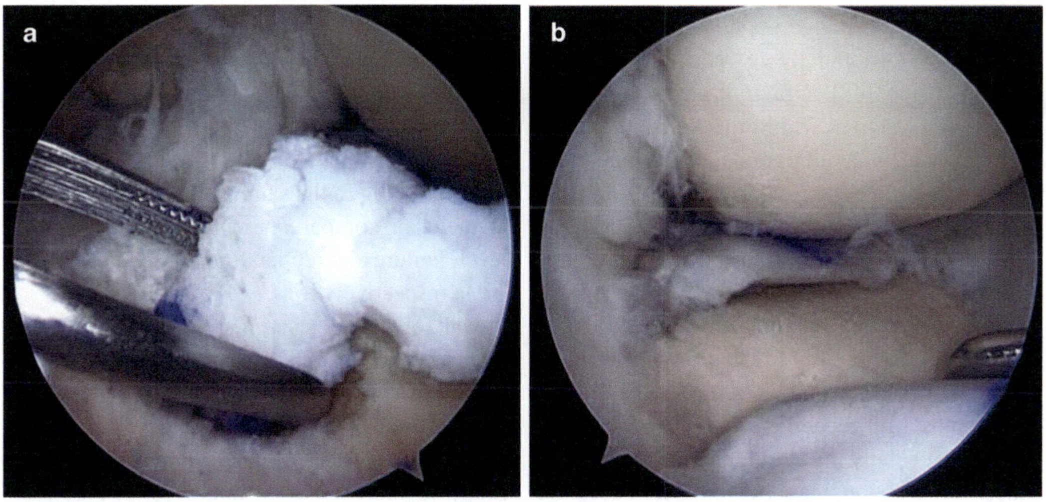

Fig. 18.8 (**a**) Prior to seating the anterior bone-plug. (**b**) After seating the anterior bone-plug in the socket adjacent to the ACL

7. *Sutures retrieved for anterior and posterior root sockets*
8. *Lateral MAT shuttled into joint*
9. *Anterior horn/root shuttled into the anterior socket*
10. *Attachable button applied*
11. *Provisional fixation performed for the posterior root*
12. *Anterior root fixed with knotless anchor*
13. *Graft mismatch assessed*
    (a) *Too large ➔ the suspensory cortical mechanism shortened to bring posterior horn/root deeper into socket*
14. *Hybrid fixation performed (typically 6–8 fixation points)*
    (a) *All-inside posterior*
    (b) *Inside-out for mid-meniscus*
    (c) *Outside-in as needed*
15. *ROM arc after final fixation*
16. *ACL reconstruction proceeded*
17. *ACL tensioning*
18. *Direct repair of anterior horn of MAT*
19. *Final flouroscopic images*
20. *EUA*
21. *Wound closure*

Rehabilitation

Postoperative rehabilitation includes flat-foot 0% weightbearing in a hinged knee brace for approximately 6 weeks. Range of motion (ROM) progression is slow initially to reduce the risk of graft extrusion [48]. Gravity-assisted ROM or CPM may be started within the first 1–2 weeks. Early goals include full terminal extension, quadriceps activation, and passive gravity-assisted ROM to 90° by 6 weeks. After 6 weeks, patients transition to Weight bearing as tolerated (WBAT) and unlock the brace with quadriceps control. They can discontinue the brace to a knee sleeve at this time. Progressive ROM continues while avoiding closed chain squatting past 90° for 3–4 months. Mid-rehabilitation focuses on restoration of gait, daily life activities, and low impact. Linear progression may be initiated based on minimum time (~9 mos) and functional criteria. In general, complex lateral movements and impact loading are avoided in most of these patients. Select athletes (noncontact, noncollision) may progress per protocol between year 1 and year 2 as long as the joint has regained homeostasis (i.e., no effusion or pain) and regain neuromuscular strength, flexibility, and control as demonstrated on return-to-sport testing. The majority of patients are undergoing this procedure to improve previous damage, and do not progress past normal daily activites and low impact recreational sport.

Outcomes of Meniscus Allograft Transplantation

Meniscus allograft transplantation (MAT) has emerged as a viable option for treatment of meniscus deficiency, with recent studies showing improved knee function and return to activity [49–52]. Overall, there have been reliable studies demonstrating the good outcomes of MAT [49–57]. Very few studies have determined the mid- to long-term outcomes of concomitant revision ACL reconstruction and lateral MAT specifically. Zaffagnini et al. performed 50 combined ACL reconstructions with MAT (medial or lateral); 44% had primary ACL reconstruction with MAT, while 39% underwent revision ACL reconstruction and MAT. Additionally, 17% of the cohort underwent ACL reconstruction with MAT in addition to high tibial osteotomy. At 5 years post-surgery, patients reported significant improvements in outcomes (Tegner score, Lysholm score, and Visual Analog Scale [VAS]). Furthermore, 85% of patients were able to return to sport with 37% returning to the same or higher performance level when compared to pre-injury performace level. Failure and reoperation rates were 15% and 17%, respectively [58].

Saltzman et al. also prospectively followed 40 patients who underwent combined ACL reconstruction (primary or revision) and MAT (33 medial MAT, 7 lateral MAT) [59]. At a follow-up of 5.7 years, 50% of patients were able to return to sport (39% to same level of play), and patients had significantly improved outcome scores. While the re-operation rate was high at

35%, a majority were simple arthroscopic debridement procedures. The failure rate was reported at 20% with 15% undergoing total knee arthroplasty. Of note, the lateral MAT subgroup showed significantly improved patient-reported outcomes compared to the medial MAT subgroup, and the lateral MAT subgroup had no cases of reoperation or failure. This suggests that patients who undergo lateral MAT with ACL reconstruction may have better outcomes than those who undergo combined ACL reconstruction and medial MAT [59]. Table 18.1 *outlines additional studies of MAT outcomes.*

Table 18.1 Outcomes of lateral MAT and concomitant ACL reconstruction

Study	Case number (n)	Methods/fixation	Follow-up	Outcome
Saltzman et al., 2017 [59]	**27**	Bone bridge (33 medial, 7 lateral) + Anterior Cruciate Ligament Reconstruction (ACLR)	**Mean: 5.7 years**	19 concomitant procedures, including 9 HWR and 9 OCA. Significant improvements in 11/14 PRO measures at final follow-up. 50% had return to sport. No significant joint space narrowing was noted. Overall survival rate at final follow-up was 80%. Failures occurred at a mean of 7.3 years. Lateral MAT group should significantly improve PRO measures compared to medial MAT group. No failures in lateral MAT group
Marcacci et al., 2014 [50]	**16**	12 MAT in professional soccer players (6 medial, 6 lateral), soft tissue only	**36 months**	11 of 12 returned to play at semiprofessional or higher level. No significant differences in return to training/first game for medial vs. lateral or isolated vs. concomitant procedure
Chalmers et al., 2013 [52]	**18**	Bone bridge (10 lateral); bone plug (3 medial)	**Mean: 3.3 years**	10 of 13 patients (77%) returned to sporting activity at final F/U. The mean KOOS score for the sport subset was 76 (SD, 18), the mean IKDC score was 77 (SD, 14), and the mean Lysholm score was 81 (SD, 13). Of the 13 patients, 3 (23%) required further surgery, comprising one revision MAT, one partial meniscectomy, and one meniscal repair
Saltzman et al., 2012 [53]	**19**	22 MAT (13 medial with bone plug technique, 9 lateral with keyhole technique), 14 had a concomitant procedure (8 ACLR or revision ACLR)	**Mean 8.5 years**	Lateral MAT has significantly higher Overall Knee Condition and postop IKDC scores compared to medial MAT. MAT with concomitant procedure demonstrated greater improvement in most PROs than isolated transplants
Verdonk et al., 2006 [54]	**20**	Soft tissue only	**Mean: 12.1 years**	Significant improvement was seen in modified HSS pain, walking, and stair scores at final FU ($p = 0.011$, $p = 0.007$, $p = 0.018$). KOOS scores obtained at the final FU showed substantial disability/symptoms and reduced quality of life. 13/32 knees did not show any joint space narrowing. MRI showed 70% were partially extruded. There was an 18% overall failure rate. 90% of patients were satisfied with the procedure
Zaffagnini et al. 2019 [58]	**26**	50 combined ACLR-MAT	**Mean 5 years**	Significantly improved PRO measures. 85% returned to sport, 37% at same or higher performance level. Failure and reoperation rates were 15% and 17%, respectively

(continued)

Table 18.1 (continued)

Study	Case number (n)	Methods/fixation	Follow-up	Outcome
Verdonk et al., 2005 [31]	***	Soft tissue only	**Mean: 7.2 years**	11/39 (28%) of the medial allografts and 10/61 (16%) of the lateral allografts failed. Mean cumulative survival time (11.6 years) was identical for the medial and lateral allografts. The cumulative survival rates for the medial and lateral allografts at 10 years were 74.2% and 69.8%, respectively. The mean cumulative survival time and the cumulative survival rate for the medial allografts used in combination with a high tibial osteotomy were 13.0 years and 83.3% at 10 years, respectively
Yoldas et al., 2003 [60]	***	31 patients (11 isolated MAT [9 lateral, 2 medial], 20 ACLR+MAT [3 lateral, 14 medial, 3 combined]; bone plugs (medial) or bone bridge (lateral)	**Mean: 2.9 years**	No significant difference in PRO based on medial versus lateral transplant, with or without concomitant ACLR. Eighty-three percent primary ACLR+MAT and 75% revision ACLR+MAT returned to moderate sport activity
Van Arkel and de Boer, 1995 [61]	***	63 allografts (34 lateral,17 medial, 6 combined); soft tissue fixation	**Mean: 5 years**	Cumulative survival rate for lateral allografts 76% (at 11 years), medial allografts 50% (at 10 years), and combined 67% (at 9 years). Significant negative correlation between ACL rupture and successful medial MAT
Yoon et al 2020 [62]	***	31 MAT after ACLR (16 medial, 15 lateral); no concomitant ACLR-MAT; keyhole (lateral), bone plugs (medial)	**Minimum: 2 years**	Medial MAT patients had significantly greater improvement in PROs than lateral MAT patients. Significant improvements postoperatively in pivot shift test for medial MAT, but not lateral MAT. Preop side-to-side difference in anterior tibial translation was significant only in medial MAT
Sekiya et al. 2003 [63]	***	28 MAT+ACLR (21 medial [bone block], 4 lateral [bone bridge], 3 both), 19 ACLR and 9 revision ACLR	**Mean: 2.8 years**	Significantly better IKDC group rating in primary ACLR vs. revision. No significant difference in PROs based on location of MAT. No significant change in joint space narrowing. No difference in ligamentous laxity
van der Wal et al., 2020 [64]	***	109 MAT (36 medial, 73 lateral), 16 concomitant ACLR; soft tissue + suture anchor	**Median: 54 months**	MAT failure rate 10% (2 medial, 9 lateral). Mean survival 16.1 years, no significant difference between medial and lateral. Survival associated with age at baseline (greater in those <35 years old). Survival not associated with compartment treated, with or without ACLR. Less improvement in KOOS scores with concomitant CALR, greater number of knee surgeries prior to MAT

*** P values less than 0.001.

Case Example

History/Exam

Patient is a 17-year-old female, competitive soccer player, with a history of previous left knee ACL hamstring autograft reconstruction at an outside institution 3 years ago. She also underwent subtotal lateral meniscectomy in a separate procedure after return to play. Unfortunately, the athlete continued to have lateral pain, effusions, and a feeling of intermittent "giving out" of her knee with activity. She had an "episode" one day prior to presentation.

On exam, the patient had an antalgic gait, diffuse and lateral joint line tenderness, 0-0-135° range of motion, negative McMurray, grade IIIB Lachman, and explosive grade III pivot shift. Imaging studies were ordered and thoroughly evaluated. Radiographs demonstrated previous ACL with overall anatomic alignment combined with preserved joint spaces (Fig. 18.9). CT was evaluated to examine ACL tunnel position and to measure tibial slope. Tunnel widening >14 mm was demonstrated (Fig. 18.10). MRI demonstrated lateral meniscal deficiency and a disrupted ACL graft (Fig. 18.11).

Given her complex condition, inability to perform in her sport, and symptoms even with daily life activity, the patient was indicated for salvage surgical intervention. A comprehensive problem list was created. This includes failed ACL reconstruction with widened prior anatomic tunnels and lateral meniscus deficiency. Patient goals and expectations were carefully discussed including quality of life and risk/benefit and timeframe of future return to sport. A two-stage solution was proposed, as bone grafting the widened tunnels was necessary. The patient underwent diagnostic arthroscopy with bone grafting (Fig. 18.12) followed by concomitant ACL revision and lateral meniscal allograft transplantation (Fig. 18.13) once the tunnels had consolidated. Postoperative

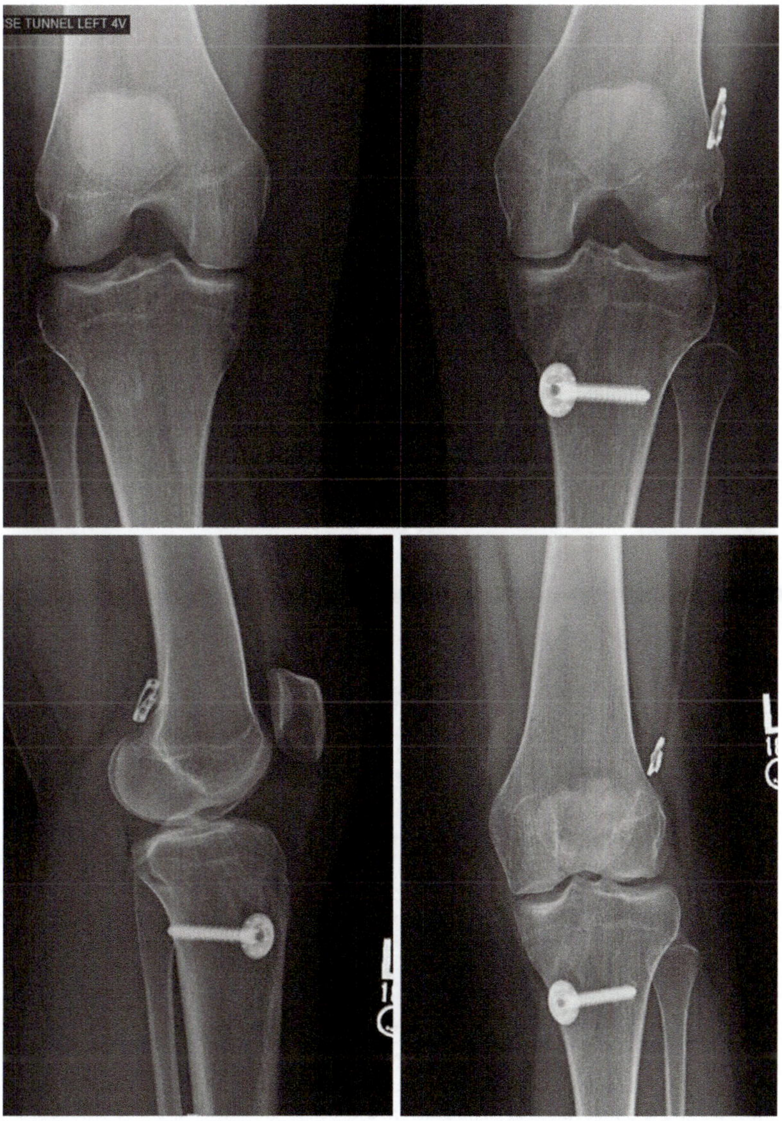

Fig. 18.9 Initial radiographs of case example demonstrating previous ACL with overall anatomic alignment combined with preserved joint spaces

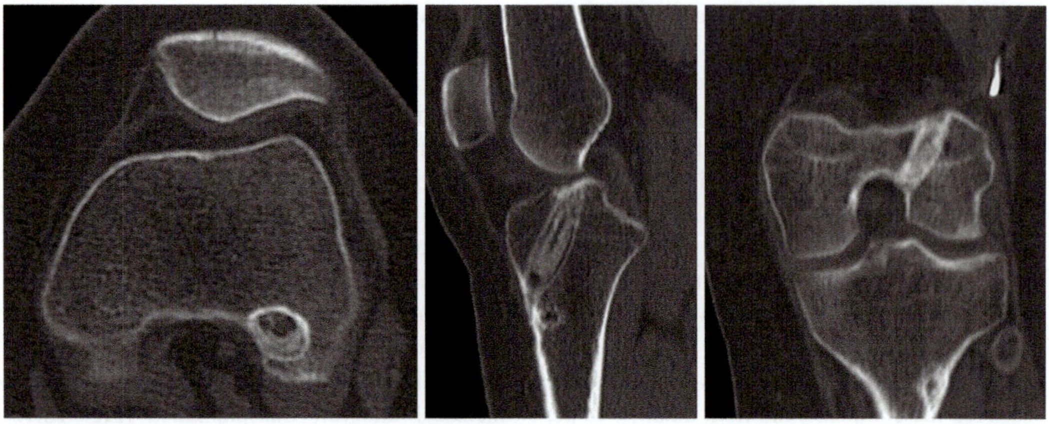

Fig. 18.10 CT revealed ACL tunnel widening of >14 mm

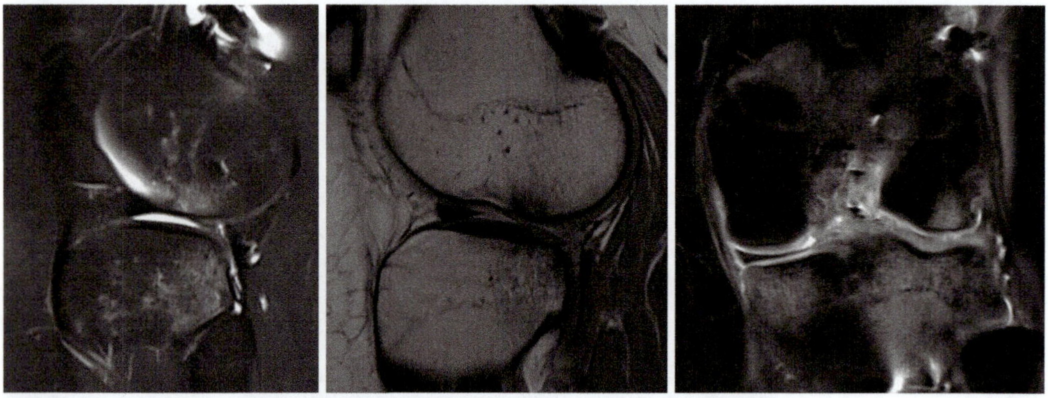

Fig. 18.11 MRI demonstrated lateral meniscal deficiency and a disrupted ACL graft

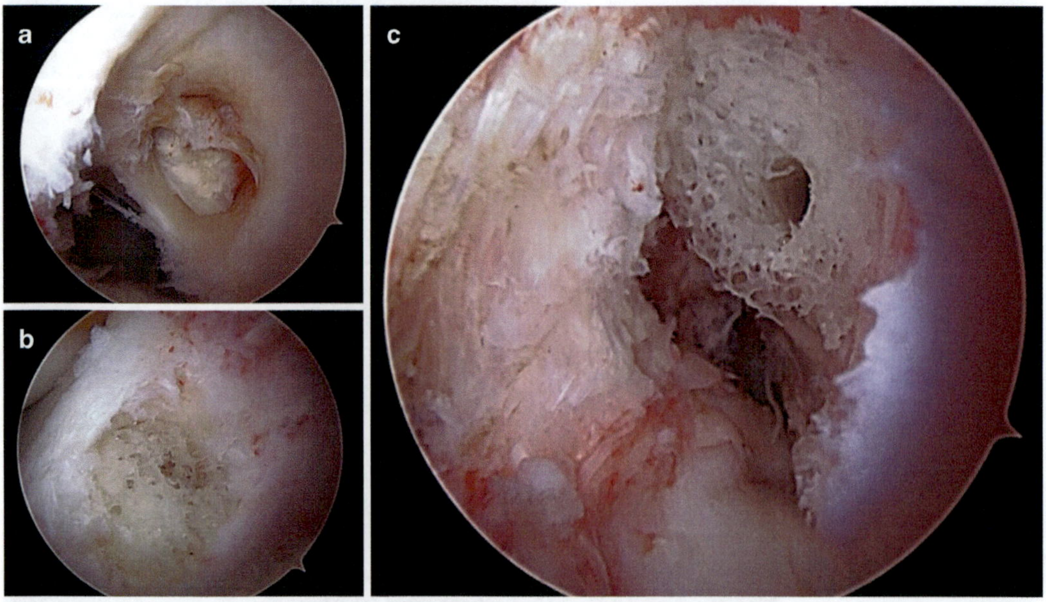

Fig. 18.12 Intraoperative arthroscopic images of diagnostic arthroscopy demonstrating disrupted ACL (**a**) and then post-removal and placement of bone graft (**b**, **c**)

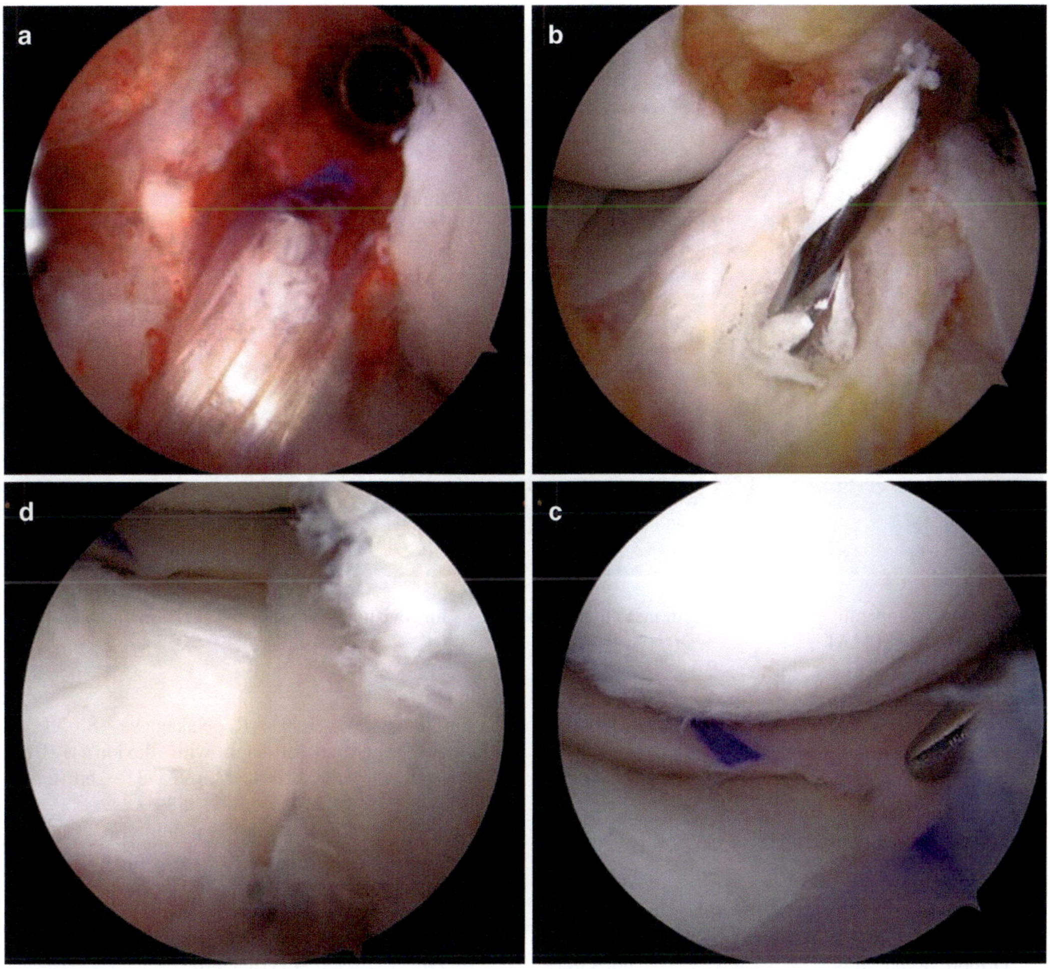

Fig. 18.13 During diagnostic arthroscopy, the patient underwent concomitant ACL revision (**a**, **b**) and lateral meniscal allograft transplantation (**c**, **d**)

radiographs demonstrate metallic screws for revision ACL autograft and buttons for concomitant lateral MAT (Fig. 18.14). The patient is doing well at short-term follow-up (<6 months) but has long recovery timeframe ahead.

Conclusion

In select patients, revision ACL reconstruction and lateral MAT can be a powerful combination to address increased rotatory instability and/or symptomatic post-meniscectomy syndrome. Appropriate indications and careful preoperative planning including staging arthroscopy are often required. Surgical precision and stepwise rehabilitation are critical. Patient expectations must be addressed to ensure optimal subjective and objective outcome. These are bridging procedures often performed in salvage. Patients should be aware of the likelihood of requiring future nonoperative or operative intervention for their challenging condition.

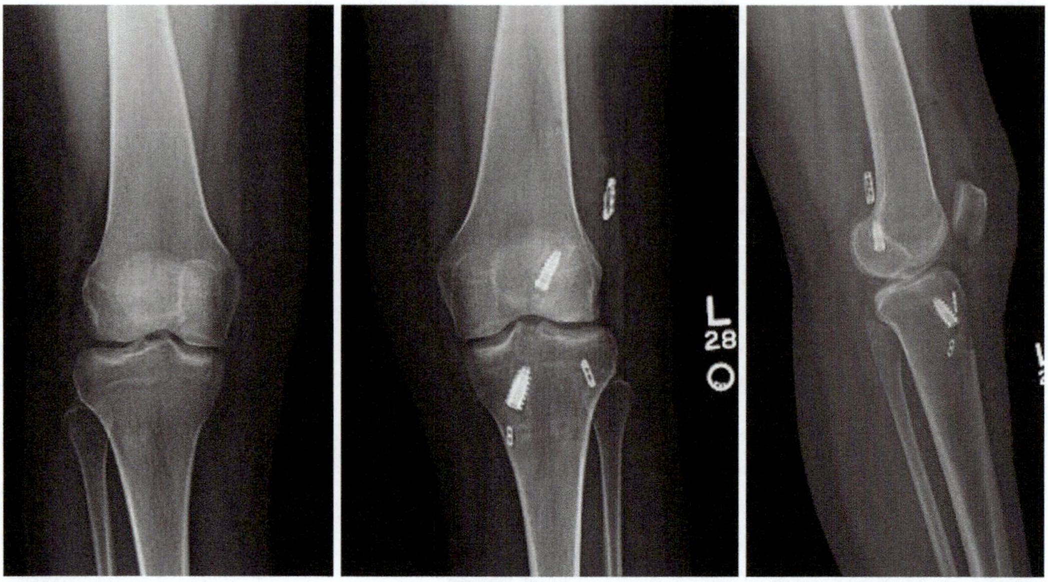

Fig. 18.14 Postoperative radiographs demonstrate metallic screws for revision ACL autograft revision and buttons for concomitant lateral MAT

Acknowledgments The authors appreciate Dr. Kristofer J. Jones, for the case example.

References

1. Walker PS, Erkman MJ. The role of the menisci in force transmission across the knee. Clin Orthop Relat Res. 1975;109:184–92. https://doi.org/10.1097/00003086-197506000-00027.
2. Spang JT, Dang AB, Mazzocca A, et al. The effect of medial meniscectomy and meniscal allograft transplantation on knee and anterior cruciate ligament biomechanics. Arthroscopy. 2010;26(2):192–201. https://doi.org/10.1016/j.arthro.2009.11.008.
3. Ahmed AM, Burke DL. In-vitro measurement of static pressure distribution in synovial joints–part I: tibial surface of the knee. J Biomech Eng. 1983;105(3):216–25. https://doi.org/10.1115/1.3138409.
4. Makris EA, Hadidi P, Athanasiou KA. The knee meniscus: structure-function, pathophysiology, current repair techniques, and prospects for regeneration. Biomaterials. 2011;32(30):7411–31. https://doi.org/10.1016/j.biomaterials.2011.06.037.
5. Seedhom BB, Dowson D, Wright V. Proceedings: functions of the menisci. A preliminary study. Ann Rheum Dis. 1974;33(1):111. https://doi.org/10.1136/ard.33.1.111.
6. Kurosawa H, Fukubayashi T, Nakajima H. Load-bearing mode of the knee joint: physical behavior of the knee joint with or without menisci. Clin Orthop Relat Res. 1980;149:283–90.
7. Pinskerova V, Johal P, Nakagawa S, et al. Does the femur roll-back with flexion? J Bone Joint Surg Br. 2004;86(6):925–31. https://doi.org/10.1302/0301-620x.86b6.14589.
8. Musahl V, Citak M, O'Loughlin PF, Choi D, Bedi A, Pearle AD. The effect of medial versus lateral meniscectomy on the stability of the anterior cruciate ligament-deficient knee. Am J Sports Med. 2010;38(8):1591–7. https://doi.org/10.1177/0363546510364402.
9. Levy IM, Torzilli PA, Warren RF. The effect of medial meniscectomy on anterior-posterior motion of the knee. J Bone Joint Surg Am. 1982;64(6):883–8.
10. Simonian PT, Sussmann PS, Wickiewicz TL, et al. Popliteomeniscal fasciculi and the unstable lateral meniscus: clinical correlation and magnetic resonance diagnosis. Arthroscopy. 1997;13(5):590–6. https://doi.org/10.1016/s0749-8063(97)90185-7.
11. Krinsky MB, Abdenour TE, Starkey C, Albo RA, Chu DA. Incidence of lateral meniscus injury in professional basketball players. Am J Sports Med. 1992;20(1):17–9. https://doi.org/10.1177/036354659202000105.
12. Jones JC, Burks R, Owens BD, Sturdivant RX, Svoboda SJ, Cameron KL. Incidence and risk factors associated with meniscal injuries among active-duty US military service members. J Athl Train. 2012;47(1):67–73. https://doi.org/10.4085/1062-6050-47.1.67.
13. Petty CA, Lubowitz JH. Does arthroscopic partial meniscectomy always cause arthritis? Sports Med Arthrosc Rev. 2012;20(2):58–61. https://doi.org/10.1097/JSA.0b013e31824fbf3a.

14. Hede A, Larsen E, Sandberg H. Partial versus total meniscectomy. A prospective, randomised study with long-term follow-up. J Bone Joint Surg Br. 1992;74(1):118–21. https://doi.org/10.1302/0301-620X.74B1.1732238.
15. Shelbourne KD, Gray T. Results of anterior cruciate ligament reconstruction based on meniscus and articular cartilage status at the time of surgery. Five- to fifteen-year evaluations. Am J Sports Med. 2000;28(4):446–52. https://doi.org/10.1177/03635465000280040201.
16. Matheny LM, Ockuly AC, Steadman JR, LaPrade RF. Posterior meniscus root tears: associated pathologies to assist as diagnostic tools. Knee Surg Sports Traumatol Arthrosc. 2015;23(10):3127–31. https://doi.org/10.1007/s00167-014-3073-7.
17. Feucht MJ, Salzmann GM, Bode G, et al. Posterior root tears of the lateral meniscus. Knee Surg Sports Traumatol Arthrosc. 2015;23(1):119–25. https://doi.org/10.1007/s00167-014-2904-x.
18. Brody JM, Lin HM, Hulstyn MJ, Tung GA. Lateral meniscus root tear and meniscus extrusion with anterior cruciate ligament tear. Radiology. 2006;239(3):805–10. https://doi.org/10.1148/radiol.2393050559.
19. De Smet AA, Blankenbaker DG, Kijowski R, Graf BK, Shinki K. MR diagnosis of posterior root tears of the lateral meniscus using arthroscopy as the reference standard. AJR Am J Roentgenol. 2009;192(2):480–6. https://doi.org/10.2214/AJR.08.1300.
20. Forkel P, Reuter S, Sprenker F, et al. Different patterns of lateral meniscus root tears in ACL injuries: application of a differentiated classification system. Knee Surg Sports Traumatol Arthrosc. 2015;23(1):112–8. https://doi.org/10.1007/s00167-014-3467-6.
21. Krych AJ, LaPrade MD, Cook CS, et al. Lateral meniscal oblique radial tears are common with ACL injury: a classification system based on arthroscopic tear patterns in 600 consecutive patients. Orthop J Sports Med. 2020;8(5):2325967120921737. https://doi.org/10.1177/2325967120921737.
22. Feucht MJ, Bigdon S, Mehl J, et al. Risk factors for posterior lateral meniscus root tears in anterior cruciate ligament injuries. Knee Surg Sports Traumatol Arthrosc. 2015;23(1):140–5. https://doi.org/10.1007/s00167-014-3280-2.
23. Raines BT, Naclerio E, Sherman SL. Management of anterior cruciate ligament injury: what's in and what's out? Indian J Orthop. 2017;51(5):563–75. https://doi.org/10.4103/ortho.IJOrtho_245_17.
24. Parkinson B, Robb C, Thomas M, Thompson P, Spalding T. Factors that predict failure in anatomic single-bundle anterior cruciate ligament reconstruction. Am J Sports Med. 2017;45(7):1529–36. https://doi.org/10.1177/0363546517691961.
25. Robb C, Kempshall P, Getgood A, et al. Meniscal integrity predicts laxity of anterior cruciate ligament reconstruction. Knee Surg Sports Traumatol Arthrosc. 2015;23(12):3683–90. https://doi.org/10.1007/s00167-014-3277-x.
26. Trojani C, Sbihi A, Djian P, et al. Causes for failure of ACL reconstruction and influence of meniscectomies after revision. Knee Surg Sports Traumatol Arthrosc. 2011;19(2):196–201. https://doi.org/10.1007/s00167-010-1201-6.
27. Wu WH, Hackett T, Richmond JC. Effects of meniscal and articular surface status on knee stability, function, and symptoms after anterior cruciate ligament reconstruction: a long-term prospective study. Am J Sports Med. 2002;30(6):845–50. https://doi.org/10.1177/03635465020300061501.
28. Milachowski KA, Weismeier K, Wirth CJ. Homologous meniscus transplantation. Experimental and clinical results. Int Orthop. 1989;13(1):1–11. https://doi.org/10.1007/bf00266715.
29. Elattar M, Dhollander A, Verdonk R, Almqvist KF, Verdonk P. Twenty-six years of meniscal allograft transplantation: is it still experimental? A meta-analysis of 44 trials. Knee Surg Sports Traumatol Arthrosc. 2011;19(2):147–57. https://doi.org/10.1007/s00167-010-1351-6.
30. LaPrade RF, Wills NJ, Spiridonov SI, Perkinson S. A prospective outcomes study of meniscal allograft transplantation. Am J Sports Med. 2010;38(9):1804–12. https://doi.org/10.1177/0363546510368133.
31. Verdonk PC, Demurie A, Almqvist KF, Veys EM, Verbruggen G, Verdonk R. Transplantation of viable meniscal allograft. Survivorship analysis and clinical outcome of one hundred cases. J Bone Joint Surg Am. 2005;87(4):715–24. https://doi.org/10.2106/JBJS.C.01344.
32. Shybut TB, Vega CE, Haddad J, et al. Effect of lateral meniscal root tear on the stability of the anterior cruciate ligament-deficient knee. Am J Sports Med. 2015;43(4):905–11. https://doi.org/10.1177/0363546514563910.
33. Forkel P, von Deimling C, Lacheta L, et al. Repair of the lateral posterior meniscal root improves stability in an ACL-deficient knee. Knee Surg Sports Traumatol Arthrosc. 2018;26(8):2302–9. https://doi.org/10.1007/s00167-018-4949-8.
34. Frank JM, Moatshe G, Brady AW, et al. Lateral meniscus posterior root and meniscofemoral ligaments as stabilizing structures in the ACL-deficient knee: a biomechanical study. Orthop J Sports Med. 2017;5(6):2325967117695756. https://doi.org/10.1177/2325967117695756.
35. Group M, Group M. Effect of graft choice on the outcome of revision anterior cruciate ligament reconstruction in the Multicenter ACL Revision Study (MARS) Cohort. Am J Sports Med. 2014;42(10):2301–10. https://doi.org/10.1177/0363546514549005.
36. Getgood A, LaPrade RF, Verdonk P, et al. International meniscus reconstruction experts forum (IMREF) 2015 consensus statement on the practice of meniscal allograft transplantation. Am J Sports Med. 2017;45(5):1195–205. https://doi.org/10.1177/0363546516660064.

37. Trentacosta N, Graham WC, Gersoff WK. Meniscal allograft transplantation: state of the art. Sports Med Arthrosc Rev. 2016;24(2):e23–33. https://doi.org/10.1097/JSA.0000000000000107.
38. Gelber PE, Verdonk P, Getgood AM, Monllau JC. Meniscal transplantation: state of the art. J ISAKOS. 2017;2(6):339–49. https://doi.org/10.1136/jisakos-2017-000138.
39. Yoon JR, Kim TS, Lim HC, Lim HT, Yang JH. Is radiographic measurement of bony landmarks reliable for lateral meniscal sizing? Am J Sports Med. 2011;39(3):582–9. https://doi.org/10.1177/0363546510390444.
40. Lee BS, Chung JW, Kim JM, Kim KA, Bin SI. Width is a more important predictor in graft extrusion than length using plain radiographic sizing in lateral meniscal transplantation. Knee Surg Sports Traumatol Arthrosc. 2012;20(1):179–86. https://doi.org/10.1007/s00167-011-1712-9.
41. Prodromos CC, Joyce BT, Keller BL, Murphy BJ, Shi K. Magnetic resonance imaging measurement of the contralateral normal meniscus is a more accurate method of determining meniscal allograft size than radiographic measurement of the recipient tibial plateau. Arthroscopy. 2007;23(11):1174–1179.e1. https://doi.org/10.1016/j.arthro.2007.06.018.
42. Shaffer B, Kennedy S, Klimkiewicz J, Yao L. Preoperative sizing of meniscal allografts in meniscus transplantation. Am J Sports Med. 2000;28(4):524–33. https://doi.org/10.1177/03635465000280041301.
43. Rosso F, Bisicchia S, Bonasia DE, Amendola A. Meniscal allograft transplantation: a systematic review. Am J Sports Med. 2015;43(4):998–1007. https://doi.org/10.1177/0363546514536021.
44. Yoon KH, Lee SH, Park SY, Kim HJ, Chung KY. Meniscus allograft transplantation: a comparison of medial and lateral procedures. Am J Sports Med. 2014;42(1):200–7. https://doi.org/10.1177/0363546513509057.
45. Myers P, Tudor F. Meniscal allograft transplantation: how should we be doing it? A systematic review. Arthroscopy. 2015;31(5):911–25. https://doi.org/10.1016/j.arthro.2014.11.020.
46. Masferrer-Pino A, Monllau JC, Ibanez M, Erquicia JI, Pelfort X, Gelber PE. Capsulodesis versus bone trough technique in lateral meniscal allograft transplantation: graft extrusion and functional results. Arthroscopy. 2018;34(6):1879–88. https://doi.org/10.1016/j.arthro.2018.01.017.
47. Masferrer-Pino A, Monllau JC, Abat F, Gelber PE. Capsular fixation limits graft extrusion in lateral meniscal allograft transplantation. Int Orthop. 2019;43(11):2549–56. https://doi.org/10.1007/s00264-019-04398-8.
48. Lee DW, Lee JH, Kim DH, Kim JG. Delayed rehabilitation after lateral meniscal allograft transplantation can reduce graft extrusion compared with standard rehabilitation. Am J Sports Med. 2018;46(10):2432–40. https://doi.org/10.1177/0363546518783732.
49. Zaffagnini S, Grassi A, Marcheggiani Muccioli GM, et al. Is sport activity possible after arthroscopic meniscal allograft transplantation? Midterm results in active patients. Am J Sports Med. 2016;44(3):625–32. https://doi.org/10.1177/0363546515621763.
50. Marcacci M, Marcheggiani Muccioli GM, Grassi A, et al. Arthroscopic meniscus allograft transplantation in male professional soccer players: a 36-month follow-up study. Am J Sports Med. 2014;42(2):382–8. https://doi.org/10.1177/0363546513508763.
51. Alentorn-Geli E, Vázquez RS, Díaz P, Cuscó X, Cugat R. Arthroscopic meniscal transplants in soccer players: outcomes at 2- to 5-year follow-up. Clin J Sport Med. 2010;20(5):340–3. https://doi.org/10.1097/JSM.0b013e3181f207dc.
52. Chalmers PN, Karas V, Sherman SL, Cole BJ. Return to high-level sport after meniscal allograft transplantation. Arthroscopy. 2013;29(3):539–44. https://doi.org/10.1016/j.arthro.2012.10.027.
53. Saltzman BM, Bajaj S, Salata M, et al. Prospective long-term evaluation of meniscal allograft transplantation procedure: a minimum of 7-year follow-up. J Knee Surg. 2012;25(2):165–75. https://doi.org/10.1055/s-0032-1313738.
54. Verdonk PC, Verstraete KL, Almqvist KF, et al. Meniscal allograft transplantation: long-term clinical results with radiological and magnetic resonance imaging correlations. Knee Surg Sports Traumatol Arthrosc. 2006;14(8):694–706. https://doi.org/10.1007/s00167-005-0033-2.
55. Wirth CJ, Peters G, Milachowski KA, Weismeier KG, Kohn D. Long-term results of meniscal allograft transplantation. Am J Sports Med. 2002;30(2):174–81. https://doi.org/10.1177/03635465020300020501.
56. Vundelinckx B, Vanlauwe J, Bellemans J. Long-term subjective, clinical, and radiographic outcome evaluation of meniscal allograft transplantation in the knee. Am J Sports Med. 2014;42(7):1592–9. https://doi.org/10.1177/0363546514530092.
57. van der Wal RJ, Thomassen BJ, van Arkel ER. Long-term clinical outcome of open meniscal allograft transplantation. Am J Sports Med. 2009;37(11):2134–9. https://doi.org/10.1177/0363546509336725.
58. Zaffagnini S, Grassi A, Romandini I, Marcacci M, Filardo G. Meniscal allograft transplantation combined with anterior cruciate ligament reconstruction provides good mid-term clinical outcome. Knee Surg Sports Traumatol Arthrosc. 2019;27(6):1914–23. https://doi.org/10.1007/s00167-018-5078-0.
59. Saltzman BM, Meyer MA, Weber AE, Poland SG, Yanke AB, Cole BJ. Prospective clinical and radiographic outcomes after concomitant anterior cruciate ligament reconstruction and meniscal allograft transplantation at a mean 5-year follow-up. Am J Sports Med. 2017;45(3):550–62. https://doi.org/10.1177/0363546516669934.
60. Yoldas EA, Sekiya JK, Irrgang JJ, Fu FH, Harner CD. Arthroscopically assisted meniscal allograft

transplantation with and without combined anterior cruciate ligament reconstruction. Knee Surg Sports Traumatol Arthrosc. 2003;11(3):173–82. https://doi.org/10.1007/s00167-003-0362-y.
61. van Arkel ER, de Boer HH. Survival analysis of human meniscal transplantations. J Bone Joint Surg Br. 2002;84(2):227–31. https://doi.org/10.1302/0301-620x.84b2.12443.
62. Yoon KH, Lee HW, Park SY, Yeak RDK, Kim JS, Park JY. Meniscal allograft transplantation after anterior cruciate ligament reconstruction can improve knee stability: a comparison of medial and lateral procedures. Am J Sports Med. 2020;48(10):2370–5. https://doi.org/10.1177/0363546520938771.
63. Sekiya JK, Giffin JR, Irrgang JJ, Fu FH, Harner CD. Clinical outcomes after combined meniscal allograft transplantation and anterior cruciate ligament reconstruction. Am J Sports Med. 2003;31(6):896–906. https://doi.org/10.1177/03635465030310062701.
64. van der Wal RJP, Nieuwenhuijse MJ, Spek RWA, Thomassen BJW, van Arkel ERA, Nelissen R. Meniscal allograft transplantation in The Netherlands: long-term survival, patient-reported outcomes, and their association with preoperative complaints and interventions. Knee Surg Sports Traumatol Arthrosc. 2020;28(11):3551–60. https://doi.org/10.1007/s00167-020-06276-y.

Management of the Stiff ACL Reconstruction

19

Michael J. Sayegh, Colin Burgess, Franklin Paulino, and Nicholas A. Sgaglione

Case Presentation

An 18-year-old female who is a collegiate lacrosse player presented 3 days after injuring her right knee during a game in which she pivoted and felt a "pop" in her right knee. Physical examination revealed an antalgic gait and a right knee effusion with 10–75 degrees of range of motion (ROM). On presentation, 30 cubic centimeters (cc) of serosanguineous fluid was aspirated from the knee. Weight-bearing plain radiographs were noncontributory. The patient was referred for magnetic resonance imaging (MRI) and physical therapy to regain motion and begin strengthening and modalities to decrease pain and swelling. MRI revealed a complete mid-substance ACL tear and a tear of the posterior horn of the lateral meniscus (Fig. 19.1). There was no sprain/injury of the medial collateral ligament (MCL). Surgery was provisionally scheduled 19 days after her injury.

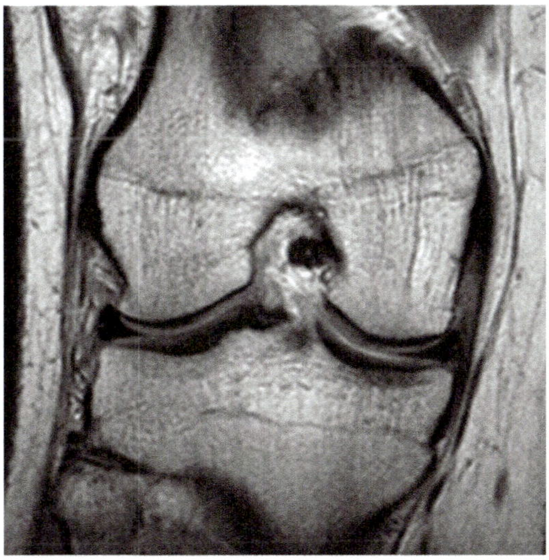

Fig. 19.1 Pre-operative MRI of presented case

The patient underwent a right knee arthroscopic-assisted ACL reconstruction with a bone-patellar tendon-bone autograft and meniscus repair 19 days after her injury. She tolerated the procedure well without complications and was prescribed hydrocodone/acetaminophen post-operatively. She was made partial weight-bearing in a hinged brace orthosis. Post-operative

M. J. Sayegh · F. Paulino
Department of Orthopaedic Surgery, Northwell Health System, Donald and Barbara Zucker School of Medicine at Hofstra/Northwell, Long Island Jewish Medical Center, New Hyde Park, NY, USA

C. Burgess
Department of Orthopaedic Surgery, Northwell Health System, Donald and Barbara Zucker School of Medicine at Hofstra/Northwell, Huntington Hospital, Huntington, NY, USA

N. A. Sgaglione (✉)
Department of Orthopaedic Surgery, Northwell Health System, Donald and Barbara Zucker School of Medicine at Hofstra/Northwell, Great Neck, NY, USA

M. J. Alaia, K. J. Jones (eds.), *Revision Anterior Cruciate Ligament Reconstruction*, https://doi.org/10.1007/978-3-030-96996-7_19

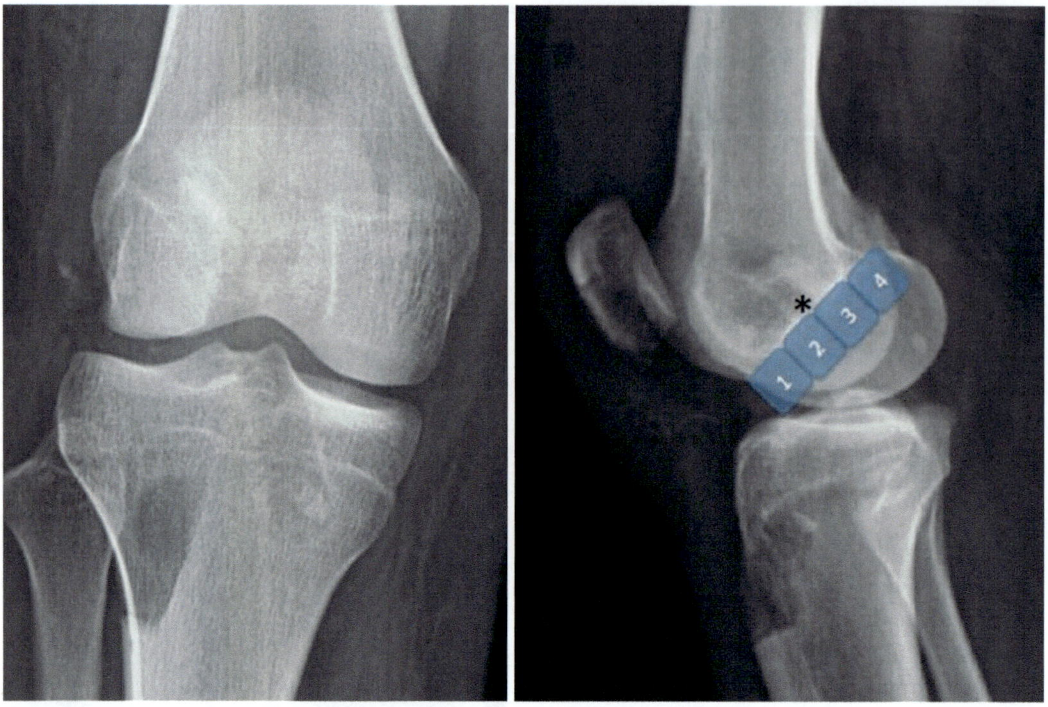

Fig. 19.2 Post-operative radiographs of presented case. The asterisk denotes the femoral tunnel position on the lateral view and illustration of radiographic quadrant method for identification of the anatomic site for femoral insertion of the graft during ACL reconstruction. It is noted that the femoral tunnel placement may be slightly anterior; however, the authors acknowledge that this is not a true lateral radiograph

radiographs were performed (Fig. 19.2). Upon evaluation of the radiographs, it was suggested that the femoral tunnel was placed slightly anterior to the normal anatomic site using the radiographic quadrant method [1]. She presented to the emergency department on post-operative day (POD) 3 with complaints that her pain was not under control. She was discharged home after workup revealed no evidence of infection or thromboembolic disorders.

The patient was seen on POD 12 without concerns, and an evaluation revealed an otherwise routine post-operative course. On POD 37, she complained that her knee was increasing in stiffness, and on exam her ROM was 15–75 degrees (Fig. 19.3). At this time, the patient was fitted for a dynamic-hinged brace that allowed dynamic progressive stretching, started on nonsteroidal anti-inflammatory drugs, and instructed to continue aggressive physical therapy. Possible arthroscopic adhesiolysis in the future was discussed. At 9 weeks post-operatively, the patient's ROM improved to 5–115 degrees after aggressive physical therapy. At 15 weeks post-operatively, the ROM of her right knee was 10–130 degrees compared to 0–155 degrees on

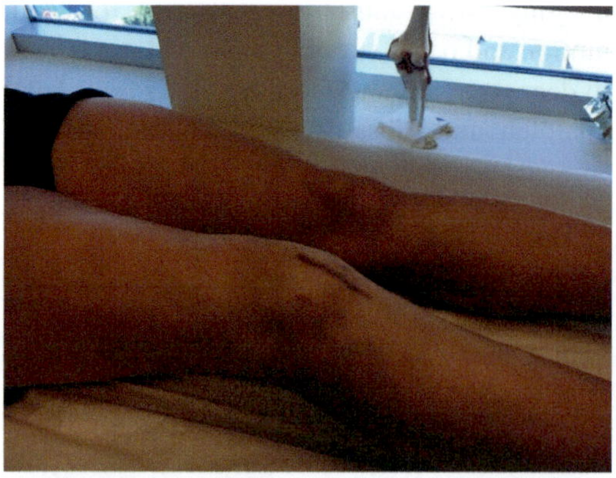

Fig. 19.3 Demonstrating lack of extension on POD 37 of presented case

the contralateral leg. She was instructed to continue aggressive physical therapy and to wear a static extension brace. At 17 weeks post-operatively, the patient's ROM was 10–135 degrees, and she continued aggressive physical therapy. At 21 weeks post-operatively, her ROM improved to 5–140 degrees and was able to achieve near full extension with physical therapy. The patient continued to participate in physical therapy.

The potential problems that may raise concern as to the patient's development of post-operative stiffness following ACL reconstruction include the following:

1. Pre-operative loss of extension
2. A short interval from time of injury to time of surgery (19 days)
3. Increased perioperative pain
4. A concomitant meniscus repair
5. A non-anatomical anterior femoral tunnel (Fig. 19.2)

This chapter addresses these potential problems associated with the presented case and appropriate treatment strategies.

Introduction

ACL injuries remain one of the most frequently injured ligaments that require surgery. With about 120,000–150,000 primary reconstructions being performed annually in the United States, the incidence of revisions will likely continue to increase [2, 3]. One of the primary goals of ACL reconstruction is to recreate native biomechanics of the knee while also restoring symmetric ROM [4]. Arthrofibrosis following primary ACL reconstruction is a well-defined complication with an incidence of 4–38% [5–8]. Patient-reported stiffness can be more common following revision ACL reconstruction when compared to primary ACL reconstruction [9]. Significant etiologic variability exists regarding the precise causes, ideal rehabilitation protocol, and optimal treatment. If not recognized, post-operative arthrofibrosis causing loss of motion can be more debilitating than an ACL-deficient knee [8]. Decreased knee ROM may lead to quadriceps atrophy, increased patellofemoral forces with loss of patellar mobility, patellar tendon shortening, and eventual articular cartilage damage [10–13]. Therefore, it is important to properly identify these patients early in the post-operative period to manage loss of motion appropriately.

Definition and Classification

Loss of motion remains one of the challenging complications faced by orthopedic surgeons following ACL reconstruction. While there is lack of clear evidence on the definition of arthrofibrosis, there is a consensus that arthrofibrosis requiring surgery is based upon a clinical limitation in knee ROM compared to the contralateral side that is symptomatic and refractory to non-operative treatment [8]. Arthrofibrosis has been previously defined as "abnormal proliferation of fibrous tissue in a joint with an unclear etiopathogenesis that leads to loss of motion, pain, muscle weakness, swelling, and functional limitation" [14]. Clinically it is identified as a loss of motion in comparison to the contralateral extremity [15]. Shelbourne et al. classified this loss of motion into four separate types. Type 1 is a <10 degree extension loss and normal flexion. Type 2 is a >10 degree extension loss and normal flexion. Type 3 is a >10 degree extension loss and >25 degree flexion loss with a tight patella. Type 4 is a >10 degree extension loss, 30 degrees or more flexion loss, and patella infera with marked patellar tightness [15]. A simpler classification of arthrofibrosis was proposed by Mayr et al., who defined it as abnormal scar tissue within at least one compartment that caused restricted ROM [16]. Asymmetric motion of the operative leg compared to the contralateral knee should be noted clinically and addressed appropriately.

Patients typically do not handle loss of extension as well as a flexion deficit [17]. A loss of 5° of extension can lead to abnormal forces in the knee joint. This can cause increased joint loading, quadriceps weakness, and patellofemoral pain [18]. A recent definition for loss of extension following

ACL reconstruction is a difference of greater than 5° loss of extension compared to the contralateral knee [10]. In addition, this seemingly minimal lack of motion can have long-term effects on patient outcomes. A study by Shelbourne et al. with 10-year follow-up found a loss of as low as 3° of knee extension leads to adverse results on both subjective and objective measurements [19]. These adverse outcomes were significantly greater in association with concurrent meniscal and/or articular cartilage procedures.

When evaluating a patient to determine their ROM after undergoing ACL reconstruction, another important consideration is whether the presentation is acute or chronic. Patients should be monitored closely in the acute post-operative period to ensure adequate rehabilitation and that motion is regained. Many rehabilitation programs consist of a combination of ROM and quad strengthening to prevent both weakness and ROM loss [10, 17, 20]. Despite the quantity of research regarding ACL reconstruction, there remains no definitive time period defining ROM loss post-operatively. Noll et al. of motion following ACL reconstruction at initial post-op visit up to 12 compared knee extension range weeks. They found a statistically significant correlation with loss of extension at 4 weeks post-op compared to 12 weeks [17]. Another study found that 48% of patients with a loss of extension at 4 weeks post-operatively eventually underwent an arthroscopic lysis of adhesions [10]. It is important for clinicians to identify an asymmetric ROM early in the rehabilitation phase (within 4 weeks) to ensure adequate motion is restored to prevent poor patient outcomes.

Risk Factors and Etiology

Risk factors for loss of ROM include pre-operative stiffness. One of the major focuses prior to undergoing ACL reconstruction is "prehab." Physical therapy is prescribed after injury but before surgery with a goal to regain similar side-to-side ROM prior to surgery. Patients who did not have full extension at the time of surgery were at a statistically significant higher risk for loss of extension after ACL reconstruction [10]. Having symmetric side-to-side ROM preoperatively is an important checkpoint for any patient undergoing ACL reconstruction.

Timing of ACL Reconstruction

Historically timing between initial injury and surgery has always been a debate. Previous studies have found a significant relationship in post-operative complications, including stiffness, in patients who undergo ACL reconstruction more acutely [10, 16, 21]. These studies found an increased risk for arthrofibrosis in patients who had surgery less than 3 weeks from time of injury. There is recent literature, however, showing that timing may not be a factor in the development of arthrofibrosis. Deabate et al. performed a meta-analysis of multiple randomized control trials, which showed ACL reconstruction within 3 weeks of injury had no influence on stiffness and other complications [22]. Another systematic review found similar results, with no difference in clinical outcomes in patients undergoing ACL reconstruction within 3 weeks of injury compared to delayed surgery [23]. Undergoing ACL reconstruction acutely may not have as much of an impact on stiffness post-operatively as previously believed.

Associated MCL Injury

Patients with an ACL injury requiring reconstruction that also have a MCL injury may be at higher risk of post-operative stiffness requiring surgery, regardless of whether the MCL injury is treated non-operatively or operatively [24]. In a prospective study, Noyes et al. showed that 22% of patients with MCL repair during ACL reconstruction lost ROM after surgery which was significant when compared with ACL reconstruction alone [25]. Patients should be counseled about post-operative stiffness and potential increased reoperation risks if there is an associated MCL injury in patients also undergoing ACL reconstruction. In addition, delaying ACL reconstruction until MCL healing occurs is an important consideration.

Graft Choice

Surgical reconstruction graft choice and harvest morbidity have a potential impact on post-operative ROM. While bone-patellar-tendon bone (BTBP) and hamstring tendon autografts remain the most popular autograft choices, others such as quadriceps tendon autografts and allografts such as Achilles tendons and tibialis anterior tendons are commonly used [26]. A prospective analysis comparing BTBP and hamstring autograft found no significant difference in outcomes related to stiffness [27]. They did, however, find a higher incidence of "cyclops" lesions in the hamstring group, although this had no statistically significant impact on ROM. In several studies, no significant differences have been found in post-operative ROM comparing bone-patellar-tendon bone and hamstring autograft [28, 29]. Huleatt et al. found a higher incidence rate of manipulation under anesthesia and/or lysis of adhesions in patients with a quadriceps tendon autograft compared to other graft types [30]. In the pediatric population, studies have bone bone-patellar-tendon bone tendons to have a higher incidence of stiffness compared to hamstring autograft [31]. Additionally, graft size may have an impact on arthrofibrosis following ACL reconstruction. Su et al. found a 3.2 times increase in odds of arthrofibrosis with an increase in graft diameter by 1 millimeter (mm) in their cohort of 1121 patients [32]. Graft choice and size can play a significant role in ROM-related outcomes following ACL reconstruction.

Concomitant Procedures

It is common for additional procedures to be performed concomitantly with ACL reconstruction. Often an ACL tear is associated with meniscal injury, articular cartilage damage, or other intra-/extra-articular ligament pathology. Huleatt et al. found an increased rate of arthrofibrosis in patients who underwent concomitant procedures at the time of ACL reconstruction [30]. They found an increase in incidence of manipulation under anesthesia (MUA) and lysis of adhesions (LOA) from 3.7% in isolated ACL reconstruction to 5.2% with additional procedures. A similar study found an increase of 1.8–8.0% compared to 0.3–0.5% in MUA/LOA in patients with multiple procedures done simultaneously compared to isolated ACL reconstruction, respectively [33]. Noyes et al. showed that in patients who underwent MCL repair during ACL reconstruction, there is an increased risk of arthrofibrosis [25]. Associated pathology that is addressed with ACL reconstruction clearly plays a role in motion restriction post-operatively.

Tunnel Position

Position of both femoral and tibial tunnels in ACL reconstruction is a critical part in the success of the operation. Restoring normal knee kinematics and biomechanics through an anatomic ACL footprint is a goal of every ACL reconstruction. Therefore, positioning the tunnels as close to their anatomic location as possible should be the objective for all surgeons. Intercondylar roof impingement is a leading cause of extension loss related to graft position post-ACL reconstruction [34, 35]. A tibial tunnel too anterior can lead to impingement on the intercondylar notch and loss of extension [35]. In addition, Maak et al. reviewed femoral tunnel position and its relationship to impingement [36]. They found that creating a femoral tunnel as close to the center of the ACL footprint had lower rates of impingement as opposed to higher and/or more anteromedial placement. A femoral tunnel placed too anterior may result in graft/notch impingement and result in loss of flexion and extension.

Impingement against the native PCL can also be a cause of post-operative stiffness. This can lead to a mechanical block in flexion. If the tibia tunnel is placed too posteriorly, the graft is more likely to impinge on the PCL during flexion [37].While this may lead to a mechanical block, it can also cause pain with flexion and secondarily lead to loss of motion in the rehabilitation period. This apparent proprioceptive pain can be caused by a vertical "high noon" femoral tunnel placement and lead to a reflex loss of extension [38]. Tunnel position during the index procedure remains a key factor in preventing stiffness after ACL reconstruction.

Other Risk Factors

Other clinical factors have been shown to lead to arthrofibrosis in the post-operative ACL reconstruction period. Post-operative infection remains a relatively less common but potentially devastating complication following ACL reconstruction. The incidence of infection after ACL surgery is reported to be less than 1% [39]. Infection and/or hematoma was found to be an independent risk of stiffness following ACL reconstruction [30]. As seen with risk for initial ACL tear, females are also seemingly at increased risk for developing arthrofibrosis following reconstruction [30]. Additionally, it has been suggested that patients below the age of 18 also are associated with higher rates of stiffness in the post-operative period [30]. Tourniquet use may also have an influence on post-operative ROM. A recent study found increased tourniquet time to have an increased risk of return to the operating room for motion loss following ACL reconstruction [11].

Non-operative Management

Aggressive non-operative management of stiffness following ACL reconstruction is critical, and therefore early diagnosis is essential in the post-operative period. There should be an immediate focus on adequate pain control that starts at surgery with a planned pre-emptive multi-modal protocol. A supervised physical therapy program beginning on post-operative day 1 is important to ensure adequate early motion and stretching. Static or dynamic splinting methods may be helpful as an adjunct, and there may be a role in oral corticosteroids and/or biologics in the post-operative period to prevent stiffness.

Pain Control

Non-operative treatment during the post-operative period after ACL reconstruction must be aimed at addressing the etiology for the individual patient. The fear of movement, or kinesiophobia, and pain catastrophizing are associated with decreased return to sport [40]. For stiff kinesiophobic patients, providers must ensure pain is properly controlled to facilitate adequate participation in physiotherapy in order to prevent stiffness. Pain therapy must be directed at achieving maximum therapeutic benefit while minimizing systemic side effects. In the author's experience, a single shot of intra-articular bupivacaine has been effective in treating immediate post-operative pain. Regional nerve blocks, specifically adductor canal blocks and femoral nerve blocks, are also frequently used in the management of pain in the immediate post-operative period. Abdallah et al. showed that adductor canal blocks and femoral nerve blocks are equally effective in treating pain; however, adductor canal blocks result in greater quadriceps strength which is essential for active participation in physical therapy [41]. It is also in the author's experience that use of IV acetaminophen and intra-articular injection of ketorolac are effective at treating pain associated with stiffness.

Physical Therapy

The primary goal of early physical therapy is to prevent joint stiffness and potential arthrofibrosis. Most surgeons initiate formal supervised therapy 1–10 days after ACL reconstruction. Patients are instructed to use crutches for ambulation with weight-bearing as tolerated. Many surgeons prefer the use of a post-operative knee brace. Ice is essential to manage swelling and pain. Ideally patients will obtain full active and passive ROM by 2 weeks post-operatively. Patient education is essential as home exercises are a key component of successful therapy. Special consideration should be paid to dosage of exercises with respect to frequency, duration, and intensity. Lack of progress signifies that a patient might require an increase in dose of physical therapy. In contrast worsening pain, loss of ROM, and swelling could demonstrate a need to decrease dosing of physical therapy. Bracing and in certain cases casting may serve as augments to physical therapy in patients with stiffness refractory to conventional physical therapy.

Casting and Dynamic Splinting

Serial casting and drop-out casting have been utilized as a non-operative treatment for arthrofibrosis following ACL reconstruction, although limited results have been reported only by case series [8, 15, 42–45]. This method of static splinting is explained by the theory of low-load long-duration stretching to improve knee extension in patients that do not respond to standard physical therapy interventions. Biologically, there is an increase in remodeling of periarticular connective tissue in response to stretch and stress relaxation through elongation [46]. Potential benefits of drop-out casting compared to serial casting are that it is less cumbersome and it provides the option of removing the cast to perform other functional activities [42]. In a systematic review of 13 patients treated by drop-out casting, there was a 6.2-degree improvement in extension which as a treatment option provided the greatest improvement of extension loss [8]. Casting has also been proposed to be significantly more cost-effective than dynamic splinting as a means of stretching to improve terminal extension [42].

Although dynamic splinting devices have been most frequently been described in the arthroplasty literature with varied success, there may be a role in patients with arthrofibrosis following ACL reconstruction [47]. Dynamic splinting capitalizes upon the "creep" mechanical property of tissue. By applying a constant force, typically through a spring-loaded coil, these splints gradually stretch tissue [48]. In the pediatric population, Pace et al. demonstrated in their retrospective study that there was an 84% improvement in knee ROM with dynamic splinting in patients with arthrofibrosis following ACL reconstruction or meniscal repair [49]. Additionally, 58% of these patients avoided the need for surgery.

Anti-Inflammatory Agents

Post-operative inflammation contributes to stiffness and the struggle to regain full ROM post-operative. Short-term low-dose oral corticosteroids are a viable option for non-surgical management of loss of ROM after ACL reconstruction. Rue et al. conducted a study to evaluate the effectiveness of treatment with a short course of tapered methylprednisolone in the early post-operative period for loss of flexion [50]. Their study included 252 patients who underwent primary ACL reconstruction of which 28 (11%) had early post-operative loss of ROM. Mean flexion deficit in these patients was of 31 degrees compared to contralateral side. The oral corticosteroid was initiated at an average of 6 weeks. Patients demonstrated a mean improvement of 29.2 degrees. Treatment with oral corticosteroids utilizing a short course of tapered methylprednisolone was correlated with a return to normal ROM in 78% of patients with early post-operative loss of flexion after ACL reconstruction. There were no associated complications or associated decrease in knee stability as measured using objective stability measurements.

Intra-articular injection of anakinra, an interleukin-1 (IL-1) receptor antagonist, presents another viable option to reduce post-operative inflammation. Interleukin-1 is a key mediator of the inflammatory response and the maintenance of chronic inflammation. In a retrospective trial by Brown et al., they hypothesized that intra-articular anakinra would lead to sustained attenuation of chronic refractory arthrofibrosis and limited arthrofibrosis of the knee [51]. They reviewed eight patients who were injected with 200 mg of intra-articular anakinra. Six of these patients returned to prior activity levels and reported improvement in pain levels. Additionally, four of these patients reported an improvement in ROM between 20 and 45 degrees.

Operative Management

Aggressive management for the stiff knee following ACL reconstruction with arthroscopy, adhesiolysis +/− scar excision and/or notchplasty, and MUA has consistently been a gold standard in the operative management. Shelbourne et al. defined a classification system based on loss of motion compared to the contralateral knee, which has since guided surgeons in the evaluation and treatment of arthrofibrosis [15]. Mayr et al. defined arthrofibrosis following ACL reconstruction as scar tissue within the knee that limited ROM [16]. There is a general consensus that arthrofibrosis requiring surgery is based upon a clinical limitation in knee ROM compared to the contralateral side that is symptomatic, persistent, and refractory to aggressive non-operative treatment [8].

Surgical Indications

Surgical indications include a loss of extension or asymmetric terminal flexion in a patient that has failed to improve with non-operative treatments. The etiology as to why stiffness has occurred must first be identified. Reasons may include primary arthrofibrosis, pain syndromes (such as complex regional pain syndrome), post-operative infection (especially within the first month), other associated ligamentous injuries, suboptimal post-operative rehabilitation (which may include inadequate patient compliance), tunnel malposition, and/or prior surgery.

Classically, timing for operative management of arthrofibrosis is within 3 months post-operatively and with a failure to progress during rehabilitation. This timing is based upon the clinical observation that the knee should be beyond the inflammatory state and that there must be a strengthening of the quadriceps muscles before proceeding with surgery [45].

Tunnel malposition rather than arthrofibrosis may be a cause of stiffness following ACL reconstruction. If the tunnel is anterior on the femur, the graft may impinge in extension and/or be stretched in flexion. If the tunnel is posterior on the femur, there will be laxity in flexion. If the tunnel is anterior on the tibia, there may also be graft impingement in extension. Lastly, as commonly seen in vertical tunnels, if the tunnel is placed posteriorly on the tibia, it will be stretched in extension, there will be laxity in flexion, and the graft may impinge on the posterior cruciate ligament (PCL). Careful analysis of the patient's anatomy and tunnel placement is therefore very important, and using computed tomography if needed to identify this may be necessary.

Surgical Management

Arthroscopic adhesiolysis is the most common technique used today; however, open or combined open and arthroscopic procedures may be necessary. Paulos et al. described an open technique for infrapatellar contracture syndrome which involves intra-articular and extra-articular release of lateral retinacular, hypertrophied fat pad, and the lateral and medial patellomeniscal ligaments [45]. Combined arthroscopic and open techniques have been described in which adhesions are lysed arthroscopically in the suprapatellar pouch, medial and lateral gutters, and intercondylar notch. If necessary, open releases of anterior extra-articular scar tissue and posterolateral and posteromedial capsule releases may be performed [52]. In addition to the need of open releases in cases of severe arthrofibrosis, there are instances that tibial tubercle osteotomy and fixation proximally may be necessary with patella baja [45].

Today, most surgeons describe arthroscopic adhesiolysis combined with MUA as the most common surgical treatment for arthrofibrosis following ACL reconstruction (Fig. 19.4). *Author's (NAS) preferred surgical treatment*: A standard knee arthroscopy setup with a lateral post and tourniquet is used. A regional nerve block either femoral nerve or adductor canal block is performed, and a careful exam under anesthesia is utilized to better measure the patient's knee ROM which may have been limited by pain in the office. A well-padded thigh tourniquet is commonly utilized and then deflated following completion of all releases to ensure adequate hemostasis and to avoid postoperative hematomas. Diagnostic arthroscopy using a powered fluid irrigation pump is then performed followed by MUA as needed with the purpose of limiting chondrolysis. Then, intra-articular adhesions are lysed using a proprietary controlled radiofrequency temperature – monitored ablation in the suprapatellar pouch, medial and lateral gutters,

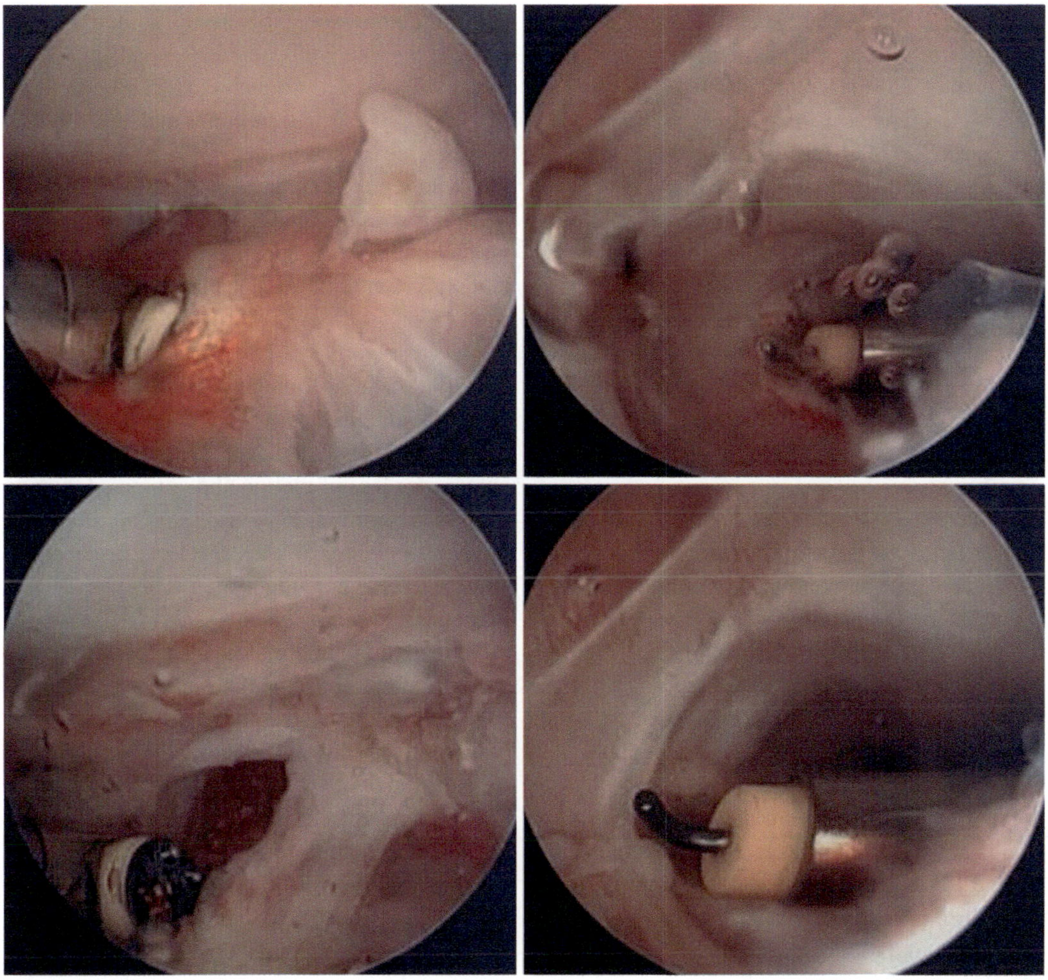

Fig. 19.4 Arthroscopic adhesiolysis for arthrofibrosis following ACL reconstruction

and intercondylar notch (Fig. 19.4). Accessory portals may also be utilized. Following precise intra-articular arthroscopic adhesiolysis, arthroscopic retinacular releases are performed under direct visualization, particularly if peripatellar fibrosis is pronounced. A MUA may then be gently performed which is often successful at gaining adequate extension and flexion. If there is lack of terminal extension, scar excisions, posterior capsular releases, and/or bony notchplasty may be also required. Open techniques may be utilized at this point if arthroscopic releases are found to be inadequate, but that is less commonly needed.

Shelbourne et al. described arthroscopic methods based on their classification system which may be helpful in guiding surgeons [15]. With the goal of achieving full extension, the hypertrophied "cyclops" lesion can be removed from the base of the ACL, anterior intra-synovial and extra-synovial scar tissue can be resected, and the graft may be "debrided." Also, a notchplasty and/or fibrotic capsule excision up to the vastus medialis and lateralis insertion to free the patella and patellar tendon completely may be required. MUA is again used after scar resection to achieve as much flexion as possible.

Lastly, during arthroscopic evaluation, revision ACL reconstruction may be considered at the index adhesiolysis or as a staged procedure if the graft is malpositioned. However, preoperative workup, computerized tomography scan evaluation, and confirmation of non-anatomic graft positioning in addition to patient counseling are essential. Anterior fibers may also be resected with an anterolateral notchplasty at the time of arthroscopic adhesiolysis. It is the author's preference to perform a revision ACL reconstruction in a staged fashion if the graft is noted to be non-anatomic as a cause of stiffness and all else fails. This allows the patient to pursue post-operative rehabilitation after arthroscopic adhesiolysis with appropriate patient counseling. It is important to set realistic patient expectations.

Post-Operative Rehabilitation

Post-operatively, bracing and an immediate rehabilitation program are required to ensure success. This includes an emphasis on achieving adequate extension before aggressive measures are taken to improve flexion. This requires patient compliance and diligence with aggressive post-operative protocols. It is the author's preference to more recently not routinely use continuous passive motion (CPM) machines and to selectively use dynamic splinting only in cases where full extension is not achieved after arthroscopic adhesiolysis and MUA. To limit pain and swelling in the immediate post-operative period, regional anesthesia and intra-articular ketorolac, as well as cryotherapy compression cuffs, are routinely utilized. An opioid-limited, multimodal pain control regimen is prescribed including acetaminophen and nonsteroidal anti-inflammatory drugs (NSAIDs). More recently, we have had success with current pain management methodologies and the above protocol and have not found it necessary to routinely admit the patient overnight for epidural analgesia and continuous passive motion, given the desire to discharge the patient home on the same day as surgery and with adequate pain control.

Outcomes

Surgery generally can lead to a significant improvement in ROM post-operatively according to a recent systematic review [8]. The surgical outcomes of arthroscopic adhesiolysis reported by Shelbourne et al. were adequate, and patients showed improvements in ROM, mean stiffness, self-evaluation, functional activity, and Noyes knee scores [15]. Dodds et al. were the first who reported significant improvements both flexion and extension in 86% of patients treated with MUA who had persistent flexion or extension deficits after intra-articular ACL reconstructions [53].

Recent reports indicate that arthroscopic surgery for stiffness following ACL reconstruction does not affect patient function at 2-year follow-up. Worsham et al. reviewed 29 patients requiring surgery for loss of motion and compared them to matched controls [11]. They found no difference in time to release to play, level of participation, and subjective function scores. This was despite higher International Knee Disability Committee (IKDC) scores and single-legged hop testing in the control group, although not significant. This may be important as other authors found that patients following ACL reconstruction who had post-operative stiffness had significantly lower IKDC scores than those with normal ROM [54].

Regarding appropriate timing of operative intervention for arthrofibrosis, a recent study by Mayr et al. found that patients who underwent arthrolysis greater than 1 year after ACL reconstruction had more severe osteoarthritis and a lower IKDC score compared to those who underwent arthrolysis within 1 year [12]. This further emphasizes the importance of early diagnosis and aggressive management.

Conclusion

The keys to preemptive management for stiffness following ACL reconstruction include early diagnosis of loss of motion post-operatively with a defined etiology, aggressive non-operative treatments and surgical intervention with arthroscopic adhesiolysis, and MUA for failure of improvement after 3 months. Prevention of arthrofibrosis is critical, and we must educate patients, prescribe early motion, and work closely with physical therapists to improve perioperative rehabilitation. As surgeons, we also must improve surgical techniques which include reducing harvest morbidity and optimizing anatomic tunnel placement.

References

1. Bernard M, Hertel P, Hornung H, Cierpinski T. Femoral insertion of the ACL. Radiographic quadrant method. Am J Knee Surg. 1997;10:12–4.
2. Mall NA, Chalmers PN, Moric M, Tanaka MJ, Cole BJ, Bach BR, Paletta GA. Incidence and trends of anterior cruciate ligament reconstruction in the United States. Am J Sports Med. 2014;42:2363–70.
3. Kraeutler MJ, Welton KL, McCarty EC, Bravman JT. Revision anterior cruciate ligament reconstruction. J Bone Jt Surg Am Vol. 2017;99:1689–96.
4. Eckenrode BJ, Carey JL, Sennett BJ, Zgonis MH. Prevention and management of post-operative complications following ACL reconstruction. Curr Rev Musculoskelet Med. 2017;10:315–21.
5. Whitehead TS. Failure of anterior cruciate ligament reconstruction. Clin Sports Med. 2013;32:177–204.
6. Petsche TS, Hutchinson MR. Loss of extension after reconstruction of the anterior cruciate ligament. J Am Acad Orthop Surg. 1999;7:119–27.
7. Kartus J, Magnusson L, Stener S, Brandsson S, Eriksson BI, Karlsson J. Complications following arthroscopic anterior cruciate ligament reconstruction. Knee Surg Sports Traumatol Arthrosc. 1999;7:2–8.
8. Ekhtiari S, Horner NS, de Sa D, Simunovic N, Hirschmann MT, Ogilvie R, Berardelli RL, Whelan DB, Ayeni OR. Arthrofibrosis after ACL reconstruction is best treated in a step-wise approach with early recognition and intervention: a systematic review. Knee Surg Sports Traumatol Arthrosc. 2017;25:3929–37.
9. Lefevre N, Klouche S, Mirouse G, Herman S, Gerometta A, Bohu Y. Return to sport after primary and revision anterior cruciate ligament reconstruction. Am J Sports Med. 2017;45:34–41.
10. Mauro CS, Irrgang JJ, Williams BA, Harner CD. Loss of extension following anterior cruciate ligament reconstruction: analysis of incidence and etiology using IKDC criteria. Arthrosc J Arthrosc Relat Surg. 2008;24:146–53.
11. Worsham J, Lowe WR, Copa D, Williams S, Kleihege J, Lauck K, Mascarenhas R, Bailey L. Subsequent surgery for loss of motion after anterior cruciate ligament reconstruction does not influence function at 2 years: a matched case-control analysis. Am J Sports Med. 2019;47:2550–6.
12. Mayr HO, Brandt CM, Weig T, Koehne M, Bernstein A, Suedkamp NP, Hube R, Stoehr A. Long-term results of arthroscopic arthrolysis for arthrofibrosis after anterior cruciate ligament reconstruction. Arthrosc J Arthrosc Relat Surg. 2017;33:408–14.
13. Widuchowski W, Widuchowska M, Ko Czy B, Dragan S, Czamara A, Tomaszewski W, Widuchowski J. Femoral press-fit fixation in ACL reconstruction using bone-patellar tendon-bone autograft: results at 15years follow-up. BMC Musculoskelet Disord. 2012;13:1–8.
14. Magit D, Wolff A, Sutton K, Medvecky MJ. Arthrofibrosis of the knee. J Am Acad Orthop Surg. 2007;15:682–94.
15. Shelbourne KD, Patel DV, Martini DJ. Classification and management of arthrofibrosis of the knee after anterior cruciate ligament reconstruction. Am J Sports Med. 1996;24:857–62.
16. Mayr HO, Weig TG, Plitz W. Arthrofibrosis following ACL reconstruction - reasons and outcome. Arch Orthop Trauma Surg. 2004;124:518–22.
17. Noll S, Craig Garrison J, Bothwell J, Conway JE. Knee extension range of motion at 4 weeks is related to knee extension loss at 12 weeks after anterior cruciate ligament reconstruction. Orthop J Sports Med. 2015;3:1–6.
18. Perry J, Antonelli D, Ford W. Analysis of knee-joint forces during flexed-knee stance. J Bone Joint Surg Am. 1975;57:961–7.
19. Shelbourne KD, Gray T. Minimum 10-year results after anterior cruciate ligament reconstruction: how the loss of normal knee motion compounds other factors related to the development of osteoarthritis after surgery. Am J Sports Med. 2009;37:471–80.
20. Ektas N, Scholes C, Kulaga S, Kirwan G, Lee B, Bell C. Recovery of knee extension and incidence of extension deficits following anterior cruciate ligament injury and treatment: a systematic review protocol. J Orthop Surg Res. 2019;14:1–7.
21. Shelbourne KD, Wilckens JH, Mollabashy A, Decarlo M. Arthrofibrosis in acute anterior cruciate ligament reconstruction: the effect of timing of reconstruction and rehabilitation. Am J Sports Med. 1991;19:332–6.
22. Deabate L, Previtali D, Grassi A, Filardo G, Candrian C, Delcogliano M. Anterior cruciate ligament reconstruction within 3 weeks does not increase stiffness and complications compared with delayed reconstruction: a meta-analysis of randomized controlled trials. Am J Sports Med. 2019:48:1–10.
23. Smith TO, Davies L, Hing CB. Early versus delayed surgery for anterior cruciate ligament reconstruction: a systematic review and meta-analysis. Knee Surg Sports Traumatol Arthrosc. 2010;18:304–11.
24. Westermann RW, Spindler KP, Huston LJ, et al. Outcomes of grade III medial collateral ligament injuries treated concurrently with anterior cruciate ligament reconstruction: a multicenter study. Arthrosc J Arthrosc Relat Surg. 2019;35:1466–72.
25. Noyes FR, Berrios-Torres S, Barber-Westin SD, Heckmann TP. Prevention of permanent arthrofibrosis after anterior cruciate ligament reconstruction alone or combined with associated procedures: a prospective study in 443 knees. Knee Surg Sports Traumatol Arthrosc. 2000;8:196–206.

26. Richmond JC. Anterior cruciate ligament reconstruction. Sports Med Arthrosc. 2018;26:165–7.
27. Rousseau R, Labruyere C, Kajetanek C, Deschamps O, Makridis KG, Djian P. Complications after anterior cruciate ligament reconstruction and their relation to the type of graft: a prospective study of 958 cases. Am J Sports Med. 2019;47:2543–9.
28. Spindler KP, Wright RW. Clinical practice. Anterior cruciate ligament tear. N Engl J Med. 2008;359:2135–42.
29. Sajovic M, Stropnik D, Skaza K. Long-term comparison of semitendinosus and gracilis tendon versus patellar tendon autografts for anterior cruciate ligament reconstruction: a 17-year follow-up of a randomized controlled trial. Am J Sports Med. 2018;46:1800–8.
30. Huleatt J, Gottschalk M, Fraser K, Boden A, Dalwadi P, Xerogeanes J, Hammond K. Risk factors for manipulation under anesthesia and/or lysis of adhesions after anterior cruciate ligament reconstruction. Orthop J Sports Med. 2018;6:1–7.
31. Nwachukwu BU, McFeely ED, Nasreddine A, Udall JH, Finlayson C, Shearer DW, Micheli LJ, Kocher MS. Arthrofibrosis after anterior cruciate ligament reconstruction in children and adolescents. J Pediatr Orthop. 2011;31:811–7.
32. Su AW, Storey EP, Lin SC, Forst B, Lawrence JT, Ganley TJ, Wells L. Association of the graft size and arthrofibrosis in young patients after primary anterior cruciate ligament reconstruction. J Am Acad Orthop Surg. 2018;26:e483–9.
33. Werner BC, Cancienne JM, Miller MD, Gwathmey FW. Incidence of manipulation under anesthesia or lysis of adhesions after arthroscopic knee surgery. Am J Sports Med. 2015;43:1656–61.
34. Howell SM, Taylor MA. Failure of reconstruction of the anterior cruciate ligament due to impingement by the intercondylar roof. J Bone Jt Surg Ser A. 1993;75:1044–55.
35. Iriuchishima T, Shirakura K, Fu FH. Graft impingement in anterior cruciate ligament reconstruction. Knee Surg Sports Traumatol Arthrosc. 2013;21:664–70.
36. Maak TG, Bedi A, Raphael BS, Citak M, Suero EM, Wickiewicz T, Pearle AD. Effect of femoral socket position on graft impingement after anterior cruciate ligament reconstruction. Am J Sports Med. 2011;39:1018–23.
37. Astur DC, Santos CV, Aleluia V, Astur Neto N, Arliani GG, Kaleka CC, Skaf A, Cohen M. Characterization of cruciate ligament impingement: the influence of femoral or tibial tunnel positioning at different degrees of knee flexion. Arthrosc J Arthrosc Relat Surg. 2013;29:913–9.
38. Strobel MJ, Castillo RJ, Weiler A. Reflex extension loss after anterior cruciate ligament reconstruction due to femoral "high noon" graft placement. Arthroscopy. 2001;17:408–11.
39. Cvetanovich GL, Chalmers PN, Verma NN, Cole BJ, Bach BR. Risk factors for short-term complications of anterior cruciate ligament reconstruction in the United States. Am J Sports Med. 2016;44:618–24.
40. Hartigan EH, Lynch AD, Logerstedt DS, Chmielewski TL, Snyder-Mackler L. Kinesiophobia after anterior cruciate ligament rupture and reconstruction: noncopers versus potential copers. J Orthop Sports Phys Ther. 2013;43:821–32.
41. Abdallah FW, Whelan DB, Chan VW, Prasad GA, Endersby RV, Theodoropolous J, Oldfield S, Oh J, Brull R. Adductor Canal Block Provides Noninferior Analgesia and Superior Quadriceps Strength Compared with Femoral Nerve Block in Anterior Cruciate Ligament Reconstruction. Anaesthesiology. 2016:124:1053–64.
42. Logerstedt D, Sennett BJ. Case series utilizing drop-out casting for the treatment of knee joint extension motion loss following anterior cruciate ligament reconstruction. J Orthop Sports Phys Ther. 2007;37:404–11.
43. Shelbourne KD, Patel DV. Treatment of limited motion after anterior cruciate ligament reconstruction. Knee Surg Sports Traumatol Arthrosc. 1999;7:85–92.
44. Shelbourne KD, Johnson GE. Outpatient surgical management of arthrofibrosis after anterior cruciate ligament surgery. Am J Sports Med. 1994;22:192–7.
45. Paulos LE, Wnorowski DC, Greenwald AE. Infrapatellar contracture syndrome. Am J Sports Med. 1994;22:440–9.
46. Flowers KR. A proposed decision hierarchy for splinting the stiff joint, with an emphasis on force application parameters. J Hand Ther. 2002;15:158–62.
47. Bonutti PM, McGrath MS, Ulrich SD, McKenzie SA, Seyler TM, Mont MA. Static progressive stretch for the treatment of knee stiffness. Knee. 2008;15:272–6.
48. Glasgow C, Tooth LR, Fleming J, Peters S. Dynamic splinting for the stiff hand after trauma: predictors of contracture resolution. J Hand Ther. 2011;24:195–206.
49. Pace JL, Nasreddine AY, Simoni M, Zurakowski D, Kocher MS. Dynamic splinting in children and adolescents with stiffness after knee surgery. J Pediatr Orthop. 2016;38:38–43.
50. Rue JPH, Ferry AT, Lewis PB, Bach BR. Oral corticosteroid use for loss of flexion after primary anterior cruciate ligament reconstruction. Arthrosc J Arthrosc Relat Surg. 2008;24:554–9.
51. Brown CA, Toth AP, Magnussen B. Clinical benefits of intra-articular anakinra for arthrofibrosis. Orthopedics. 2010;33:877.
52. Cosgarea AJ, DeHaven KE, Lovelock JE. The surgical treatment of arthrofibrosis of the knee. Am J Sports Med. 1994;22:184–91.
53. Dodds JA, Keene JS, Graf BK, Lange RH. Results of knee manipulations after anterior cruciate ligament reconstructions. Am J Sports Med. 1991;19:283–7.
54. Biggs-Kinzer A, Murphy B, Shelbourne KD, Urch S. Perioperative rehabilitation using a knee extension device and arthroscopic debridement in the treatment of arthrofibrosis. Sports Health. 2010;2:417–23.

Surgical Management of the Failed Pediatric ACL Reconstruction

20

Cordelia W. Carter and Philip L. Wilson

Introduction

The "epidemic" of anterior cruciate ligament (ACL) injuries in young athletes has prompted a wealth of research dedicated to ACL injury prevention, to the development and study of pediatric-friendly surgical techniques for ligament reconstruction, and to rehabilitation and return to sport protocols that successfully get children and adolescents back to athletic participation. A significant part of the scientific discussion of pediatric ACL injury centers around surgical techniques that spare the physis of a still-growing child. However, while growth disturbances related to ACL reconstruction (ACL-R) are a reported complication, perhaps the most common complication of ACL-R in the young athletic population is re-injury, with rates of ACL graft rupture reported to be as high as 19% for patients under 18 years [1]. When ACL re-injury occurs, the patient is typically still young and active with aspirations to return once again to high levels of physical activity and frequently to competitive sports. In the United States, revision ACL-R remains the standard of care for returning young athletes who sustain ACL graft ruptures to play. Just as with adult ACL graft tears, it is important to understand the key factors underlying failure of the primary reconstruction and to address each systematically in the revision setting. In addition, understanding a young athlete's unique anatomy, physeal status, and cognitive/behavioral stage of development is essential for optimizing chances of return to sport and remaining injury-free following revision ACL-R.

C. W. Carter (✉)
Department of Orthopedic Surgery, Division of Sports Medicine, NYU Langone Health, New York, NY, USA

P. L. Wilson
Department of Orthopedic Surgery, Scottish Rite for Children, University of Texas Southwestern Medical Center, Frisco, TX, USA

Assessment of the Pediatric Patient with a Failed ACL-R

Factors Contributing to ACL Graft Tear

There are myriad reasons why primary ACL-R fails in children and adolescents, and a thorough assessment of the factors contributing to an individual young athlete's risk of ACL injury and re-injury is critical for planning revision reconstruction. Underlying reasons for graft failure may be patient-specific (e.g., diffuse ligamentous laxity or an elevated posterior tibial slope [2, 3]); surgery-specific (e.g., allograft used for reconstruction [4]); or situation-specific (e.g., the athlete returned to a cutting/pivoting sport or

M. J. Alaia, K. J. Jones (eds.), *Revision Anterior Cruciate Ligament Reconstruction*,
https://doi.org/10.1007/978-3-030-96996-7_20

Table 20.1 Factors contributing to failure of a primary ACL-R in children and adolescents

Patient-specific	
Anatomic	Diffuse ligamentous laxity Valgus knee deformity Elevated posterior tibial slope Notch stenosis

Other	Young age
	Female sex
	Psychological factors
	  Kinesiophobia
	  Impaired psychological readiness
	Developmental level
	  Childhood (does not remember to comply with restrictions)
	  Adolescence (does not choose to comply with restrictions)

Surgery-specific	

	Allograft use
	Tunnel placement
	  Non-anatomic tunnels
	  Over-verticalized tunnels

Situation-specific	
	Return to cutting/pivoting sport Earlier return to sport

did not comply with rehab guidelines [5]). Additionally, recent studies have demonstrated an increased risk of ACL graft tear for patients who have higher levels of self-reported kinesiophobia at the time of return to sport following primary reconstruction [6, 7]. A factor that may play a particular role in re-injury for young athletes is their developmental level: adolescence is characterized by impulsive, risk-taking behavior and an inability to consider consequences of actions taken. Table 20.1 provides a list of potential factors contributing to ACL re-injury in this population.

Common Primary Pediatric ACL-R Techniques

Unlike revision ACL-R in adult patients, pediatric athletes who sustain ACL graft tears will frequently have undergone a primary surgical reconstruction using a physeal-sparing and/or physeal-respecting technique, and a working knowledge of each is useful. There are two principal methods of physeal-sparing ACL-R. The first is commonly called the "ITB," the "Micheli," or the "modified MacIntosh" technique and is unique in that no tunnels are created. In this technique, the central aspect of the child's iliotibial band (ITB) is used for graft. During graft harvest, the desired width of ITB is detached proximally and left attached to Gerdy's tubercle distally. Using a combination of open and arthroscopic incisions, the graft is looped over the posterior femur in the "over-the-top" position and secured to the periosteum over the posterolateral distal femur with sutures. The free end is then brought into the knee where it recreates the bicruciate appearance of the native ACL. Lastly, the graft is shuttled under the intermeniscal ligament anteriorly and secured with sutures to the periosteum of the proximal medial tibial metaphysis [8]. A recent study reporting long-term outcomes of this technique performed in 237 patients with an average age of 11.2 years found a 6.6% rate of retear at an average follow-up of 6.2 years without any significant growth disturbance noted [9].

The second physeal-sparing technique for ACL reconstruction in skeletally immature patients does require tunnel drilling, but unlike a standard ACL-R performed in older adolescents and adults, the tunnels created are all-epiphyseal and thus theoretically spare the growth plate [10]. This nontraditional tunnel placement may pose a particular challenge in the revision setting, which is further discussed below. The largest reported series to date of all-epiphyseal ACL-R retrospectively evaluated 103 patients who had undergone this procedure at an average age of 12.1 years. The rate of re-tear for this technique was found to be 10.7% at a mean of 21 months following surgery, with <1% noted to have significant growth disturbance [11].

Physeal-sparing ACL-R techniques are typically reserved for patients who have a significant amount of growth remaining, as predicted from bone age films, Tanner staging, and (in females) menarchal status. For young adolescents who have some growth remaining but are not completely skeletally immature, a hybrid technique (e.g., avoiding the femoral physis and drilling through the tibial physis) or trans-physeal reconstruction may be performed in which "physeal-respecting" strategies are employed. The goal of the latter is to perform an ACL-R that uses osseous tunnels drilled across the physis to simulate an adult-type reconstruction but seeks to minimize the risk of iatrogenic physeal injury. Physeal-respecting considerations include use of soft tissue graft, cautious dissection near the perichondrial ring of LaCroix, avoidance of overtensioning of the graft, and use of metaphyseal methods of graft fixation. Verticalizing the tunnels has been shown to decrease volumetric injury to the growth plate and is therefore another method by which the risk of iatrogenic growth disturbance may be mitigated [12]; however, tunnels are drilled more vertically than those for a standard adult-type ACL risk loss of rotational control and may require revision in the setting of graft tear.

Suggested Checklist for Preoperative Planning

As outlined above, understanding the patient-specific, surgery-specific, and situation-specific factors contributing to a pediatric patient's failed primary ACL-R is essential for planning surgical revision. Additionally, a thorough preoperative evaluation should include an assessment of (1) skeletal maturity; (2) bony alignment; (3) prior surgical technique used including graft and any tunnels created; and (4) concomitant injuries of the meniscus, cartilage, posterior cruciate and collateral ligaments, and posterolateral and posteromedial corners of the knee. A suggested checklist for the preoperative assessment of the pediatric patient with a failed ACL-R is found in Table 20.2.

Table 20.2 Recommended checklist for preoperative assessment of the young athlete with a prior, failed ACL-R

Is the patient still skeletally immature?	
Info needed:	Chronologic age Bone age Menarchal status (for females)
Is bony alignment contributing to the risk of ACL injury?	
Info needed:	Standing coronal alignment film To assess valgus/varus deformity Sagittal imaging (plain radiographs or magnetic resonance imaging (MRI)) To assess tibial slope Physeal imaging (plain radiographs, MRI, and/or computed tomography (CT)) To assess for growth arrest ***if yes***: Can guided growth techniques be employed? E.g., hemiepiphysiodesis, epiphysiodesis, and/or bar resection Is osteotomy required to improve alignment?
Were tunnels previously created?	
Info needed:	Operative report Diagnostic imaging (plain radiographs, MRI, and/or (CT) ***if yes***: Are the tunnels anatomically placed? Are the tunnels useable? Is osteolysis present? Are tunnel angles too acute? Are tunnels too vertical?
What graft was previously used and what grafts are still available?	
Info needed:	Operative report Physical examination ***Considerations:*** Autograft preferred Bone plugs should not be placed across open physes
Are untreated or inadequately treated concomitant injuries present?	
Info needed:	History Physical examination Diagnostic imaging (plain radiographs, MRI, and/or (CT) ***if yes***: Additional injuries should be treated as part of single or staged revision

Surgical Decision-Making and Illustrative Cases

As previously noted, the variable techniques used in ACL reconstruction for the skeletally immature may pose unique challenges when encountering the need for revision reconstruction. The tissue used for the graft at the time of primary reconstruction, the presence and position of prior bone tunnels, and the current status of the physis are important considerations. At all ages, just as in revision ACL reconstruction in the skeletally mature, consideration and treatment of collateral ligament instability (most commonly occult medial collateral residual laxity) and subtotal meniscal loss (with possible meniscal allograft reconstruction) may be important additional interventions to improve outcomes and reduce the risk of revision graft failure. Alignment should be evaluated with standing hip to ankle radiographs (EOS if available for lower-dose radiation), and if significant growth remains, guided growth should be considered for grade 3 coronal plane malalignment or possibly excessive posterior tibial slope (Figs. 20.1 and 20.2). Consideration of the possibility of inadequate

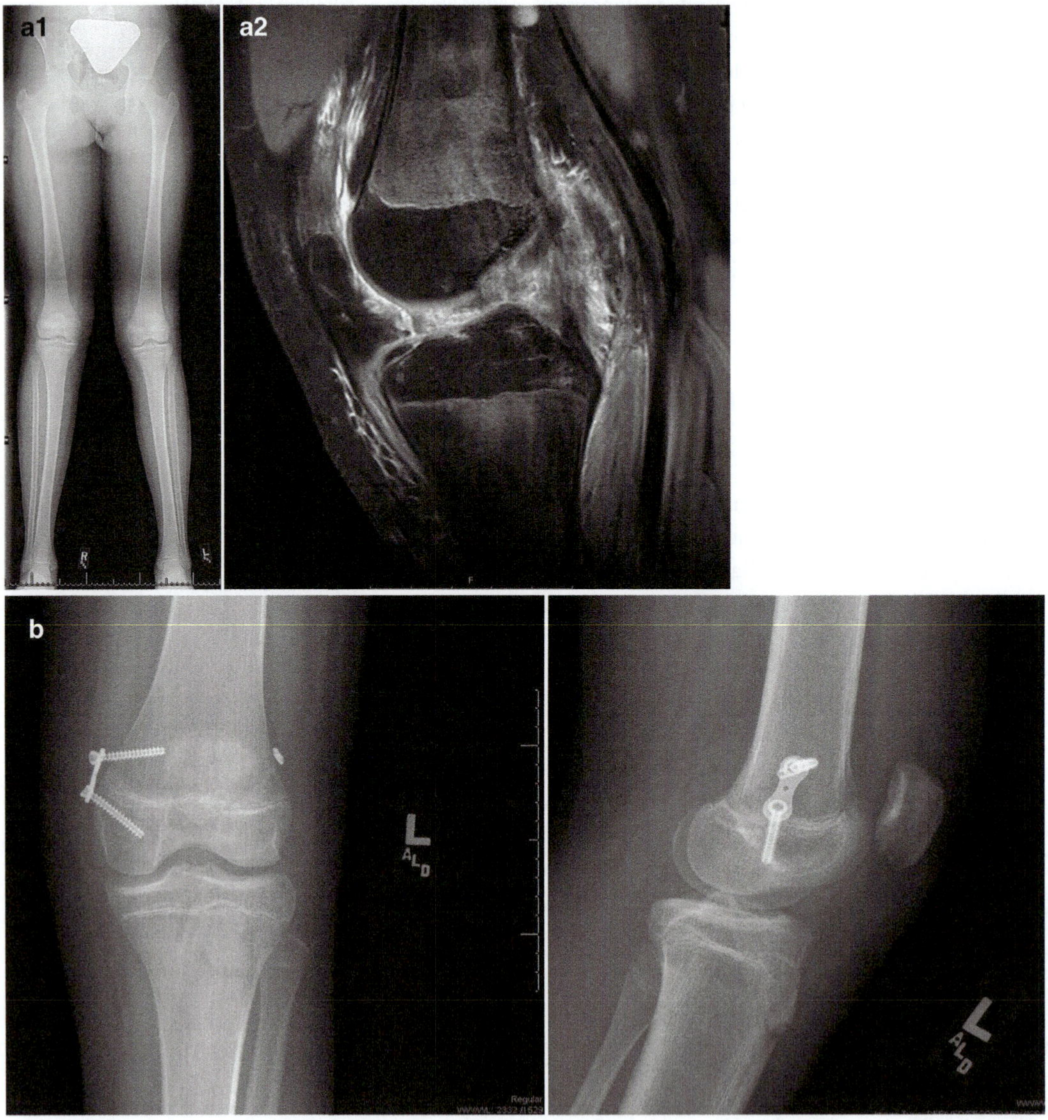

Fig. 20.1 (**a**) Anterior-posterior standing alignment (EOS) of failed primary left extra-osseous ACL graft with minor leg length inequality and significant genu valgum. Sagittal MRI demonstrating graft rupture. (**b**) Anterior-posterior and lateral radiographs demonstrating medial plate and screw device for guided-growth hemi-epiphysiodesis in conjunction with trans-physeal revision ACL reconstruction. (**c**) Anterior-posterior standing alignment (EOS) demonstrating achievement of neutral coronal alignment with no additional leg length inequality. Fluoroscopic anterior-posterior images of guided growth implant removal to allow symmetric completion of growth remaining

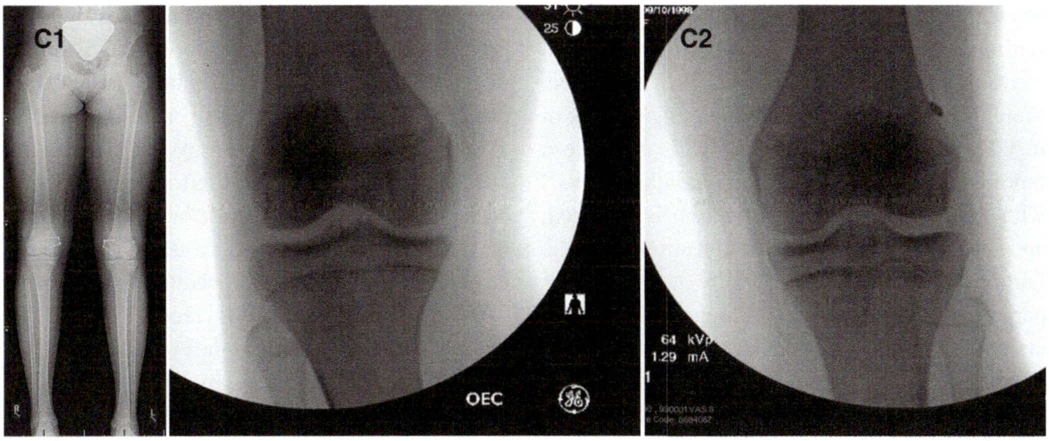

Fig. 20.1 (continued)

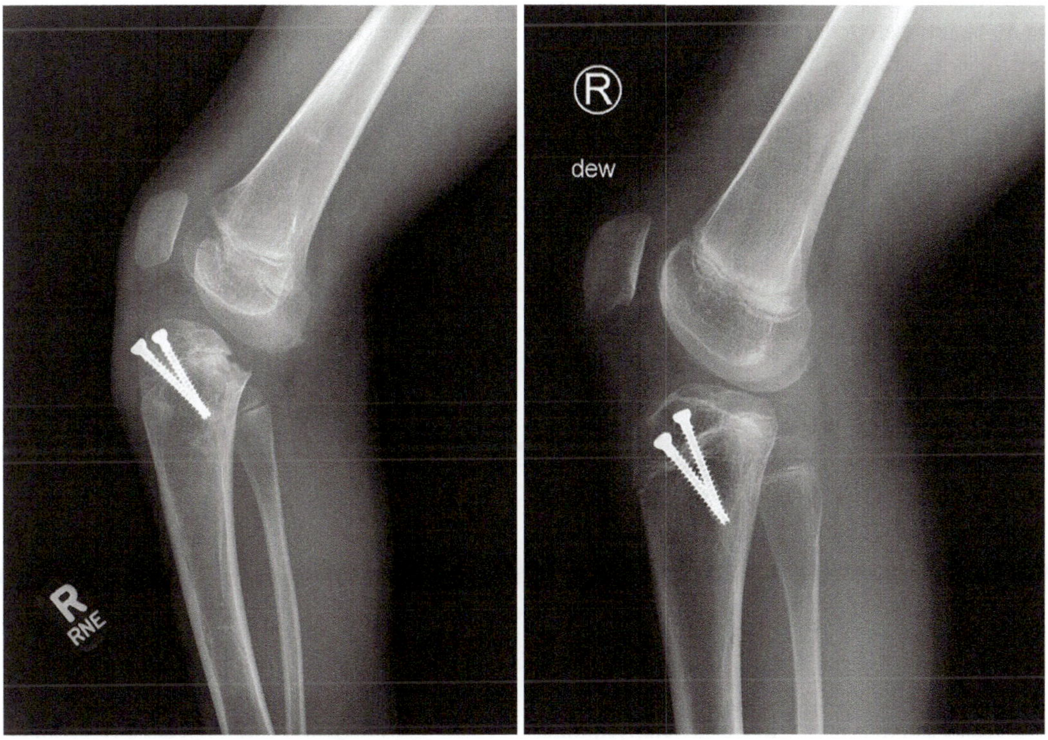

Fig. 20.2 Lateral radiographs demonstrating progressive correction of excessive posterior tibial slope with anterior tibial percutaneous trans-physeal screw guided growth. This technique may be considered in cases of excessive posterior slope with significant growth remaining. Close radiographic follow-up to ensure iatrogenic physeal arrest is identified early and treated if it should occur due to the multiple implants and possible tunnels present in the setting of revision ACL reconstruction

physeal growth and subsequent deformity in the setting of combined guided growth and trans-physeal tunnel placement must be considered. Weighing these risks, versus accepting the risk of malalignment, is required. In all cases, close monitoring of alignment at 6-month intervals with the possibility of intervention is required; and significant preoperative education with the family surrounding the possibility of deformity is paramount. Additionally, the higher activity levels and significant prevalence of both ligamentous laxity and increased posterior tibial slope in the skeletally immature merit consideration of an added lateral extra-articular tenodesis to support rotation in the setting of revision ACL reconstruction [13–21]. A version of the modified MacIntosh iliotibial band ACL reconstruction may be utilized to achieve this lateral extra-articular tenodesis without the requirement for bony fixation on the lateral distal femur and may allow for continued growth in the skeletally immature [22] (Fig. 20.3). The cases that follow serve to illustrate a variety of situations that may be encountered in the setting of revision ACL-R in the pediatric patient.

Case #1: Revision of a Primary Extra-osseous Iliotibial Band ACL Reconstruction

When revising a primary extra-osseous iliotibial band ACL reconstruction, the bony structures are largely native without prior bone tunnels which may decrease the technical complexity of the reconstruction. In this setting however, as an extra-osseous reconstruction is often performed in the most immature patients, the patient requiring reconstruction may still be skeletally immature. If the patient is mature, a standard ACL reconstruction technique of the author's choice would be appropriate and would be similar to a primary reconstruction.

If the patient is still immature, ipsilateral hamstrings or quadriceps soft tissue grafts would be considerations for either all epiphyseal or trans-physeal ACL reconstruction. As a lateral tenodesis may be a desired additional stabilizing procedure in a patient undergoing revision, in this setting the surgeon would need to be aware that the iliotibial band will be significantly altered in its anatomy and may not be an autograft choice for this lateral extra-articular tenodesis. Therefore, an allograft or other autograft may need to be considered should a supplementary lateral stabilizing procedure (e.g., lateral extra-articular ligamentous reconstruction) be planned. While use of allograft to reconstruct an ACL in an "over the top" manner, similar to a modified Macintosh procedure, has been described for adults undergoing revision ACL-R complicated by excessive tunnel osteolysis, this is not typically considered in the pediatric population given the significantly higher rates of graft rupture reported when an intraarticular allograft is used [4].

- *Authors' preferred approach* (Fig. 20.4):
  - *9 mm autograft quadriceps tendon soft tissue trans-physeal ACL graft (hamstring autograft may be considered; however deficient graft size may be encountered)*
  - *Concurrent meniscal repair if required*
  - *Concurrent guided growth of the distal femur or proximal tibia if zone 3 coronal plane malalignment is present*
  - *Concurrent lateral extra-articular tenodesis*
    - *Use of existing lateral incision and an appropriate band of residual iliotibial band for bony socket or suture anchor fixation at the appropriate lateral tenodesis point on lateral femoral epiphysis*
    - *Preparation for use of hamstring autograft or allograft tibial epiphyseal to lateral femoral epiphyseal lateral extra-articular ligament reconstruction if adequate iliotibial band is not present during surgical inspection*
  - *Standing alignment radiographs at 6-month intervals to monitor for deformity and possible intervention with guided growth or completion epiphysiodesis if required*

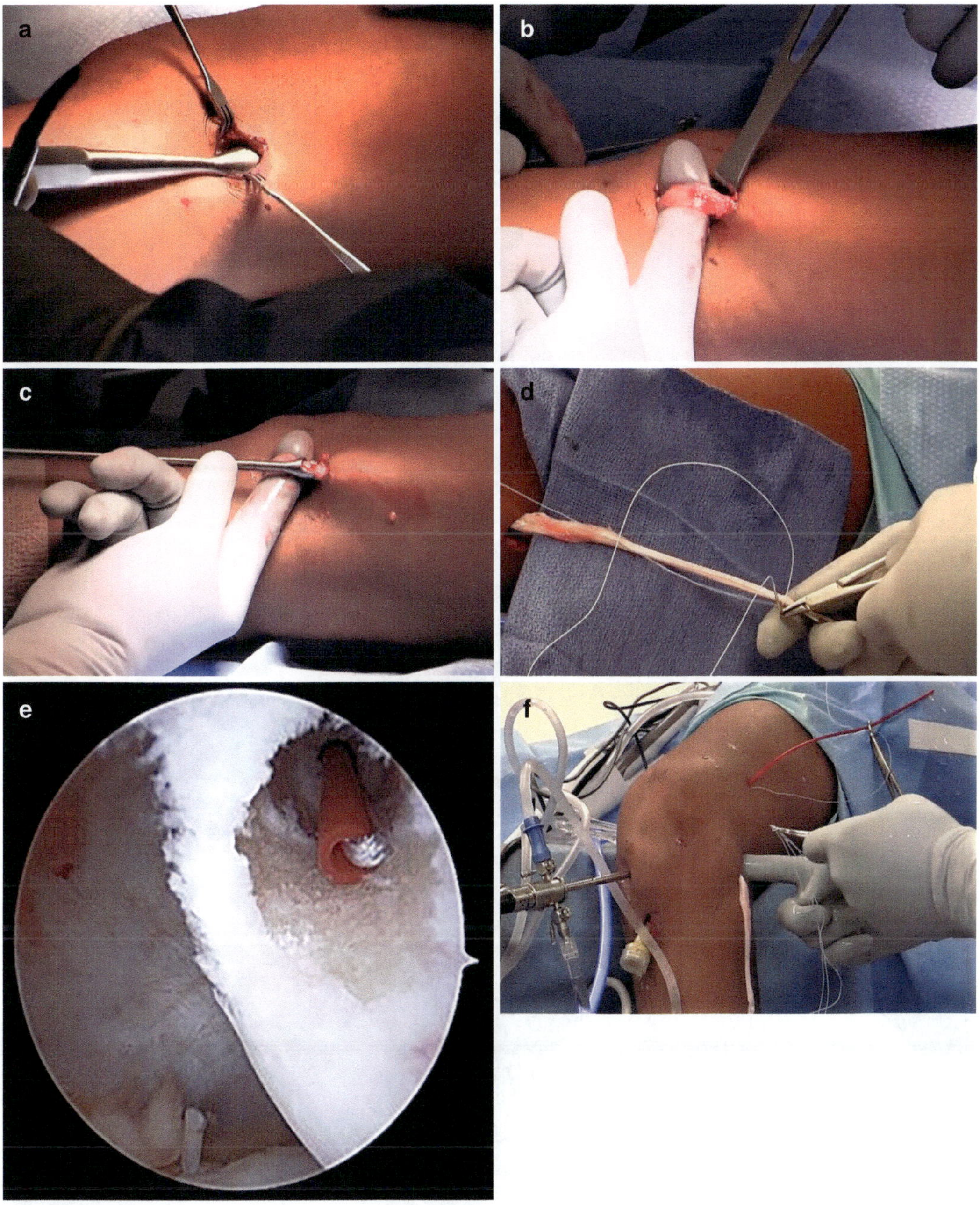

Fig. 20.3 Technique for modified MacIntosh iliotibial band lateral extra-articular tenodesis to be utilized in conjunction with ACL revision grafting. (**a**) Cobb elevator dissection overlying the iliotibial band. (**b**) Isolation of a section of the direct branch of the iliotibial band. (**c**) Large-caliber open tendon stripper harvest of the iliotibial band. (**d**) Whipstitch of the iliotibial band proximally after percutaneous release at approximately 13 cm from Gerdy's tubercle. (**e**) Arthroscopic view of ACL transphyseal tunnel. (**f**) External view of preparation for graft passage posterior to lateral femoral metaphyseal-condylar junction. (**g**) Intra-articular view of hemostat over the posterior lateral fold directly behind the lateral femoral condyle. (**h**) Arthroscopic view of suture passage for the iliotibial band graft. (**i**) Arthroscopic view of the iliotibial band graft in place traversing past the femoral ACL tunnel. (**j**) External view of the lateral extra-articular tenodesis portion of the iliotibial band. (**k**) Arthroscopic view of the iliotibial band entering the tibial tunnel with the sutures prepared for passage of the ACL graft anterior to this graft. (**l**) Arthroscopic view of ACL graft and iliotibial band graft within the notch and tibial tunnel. (**m**) Artist rendering combined lateral extra-articular tenodesis and ACL augmentation using the modified MacIntosh iliotibial band technique

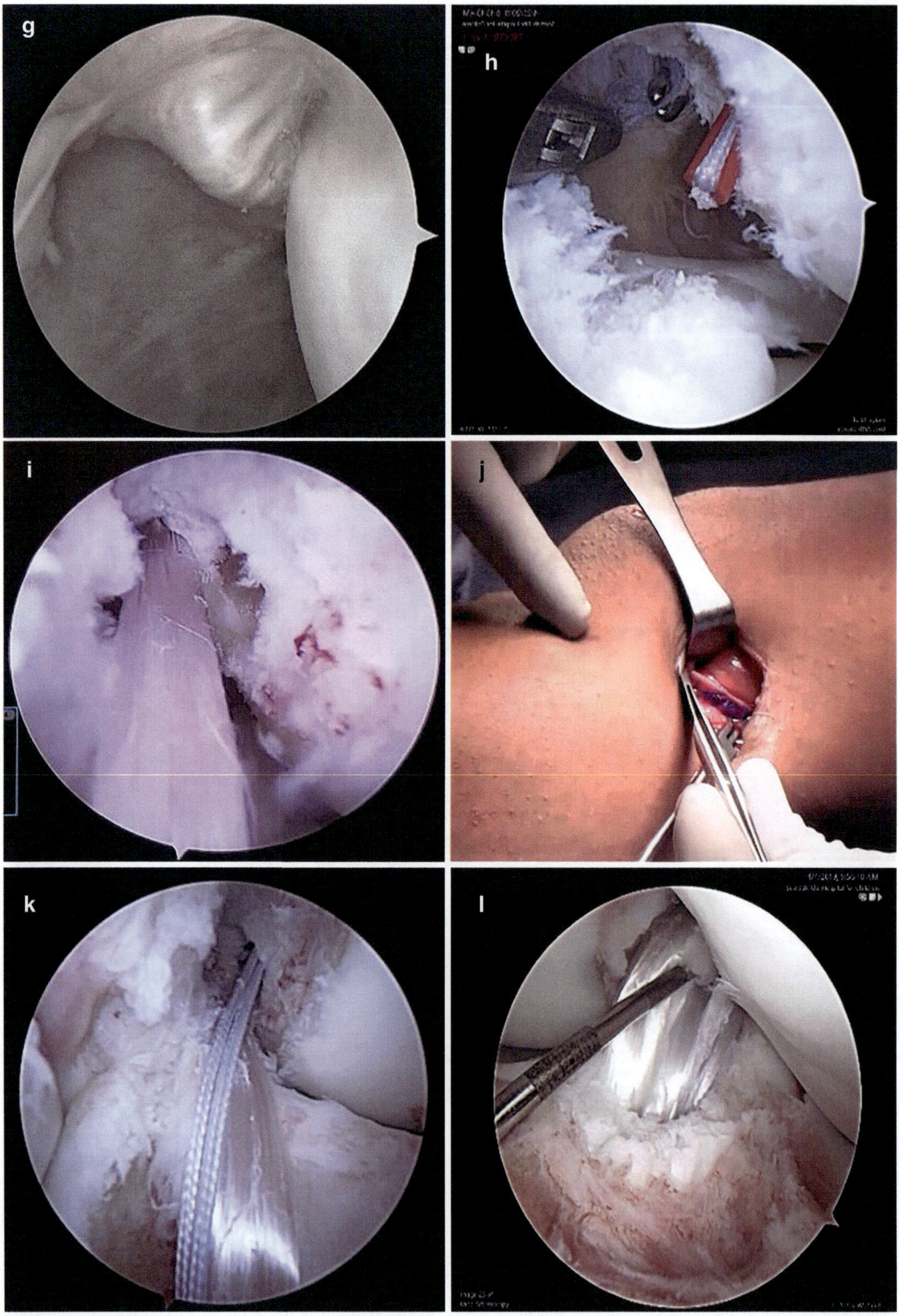

Fig. 20.3 (continued)

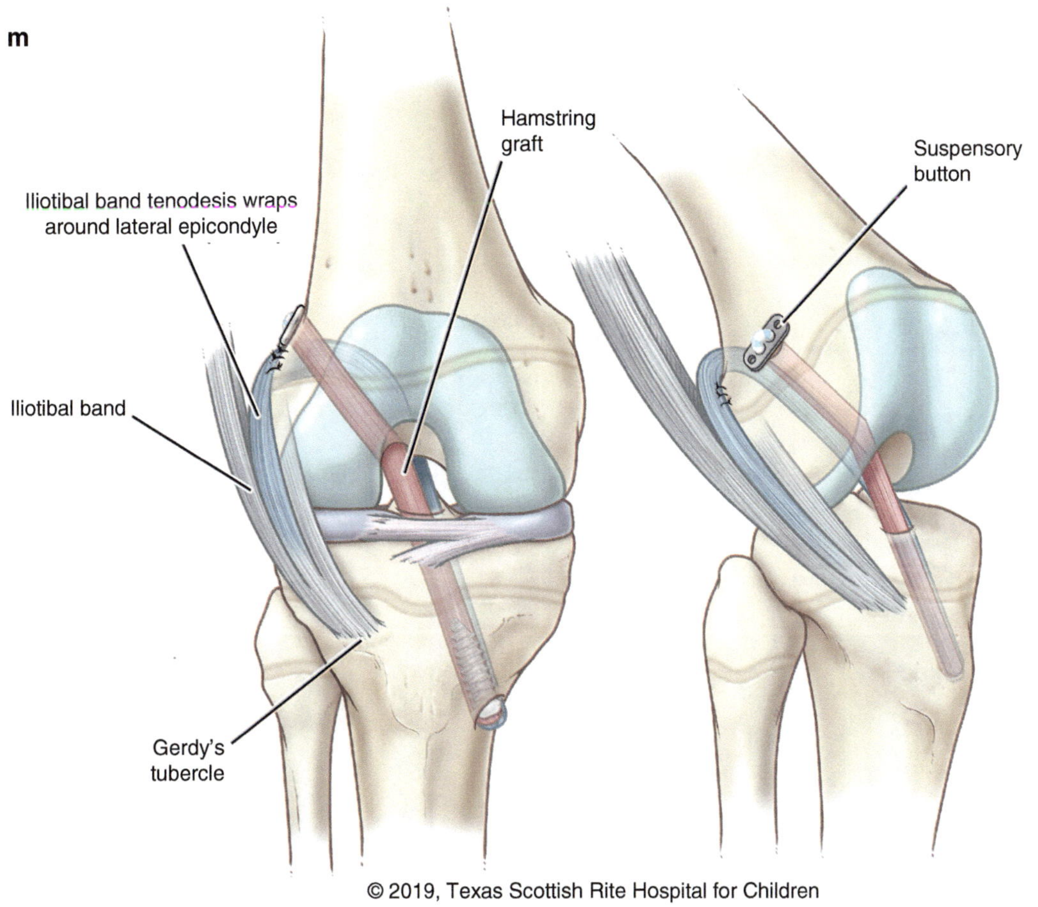

Fig. 20.3 (continued)

Case #2: Revision of a Primary All-Epiphyseal ACL Reconstruction

When revising a primary all epiphyseal ACL reconstruction, the femoral tunnel will be present on the lateral wall of the femur and may or may not be in a position that may be incorporated in the revision graft setting. This tunnel in some cases may be significantly anterior and may occasionally be left in situ without any need to address the structure, and a revision tunnel can be placed posteriorly. In other cases, the aperture of the tunnel will be in an ideal position for the revision graft, and a new trajectory of the revision tunnel may be obtained from this aperture, and the more lateral portions of the prior epiphyseal tunnel may not interfere with stability or incorporation of the revision graft. In rare cases, the aperture and tunnel of the primary all epiphyseal graft may need to be grafted with a cancellous dowel or bulk cancellous graft with techniques described elsewhere in this text.

The tibial tunnel may be either all epiphyseal or trans-physeal depending upon the technique used at the primary reconstruction. In the case of an all epiphyseal tunnel, grafting may be required, or the aperture may be utilized for a trans-physeal graft with no need to address the primary tunnel, similar to the femoral side. In the setting of a trans-physeal tibial tunnel, if the primary tunnel location was appropriately placed, this may be utilized in the revision setting.

As noted in the previous case, the patient requiring reconstruction in this setting may still be skeletally immature. Therefore, assessment of physeal status and a revision technique allowing

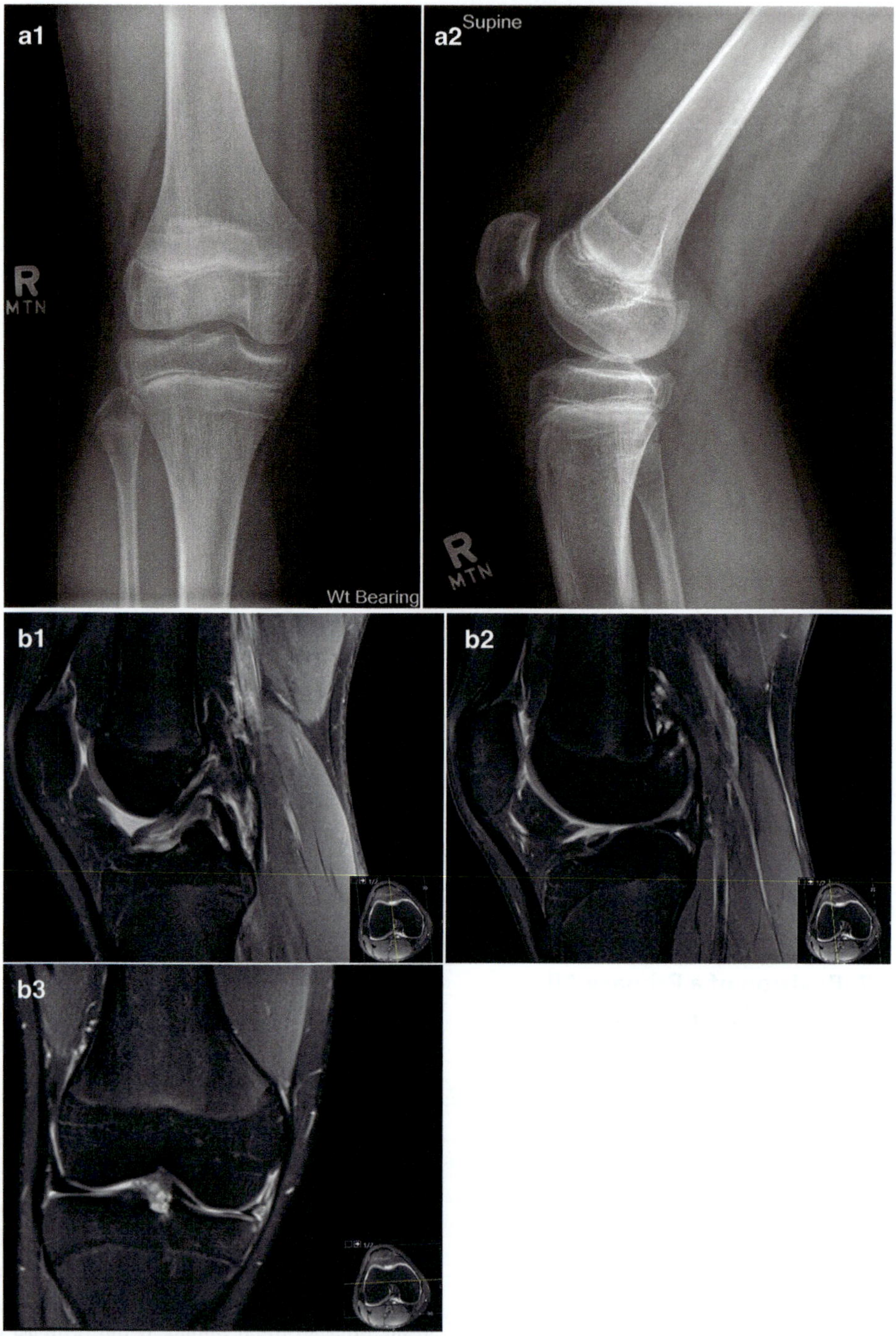

Fig. 20.4 (**a**) Anterior-posterior and lateral radiographs of a knee demonstrating symmetric Park Harris growth arrest lines after failed extra-osseous iliotibial band ACL reconstruction. (**b**) Sagittal and coronal MRI demonstrating extra-osseous graft failure and red arrows demonstrating femoral path of prior ACL graft and shallow tibial trough without tunnel from prior reconstruction. (**c**) Arthroscopic views demonstrating iliotibial band graft failure, tibial surface with altered surface anatomy, but no tunnel. Femoral arthroscopic view of native lateral wall with prior graft in the over-the-top position. (**d**) Arthroscopic view of femoral trans-phi seal tunnel with cartilaginous phi seal ring visible, transphyseal quadriceps soft tissue autograft in place, and radiographic anterior-posterior and lateral views of tunnels and implants following reconstruction

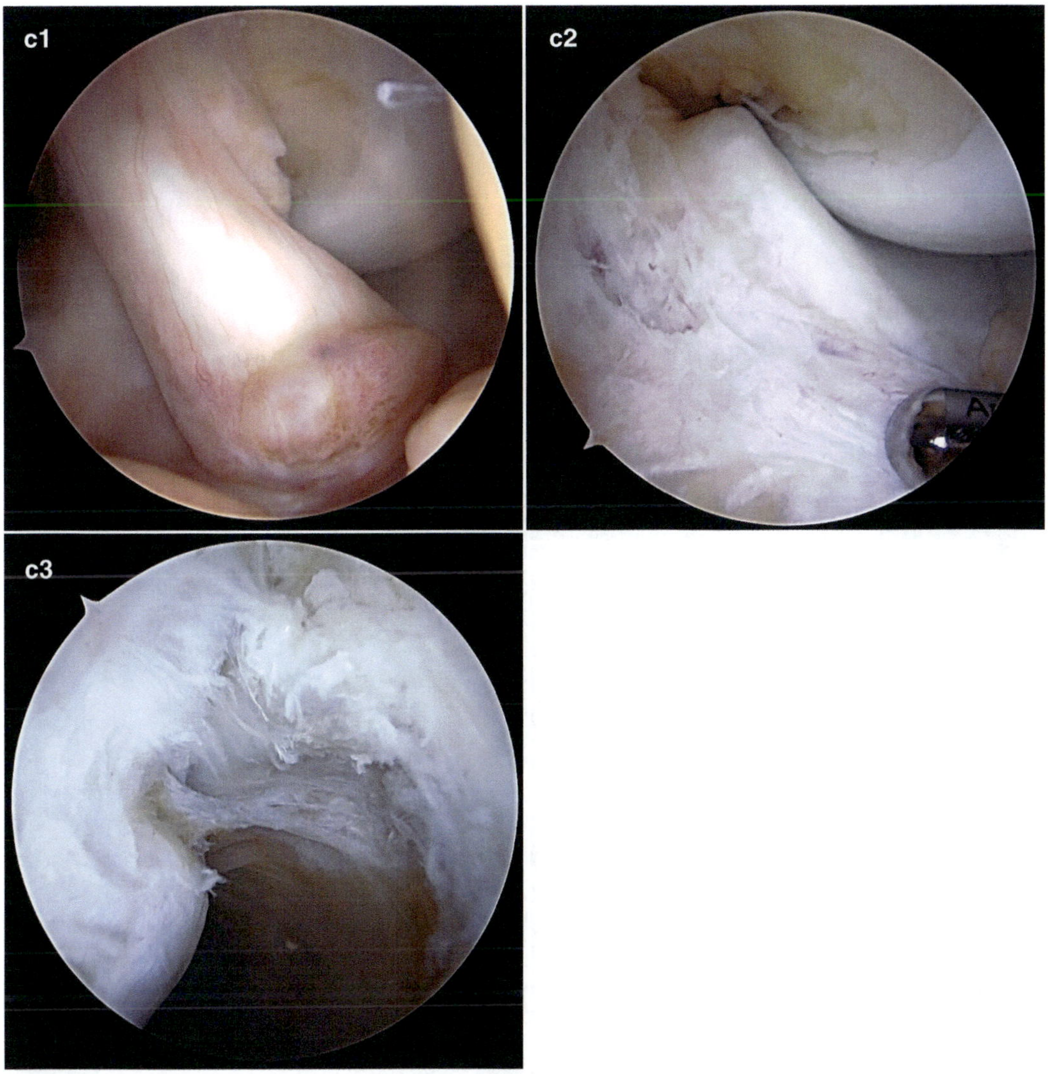

Fig. 20.4 (continued)

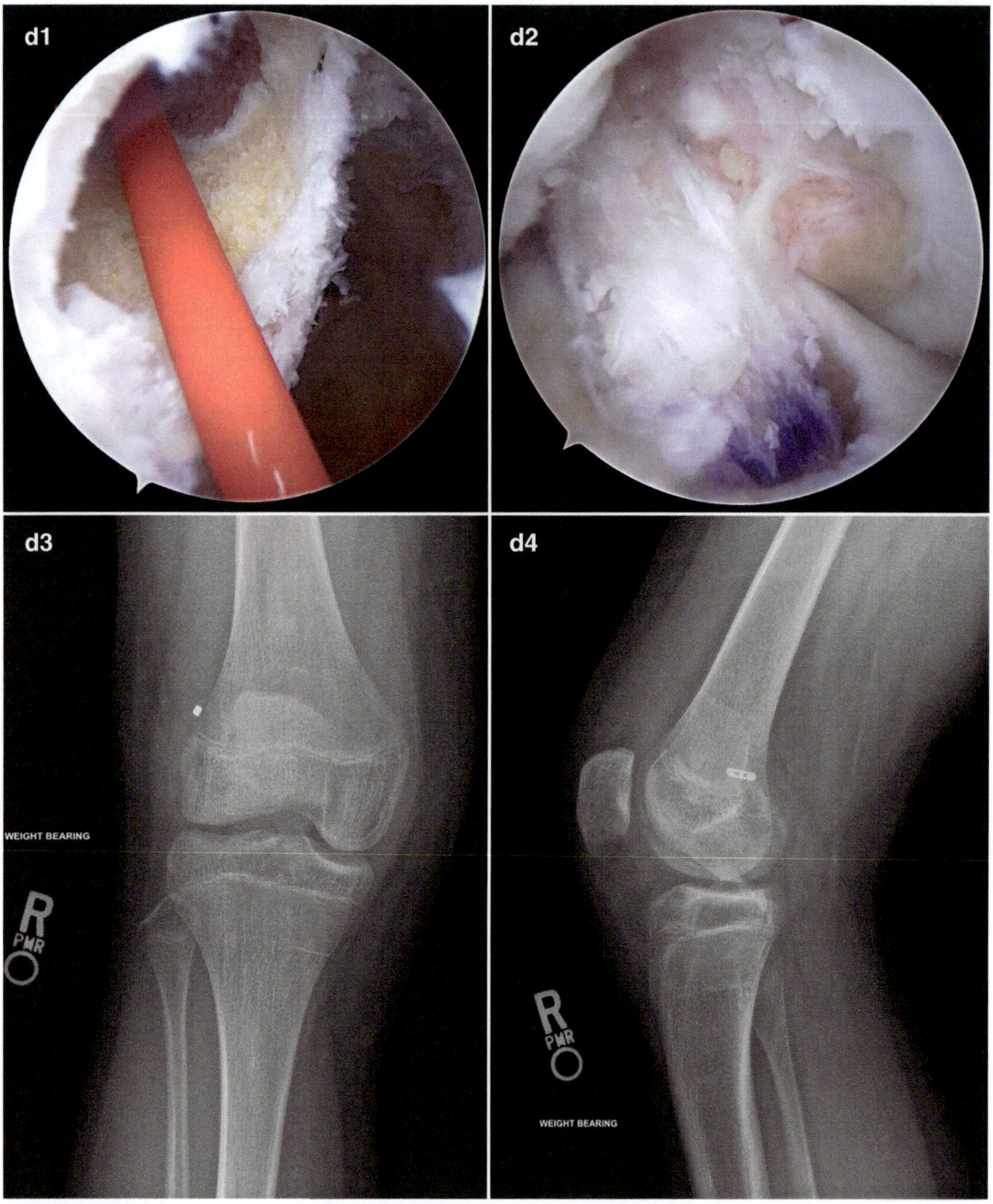

Fig. 20.4 (continued)

for completion of growth may be required. Ipsilateral hamstrings or quadriceps soft tissue grafts would be first-line considerations for transphyseal ACL reconstruction, and the surgeon performing the revision may be faced with utilizing the remainder of these two choices if one was used in the primary surgery.

- *Authors' preferred approach* (Fig. 20.5):
  - *9 mm autograft quadriceps tendon soft tissue trans-physeal ACL graft. The surgeon may be limited by the tissue utilized as the primary graft. Ipsilateral hamstring autograft may also be considered; however deficient graft size may be encountered. An*

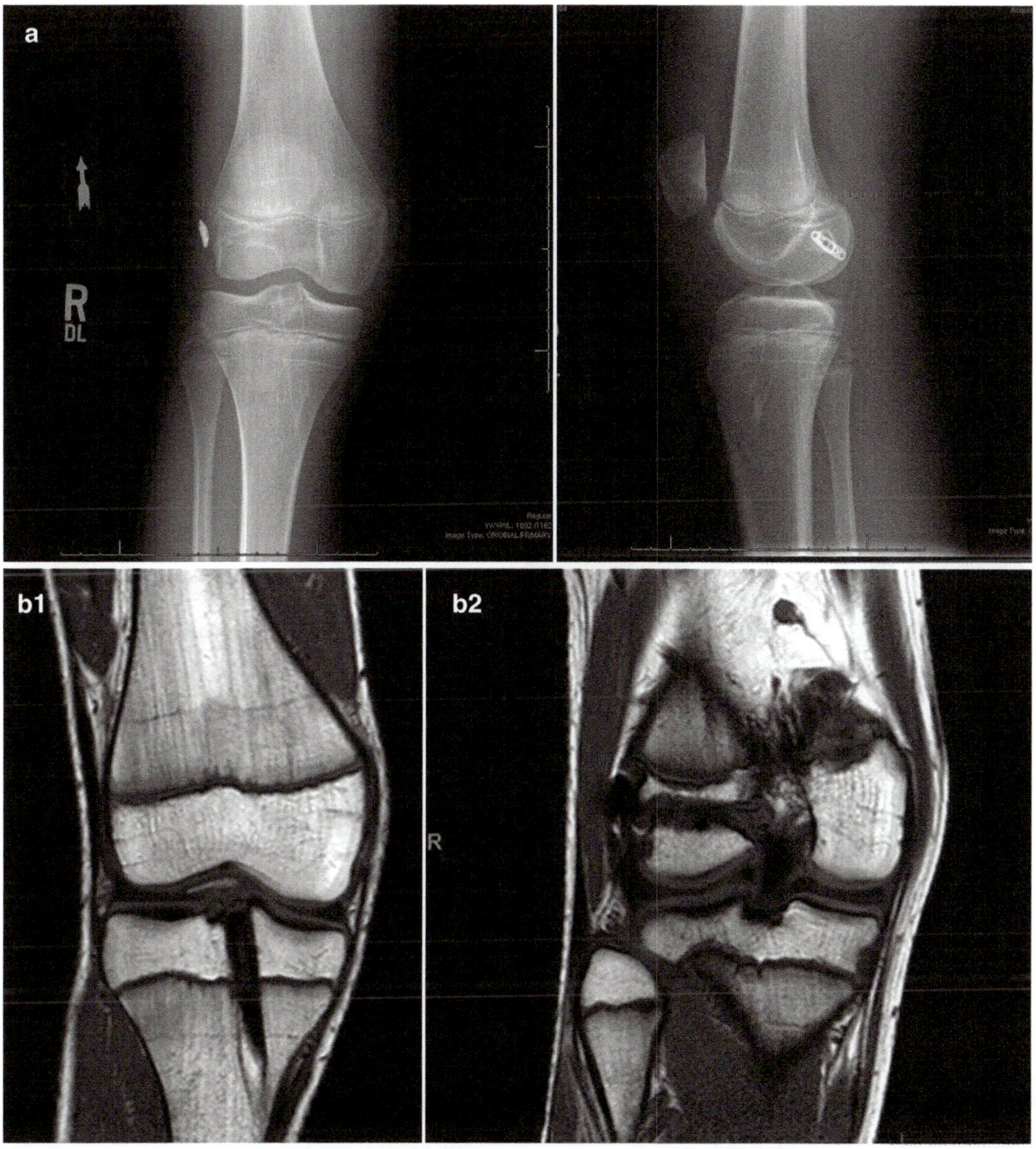

Fig. 20.5 (**a**) Anterior-posterior and lateral radiographs of a knee following hybrid all epiphyseal femoral reconstruction and trans-physeal tibial reconstruction. (**b**) Coronal MRI demonstrating the location of tibial and femoral tunnels, respectively. (**c**) Sagittal MRI demonstrating tibial and femoral tunnels with locations appropriate for new trans-physeal tunnel trajectories with shared-aperture entrance and exit locations into the knee using the current native apertures of the primary tunnels present. The tibial implant would not be removed

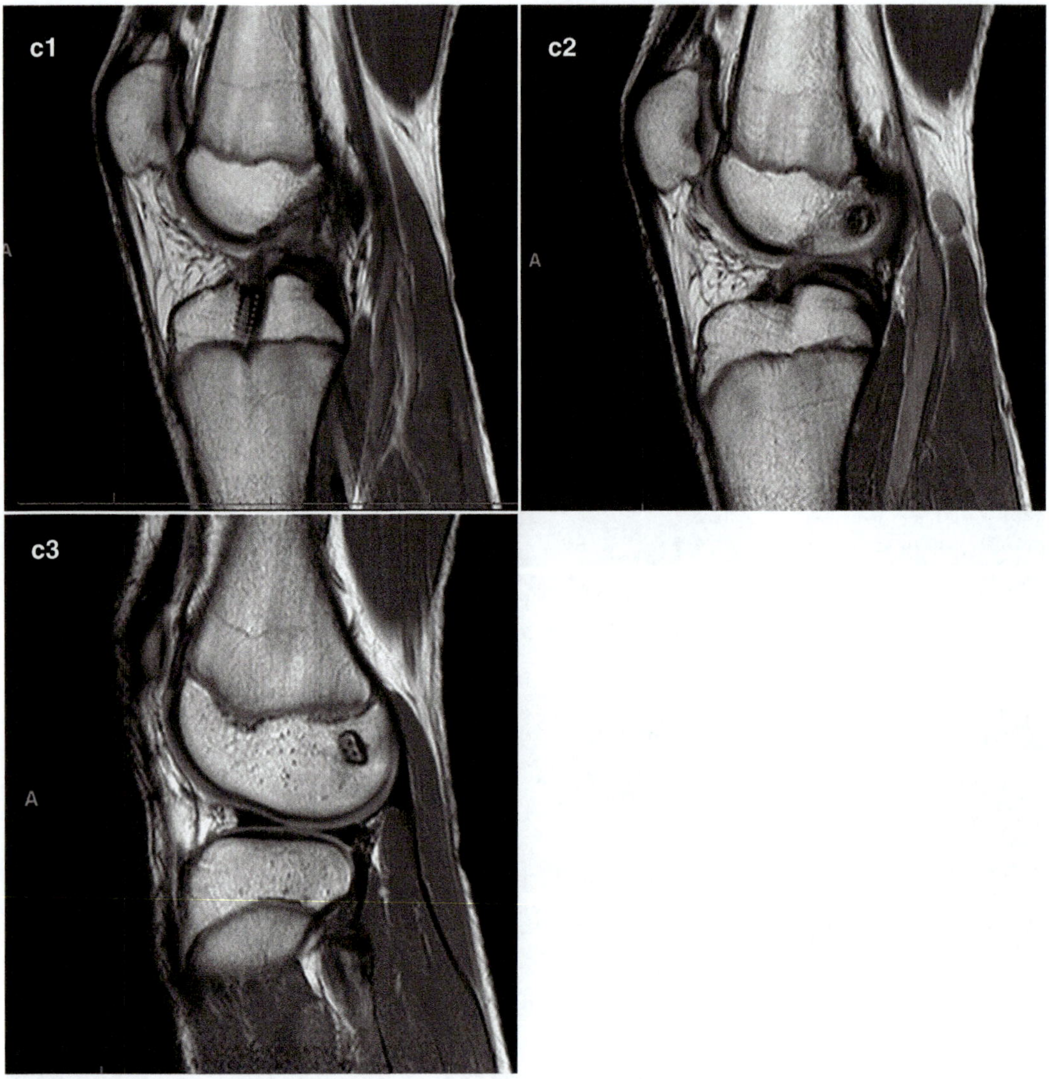

Fig. 20.5 (continued)

additional option in this setting is the addition of contralateral hamstrings to augment ipsilateral hamstring size if required.

- *Concurrent meniscal repair if required.*
- *Concurrent guided growth of the distal femur or proximal tibia if zone 3 coronal plane malalignment is present.*
- *Concurrent lateral extra-articular tenodesis.*

  Use of modified MacIntosh iliotibial band lateral tenodesis with incorporation of the graft in the tibial tunnel
- *Standing alignment radiographs at 6-month intervals to monitor for deformity and possible intervention with guided growth or completion epiphysiodesis if required.*

Case #3: Revision of a Primary Trans-physeal ACL Reconstruction

When revising a primary trans-physeal ACL reconstruction, the femoral tunnel will be present on the lateral wall of the femur, and this tunnel and aperture may or may not be in a position that may be used directly in the revision graft setting. This tunnel in some cases may be significantly anterior and may occasionally be left in situ without any need to address the structure, and a revision tunnel can be placed posteriorly. In other cases, the aperture of the tunnel will be in an ideal position for the revision graft, and a new trajectory of the revision tunnel may be obtained from this aperture, and the more lateral portions of the prior epiphyseal tunnel may not interfere with stability or incorporation of the revision graft. The trans-physeal tibial tunnel may be addressed in a similar fashion.

In cases in which the patient has significant growth remaining and one or both trans-physeal tunnels cannot be either used or completely avoided, the surgeon is faced with a difficult choice. The patient may be braced until he/she/they are mature enough to perform bony grafting of the tunnel without risking resultant deformity and thereby staged for a subsequent ACL reconstruction. Alternatively, a bio-absorbable screw may be placed within the inappropriate primary trans-physeal tunnel, and a new revision tunnel may be created. This allows support for the revision tunnel and even the ability to drill through a portion of the screw during creation of a more desirable tunnel; however the additional defect and implant placement across the physis may risk growth alteration or arrest. This may be a preferable strategy, with combined close observation of growth, if the patient has significant instability risking further intra-articular damage. In this setting, extensive education with the family that completion epiphysiodesis could be required if growth alteration occurs should be conducted. In practice, this may be an uncommon situation as the amount of growth remaining at the time of revision is often negligible, and principles of adult revision reconstruction may be followed. In the extremely uncommon case of a skeletally immature child with significant growth remaining who has previously undergone a trans-physeal ACL-R and requires revision surgery, an isolated physeal-sparing, extra-osseous reconstruction technique (e.g., ITB ACL-R) may be considered; it is more common, however, for the native ITB to be used as autograft for a lateral extra-articular tenodesis which supplements a revision trans-physeal ACL-R (see authors' preferred approach).

Ipsilateral hamstrings or quadriceps soft tissue grafts would be considerations for trans-physeal ACL reconstruction, and the surgeon performing the revision may be faced with utilizing the remainder of these two choices if one was used in the primary surgery.

- *Authors' preferred approach* (Fig. 20.6):
  - *9–10 mm autograft quadriceps tendon soft tissue trans-physeal ACL graft. The surgeon may be limited by the tissue utilized as the primary graft. Ipsilateral hamstring autograft may also be considered; however deficient graft size may be encountered. An additional option in this setting is the addition of contralateral hamstrings to augment ipsilateral hamstring size if required.*
  - *Use of the prior tunnels if appropriate.*
  - *Placement of a bio-absorbable screw in a poorly positioned but infringing prior tunnel. Bone graft cannot be utilized in this setting if significant growth remains.*
  - *Concurrent meniscal repair if required.*
  - *Concurrent lateral extra-articular tenodesis.*

    Use of modified MacIntosh iliotibial band lateral tenodesis with incorporation of the graft in the tibial tunnel
  - *Standing alignment radiographs at 6-month intervals to monitor for deformity and possible intervention with completion epiphysiodesis if required.*

Outcomes of Revision ACL-R in the Pediatric Population

The existing outcomes data for revision ACL-R in children and adolescents are grim. One recent retrospective case series examined outcomes for 90 patients who sustained ACL graft ruptures and underwent revision ACL-R at an average age of 16.6 years. Approximately 20% of these patients sustained a new injury to the graft following revision reconstruction, and 25% of patients required additional surgical procedures. An alarming 20% sustained ACL injuries of the contralateral knees. Only 55% of these young athletes returned to

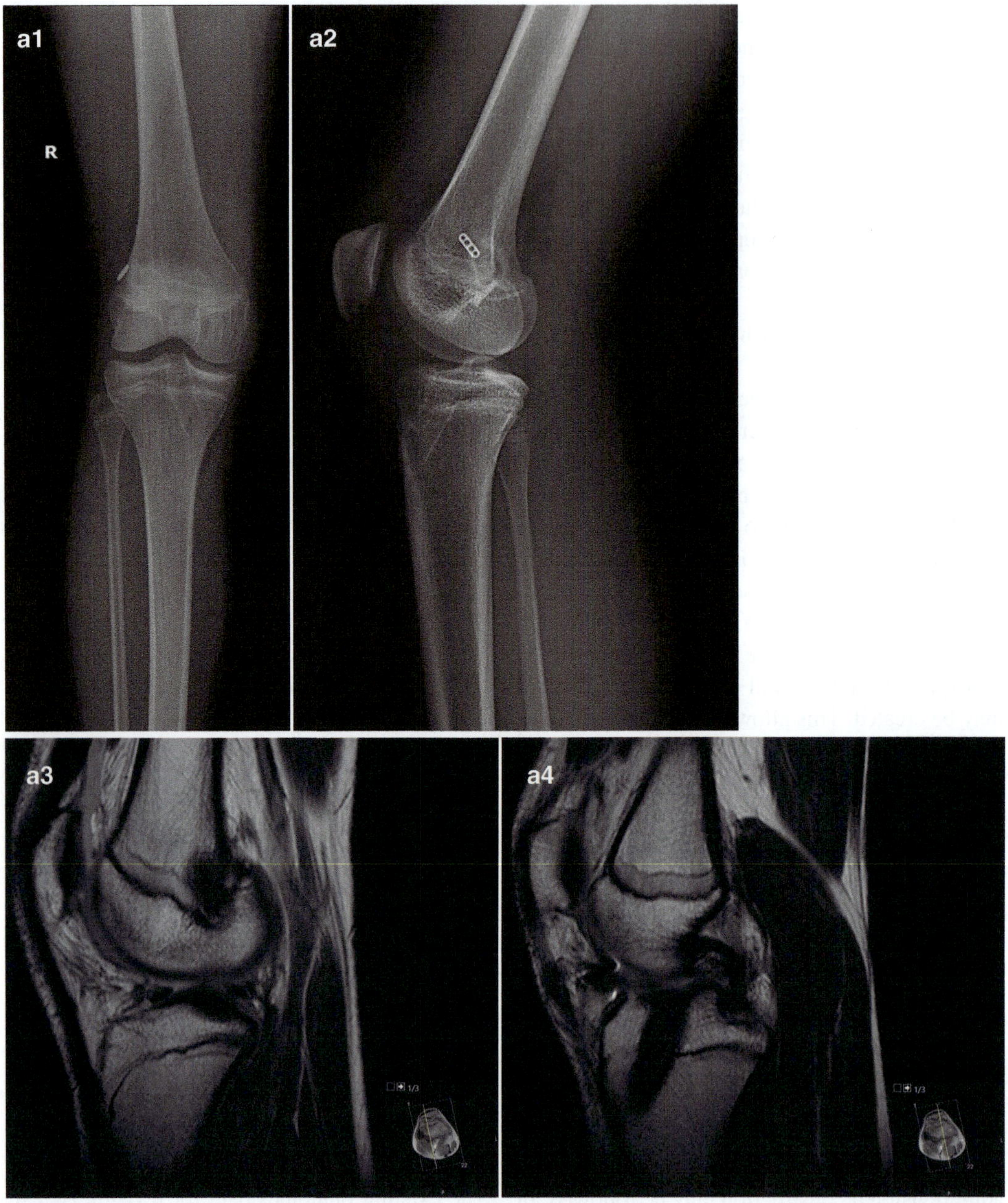

Fig. 20.6 (**a**) Anterior-posterior and lateral radiographs with coronal and sagittal MRI slices following failed trans-physeal soft tissue allograft ACL reconstruction. An appropriate tibial tunnel position and an anterior femoral position are demonstrated. (**b**) Standing alignment (EOS) radiograph demonstrating symmetry and skeletal immaturity, with hand radiograph demonstrating open phalangeal physes representative of further growth remaining. (**c**) Arthroscopic images of an appropriate anterior femoral tunnel and appropriate positioning of tibial tunnel with failed torn allograft present. (**d**) Arthroscopic visualization of the primary femoral ACL tunnel position (red circle) and a cautery mark (green circle) indicating a more appropriate desired ACL femoral tunnel position. (**e**) Arthroscopic view of new revision ACL femoral tunnel posterior and free from convergence with the prior inappropriate primary ACL femoral position (red circle). Physeal cartilage ring in the revision femoral tunnel is noted. (**f**) Arthroscopic view of removal of implant and graft from the primary appropriately positioned tibial tunnel with arthroscopic view of the appropriate tunnel walls and healthy cancellous bone prior to use for the revision reconstruction. (**g**) Arthroscopic view of autologous quadriceps tendon ACL revision graft and anterior-posterior and lateral radiographs of revision tunnel positions and implants. (**h**) Anterior-posterior and lateral radiographs demonstrating mature tunnel incorporation and completion of symmetric growth following revision trans-physeal ACL reconstruction

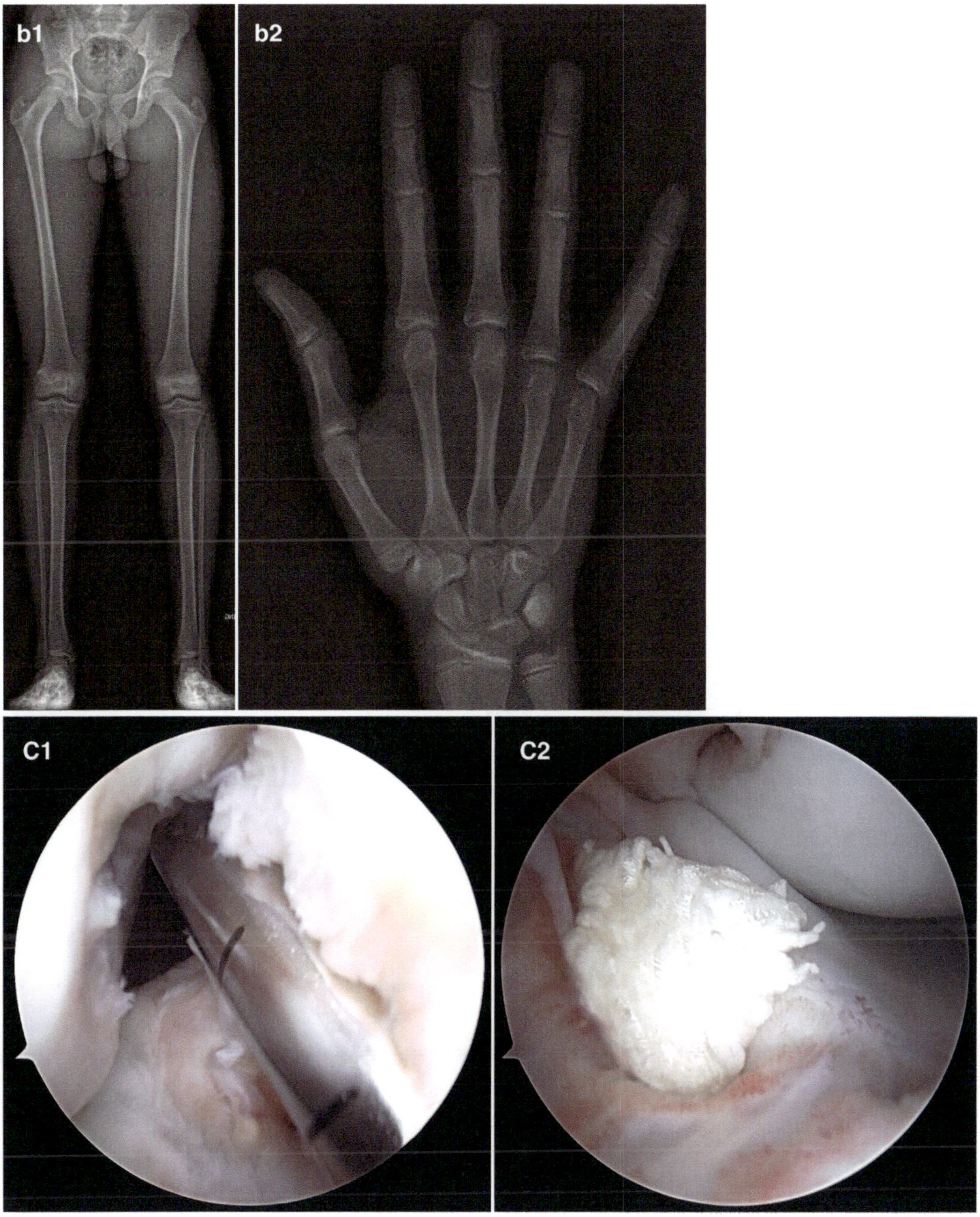

Fig. 20.6 (continued)

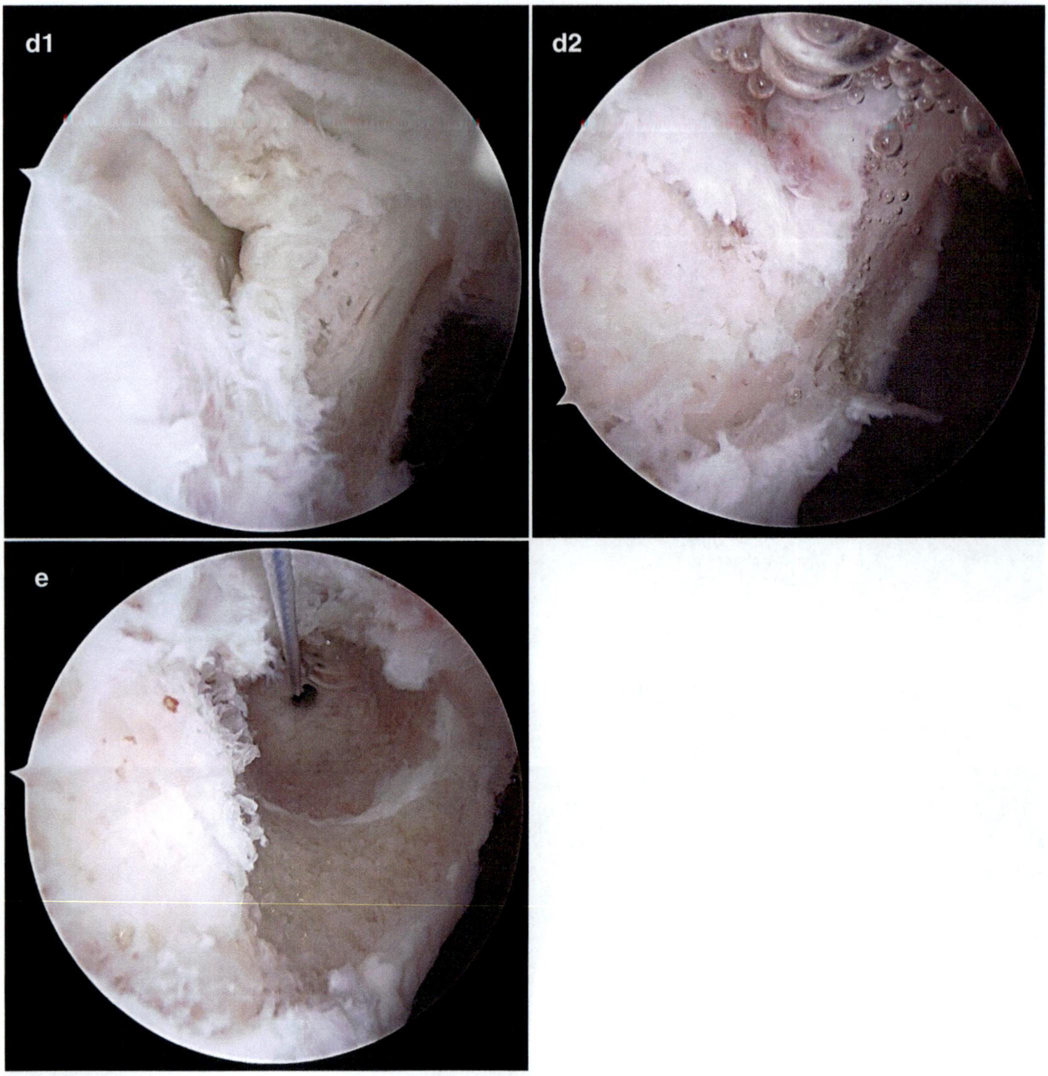

Fig. 20.6 (continued)

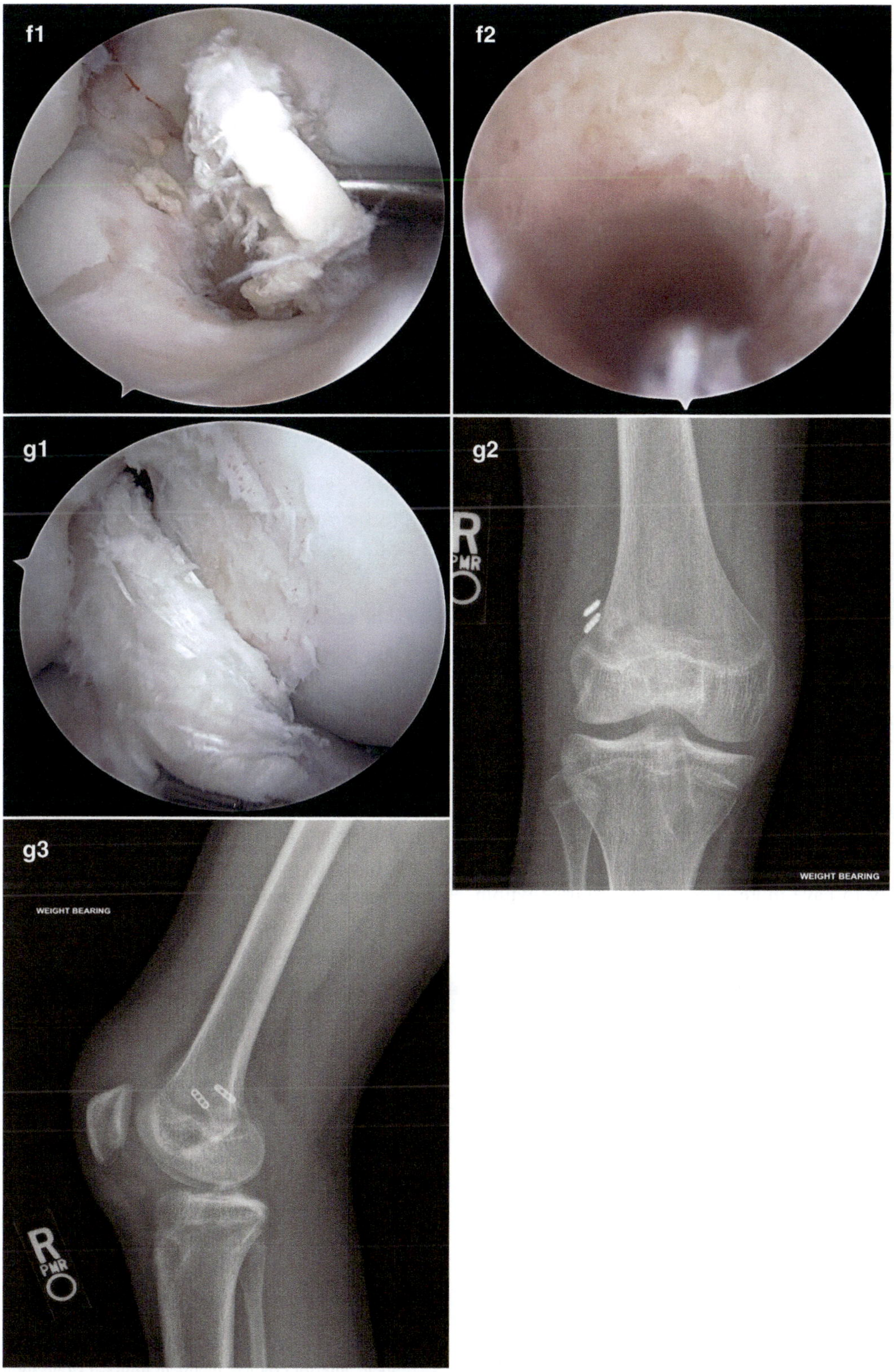

Fig. 20.6 (continued)

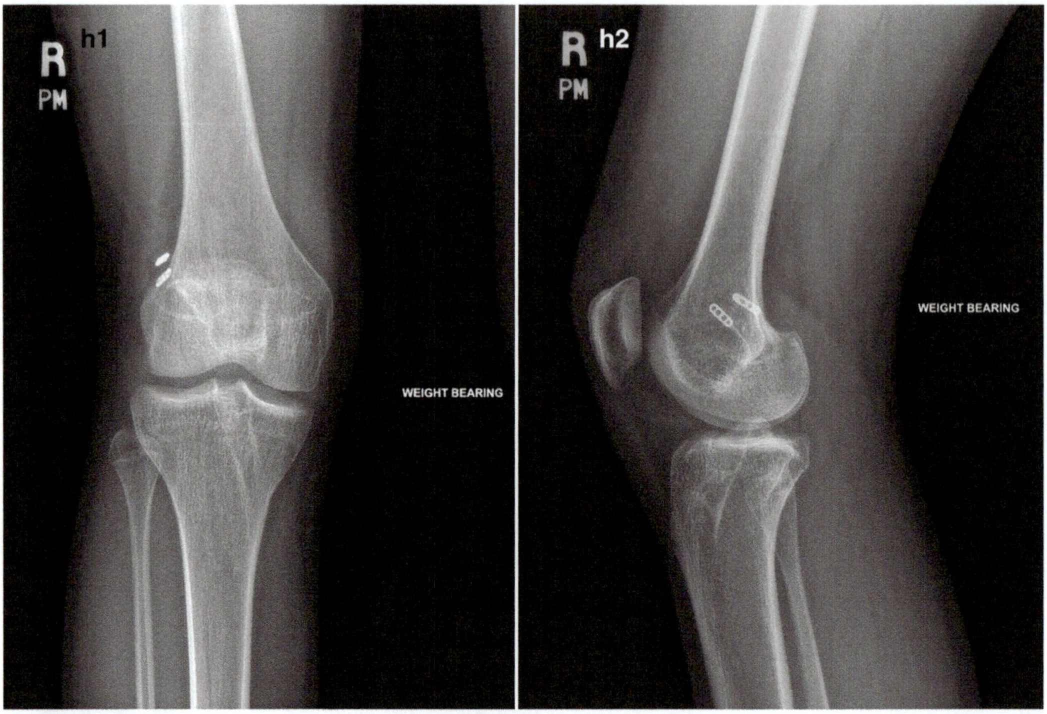

Fig. 20.6 (continued)

sport at their preinjury level of play [23]. The authors of a second recent study compared the outcomes of primary ACL-R with those for revision ACL-R in young athletes and had similar findings. Specifically, young patients who underwent revision ACL-R were significantly more likely to have more concomitant injuries within the operative knee, to have lower return to sport rates, and to sustain higher rates of graft re-tear than those undergoing primary ACL-R [24]. Taken together, these studies demonstrate underwhelming clinical outcomes for young patients undergoing revision ACL-R and make a powerful argument for managing all factors contributing to ACL injury risk as well as for managing the expectations of young athletes and their parents.

Conclusion

Failure of a primary ACL-R in the young athlete is a devastating complication that may be a season-ending or even career-ending injury. Revision ACL-R is typically recommended for patients with ACL graft tears who have functional instability and wish to pursue continued participation in sports. Prior to performing revision reconstruction, a comprehensive assessment of the factors contributing to an individual athlete's risk of re-injury should be performed, and each factor that is identified should be systematically addressed, just as with an adult patient. Key considerations for young athletes in this setting include the status of the growth plates as well as the possibility that a physeal-sparing or physeal-respecting surgical technique may have been previously employed. In addition, understanding how a young athlete's psychological state and developmental level may affect his/her/their risk is essential for achieving a safe and injury-free return to sport.

References

1. Dekker TJ, Godin JA, Dale KM, Garrett WE, Taylor DC, Riboh JC. Return to sport after pediatric anterior cruciate ligament reconstruction and its effect on subsequent anterior cruciate ligament injury. J Bone Joint Surg Am. 2017;99:987–04.

2. O'Malley MP, Milewski MD, Solomito MJ, Erwteman AS, Nissen CW. The association of tibial slope and anterior cruciate ligament rupture in skeletally immature patients. Arthroscopy. 2015;31(1):77–82.
3. Dare DM, Fabricant PD, McCarthy MM, et al. Increased lateral tibial slope is a risk factor for pediatric anterior cruciate ligament injury. Am J Sports Med. 2015;43(7):1632–9.
4. Engelman GH, Carry PM, Hitt KG, Polousky JD, Vidal AF. Comparison of allograft versus autograft anterior cruciate ligament reconstruction graft survival in an active adolescent cohort. Am J Sports Med. 2014;42(10):2311–8.
5. Webster KE, Feller JA, Leigh WB, Richmond AK. Younger patients are at increased risk for graft rupture and contralateral injury after anterior cruciate ligament reconstruction. Am J Sports Med. 2014;42(3):641–7.
6. McPherson AL, Feller JA, Hewett TE, Webster KE. Smaller change in psychological readiness to return to sport is associated with second anterior cruciate ligament injury among younger patients. Am J Sports Med. 2019;47(5):1209–15.
7. Paterno MV, Flynn K, Thomas S, Schmitt LC. Self-reported fear predicts functional performance and second ACL injury after ACL reconstruction and return to sport: a pilot study. Sports Health. 2018;10(3):228–33.
8. Kocher MS, Garg S, Micheli LJ. Physeal sparing reconstruction of the anterior cruciate ligament in skeletally immature prepubescent children and adolescents. Surgical technique. J Bone Joint Surg Am. 2006;88 Suppl 1 Pt 2:283–93.
9. Kocher MS, Heyworth BE, Fabricant PD, Tepolt FA, Micheli LJ. Outcomes of physeal-sparing ACL reconstruction with iliotibial band autograft in skeletally immature prepubescent children. J Bone Joint Surg Am. 2018;100:1087–94.
10. Fabricant PD, McCarthy MM, Cordasco FA, Green DW. All-inside, all-epiphyseal autograft reconstruction of the anterior cruciate ligament in the skeletally immature athlete. JBJS Essent Surg Tech. 2013;3(2):e9.
11. Cruz AI, Fabricant PD, McGraw M, Rozell JC, Ganley TJ, Wells L. All-epiphyseal ACL reconstruction in children: review of safety and early complications. J Pediatr Orthop. 2017;37(3):204–9.
12. Kercher J, Xerogeanes J, Tannenbaum A, Al-Hakim R, Black JC, Zhao J. Anterior cruciate ligament reconstruction in the skeletally immature: an anatomical study utilizing 3- dimensional magnetic resonance imaging reconstructions. J Pediatr Orthop. 2009;29(2):124–7.
13. Christensen JJ, Krych AJ, Engasser WM, Vanhees MK, Collins MS, Dahm DL. Lateral tibial posterior slope is increased in patients with early graft failure after anterior cruciate ligament reconstruction. Am J Sports Med. 2015;43(10):2510–4.
14. Grassi A, Signorelli C, Urrizola F, et al. Patients with failed anterior cruciate ligament reconstruction have an increased posterior lateral tibial plateau slope: a case-controlled study. Arthroscopy. 2019;35(4):1172–82.
15. Hewison CE, Tran MN, Kaniki N, Remtulla A, Bryant D, Getgood AM. Lateral extra-articular tenodesis reduces rotational laxity when combined with anterior cruciate ligament reconstruction: a systematic review of the literature. Arthroscopy. 2015;31(10):2022–34.
16. Kaeding CC, Pedroza AD, Reinke EK, Huston LJ, Consortium M, Spindler KP. Risk factors and predictors of subsequent ACL injury in either knee after ACL reconstruction: prospective analysis of 2488 primary ACL reconstructions from the MOON cohort. Am J Sports Med. 2015;43(7):1583–90.
17. Paterno MV, Huang B, Thomas S, Hewett TE, Schmitt LC. Clinical factors that predict a second ACL injury after ACL reconstruction and return to sport: preliminary development of a clinical decision algorithm. Orthop J Sports Med. 2017;5(12):2325967117745279.
18. Rosenstiel N, Praz C, Ouanezar H, et al. Combined anterior cruciate and anterolateral ligament reconstruction in the professional athlete: clinical outcomes from the Scientific Anterior Cruciate Ligament Network International Study Group in a series of 70 patients with a minimum follow-up of 2 years. Arthroscopy. 2019;35(3):885–92.
19. Sonnery-Cottet B, Saithna A, Cavalier M, et al. Anterolateral ligament reconstruction is associated with significantly reduced ACL graft rupture rates at a minimum follow-up of 2 years: a prospective comparative study of 502 patients from the SANTI Study Group. Am J Sports Med. 2017;45(7):1547–57.
20. Vundelinckx B, Herman B, Getgood A, Litchfield R. Surgical indications and technique for anterior cruciate ligament reconstruction combined with lateral extra-articular tenodesis or anterolateral ligament reconstruction. Clin Sports Med. 2017;36(1):135–53.
21. Webster KE, Feller JA. Exploring the high reinjury rate in younger patients undergoing anterior cruciate ligament reconstruction. Am J Sports Med. 2016;44(11):2827–32.
22. Wilson PL, Wyatt CW, Wagner KJ 3rd, Boes N, Sabatino MJ, Ellis HB Jr. Combined transphyseal and lateral extra-articular pediatric anterior cruciate ligament reconstruction: a novel technique to reduce ACL reinjury while allowing for growth. Am J Sports Med. 2019;47(14):3356–64.
23. Christino MA, Tepolt FA, Sugimoto D, Micheli LJ, Kocher MS. Revision ACL reconstruction in children and adolescents. J Pediatr Orthop. 2020;40(3):129–34.
24. Ouillette R, Edmonds E, Chambers H, Bastrom T, Pennock A. Outcomes of revision anterior. Cruciate ligament surgery in adolescents. Am J Sports Med. 2019;47(6):1346–52.

Management of Cartilage Defects in the Setting of Revision ACL Reconstruction

21

Ignacio Garcia-Mansilla, Brian M. Cash, Evan E. Vellios, and Kristofer J. Jones

Introduction

One of the many challenges associated with revision anterior cruciate ligament reconstruction (rACLR) is the management of associated chondral injuries. Patients undergoing rACLR have a significantly higher prevalence of cartilage injuries as well as higher-grade defects in comparison to patients undergoing primary ACLR. Moreover, the status of the articular cartilage at the time of rACLR is one of the most significant contributors to successful patient outcomes.

Cartilage injuries are present in roughly 30–70% of patients undergoing rACLR, and the medial femoral condyle (MFC) is the most common location of injury [1–4]. Borchers et al. compared intra-articular findings in the MOON and MARS study groups and found an increased odds ratio of Outerbridge grade 3 and 4 chondral lesions in rACLR compared with primary ACLR in the lateral and patellofemoral compartments, but not in the medial compartment regardless of prior meniscal treatment [5].

Although studies evaluating long-term outcomes of combined rACLR and cartilage procedures are limited, most report that the status of the articular cartilage has a significant effect on clinical outcomes [6–8]. The MARS group reported that previous meniscal injury and current articular cartilage damage are associated with the poorest outcomes. Specifically, patients with high-grade trochlear lesions were 1.6 to 2.7 times more likely to report significantly worse 2-year outcomes than those without chondral pathology. Interestingly, activity levels at 2 years were not affected by meniscal or articular cartilage pathology [9]. Only a few studies have compared different cartilage procedures in the setting of primary or rACLR, and there is no consensus on the optimal treatment of full-thickness cartilage lesions in ACL-injured knees [10]. Røtterud et al. performed a nationwide cohort study in Sweden/Norway of 357 patients with concomitant primary ACLR and full-thickness cartilage lesions treated with microfracture (MFx), chondroplasty/debridement, or benign neglect. At 2-year follow-up, those patients treated with MFx showed significantly worse outcome scores compared to those patients who underwent chondroplasty/debridement or no treatment at all. Furthermore, chondroplasty/debridement showed no positive or negative effects on patient-reported outcomes after primary ACLR at 2- year follow-

I. Garcia-Mansilla · B. M. Cash
Division of Sports Medicine and Shoulder Surgery, Department of Orthopaedic Surgery, David Geffen School of Medicine at UCLA, Los Angeles, CA, USA

K. J. Jones (✉)
Department of Orthopaedic Surgery, Division of Sports Medicine, David Geffen School of Medicine at UCLA, Los Angeles, CA, USA

E. E. Vellios
Sports Medicine and Shoulder Surgery Service, Sports Medicine Institute, Hospital for Special Surgery, New York, NY, USA

M. J. Alaia, K. J. Jones (eds.), *Revision Anterior Cruciate Ligament Reconstruction*,
https://doi.org/10.1007/978-3-030-96996-7_21

up [11]. In contrast, Johnson et al. reviewed 78 patients who underwent rACLR and found no significant differences in subjective outcome scores for patients who underwent concurrent partial meniscectomy, MFx, or chondroplasty at an average of 52 months post-op [12].

A comprehensive preoperative evaluation is important when treating chondral injuries combined with ACLR failures. Attention should be given to patient age, activity level, symptoms, physical examination findings (malalignment, ligament instability, hyperlaxity), and imaging studies (tibial/femoral tunnel placement and size, articular cartilage/meniscus integrity, and coronal plane/sagittal plane alignment). In a cohort study of 246 patients undergoing rACLR with articular cartilage injuries and lower extremity alignment films, Brophy et al. demonstrated that articular cartilage lesions correlated directly with meniscus integrity. Medial compartment lesions were associated with varus malalignment, medial meniscus deficiency, and increased BMI, while lateral compartment lesions were associated with increased age and lateral meniscal deficiency. However, activity level, number of revision procedures, and previous ACL graft type were not associated with cartilage changes in the tibiofemoral compartments at the time of rACLR [13].

The following two cases illustrate the potential management of concomitant chondral injuries in the setting of rACLR. The authors would like to emphasize that despite chondral lesions being relatively common at the time of rACLR, a large majority do not require formal surgical treatment, and final treatment decisions should rely on a comprehensive evaluation of the patient.

Case 1

History and Physical Exam

The patient is a 21-year-old female collegiate soccer player who complained of left knee instability. She denied any pain or mechanical symptoms. She previously underwent a primary ACLR utilizing bone-patellar tendon-bone (BTB) autograft 3 years ago and sustained a repeat injury to her left knee while playing soccer. She presented with a small left knee effusion but full range of motion. Physical examination revealed a grade 2B Lachman and a grade 1+ pivot shift test consistent with a recurrent ACL injury. Her left lower extremity alignment was neutral.

Imaging and Other Diagnostic Studies

Radiographic (Fig. 21.1) and MRI images (Fig. 21.2) reveal a torn ACL graft with bioabsorbable screw fixation. Tunnel positioning is satisfactory, and there is no evidence of significant tunnel widening. The lateral meniscus shows irregularity along the posterior root and posterior horn, suggestive of a lateral root tear. A deep chondral fissure was visualized along the posterior weightbearing portion of the medial femoral condyle (MFC) with chondral delamination and associated bone edema.

Preoperative Planning

In this case, a decision was made to proceed with a one-stage rACLR with treatment of concomitant meniscal/chondral pathology. Given the patient's activity level, and desire to return to collegiate soccer, the decision was made to proceed with rACLR using BTB autograft from the contralateral knee. Additionally, we planned to perform a lateral meniscus root repair and a chondroplasty of the MFC chondral lesion. Given the acute nature of this injury, we elected to not treat the MFC lesion with any formal cartilage restoration procedure. Intraoperatively, the decision would be made to proceed with an articular cartilage biopsy for future cell-based treatment of the chondral lesion using matrix-associated autologous chondrocyte implantation (MACI) if necessary.

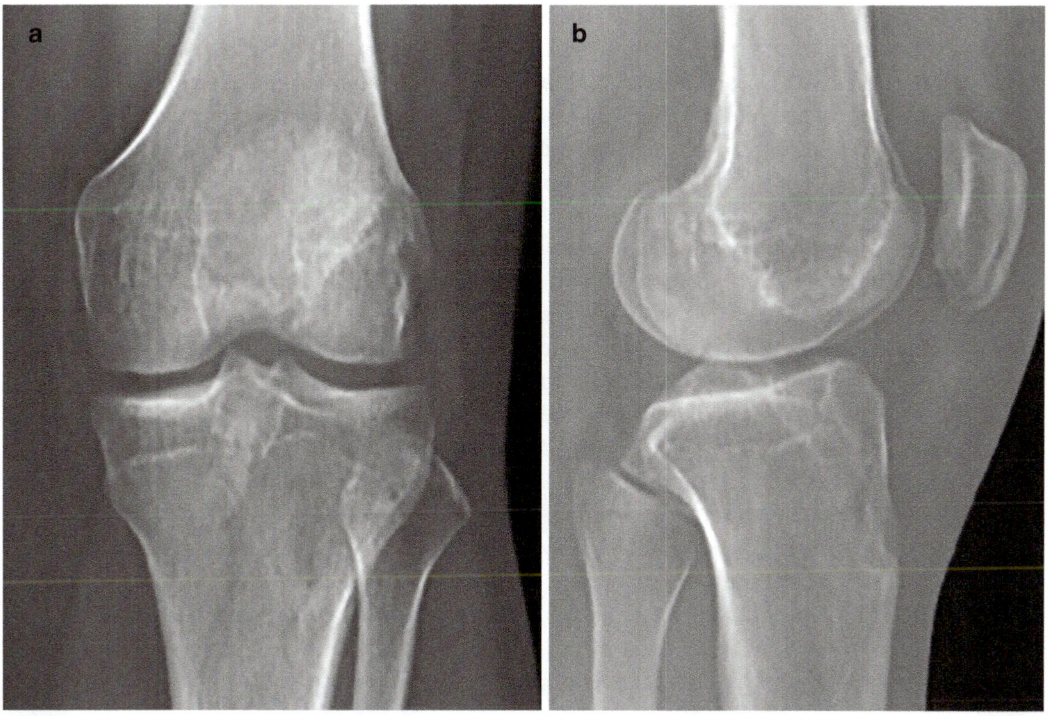

Fig. 21.1 Preoperative X-rays of the left knee. AP (**a**) and lateral (**b**) views show appropriate tunnel positioning and no evidence of tunnel osteolysis

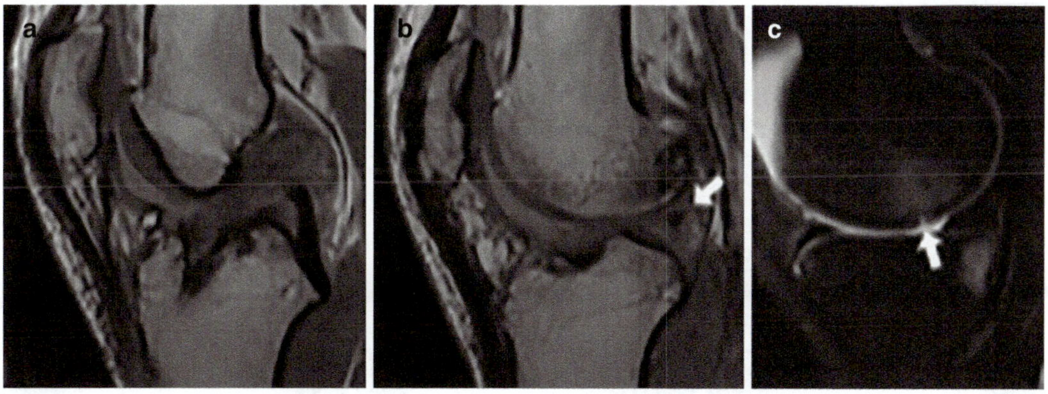

Fig. 21.2 Preoperative MRI of the left knee. Sagittal views show a torn ACL graft (**a**) and a posterior root tear of the lateral meniscus (**b**). Sagittal T2 fat-sat (**c**) reveals a cartilage lesion in the medial femoral condyle with associated bone edema

Surgical Procedure

To begin, the BTB autograft was harvested from the right leg and prepared on the back table. Next, a diagnostic arthroscopy was performed using standard anterolateral and anteromedial portals. If previous incisions are adequately positioned, they may be used, but the appropriate placement of incisions should not be compromised for the sole purpose of cosmesis. Figure 21.3 depicts intraoperative findings. Inspection of the medial compartment revealed a small focal grade 3/4 chondral lesion along the weightbearing aspect of the medial femoral condyle. The surrounding cartilage was unstable to probing, revealing a small delaminated chondral flap (Fig. 21.3a). Examination of the intercondylar notch showed an intact PCL and a complete mid-substance tear of the ACL graft (Fig. 21.3b). The lateral compartment demonstrated intact chondral surfaces, but there was a complete tear of the lateral meniscus near the root attachment (type 2 tear) that was unstable to probing (Fig. 21.3c). A ring curette and 4.5 mm arthroscopic shaver were used to debride the loose cartilage flap overlying the medial femoral condyle resulting in a stable and well-shouldered lesion of 10 × 8 mm (Fig. 21.4). Given the small size of the lesion, a decision was made to proceed with an abrasion arthroplasty (marrow stimulation procedure). A 5.5 bone cutter was then used to abrade the subchondral bone, thereby resulting in visible bleeding of the bony surface. We prefer this technique relative to other marrow stimulation procedures such as microfracture, as it does not significantly compromise the underlying subchondral bone, an important factor that affects clinical outcomes for future cell-based procedures. The residual ACL graft was debrided. Both the tibial and femoral ACL tunnels were found to be in adequate position. The prior femoral tunnel was fully incorporated with bone from the prior BTB autograft. Attention was then turned to the type 2 root tear. Using a 4.5 mm arthroscopic shaver, the root attachment was debrided removing any residual soft tissue to expose the underlying bone. Using an all-inside meniscal repair device, two luggage tag sutures were placed through the root of the lateral meniscus. These sutures were then docked through a separate portal for later repair (Fig. 21.5a).

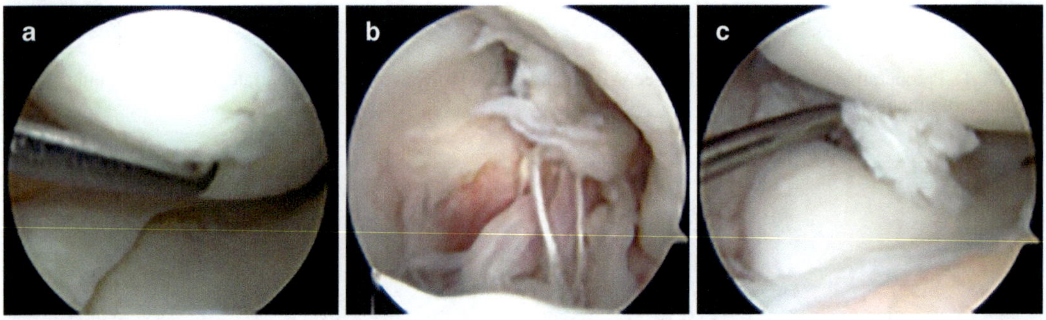

Fig. 21.3 (**a**) Focal grade 3/4 chondral lesion along the weightbearing aspect of the medial femoral condyle. Surrounding cartilage is unstable to probing. (**b**) Mid-substance tearing of existing ACL graft. (**c**) Complete radial tear of the posterior root of the lateral meniscus (type 2 tear) with displacement into the lateral compartment

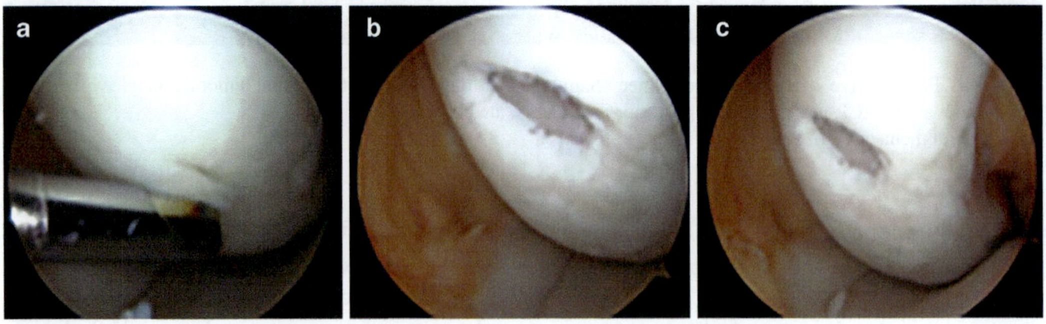

Fig. 21.4 Debridement of medial femoral condyle cartilage lesion. (**a**) 4.5 mm arthroscopic shaver is used to remove the loose chondral flap. (**b**, **c**) A stable and well-shouldered lesion of approximately 10 × 8 mm is observed following formal debridement

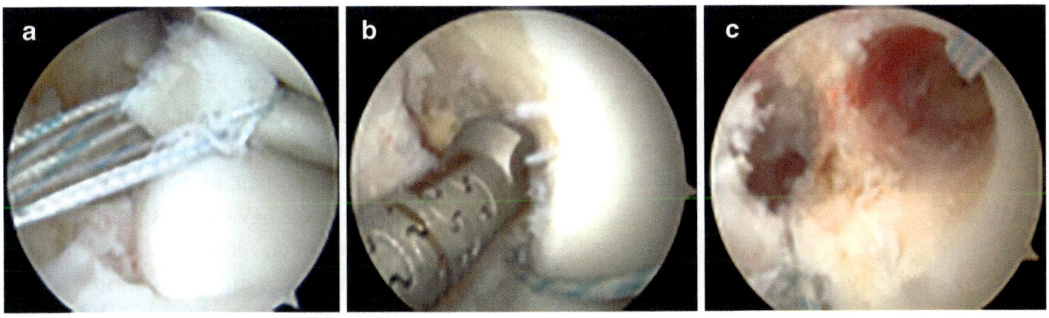

Fig. 21.5 (**a**) Lateral meniscus posterior root repair. (**b**) Flexible reamer is inserted to drill the femoral ACL tunnel. (**c**) Completed ACL femoral tunnel with an intact, 2 mm posterior wall

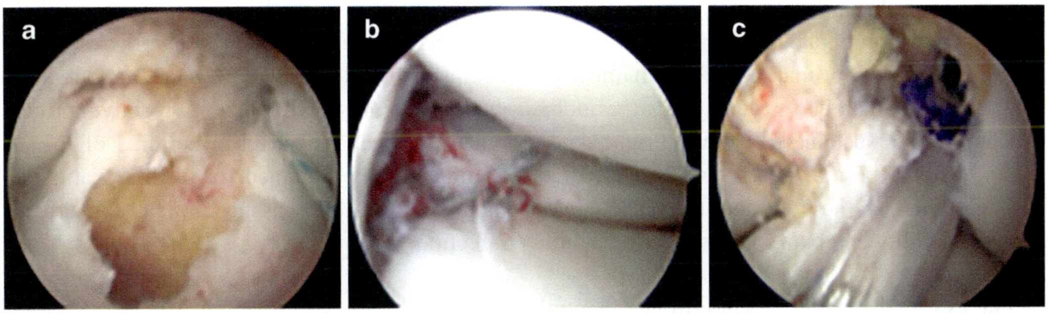

Fig. 21.6 (**a**) Tibial tunnel drilled. (**b**) Lateral meniscal root repair with sutures docked in tibial tunnel. (**c**) Graft secured in place

The new ACL tunnels were then drilled using a flexible reamer and a free hand femoral guide (Figs. 21.5b, c and 21.6a). The meniscal root repair sutures were then shuttled through the tibial ACL tunnel to anatomically approximate the root to its native footprint (Fig. 21.6b). The ACL graft was then passed through the tibial tunnel and docked into the femoral tunnel. The graft was fixed with a 7 × 20 mm metal interference screw inserted over a guidewire (Fig. 21.6c). The knee was then placed in full extension, and a size 9 × 20 mm metal interference screw was inserted over a guidewire into the tibial tunnel. The meniscal root repair sutures were tensioned and then secured to a 4.75 mm bio-composite swivel-lock within the proximal tibia, approximately 1 cm distal to the aperture of the tibial tunnel.

Post-Operative Protocol

In this case, post-operative management was guided by the meniscal root repair. Weightbearing in full extension was limited to toe touch (20%) in a hinged knee brace, and knee flexion was limited to 90 degrees until 4 weeks after surgery. After 4 weeks, the patient was allowed to discontinue use of the brace and begin full weightbearing and full knee range of motion. Supervised physical therapy was initiated as soon as possible, with an emphasis on range of motion and isometric strengthening. When available, blood flow restriction (BFR) exercises are initiated early to mitigate muscle atrophy. Loading of the knee at angles greater than 90 degrees was not permitted until 4 months post-operatively. Return to sport is typically permitted approximately 8–10 months post-operatively if a functional testing algorithm demonstrates the athlete is at low risk for reinjury.

Case 2

History and Physical Exam

The patient is a 33-year-old male personal trainer who presented with a longstanding history of right knee instability and lateral knee pain. He sustained a right knee ACL tear approximately 2 years ago while playing soccer and subsequently underwent primary ACLR with allograft tissue. Approximately 1.5 years after the index procedure, he sustained a repeat right knee injury. After a period of rest and self-directed physical therapy, he returned to activity, but noted instability and pain localized to the lateral joint line.

On exam, the patient demonstrated neutral alignment. There was no suggestion of a medial or lateral thrust with ambulation. There was a mild knee effusion. He had moderate lateral joint line tenderness. Lachman exam was 2B, and pivot shift was 1+. Anterior drawer was positive and posterior drawer was negative. The knee was stable to varus and valgus stress in extension and at 30 degrees of flexion with a negative dial test. His neurovascular exam was normal.

Imaging and Other Diagnostic Studies

Radiographs of the right knee revealed implants from the previous ACLR, as well as notable widening of the femoral and tibial tunnels (Fig. 21.7). In this patient with a soft tissue allograft used for his index ACL reconstruction, as well as fixation at the proximal end of the femoral tunnel and distal end of the tibial tunnel, tunnel widening is a consequence of the "windshield wiper" effect, a concept originally described by L'insalata and corroborated by others [14–16]. With tunnel widening evident on routine radiographs, a CT scan was obtained for further evaluation of tunnel size, position, and orientation (Fig. 21.8) [17]. An MRI was obtained to evaluate the ACL graft and investigate for concomitant meniscal or chondral pathology. It is important to note that metallic graft fixation devices may create significant artifact on MRI, and metal suppression sequences may be useful in these clinical scenarios. In this case, the MRI revealed a focal grade 3/4 chondral lesion of the lateral femoral condyle (LFC) (Fig. 21.8d).

If there is clinical suspicion for infection, especially in cases with significant osteolysis of previous tunnels, then bloodwork including complete blood count (CBC), erythrocyte sedimentation rate (ESR), and C-reactive protein (CRP), as well as bacterial cultures of a knee aspirate, can be obtained for further evaluation. In this case, there was no clinical concern for infection.

Preoperative Planning

A number of factors must be considered when deciding to move forward with a one- or two-stage revision procedure. These factors include tunnel anatomy (size, position, and orientation), preoperative knee range of motion, and concomitant intra-articular injuries. The size of the tunnels should be measured at their apertures within the knee joint, as well as at their widest mid-tunnel diameter on coronal or sagittal CT imaging [18]. In this case, due to widening of the femoral and tibial tunnels >15 millimeters, the decision was made to proceed with a two-stage revision ACL reconstruction [19]. In the setting of recurrent ACL injuries with cartilage pathology, a two-stage procedure affords an opportunity to examine the cartilage lesion and determine optimal management. If a two-stage cartilage restoration procedure – such as MACI – is planned, the harvest of autologous chondrocytes can be performed at the same time as bone grafting of the tunnels. Additionally, if a fresh tissue transfer procedure such as osteochondral allograft (OCA)

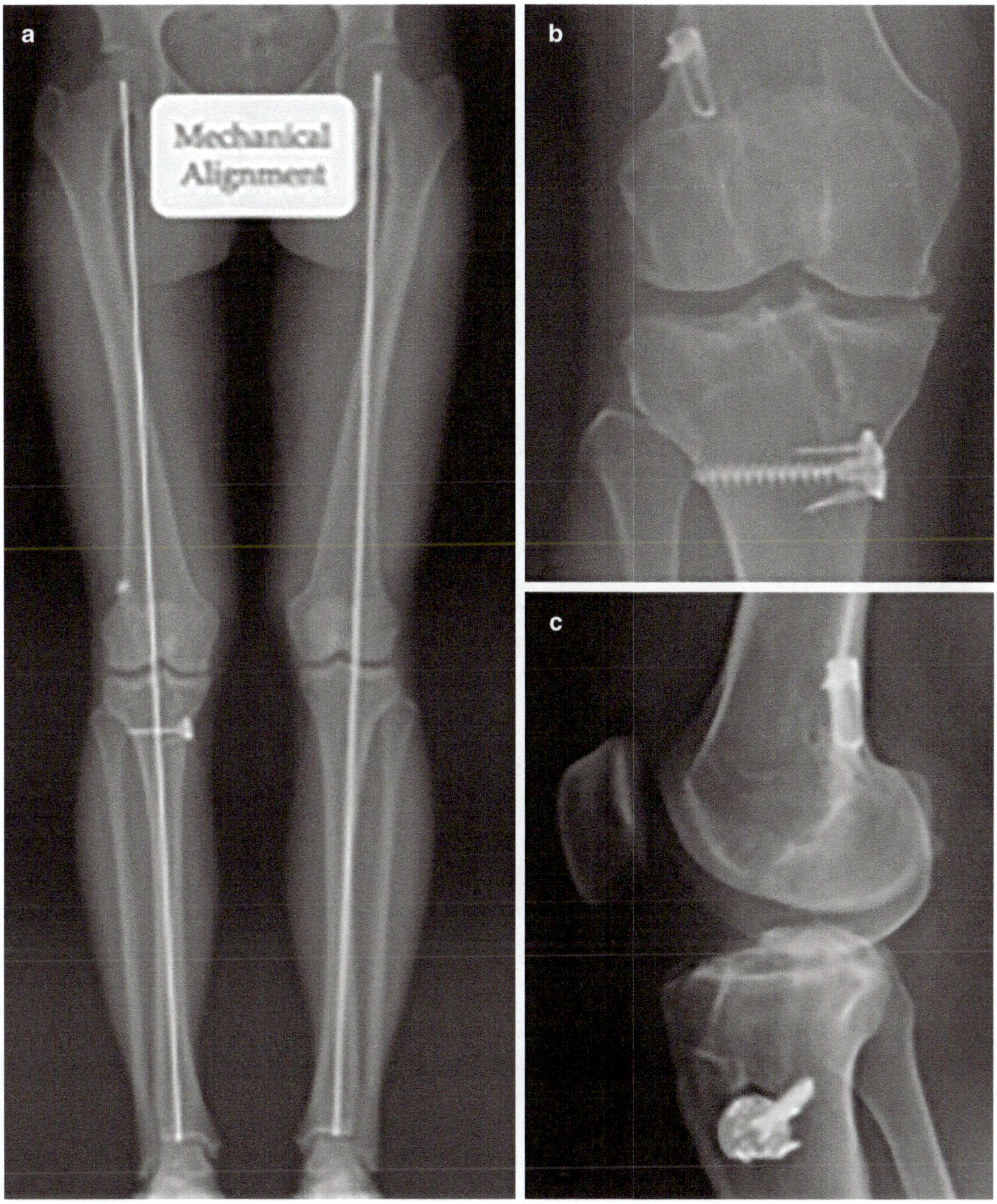

Fig. 21.7 Preoperative X-rays of the right knee. Alignment films (**a**) show neutral alignment of the right knee. AP (**b**) and lateral (**c**) radiographs reveal implants from previous ACL reconstruction. Anterior translation of the tibia relative to the femur can be noted on the lateral radiograph, suggesting failure of the ACL graft. Additionally, both radiographs reveal tunnel widening

transplantation is indicated after arthroscopic evaluation of the lesion, it is possible to arrange for accurate OCA graft matching, while the bone graft heals within the tunnels.

First-Stage Surgery

At the time of the first stage, a standard diagnostic arthroscopy was performed through anterolat-

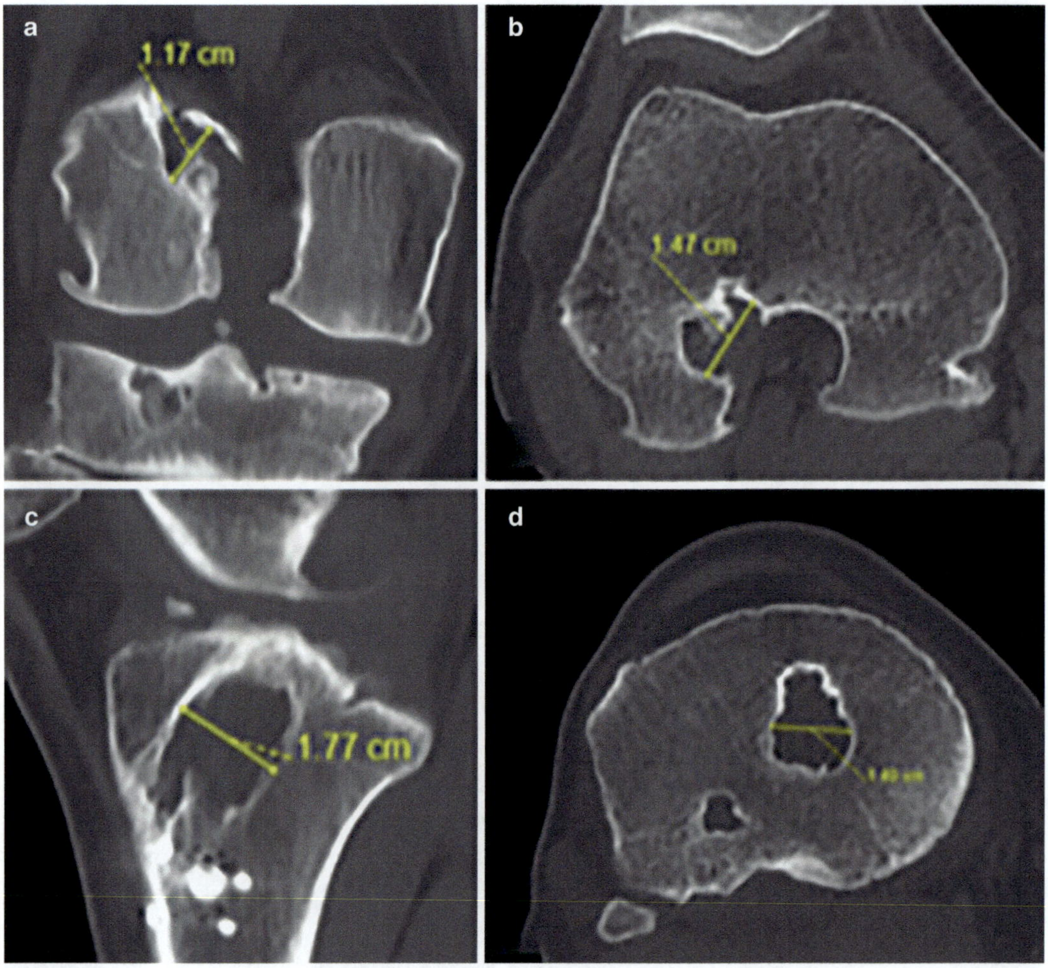

Fig. 21.8 Preoperative CT scan images of the right knee. For the femoral tunnel, the diameter is measured at the aperture, seen on the axial view (**b**), as well as the widest portion of the mid-tunnel, seen here on the coronal view (**a**). For the tibial tunnel, the widest portion of the tunnel is measured on the sagittal (**c**) and axial views. Sagittal MRI reveals a focal grade 3/4 chondral lesion along the weightbearing aspect of the LFC (**d**)

eral and anteromedial portals. In this case, an incompetent ACL graft was noted (Fig. 21.9a). Inspection of the lateral compartment revealed a 15 × 15 mm grade IV osteochondral lesion of the lateral femoral condyle (Fig. 21.9b). With a symptomatic lesion of this size in the setting of a rACLR, we prefer to use an osteochondral allograft, which is performed during the second stage of a two-stage ACL reconstruction. At the time of this procedure, any other intra-articular pathology should be inspected and addressed as needed. In this case, a loose osteochondral body was also found in the lateral compartment and removed (Fig. 21.9c). Additionally, a small horizontal tear of the lateral meniscus was present, and a partial lateral meniscectomy was performed with a 4.5 mm arthroscopic shaver (Fig. 21.9d).

The implants securing the ACL graft were removed, the graft was debrided, and the femoral/tibial tunnels were identified to remove all soft tissue using arthroscopic shavers and curved curettes (Fig. 21.10a). Next, the tibial tunnel was reamed and sequentially dilated to a final size of 16 mm, and a 16 × 35 mm bone dowel allograft was press-fit into the tibial tunnel (Fig. 21.10d). Allograft dowels are available from various com-

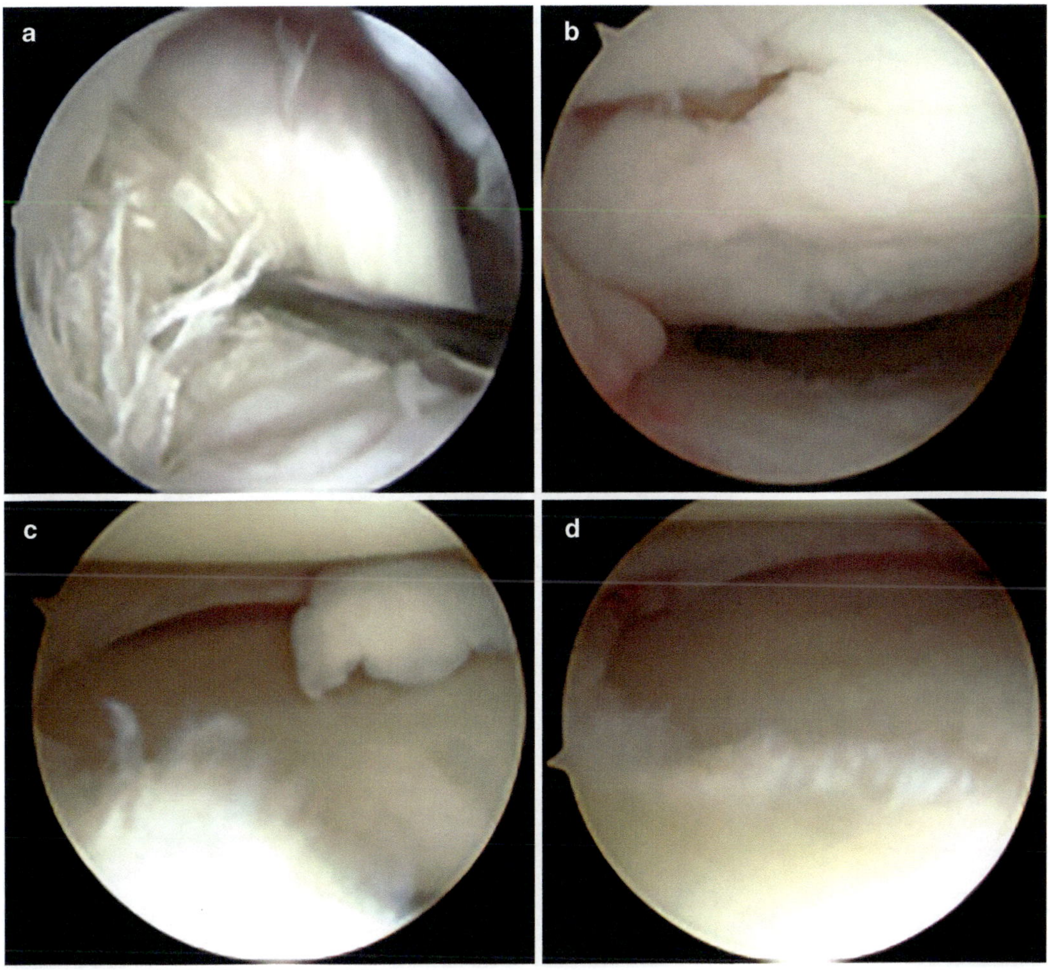

Fig. 21.9 First-stage intraoperative findings. (**a**) The previous ACL graft was noted to be incompetent. (**b**) A 15 × 15 mm, grade 3/4 osteochondral lesion of the lateral femoral condyle was noted. (**c**) A loose body was found in the lateral compartment and was removed. (**d**) There was a horizontal tear of the lateral meniscus, from the midbody to posterior horn, which was treated with debridement using an arthroscopic shaver

mercial vendors. Finally, the femoral tunnel aperture was measured to corroborate the findings from the preoperative CT scan and confirm that bone grafting was necessary. In this case, the femoral tunnel aperture measured 16 mm. The femoral tunnel was grafted with 10 cc of cortical fibers and 10 cc of demineralized bone matrix (DBM) putty mixed with platelet-rich plasma (PRP). The bone graft was then inserted via a commercial graft delivery system after all arthroscopic fluid was evacuated from the knee (Fig. 21.10b, c).

Clinical Management

After stage one, the patient was kept toe-touch weightbearing (20%) in a hinged knee brace for approximately 2 weeks post-operatively. Supervised physical therapy was initiated with a focus on range of motion and isometric strengthening exercises. Around 5–6 weeks post-operatively, the patient may begin low-impact exercises such as stationary biking or swimming. A CT scan of the knee is obtained around 4 months post-operatively, and if the bone graft is

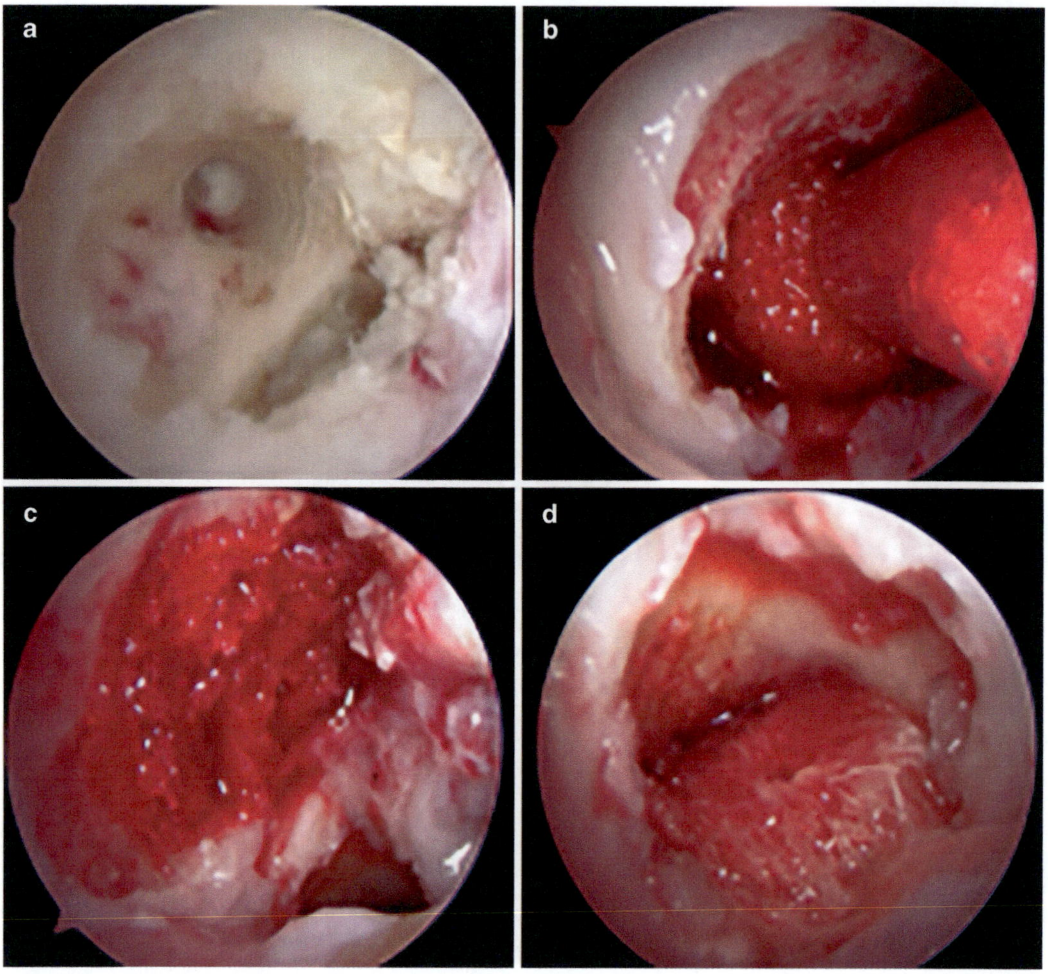

Fig. 21.10 (**a**) Femoral tunnel after debridement and removal of soft tissue. (**b**, **c**) Femoral tunnel was grafted with 10 cc of cortical fibers and 10 cc of DBM putty mixed with PRP and inserted via a commercial graft delivery system. (**d**) Tibial tunnel grafted with a 16 × 35 mm bone dowel allograft

sufficiently incorporated, we proceed with the second stage of the rACLR procedure.

Second-Stage Surgery

Given recent literature that suggests biologic augmentation may improve OCA graft incorporation, we prefer to treat these grafts with bone marrow aspirate concentrate (BMAC) prior to implantation [20]. Prior to formal preparation and draping, the patient is placed in the supine position on the operating room table, and a large Jamshidi needle is percutaneously inserted to aspirate bone marrow from the anterior iliac crest. The bone marrow aspirate is then placed in a centrifuge for preparation and later use during the procedure.

Next, we proceed with rACLR. The intended ACL autograft can be harvested from the ipsilateral or contralateral leg, as needed. In this case, we harvested a BTB autograft from the ipsilateral leg. A diagnostic arthroscopy was then performed through standard anterolateral and anteromedial portals, allowing the surgeon to re-examine the cartilage injury and ensure there has been no progression of intra-articular meniscal or cartilage pathology. With the bone graft fully incorporated

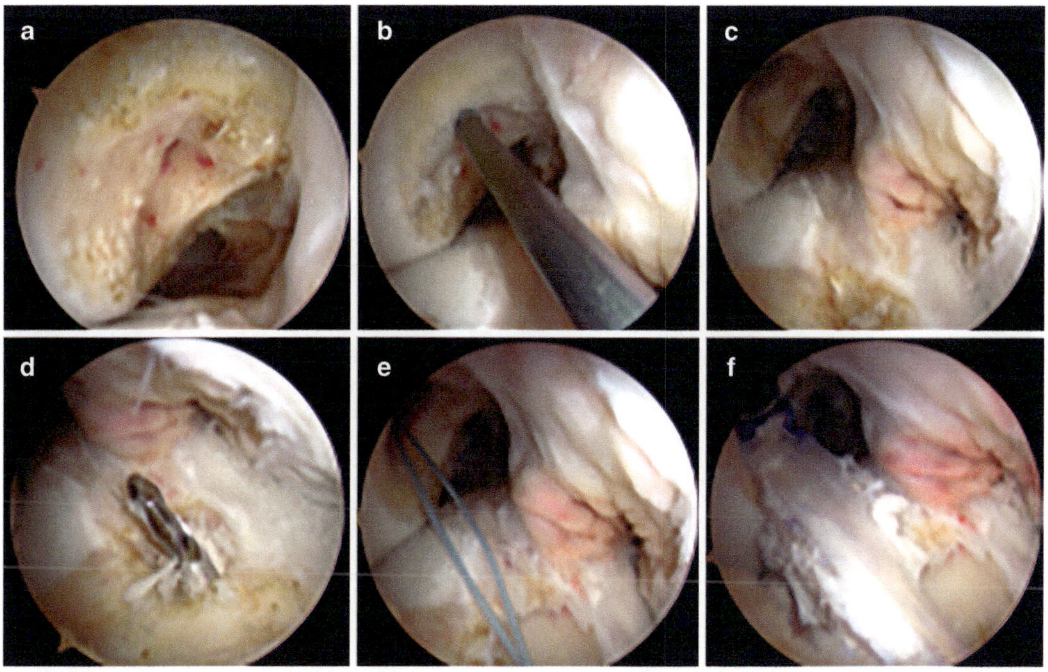

Fig. 21.11 (**a**) Inspection of the femoral condyle reveals that the previously placed bone graft is well-healed. The revision ACL reconstruction can therefore proceed similar to a primary ACL reconstruction surgery. (**b**) Using an anteromedial portal, a flexible guidewire is placed within the footprint of the native ACL. (**c**) A flexible reamer is used to drill to a depth of 20–25 mm, and the back wall is inspected to ensure it is approximately 1–2 mm without compromise. (**d**) Guide pin inserted in tibial ACL footprint. (**e**) A shuttle suture is used to pass the graft through the tibial tunnel and into the femoral tunnel. (**f**) ACL graft fixed within the femur with a metal interference screw

within the femoral and tibial tunnels, the rACLR can be completed in a similar manner as a primary ACLR (Fig. 21.11).

After the graft is fixed within the femur with a metal interference screw, we proceed with OCA transplantation. In this case, we were able to obtain accurate measurements of the cartilage defect during the first-stage procedure. The lesion measured 15 × 15 mm, thereby allowing us to proceed with OCA transplantation using a precut 15 mm OCA dowel. These pre-cut dowels are readily available from select commercial tissue banks. This approach obviates OCA graft matching and facilitates timely surgical treatment. A 6 cm vertical incision was made in line with the anterolateral portal, followed by a mini-lateral arthrotomy to expose the defect. Excision of the infrapatellar fat pad may be necessary for adequate exposure. A bent Hohmann retractor and a Z-retractor help to provide excellent exposure (Fig. 21.12b). In this case, a 15 mm sizing template was placed perpendicular to the LFC, and a 2.4 mm Kirschner wire was inserted. A 15 mm reamer is used to ream to a depth of approximately 6–7 mm based on preoperative MRI measurements (Fig. 21.12c). The resultant socket is then measured at four quadrants along a clock face to determine the subsequent size of the allograft dowel that will be implanted. The graft was marked according to these measurements, and excess bone was removed from the end of the graft using a sagittal saw. The graft was then soaked in the previously harvested BMAC (Fig. 21.12a). The allograft dowel was finally inserted into the recipient socket using a press-fit technique (Fig. 21.12d). It is important to ensure the graft sits flush to the surrounding articular surface to avoid increased contact stress that could compromise graft healing [21]. Following OCA transplantation, the ACL graft was finally

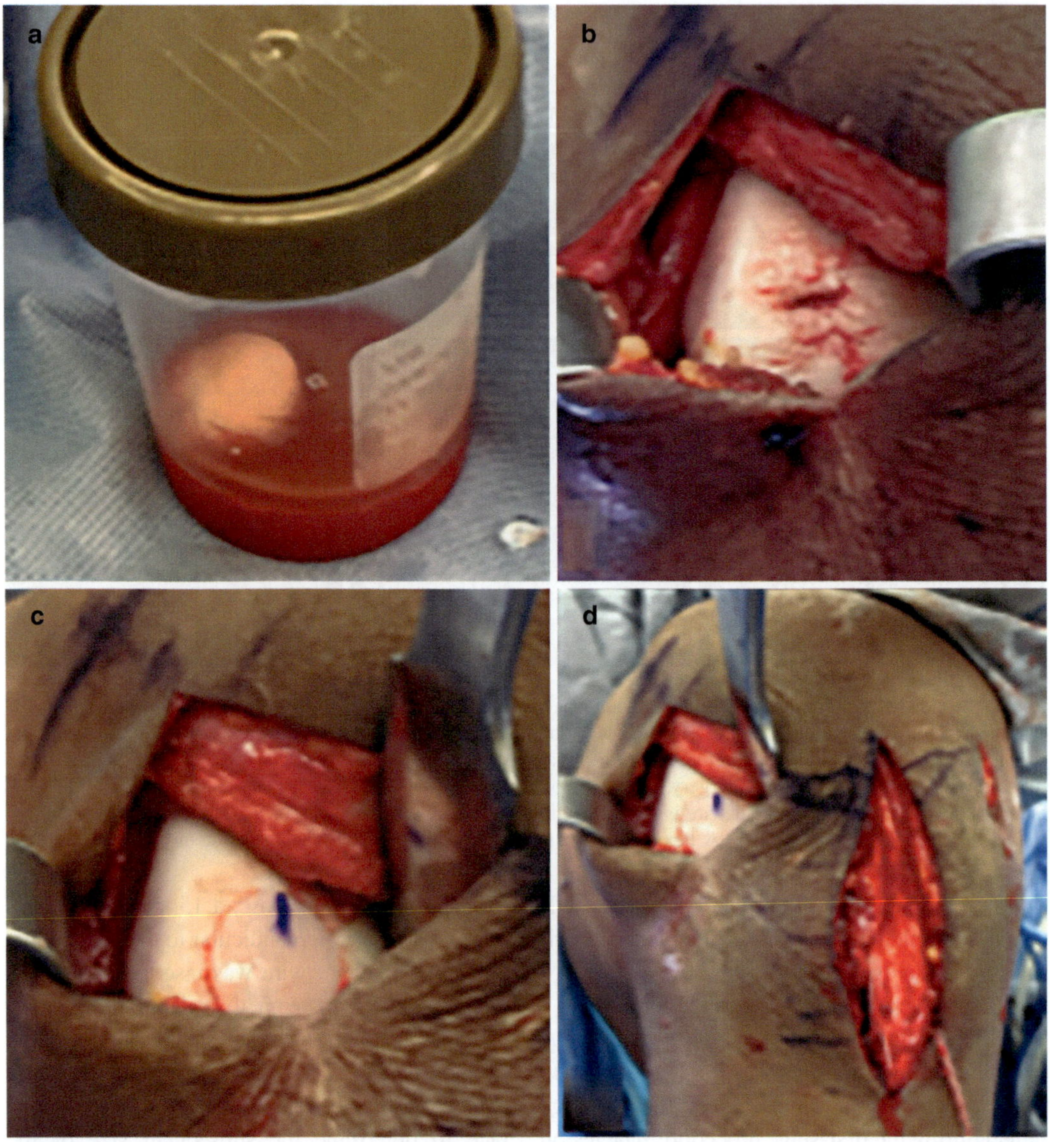

Fig. 21.12 Intraoperative images of the OCA transplantation procedure. (**a**) The allograft is soaked in the BMAC. (**b**) The lateral femoral condyle is exposed through a mini lateral arthrotomy. A bent Hohmann retractor and a Z-retractor are used to provide exposure. (**c**) The lesion is reamed to a depth of approximately 6–7 mm (**d**). The fresh, 15 mm precut allograft dowel is press-fit into the recipient socket

fixed on the tibial side with a metal interference screw. The wound was then irrigated, closed, and dressed.

Of note, while it was not an issue in this case, it is conceivable that a femoral tunnel may converge with an osteochondral graft within the lateral femoral condyle. The surgeon should consider this possibility during preoperative planning and can adjust the recipient socket depth and/or femoral tunnel angle as needed.

Post-Operative Protocol

Post-operatively, the patient was kept non-weightbearing in a hinged knee brace for approximately 2 weeks. Supervised physical therapy was initiated as soon as possible, with an emphasis on range of motion. At 2 weeks post-operatively, the patient began partial-weightbearing (50%) with the brace unlocked. At approximately 4–5 weeks post-operatively, the patient began to advance to weightbearing as tolerated and ultimately discontinued the brace, as he was progressing as expected with adequate range of motion and quadriceps strength with no significant joint effusion. The patient was advanced through a standard ACL rehabilitation protocol. The surgeon may choose to obtain a repeat MRI or CT scan at 6 months post-operatively to evaluate for osteochondral allograft integration prior to return to sport-specific training. Return to sport is not permitted until at least 9–12 months post-operatively.

Summary and Our Preferred Algorithm

The management of cartilage defects in the setting of revision ACL reconstruction can include a wide array of treatment strategies, including no treatment (benign neglect), chondroplasty, marrow stimulation with microfracture or abrasion arthroplasty, autologous chondrocyte implantation (ACI), and osteochondral autograft and allograft techniques. It is important to note that chondral lesions are quite common in the rACLR setting, and many of these lesions do not require treatment if they are not symptomatic.

In most cases, for small lesions (less than 2 cm^2) that are asymptomatic (no pain or mechanical symptoms), our preferred treatment is benign neglect, chondroplasty, or abrasion arthroplasty. When performing a marrow stimulation procedure, abrasion arthroplasty is preferred over microfracture, as it does not compromise the underlying subchondral bone. Recent studies demonstrate inferior clinical outcomes when cell-based cartilage restoration procedures are used to treat symptomatic cartilage lesions that were previously managed with a microfracture procedure [22]. Ultimately, we prefer to keep all cartilage restoration procedures available to us if future treatment is necessary, and we have largely abandoned microfracture as a potential treatment modality for this reason. For small, symptomatic lesions (up to 4 cm^2), osteochondral autograft is our treatment of choice. Osteochondral autograft is preferred for lesions of this size, as autograft plugs incorporate quickly and facilitate a faster return to athletic activity (mean 5 months) relative to other procedures [23]. For larger lesions (greater than 4 cm^2), osteochondral autograft is a less-viable option, as donor site morbidity increases. Therefore, osteochondral allograft and MACI are the preferred surgical treatments for large lesions. OCA is typically utilized if there are any signs of subchondral bone irregularities, although the MACI "sandwich" technique is also an option. MACI is particularly advantageous for defects in the patellofemoral joint, given the significant variation of individualized anatomy in this area of the knee. However, MACI techniques do have notable downsides, including increased expense, longer time for graft maturation, and the necessity of two procedures.

The treatment of chondral lesions in the rACLR setting is complex, and treatment plans hinge on several considerations including lesion size, location, and morphology; patient age and activity level; symptoms and exam findings; presence of degenerative changes throughout the knee; meniscal integrity; malalignment; instability; and involvement of subchondral bone. While there may be multiple viable treatment options for any given lesion, the nuances of these factors may push the surgeon toward a preferred strategy.

References

1. Arianjam A, Inacio MCS, Funahashi TT, Maletis GB. Analysis of 2019 patients undergoing revision anterior cruciate ligament reconstruction from a community-based registry. Am J Sports Med. 2017;45:1574–80.
2. Magnussen RA, Trojani C, Granan LP, Neyret P, Colombet P, Engebretsen L, et al. Patient demographics and surgical characteristics in ACL revision: a comparison of French, Norwegian, and North American cohorts. Knee Surg Sports Traumatol Arthrosc. 2015;23:2339–48.

3. Chen JL, Allen CR, Stephens TE, Haas AK, Huston LJ, Wright RW, et al. Differences in mechanisms of failure, intraoperative findings, and surgical characteristics between single- and multiple-revision ACL reconstructions: a MARS cohort study. Am J Sports Med. 2013;41:1571–8.
4. Mitchell JJ, Cinque ME, Dornan GJ, Matheny LM, Dean CS, Kruckeberg B, et al. Primary versus revision anterior cruciate ligament reconstruction: patient demographics, radiographic findings, and associated lesions. Arthrosc J Arthrosc Relat Surg. 2018;34:695–703.
5. Borchers JR, Kaeding CC, Pedroza AD, Huston LJ, Spindler KP, Wright RW. Intra-articular findings in primary and revision anterior cruciate ligament reconstruction surgery: a comparison of the MOON and MARS study groups. Am J Sports Med. 2011;39:1889–93.
6. Diamantopoulos AP, Lorbach O, Paessler HH. Anterior cruciate ligament revision reconstruction: results in 107 patients. Am J Sports Med. 2008;36:851–60.
7. Grossman MG, ElAttrache NS, Shields CL, Glousman RE. Revision anterior cruciate ligament reconstruction: three- to nine-year follow-up. Arthrosc J Arthrosc Relat Surg. 2005;21:418–23.
8. Salmon LJ, Pinczewski LA, Russell VJ, Refshauge K. Revision anterior cruciate ligament reconstruction with hamstring tendon autograft: 5- to 9-year follow-up. Am J Sports Med. 2006;34:1604–14.
9. Wright RW, Huston LJ, Nwosu SK, Haas AK, Allen CR, Anderson AF, et al. Meniscal and articular cartilage predictors of clinical outcome after revision anterior cruciate ligament reconstruction. Am J Sports Med. 2016;44:1671–9.
10. Brophy RH, Zeltser D, Wright RW, Flanigan D. Anterior cruciate ligament reconstruction and concomitant articular cartilage injury: incidence and treatment. Arthrosc J Arthrosc Relat Surg. 2010;26:112–20.
11. Røtterud JH, Sivertsen EA, Forssblad M, Engebretsen L, Årøen A. Effect on patient-reported outcomes of debridement or microfracture of concomitant full-thickness cartilage lesions in anterior cruciate ligament-reconstructed knees: a nationwide cohort study from Norway and Sweden of 357 patients with 2-year follow-up. Am J Sports Med. 2016;44:337–44.
12. Johnson WR, Makani A, Wall AJ, Hosseini A, Hampilos P, Li G, et al. Patient outcomes and predictors of success after revision anterior cruciate ligament reconstruction. Orthop J Sports Med. 2015;3:2325967115611660.
13. Brophy RH, Haas AK, Huston LJ, Nwosu SK, Wright RW, Harris DC, et al. Association of meniscal status, lower extremity alignment, and body mass index with chondrosis at revision anterior cruciate ligament reconstruction. Am J Sports Med. 2015;43:1616–22.
14. L'Insalata JC, Klatt B, Fu FH, Harner CD. Tunnel expansion following anterior cruciate ligament reconstruction: a comparison of hamstring and patellar tendon autografts. Knee Surg Sports Traumatol Arthrosc. 1997;5:234–8.
15. Clatworthy MG, Annear P, Bulow JU, Bartlett RJ. Tunnel widening in anterior cruciate ligament reconstruction: a prospective evaluation of hamstring and patella tendon grafts. Knee Surg Sports Traumatol Arthrosc Off J ESSKA. 1999;7:138–45.
16. Webster KE. A comparison of bone tunnel measurements made using computed tomography and digital plain radiography after anterior cruciate ligament reconstruction. Arthroscopy. 2004;20:946–50.
17. Marchant MH, Willimon CC, Vinson E, Pietrobon R, Garrett WE, Higgins LD. Comparison of plain radiography, computed tomography, and magnetic resonance imaging in the evaluation of bone tunnel widening after anterior cruciate ligament reconstruction. Knee Surg Sports Traumatol Arthrosc. 2010;18:1059–64.
18. Rizer M, Foremny GB, Rush A, Singer AD, Baraga M, Kaplan LD, et al. Anterior cruciate ligament reconstruction tunnel size: causes of tunnel enlargement and implications for single versus two-stage revision reconstruction. Skeletal Radiol. 2017;46:161–9.
19. Mayr R, Rosenberger R, Agraharam D, Smekal V, El Attal R. Revision anterior cruciate ligament reconstruction: an update. Arch Orthop Trauma Surg. 2012;132:1299–313.
20. Oladeji LO, Stannard JP, Cook CR, Kfuri M, Crist BD, Smith MJ, et al. Effects of autogenous bone marrow aspirate concentrate on radiographic integration of femoral condylar osteochondral allografts. Am J Sports Med. 2017;45(12):2797–803.
21. Du PZ, Markolf KL, Boguszewski DV, Yamaguchi KT, Lama CJ, McAllister DR, et al. Effects of proud large osteochondral plugs on contact forces and knee kinematics: a robotic study. Am J Sports Med. 2018;46(9):2122–7.
22. Pestka JM, Bode G, Salzmann G, Südkamp NP, Niemeyer P. Clinical outcome of autologous chondrocyte implantation for failed microfracture treatment of full-thickness cartilage defects of the knee joint. Am J Sports Med. 2012;40(2):325–31.
23. Krych AJ, Pareek A, King AH, Johnson NR, Stuart MJ, Williams RJ 3rd. Return to sport after the surgical management of articular cartilage lesions in the knee: a meta-analysis. Knee Surg Sports Traumatol Arthrosc. 2017;25(10):3186–96.

Revision Anterior Cruciate Ligament Reconstruction in the Elite or Professional Athlete

22

Kristofer Eastman Chenard and Kenneth Dale Montgomery

Revision anterior cruciate ligament (ACL) reconstruction in the elite or professional athlete presents a multitude of unique challenges including high demands after reconstruction, player expectations, technical challenges of revision surgery, and additional demands on the surgeon from the elite and professional sports environment including coaches, trainers, and player agents. We present several cases for discussion of the complex features of revision ACL reconstruction in elite and professional athletes.

Case 1

A 21-year-old female elite college volleyball player sustains a right anterior cruciate ligament rupture after landing awkwardly on another player's foot after making a block at the net. She previously sustained a right ACL rupture after a non-contact twisting injury in high school and underwent ACL reconstruction. She desires to return for her senior season and has aspirations to play at the professional and Olympic level. She is anxious and wants to know what her prognosis for full recovery is.

K. E. Chenard
Spine and Orthopedic Center, Plantation, FL, USA

K. D. Montgomery (✉)
New York Jets, Tri-County Orthopedics,
Cedar Knolls, NJ, USA

Discussion

A thorough history is critical for composing a plan for revision ACL reconstruction. Knowledge of previous graft type is essential for planning treatment; however, in the revision setting, many types of grafts can be used successfully. Bone patellar tendon bone grafts are frequently the standard choice for elite contact athletes in the United States; thus, BPTB grafts are often not available on the injured limb for reconstruction. In some athletes, bone patella tendon bone may not be the best choice even if available at revision. Postoperative patellofemoral pain is a particularly significant problem for jumping athletes. Most elite basketball and volleyball players are tall and tend to have very robust hamstring grafts, and successful revision after a BPTB graft can be performed with hamstring grafts in this situation.

Considering the length of time from the original operation is important and can help the surgeon understand the mode of failure and plan for future success. ACL graft tears may occur early or late and may be the result of traumatic injuries or unimpressive non-contact injuries. Early failures often occur with less dramatic mechanisms. It is important to understand why failure has occurred. Poor or incomplete rehabilitation and rush to full return to sport can put patients at risk for failure. In our practice, side to side functional ACL testing is performed at 6 months prior to

M. J. Alaia, K. J. Jones (eds.), *Revision Anterior Cruciate Ligament Reconstruction*,
https://doi.org/10.1007/978-3-030-96996-7_22

return to sport for all competitive athletes. Many athletes feel that their knee has returned to a competitive level, but functional testing often demonstrates significant deficits. Functional testing can direct the surgeon, therapist, and trainer to corrective exercises prior to return to play.

If the patient was properly rehabilitated prior to return to sport, the surgeon must look for patient-specific factors, mechanism of injury, and technical reasons for failure. The patient should be examined for hyperlaxity (knees with greater than 10 degrees hyperextension), rotatory instability, or a prominent pivot shift. In addition, the injury mechanism should be discussed with the patient. Patients who fail early with benign noncontact mechanisms may demonstrate ligamentous laxity. In our practice, these individuals will undergo an anterolateral ligament reconstruction in addition to revision ACL reconstruction. Late failures, typically at greater than 5 years from initial surgery, are less suspicious for the presence of hyperlaxity or insufficient rehabilitation. Technical reasons for failure should be examined including tunnel placement, fixation, and graft choice (auto vs allograft). Vertical tunnels, allograft reconstructions, or other technical errors may be present. A study of community ACL reconstructions at Kaiser Permanente showed that 21% of ACL reconstructions were performed by surgeons performing less than six reconstructions a year and 56% of ACL reconstructions were performed by surgeons without sports medicine fellowship training [1]. Elite athletes come from a variety of different backgrounds, and the resources and experience of surgeons performing ACL surgery at the primary reconstruction can vary widely. Patients with multiple ACL ruptures will frequently have associated knee injuries. Data from the National Hospital Discharge Survey (NHDS) and the National Survey of Ambulatory Surgery (NSAS) databases indicate that only 37% of ACL reconstructions were performed as an isolated procedure, 50.6% included concomitant meniscal surgery, and 30.9% included another concomitant knee procedure [2]. Previous injuries and associated injuries should be closely examined when planning for revision surgery.

Outcomes of revision anterior cruciate ligament reconstruction in elite athletes are generally good. Mai et al. report an 82% return to play rate for primary ACL reconstruction in National Football League (NFL) professional athletes, and Okoroha et al. report a 79.4% return to play rate in 24 NFL players undergoing revision ACL reconstruction [3, 4]. NFL players who had been drafted in the first 4 rounds, or had played in at least 55 games, or played in 4 NFL seasons prior to injury were more likely to return to play, and all players who returned to play had statistically similar subsequent career length to matched controls after revision ACL reconstruction [4]. A recent study of 24 professional soccer players undergoing revision anterior cruciate ligament reconstruction with lateral extra-articular tenodesis for patients with ACL retear with high grade pivot shift demonstrated a 91.7% rate of return to sport; further investigation is needed to assess the performance of lateral extra-articular procedures in populations of elite athletes [5].

Key Concepts

Graft Options *For recurrent ACL injuries, it is important to consider all graft options. Our general order of preference is patella tendon autograft and hamstring tendon autograft grafts, followed by quadriceps tendon grafts. A graft from the contralateral knee is an option, and allografts are chosen as a last resort or in complex multi-ligament knee injuries.*

Consider ALL Augmentation *Anterolateral ligament reconstructions (typically gracilis allograft with high-strength suture/tape augmentation) are considered for athletes who suffer early, noncontact injuries. ALL reconstruction is also considered in patients with hyperlaxity of the knee greater than 10–15 degrees of hyperextension.*

Functional Rehabilitation *Emphasis of completing a thorough rehabilitation program that can ultimately demonstrate functional symmetry, both in absolute numbers as well as biomechani-*

cal quality, is a more reliable predictor of adequate rehabilitation than is the athlete's personal assessment of their recovery.

Outcomes

Outcomes of revision ACL reconstruction in elite athletes are generally good and may be similar to the outcomes of primary ACL reconstruction. Previous ability and performance seem to correlate well with return to play. Early results of lateral extra-articular stabilization procedures for revision ACL reconstruction in elite athletes are promising and warrant further study.

Case 2

A 26-year-old professional football lineman sustains a right ACL graft rupture and MCL tear after a direct blow from a teammate on the lateral aspect of his knee while his foot was pinned to the ground. He is seen in the office, and an ACL reconstruction is recommended once full range of motion is achieved. He previously underwent primary right ACL reconstruction as a college freshman. The player and his agent inform you they are seeking a second opinion from another surgeon.

Discussion

Surgeons treating elite and professional athletes should be prepared to treat players that will seek second opinions. Professional athletes will usually seek a second opinion, and the decision on second opinion surgeon will often be dictated by the player's agent or family. If the player requests a second opinion, the team surgeon should be prepared to offer recommendations. A surgeon dealing with professional athletes should work to build a network of surgeons with good reputations and are known to him or her. An appropriate second opinion surgeon is someone of similar skill level and not affiliated with the surgeon's practice. The ideal surgeon will be someone who is well respected, known to be supportive of players and other physicians, and willing to communicate with the team physician. If the patient has a complicated injury, you may want to suggest to the patient a surgeon known to you who has particular expertise in that area. Whether the player chooses the team surgeon or not, the team surgeon should make sure to get in contact with the second opinion surgeon to learn what their opinion is on treatment. This type of communication not only assists the team surgeon in guiding the postoperative care of the player in the training room but also helps surgeons build supportive physician networks for collaborating in the treatment of elite athletes.

Although it can be difficult for a surgeon's ego, the team surgeon should not be concerned or insulted if a patient chooses to undergo surgery elsewhere. The decisions of professional athletes are heavily influenced by many factors outside of the surgeon's control. It is important for the surgeon to support the decision of a player and to communicate with the treating surgeon. Maintaining good relationships with other surgeons that treat elite athletes will grow a surgeon's experience, network, and reputation as well as help grow a surgeon's knowledge through discussion of cases with other surgeons. In addition, working relationships with other surgeons treating elite athletes will allow for a team physician and trainers successfully guide the athlete through the rehabilitation process. The relationship one develops with outside surgeons is one of the most rewarding consequences of caring for elite athletes.

If you are seeing an elite athlete as a second opinion, it is critical to be respectful of and speak well of the first opinion surgeon. If you have a difference of opinion or believe they would truly benefit more from a different type of operation that you are offering the player, the surgeon should not attempt to undermine the previous surgeon or cast doubt on their professionalism or ability. The world of medicine is very small, and the community of surgeons treating professional athletes is much smaller.

Key Concepts

Second Opinions *are frequently requested by players, families, and agents. At higher levels of competition, this should be anticipated. Welcome the concept of second opinions and even introduce the topic in cases where it seems appropriate. Having a group of surgeon colleagues whose opinions you welcome and respect allows you to provide referrals that are likely to provide an objective, supportive second opinion to the athlete. The athlete may visit the surgeon in person, or in many cases radiologic images and the clinical history can often be sent remotely to colleagues around the country. The insight of these opinions can be given to the patient directly or* via *feedback from the local orthopedic surgeon.*

Developing these professional relationships and learning from their experienced opinions is one of the most positive consequences of caring for athletes at the highest level. Embrace second opinions and learn from them. Your athletes will appreciate your openness and will be more confident in your care as a result. Athletes are more likely to seek second opinions and consider surgery outside of the team physician in situations when they have not developed a working relationship with the medical team. Young players, rookies, recently transferred or traded players, and players undergoing contract negotiations are more likely to consider surgery outside the system. When your athlete decides to pursue surgery elsewhere, be gracious and supportive of their decision, and do all you can to facilitate the process.

Case 3

A 22-year-old male professional football wide receiver sustains a contact left knee injury during special teams practice as the starting kick returner. The player had undergone previous ACL reconstruction as a college sophomore. On sideline examination, the player has a loose knee though the player is anxious and guarding throughout the exam. The player, the head coach, and the general manager are all eager to hear how severe you believe the knee injury may be.

Discussion

The team physician at the professional level will have to discuss the details of a player's injury not only with the player but also with the coach, general manager, and training staff. If the diagnosis is obvious on the field, it is important to be honest with the coach and general manager. If the physician has high certainty the player has torn their ACL, the physician should tell the coach and general manager directly and honestly that they will not be able to count on the player for the rest of the year. The coach will have to go down the roster and see who is available to fill the position, and the general manager will need to start bringing in players from around the country for physical exams. Be aware that the coach may quickly pass your findings on to other members of the team including the other players.

It is important to hedge your bets if there is uncertainty regarding the diagnosis. On occasion, it can be difficult to make the diagnosis due to player anxiety and guarding. Sometimes a player's ACL can feel stable even though rupture has occurred, for example, in the case of a concomitant displaced meniscus injury. Conversely, patients with previous ACL reconstructions, in particular, may not have complete, symmetric stability even prior to reinjury, and a moderately unstable exam may not reflect re-rupture. Do not communicate to the player or staff whether there is or is not a tear if you are uncertain. Ultimately, you will have to rely on advanced imaging to make the final decision, and it is certainly acceptable to not give a definitive answer at the time of injury. Erroneously informing the athlete, the coach, and the management that the player has re-torn the ACL and will need season-ending surgery can cause the team to lose confidence in your ability to make an accurate diagnosis and unnecessarily increase anxiety levels. Having learned from these experiences, we now tend to be more conservative and patient in presenting bad news.

Key Concepts

Communication *Be cautious with your diagnosis when evaluating the athlete on the field or in the training room. Be mindful that knees with functional ACL reconstructions may still demonstrate significant laxity compared to an uninjured knee. Considering this variability with the limited examination that can occur due to patient anxiety and guarding, reserving a definitive diagnosis until advanced imaging has been completed is often wise. Explaining to the athlete and their family that you are concerned that they may have reinjured the knee but that you need to wait for the results of advanced imaging to determine how significant the injury is allows them to begin processing the possibility of a re-injury while holding onto some hope that the injury may not be severe. This concept of "breaking the news to them slowly" allows the process to occur more humanely than a blunt immediate diagnosis. It also prevents the scenario of an incorrect diagnosis, which may cause a team to lose confidence in your ability.*

Conclusion

The treatment of professional and elite athletes with repeat ACL rupture presents several unique challenges. Surgeons should pay close attention to the history and technical details of a player's injury, similar to the evaluation of non-elite non-professional athletes. Team physicians treating professional and elite athletes should be aware of the expectations of players, coaches, general managers, and agents and how these factors can influence the course of treatment.

References

1. Inacio MCS, Paxton EW, Maletis GB, et al. Patient and surgeon characteristics associated with primary anterior cruciate ligament reconstruction graft selection. Am J Sports Med. 2012;40(2):339–45. https://doi.org/10.1177/0363546511424130.
2. Lyman S, Nakamura N, Cole BJ, Erggelet C, Gomoll AH, Farr J II. Cartilage-repair innovation at a standstill: methodologic and regulatory pathways to breaking free. J Bone Joint Surg Am. 2016;98(e63):1–8. https://doi.org/10.2106/JBJS.15.00573.
3. Mai HT, Alvarez AP, Freshman RD, et al. The NFL orthopaedic surgery outcomes database (NO-SOD): the effect of common orthopaedic procedures on football careers. Am J Sports Med. 2016;44(9):2255–62. https://doi.org/10.1177/0363546516651426.
4. Okoroha KR, Kadri O, Keller RA, Marshall N, Cizmic Z, Moutzouros V. Return to play after revision anterior cruciate ligament reconstruction in national football league players. Orthop J Sport Med. 2017;5(4). https://doi.org/10.1177/2325967117698788.
5. Alessio-Mazzola M, Formica M, Russo A, et al. Outcome after combined lateral extra-articular tenodesis and anterior cruciate ligament revision in professional soccer players. J Knee Surg. 2019;32(9):906–10. https://doi.org/10.1055/s-0038-1672120.

Special Considerations in Female Athletes with Failed ACL Reconstruction

23

Sarah N. Harangody, Wendell M. R. Heard, and Mary K. Mulcahey

Introduction

Anterior cruciate ligament (ACL) injury occurs with a four- to sixfold greater incidence in female athletes compared to male athletes playing the same landing and cutting sports [1]. The mechanism underlying gender disparity in ACL injury risk is likely multifactorial in nature. Since the passage of Title IX in 1972, there has been a significant increase in the number of girls and women participating in sports, which has led to an increase in sports-related injuries including ACL tears. The risk of ACL injury in female collegiate year-round high-level soccer and basketball players is approximately 4.4–5% per year [2, 3], compared with 1.7% for males [3]. Females are more likely than males to suffer a subsequent ACL injury following ACL reconstruction, and the injury is most likely to occur in the contralateral knee. Shelbourne et al. [4] prospectively followed 1415 patients (863 male, 552 female) for ≥5 years after ACL reconstruction. The majority of patients (79–92%) indicated that they participated in high-risk sports (sports involving jumping, twisting, or pivoting that included sports such as basketball, soccer, football, volleyball, and snow skiing) at a recreational level or higher. One hundred thirty-six patients (69 females and 67 males) incurred a subsequent ACL injury to either knee (9.6%) and females had a higher rate of subsequent ACL injuries compared with male athletes (12.5% and 7.8%, respectively; $p = 0.004$). Most subsequent knee injuries occurred playing basketball (52%) and soccer (15%). Women were more likely than men to suffer an injury to the contralateral normal knee (7.8% and 3.7%, respectively; $p < 0.001$). Both sexes had an equal risk of re-rupture of the reconstructed knee, with 4.3% in males and 4.1% in females [4]. Revision rates after ACL reconstruction ranged from 5% to 20% [5].

S. N. Harangody
Palos Northwestern Medicine, Department of Orthopaedic Surgery, Palos Heights, IL, USA

W. M. R. Heard
Department of Orthopaedic Surgery, Tulane University School of Medicine, New Orleans, LA, USA

M. K. Mulcahey (✉)
Women's Sports Medicine Program, Department of Orthopaedic Surgery, Tulane University School of Medicine, New Orleans, LA, USA

Etiology

While overall failure and re-rupture rate may be similar in males and females in the general population, female athletes have a higher re-rupture rate than their male counterparts [6]. There are multiple reasons for graft failure after ACL reconstruction including surgical technique, traumatic re-tear, lack of graft incorporation, and failure to recognize associated knee pathology/

M. J. Alaia, K. J. Jones (eds.), *Revision Anterior Cruciate Ligament Reconstruction*,
https://doi.org/10.1007/978-3-030-96996-7_23

ligamentous injuries [7]. Failure following ACL reconstruction can be grouped into different categories: (1) loss of motion or arthrofibrosis, (2) extensor mechanism dysfunction, (3) arthritis, and (4) recurrent patholaxity (graft failure) [8].

Errors in surgical technique represent one of the most common reasons for failure of ACL reconstruction, with tunnel malposition being a major cause. However, no studies have demonstrated a significant difference in tunnel malposition between males and females. Recurrent trauma can also lead to ACL graft rupture. Female athletes who return to playing soccer have a higher risk of ACL graft rupture compared to those who return to playing other sports [9]. Previous studies have shown that return to high-level activity is associated with higher risk of graft re-rupture. Salmon et al. found that the only significant predictor of graft rupture from among the measured variables was a contact mechanism of initial injury, which increased the odds of suffering a graft rupture threefold, likely a result of returning to contact sports [10]. Also, in that study, there was a trend toward an increased risk of graft rupture with return to level 1 or 2 sports, as defined by the 1993 International Knee Documentation Committee (IKDC) scale (adjusted OR = 2.1; 95% CI, 1.0–4.6) [10]. The IKDC divides activity into the following functional levels: (1) strenuous (e.g., football, hockey, basketball), (2) moderate (e.g., tennis, skiing, martial arts), (3) light recreational (e.g., jogging, cycling, swimming), and (4) sedentary, based on the demands the activity places on the knee and exposure to that functional level of at least 50 hours a year.

Risk Factors (Fig. 23.1)

Expectations

There are several risk factors to consider in the female athlete with a failed ACL reconstruction. Female athletes are less likely to return to sport after primary ACL reconstruction than male athletes and this number continues to decrease following revision ACL reconstruction [11, 12]. Webster et al. performed a cohort study of 675 patients (437 male, 238 female) undergoing primary (595 patients; 81 of whom had a prior contralateral ACLR) or revision ACL reconstruction (80 patients) to investigate return-to-sport expectations before and after ACLR and determine factors associated with changed expectations [11]. The authors found that female patients had two times the odds of giving up sport, and patients who had undergone previous ACLR had almost three times the odds. Before undergoing a revision ACLR, only 63% of athletes planned to return to their sport at their previous level [11]. When counseling female athletes with a failed ACL reconstruction, it is important to discuss their desire to return to sport and their pre-injury level of activity. In a systematic review and meta-analysis, Wiggins et al. found that athletes who returned to sport after ACLR had a higher risk of ipsilateral graft rupture and contralateral ACL rupture (20% secondary ACL injury, 8% ipsilateral, 12% contralateral) compared to those who did not return to sport [13]. The re-injury rate was even higher in the younger patient cohort, with 23% of athletes <25 years incurring a secondary ACL injury (10% ipsilateral knee and 14% contralateral knee).

Sports and Activity Level

Soccer and basketball are two of the highest risk sports for female athletes with regard to ACL injury. Previously, Arendt and Dick evaluated ACL injuries in collegiate men's and women's soccer and basketball programs over a 5 year period using the National College Athletic Association Injury Surveillance System [1]. The authors found that female soccer players had an ACL injury rate twice as high as their male counterparts and female basketball players had an injury rate three times as high as their male counterparts. In a study by Allen et al., 180 competitive (defined as being injured in a match against

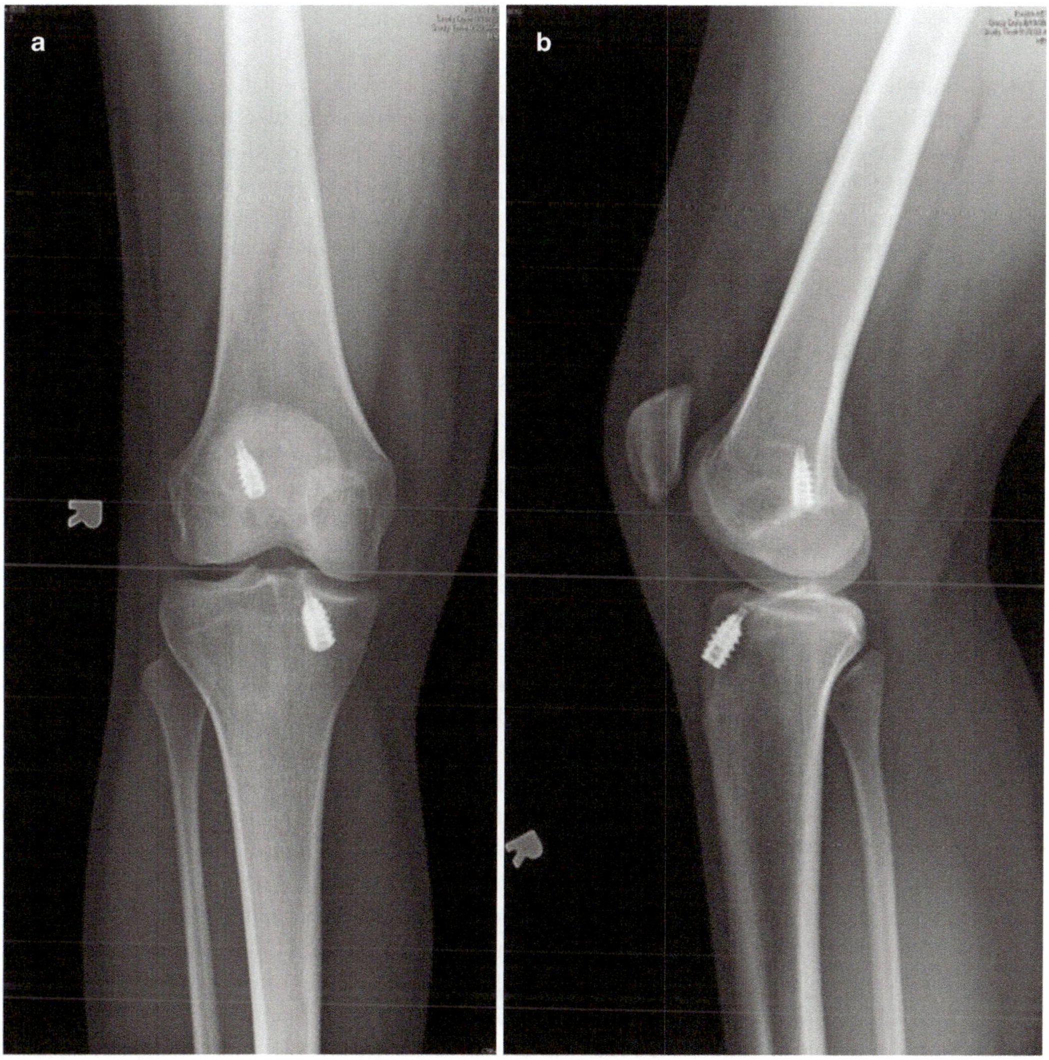

Fig. 23.1 (**a**) Preoperative AP radiograph of the right knee. (**b**) Preoperative lateral radiograph of the right knee

an opposing team) female soccer players with a mean age of 19 ± 6 years were compared to non-soccer female athletes [9]. Those soccer players who returned to sport after ACLR were more likely to rupture their graft (11% to 1%; $p < 0.01$) as well as sustain a contralateral ACL injury (17% vs 4%; $p < 0.01$) compared to non-soccer players. Of the athletes who returned to soccer, 11% (10/90) sustained a tear of their ACL graft at a mean of 24.8 ± 16.3 months [9]. Soccer is one of the sports with the highest risk of ACL tear for female athletes. Borchers et al. performed a case–control study of 21 patients with graft failure following ACL reconstruction and 42 age- and sex-matched controls to determine if activity level after reconstruction and graft type are risk factors for ACL graft failure [7]. Activity level was measured by Marx activity score with a high activity level measured as Marx ≥13 and low activity Marx < 12, Marx activity score was collected at the time of the initial injury and following graft failure. The authors found a significant increase in risk of graft failure with return to high-level activity (Marx ≥13) [7].

Age

Overall, younger age confers a higher risk of subsequent ACL injury, which is likely multifactorial. Magnussen et al. evaluated 256 patients, 53.1% male (136 male and 120 female patients) with a range in age from 11 to 52 years (mean, 25.0 years; SD, 10.5 years) to determine if younger age is a predictor of early graft revision [5]. The authors demonstrated that one revision was required in 137 patients aged 20 years or older (0.7%), but 17 revisions were required in 119 patients under age 20 years (14.3%) ($p > 0.0001$). Of the revision patients (7 males 5.1%, 11 females 9.2%, $p = 0.23$), 11 were competitive athletes and 7 were recreational athletes. Of the 18 (72.2%) athletes, 13 had returned to their prior level of sport at an average of 201 days post-surgery and 14 (77.7%) reported a traumatic re-injury [5].

Young female athletes are especially at risk for subsequent ACL injuries. Athletes under the age of 25 years have the highest risk for both primary and recurrent ACL injury [14]. This heightened risk may be due to unmodified risk factors that contributed to the first ACL injury [14]. Shelbourne et al. prospectively followed up 1415 patients (863 male, 552 female) after primary ACL reconstruction to determine if patients suffered an injury to either knee within 5 years after surgery [4]. The authors found that the rate of subsequent injuries to the ACL was age dependent: 17% for patients younger than 18 years, 7% for patients aged 18–25 years, and 4% for patients older than 25 years. Younger age may confer a higher risk secondary to higher activity level. In a prospective cohort MOON study, Kaeding et al. evaluated risk factors for ACL re-tear in 2683 subjects with average age of 27 ± 11 years (1498 men; 56%) and with varying degrees of sports participation [15]. The authors demonstrated that the risk of an ipsilateral ACL re-tear decreased by 0.09 for every yearly increase in age.

Graft Choice

Use of allograft, especially in younger patients, has been associated with a higher risk of graft failure. Kaeding et al. showed that the odds of ipsilateral ACL re-tear were 5.2 times greater ($p < 0.01$) with an allograft compared to hamstring autograft or bone-patellar tendon-bone (BTB) autograft, [15] and this was most significant in the younger age group (especially younger than age 20). For patients in their mid-30s, there was no statistically significant difference in the risk of re-tear between allograft and autograft [15]. The use of allograft is not recommended in young athletes. Noojin and Barrett evaluated 39 women (average age 23.2 years; range, 14–47 years) and 26 men (average age 29 years; range,13–48 years) who underwent quadruple-looped hamstring tendon autograft ACL reconstruction using the semitendinosus and gracilis tendons. The authors demonstrated that there was a higher failure rate among females with hamstring autograft compared to their male counterparts (sports participation was not delineated) [16]. The MOON knee group evaluated 770 patients (48% female) aged 14–22 years who underwent primary ACL reconstruction with either BTB autograft or hamstring autograft [17]. The authors showed that the incidence of ACL graft revision at 6 years after index surgery was 2.1 times higher with a hamstring autograft compared with a BTB autograft. Additionally, the authors found that young patients who underwent ACLR using hamstring autografts were more likely to undergo subsequent ACLR in their ipsilateral knee (13.0%) compared with those receiving a BTB autograft (7.1%) [17]. Therefore, in counseling the female athlete, it is necessary to discuss their desire to return to sport and to take into consideration the sport she is returning to when selecting the graft. For young athletes who desire to return to cutting or pivoting sports, a BTB autograft may be the best option for

ACLR [17]. When the ACLR has failed, it is important to consider what graft was used in the initial surgery as that may limit options for revision. Wright et al. evaluated 1205 patients (697 [58%] males) with a median age of 26 years to determine the outcomes following revision ACL reconstruction using autograft vs allograft (fresh frozen with minimal to no radiation) [18]. The authors found that at the two-year follow-up, patients who underwent ACLR using an autograft were 2.78 times less likely to sustain a subsequent graft rupture compared to patients who received an allograft ($p = 0.047$; 95% CI, 1.01–7.69). Patients who underwent revision ACLR using an autograft also had higher sports function and activity level, but no difference in activities of daily living [18].

Graft size can also contribute to the risk of re-rupture. In 2012, Magnussen et al. performed a retrospective review of 256 patients (136 male and 120 female; age range 11–52 years) who underwent ACL reconstruction with hamstring autograft [5]. The authors found that females were more likely to have a graft size of 8 mm or smaller, which has been associated with an increased revision rate compared to grafts larger than 8 mm. This is especially true with hamstring autograft. The revision rate increased even more when the patient was younger than 20 years old with a graft smaller than 8 mm. Revision was required in 1 of 22 patients (4.5%) with grafts greater than 8 mm in diameter, in 9 of 68 patients (13.2%) with grafts equal to 7.5- or 8 mm in diameter, and in 7 of 29 patients (24.1%) with grafts less than or equal to 7 mm in diameter ($p = 0.046$) [5]. Similarly, Noojin et al. demonstrated that female patients undergoing ACL reconstruction with hamstring autograft had a higher failure rate compared to males and average graft size was 2.5 mm smaller than that for the male patients ($p < 0.0001$) [16].

Anatomy

Smaller intercondylar notch widths have been shown to correlate with a higher incidence of non-contact ACL injuries; however, this has not been correlated with patient sex [19, 20]. If narrow notch width was not addressed during the first ACLR, this may contribute to graft failure and would need to be addressed in any revision surgeries [21, 22]. More recently, posterior tibial slope (PTS) has been identified as a factor contributing to the failure of ACLR. In 2013, Webb et al. evaluated 181 patients (90 female, 91 male; median age 26 years) with isolated ACL ruptures who underwent primary ACL reconstruction with hamstring tendon autografts [23]. The authors found that patients with a PTS of 12° or greater (as measured on lateral radiographs) had five times greater odds of subsequent ACL injury after reconstruction and had an ACL reinjury rate of 59%. Christensen et al. evaluated 35 patients (21 males, 14 females, mean age 21.3 years) with early ACL graft failure (within 2 years of the initial surgery) and then matched them 1:1 with a control group who had undergone ACL reconstruction with a minimum of 4 years of clinical follow-up and no evidence of graft failure [24]. The authors found that there was a much larger difference in the mean lateral tibial posterior slope (LTPS) between female patients and controls (9.1° vs 5.9°, respectively; $p = 0.015$) and the probability of graft failure increased with increasing LTPS. An increase in slope in both males and females conferred an increased risk in probability of graft failure. Interestingly, females had the greatest risk of graft failure with increased slope, with a 4° change in the LTPS increasing the risk of graft failure nearly 5 times, and a 6° change resulting in over 10 times the increased risk [24].

Ligamentous laxity is also an important consideration for the female athlete. Akhtar et al. studied 139 patients (100 male, 39 female; mean age 28 years) undergoing primary ACL reconstruction, 44 patients (29 males, 15 females; mean age 28 years) undergoing revision ACL surgery, and a control group of 70 patients without any knee ligament injury [25]. The authors found a higher rate of ligamentous laxity among those with an ACL injury and those undergoing revision ACLR ($p < 0.01$). Within the revision group, there was a subgroup who had a failure of the original surgery due to "biological failure" (no obvious cause for failure) of the primary graft. This group had a mean age of 28 years with 14 males and 9 females and an average Beighton score of 4.6. The incidence of generalized ligamentous laxity in the revision group as defined by the Beighton score was also significantly higher than for patients in the primary surgery group (4.6 vs 2.9, $p = 0.01$). All patients in the biologic failure group had ACL reconstruction performed using autografts, and the cause of failure was attributed to laxity of the autografts, causing insufficiency under load and ultimately graft failure [25].

Readiness to Return to Play (Fig. 23.2)

Female athletes have been shown to have lower psychological readiness to return to play compared to their male counterparts. Webster et al. studied a cohort of 635 athletes (389 male, 246 female; mean age of 28 years) who underwent ACLR and had been cleared to return to sport (RTS) [26]. The average follow-up time was 12 months and all athletes completed the Anterior Cruciate Ligament–Return to Sport After Injury (range 11–24 months). A positive correlation was found between psychological readiness and male sex and young age (<20 years old). The authors found that only 17% of females returned to sport versus 30% of males [26]. McPherson et al. evaluated 329 patients (118 females, 211 males with a mean age of 25.3 ± 8.7 years) who underwent primary ACLR between June 2014 and June 2016 and completed the ACL–Return to Sport After Injury (ACL-RSI) (short version) scale before their ACLR [27]. They repeated the scale at 12 months after surgery to assess psychological readiness to return to sport. Neither the type of sport nor the level of activity was specified. The authors found that 52 patients (16%) sustained a second ACL injury and trended toward lower psychological readiness at 12 months compared with non-injured patients (60.9 vs 67.2 points; $p = 0.11$). Younger (<20 years) patients with an ACL injury had significantly lower psychological readiness to return to sport than young non-injured patients (60.8 vs 71.5 points; $p = 0.02$) [27] . Fear of re-injury is also a common reason for not returning to sport after ACL reconstruction. Kvist et al. studied 62 patients (34 men and 28 women; mean age 27 years) who underwent primary ACL reconstruction [28]. Prior to injury, 47 patients (76%) were active in contact sports such as soccer, handball, ice hockey, floorball, or American football. After surgery, only 19 patients (31%) were active in the same sports ($p < 0.05$). The authors found that 46% of patients did not return to sport and 24% of those cited fear of injury as the main contributing factor [28].

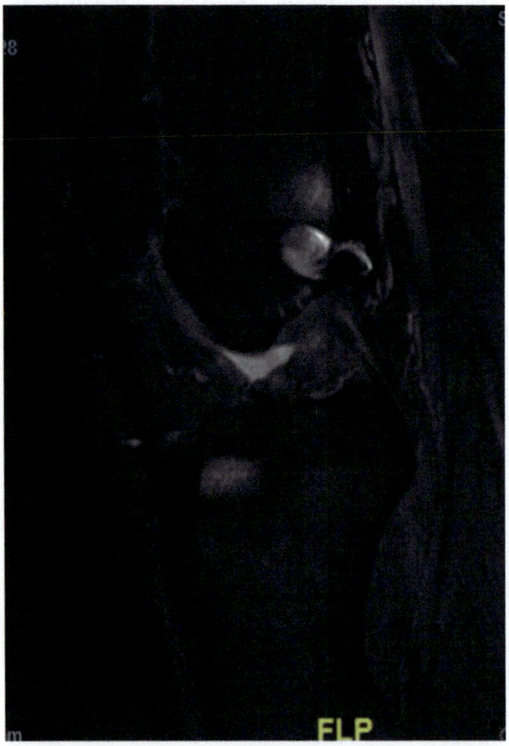

Fig. 23.2 Sagittal MRI image demonstrating a torn ACL graft

Operative Considerations in the Female Athlete

Graft choice is a significant factor in ACLR. If the female athlete already failed an allograft, autograft is the recommended choice, especially in the younger athlete. If the female athlete had a hamstring autograft and returned to cutting, pivoting sports, then a BTB autograft should be considered in the revision setting. As previously mentioned, a greater posterior tibial slope can contribute to an increased incidence of ACL graft failure. When planning revision surgery, it is important to take this into account. Dejour et al. studied nine patients (six men, three women; mean age of 28 years) who underwent second revision ACL reconstruction combined with tibial de-flexion osteotomy [29]. The authors found that all patients had healed osteotomies and stable knees, and there were no intraoperative or postoperative complications. The mean posterior tibial slope decreased from 13.2° ± 2.6° (median 13°; range 12°–18°) preoperatively to 4.4° ± 2.3° (median 4°; range 2°–8°) postoperatively [29]. If a patient has a PTS >12°, she may benefit from an osteotomy to decrease the slope [30]. Other alignment issues (coronal malalignment) should also be considered in planning revision ACLR. These topics are covered in detail in Chaps. 15 and 16.

Conclusion

The female athlete is a special subset of the population and requires unique considerations when discussing revision ACL reconstruction. Age, level of activity, sport, and graft choice can contribute to the risk of ACL graft failure and it is important to take these factors into account when counseling patients about revision surgery. In the setting of a failed ACLR in a female athlete, it is important to discuss goals and to help the female athlete understand that return to sport (especially cutting and pivoting sports) brings with it an increased risk for re-injury. Counseling young female athletes on their risk of secondary injury is important when considering return to play. Additionally, it is important to assess psychological readiness to return to sport prior to releasing athletes to full activity. In female athletes returning to cutting, pivoting sports, ACL reconstruction with BTB autograft is recommended.

Case Presentation

A 17-year-old female cheerleader and gymnast with aspirations to cheer in college presented with symptoms of right knee instability. She had a right knee ACL reconstruction with BTB autograft 1 year prior and was able to return to sport. Prior to presentation, she had twisted her knee while tumbling and felt her knee shift. The injury was associated with swelling and required crutch use for 2 days. Her knee felt unstable especially with lateral movements and her cheering activity was significantly restricted.

Her physical exam showed full range of motion with minimal effusion and soft tissue swelling. She had a Grade III Lachman and grade I anterior drawer. The patient guarded to pivot shift testing. The other ligamentous structures in the knee were stable.

Radiographic examination showed two metal interference screws from the prior ACL reconstruction with well-maintained joint spaces and no acute bony abnormality (Fig. 23.1). There was no significant tunnel osteolysis. Alignment was neutral and posterior slope was measured at approximately 5°. MRI examination showed a torn ACL graft with no obvious meniscus tear and well-maintained cartilage surfaces (Fig. 23.2).

Secondary to her symptomatic instability, she and her family elected to undergo revision ACL reconstruction with quadriceps tendon autograft. As this was a revision reconstruction, a lateral extra-articular tenodesis was performed using autologous iliotibial band (ITB).

At the time of surgery, the examination under anesthesia revealed a positive pivot shift. Arthroscopic examination showed that cartilage surfaces were intact. There was a small tear in the posterior horn of the lateral meniscus that was repaired with an all-inside technique. The medial and lateral meniscal root attachments were intact and there was no ramp lesion present. The femoral tunnel was vertical and a new tunnel was made without having to remove the previously placed screw (Figs. 23.3 and 23.4). The previously placed tibial screw was removed and a new

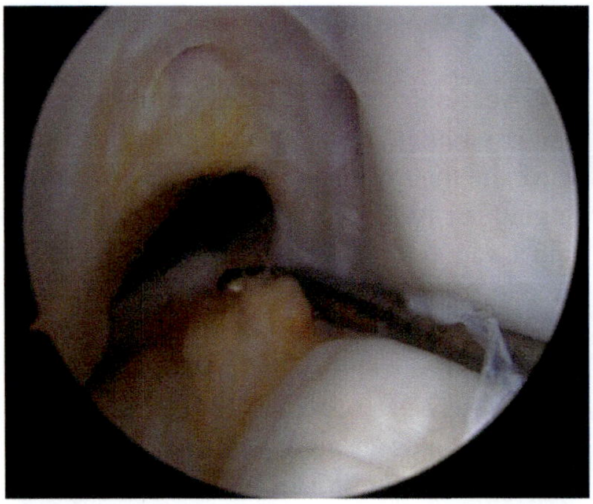

Fig. 23.3 Arthroscopic image demonstrating the previous vertical femoral tunnel

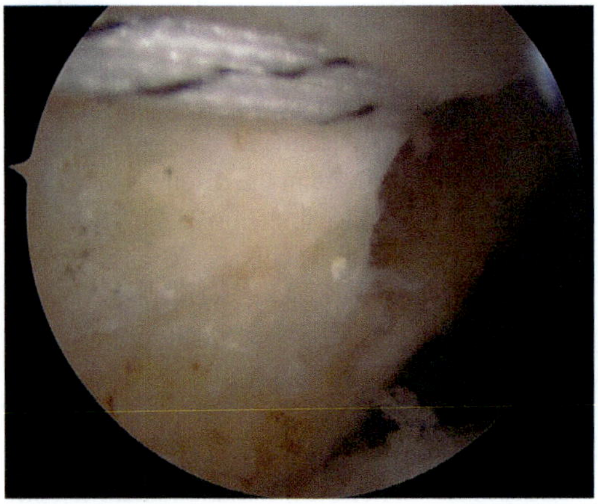

Fig. 23.4 Arthroscopic picture of the new femoral tunnel

tibial tunnel was drilled. The graft had been prepared in standard fashion and measured 9.5 mm in diameter and 70 mm in length. The graft was fixed on the femoral and tibial sides with suspensory fixation. The knee was placed in full exten-

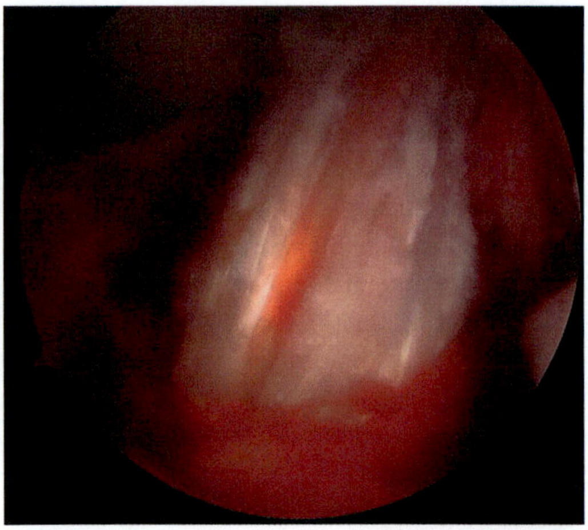

Fig. 23.5 Arthroscopic picture of the quadriceps tendon autograft after fixation

sion when fixing the graft on the tibial side and maximal manual tension was placed on the graft. A suture anchor was used as backup fixation on the tibial side. Figure 23.5 shows the intra-articular position of the quadriceps tendon autograft after fixation.

Extra-articular tenodesis was performed next. An incision was made on the lateral side of the knee from just proximal to the lateral femoral condyle to Gerdy's tubercle. The middle centimeter of the ITB was incised and left attached to Gerdy's tubercle. The proximal portion of the graft was whipstitched. A 6 mm socket was drilled to accommodate the graft in the area of the attachment of the distal Kaplan's fibers. With the knee in 20 degrees of flexion and neutral rotation, the graft was fixed with a 6 mm × 25 mm bio-absorbable screw.

Postoperative imaging showed appropriate tunnel and hardware placement (Fig. 23.6). Her recovery has been uneventful.

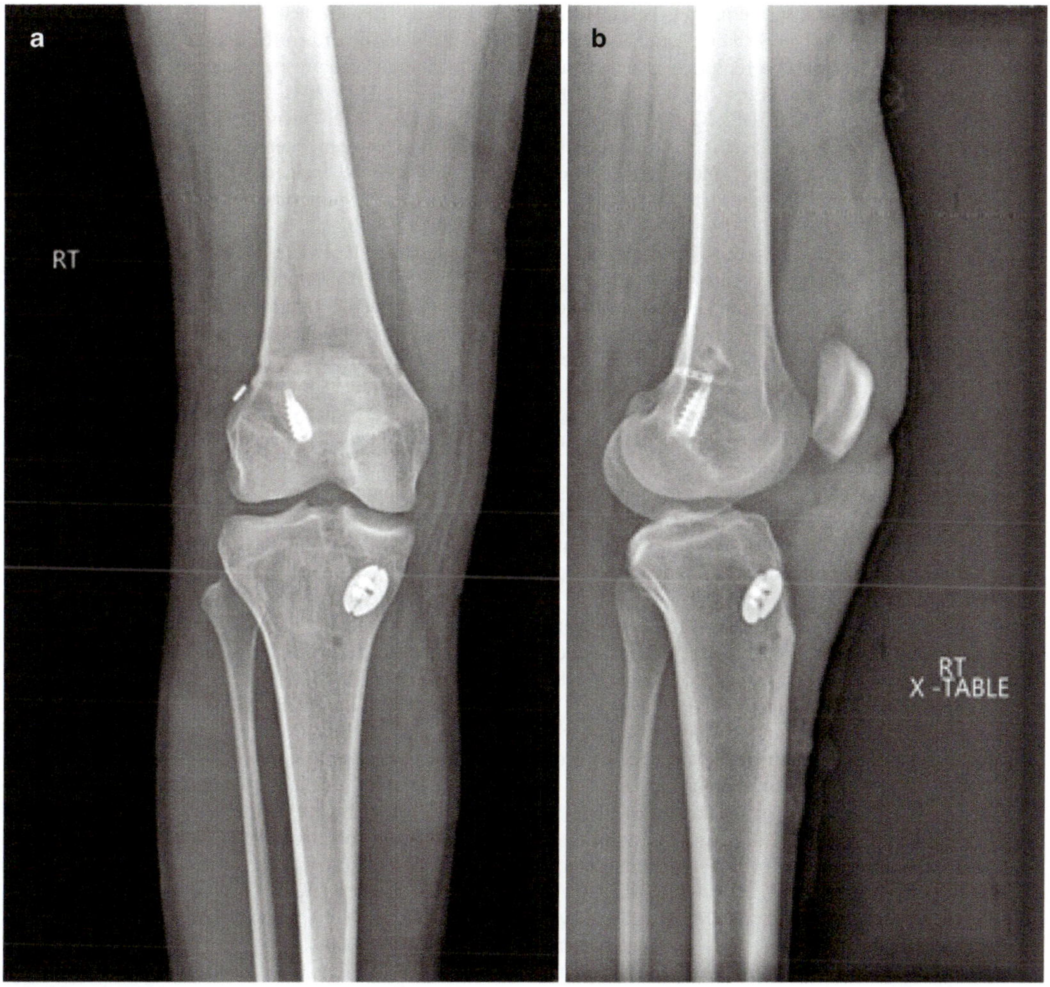

Fig. 23.6 (**a**) Postoperative AP X-ray of the right knee. (**b**) Postoperative lateral X-ray of the right knee

References

1. Arendt E, Dick R. Knee injury patterns among men and women in collegiate basketball and soccer: NCAA data and review of literature. Am J Sports Med. 1995;23(6):694–701.
2. Prodromos CC, Han Y, Rogowski J, Joyce B, Shi K. A meta-analysis of the incidence of anterior cruciate ligament tears as a function of gender, sport, and a knee injury-reduction regimen. Arthroscopy. 2007;23(12):1320–5.
3. Hewett TE, Myer GD, Ford KR, Heidt RS, Colosimo AJ, McLean SG, et al. Biomechanical measures of neuromuscular control and valgus loading of the knee predict anterior cruciate ligament injury risk in female athletes: a prospective study. Am J Sports Med. 2005;33(4):492–501.
4. Shelbourne KD, Gray T, Haro M. Incidence of subsequent injury to either knee within 5 years after anterior cruciate ligament reconstruction with patellar tendon autograft. Am J Sports Med. 2009;37(2):246–51.
5. Magnussen RA, Lawrence JTR, West RL, Toth AP, Taylor DC, Garrett WE. Graft size and patient age are predictors of early revision after anterior cruciate ligament reconstruction with hamstring autograft. Arthroscopy [Internet]. 2012;28(4):526–31. Available from: https://doi.org/10.1016/j.arthro.2011.11.024.

6. Ahldén M, Samuelsson K, Sernert N, Forssblad M, Karlsson J, Kartus J. The Swedish national anterior cruciate ligament register: a report on baseline variables and outcomes of surgery for almost 18,000 patients. Am J Sports Med. 2012;40(10):2230–5.
7. Borchers JR, Pedroza A, Kaeding C. Activity level and graft type as risk factors for anterior cruciate ligament graft failure: a case-control study. Am J Sports Med. 2009;37(12):2362–7.
8. Carson E, Anisko E, Restrepo C, Panariello R, O'Brien S, Warren R. Revision anterior cruciate ligament reconstruction – etiology of failures and clinical results. J Knee Surg. 2010;17(03):127–32.
9. Allen MM, Pareek A, Krych AJ, Hewett TE, Levy BA, Stuart MJ, et al. Are female soccer players at an increased risk of second anterior cruciate ligament injury compared with their athletic peers? Am J Sports Med. 2016;44(10):2492–8.
10. Salmon L, Russell V, Musgrove T, Pinczewski L, Refshauge K. Incidence and risk factors for graft rupture and contralateral rupture after anterior cruciate ligament reconstruction. Arthroscopy. 2005;21(8):948–57.
11. Webster KE, Feller JA. Expectations for return to preinjury sport before and after anterior cruciate ligament reconstruction. Am J Sports Med. 2019;47(3):578–83.
12. Tan SHS, Lau BPH, Khin LW, Lingaraj K. The importance of patient sex in the outcomes of anterior cruciate ligament reconstructions. Am J Sports Med. 2016;44:242–54. SAGE Publications Inc.
13. Wiggins AJ, Grandhi RK, Schneider DK, Stanfield D, Webster KE, Myer GD. Risk of secondary injury in younger athletes after anterior cruciate ligament reconstruction. Am J Sports Med. 2016;44(7):1861–76.
14. Schilaty ND, Nagelli C, Bates NA, Sanders TL, Krych AJ, Stuart MJ, et al. Incidence of second anterior cruciate ligament tears and identification of associated risk factors from 2001 to 2010 using a geographic database. Orthop J Sports Med. 2017;5(8):1–8.
15. Kaeding CC, Pedroza AD, Reinke EK, Huston LJ, Spindler KP. Risk factors and predictors of subsequent ACL injury in either knee after ACL reconstruction: prospective analysis of 2488 primary ACL reconstructions from the MOON cohort. Am J Sports Med. 2015;43(7):1583–90.
16. Noojin FK, Barrett GR, Hartzog CW, Nash CR. Clinical comparison of intraarticular anterior cruciate ligament reconstruction using autogenous semitendinosus and gracilis tendons in men versus women. Am J Sports Med. 2000;28(6):783–9.
17. Spindler KP, Huston LJ, Zajichek A, Reinke EK, Amendola A, Andrish JT, et al. Anterior cruciate ligament reconstruction in high school and college-aged athletes: does autograft choice influence anterior cruciate ligament revision rates? Am J Sports Med. 2020;48(2):298–309.
18. Wright RW. Effect of graft choice on the outcome of revision anterior cruciate ligament reconstruction in the multicenter ACL revision study (MARS) cohort. Am J Sports Med. 2014;42(10):2301–10.
19. Laprade RF, Burnett QM. Femoral intercondylar notch stenosis and correlation to anterior cruciate ligament injuries: a prospective study. Am J Sports Med. 1994;22(2):198–203.
20. Shelbourne KD, Davis TJ, Klootwyk TE. The relationship between intercondylar notch width of the femur and the incidence of anterior cruciate ligament tears: a prospective study. Am J Sports Med. 1998;26(3):402–8.
21. Anderson AF, Dome DC, Gautam S, Awh MH, Rennirt GW. Correlation of anthropometric measurements, strength, anterior cruciate ligament size, and intercondylar notch characteristics to sex differences in anterior cruciate ligament tear rates. Am J Sports Med. 2001;29(1):58–66.
22. Burnham JM, Herbst E, Pauyo T, Pfeiffer T, Johnson DL, Fu FH, et al. Technical considerations in revision anterior cruciate ligament reconstruction for operative techniques in orthopaedics. Oper Tech Orthop [Internet]. 2017;27(1):63–9. Available from: https://doi.org/10.1053/j.oto.2017.01.012.
23. Webb JM, Salmon LJ, Leclerc E, Pinczewski LA, Roe JP. Posterior tibial slope and further anterior cruciate ligament injuries in the anterior cruciate ligament-reconstructed patient. Am J Sports Med. 2013;41(12):2800–4.
24. Christensen JJ, Krych AJ, Engasser WM, Vanhees MK, Collins MS, Dahm DL. Lateral tibial posterior slope is increased in patients with early graft failure after anterior cruciate ligament reconstruction. Am J Sports Med. 2015;43(10):2510–4.
25. Akhtar MA, Bhattacharya R, Keating JF. Generalised ligamentous laxity and revision ACL surgery: is there a relation? Knee [Internet]. 2016;23(6):1148–53. Available from: https://doi.org/10.1016/j.knee.2015.11.006.
26. Webster KE, Nagelli CV, Hewett TE, Feller JA. Factors associated with psychological readiness to return to sport after anterior cruciate ligament reconstruction surgery. Am J Sports Med. 2018;46(7):1545–50.
27. McPherson AL, Feller JA, Hewett TE, Webster KE. Psychological readiness to return to sport is associated with second anterior cruciate ligament injuries. Am J Sports Med. 2019;47(4):857–62.
28. Kvist J, Ek A, Sporrstedt K, Good L. Fear of re-injury: a hindrance for returning to sports after anterior cruciate ligament reconstruction. Knee Surg Sports Traumatol Arthrosc. 2005;13(5):393–7.
29. Dejour D, Saffarini M, Demey G, Baverel L. Tibial slope correction combined with second revision ACL produces good knee stability and prevents graft rupture. Knee Surg Sports Traumatol Arthrosc. 2015;23(10):2846–52.
30. Southam BR, Colosimo AJ, Grawe B. Underappreciated factors to consider in revision anterior cruciate ligament reconstruction: a current concepts review. Orthop J Sports Med. 2018;6(1):1–11.

Outcomes After Revision Anterior Cruciate Ligament Reconstruction

24

Eoghan T. Hurley, Bogdan A. Matache, Mehul Shah, and Kirk A. Campbell

Introduction

Rupture of the anterior cruciate ligament (ACL) is one of the most common injuries in the knee, with reported age and sex adjusted incidences of 68.6 per 100,000 person-years in the general population and peak incidences of 215 per 100,000 person-years in the young athletic population [1]. ACL reconstruction (ACLR) has become the gold standard of treatment to restore knee stability, improve function, and allow for a high likelihood of return to play after an ACL tear. However, despite the advances in surgical technique, graft options, and rehabilitation protocols, rates of ipsilateral re-tear typically range from 3.8% to 10% [2]. The majority of re-tears occur within the first 2 years after the index procedure and do so as a result of a number of identifiable factors, and these patients may eventually require a revision ACLR [3].

Clinical outcomes after revision ACLR have been shown to be inferior, and re-rupture rates are higher as compared to primary reconstruction [4]. These patients often have associated pathology that needs to be addressed at the time of revision surgery, including meniscal insufficiency, unrecognized posterolateral corner injury, osteochondral injury, and excessive posterior tibial slope [5–7]. The additional procedures required to treat this associated pathology increase the complexity of the reconstruction and postoperative rehabilitation regimen, which partially accounts for the inferior outcomes observed in this population.

An important aspect of revision ACLR is setting realistic patient expectations prior to surgery. This can be achieved through a thorough understanding of the literature, which allows for appropriate patient counseling. This chapter will review the expected clinical outcomes after revision ACLR.

Outcomes: Re-rupture Rate

Re-rupture of a revision ACLR can be a devastating problem for patients who have already endured two surgical procedures and separate lengthy rehabilitation programs. The rate of graft re-rupture after a revision ACLR is three to four times higher than that of a primary ACLR and approaching 25% overall based on mid-term follow-up data [4, 8]. Patients who have had a failed revision ACLR often present with a higher rate of associated intra-articular pathology [5], which reduces their likelihood of experiencing an excellent outcome after re-revision ACLR and increases their risk of long-term arthritic change.

E. T. Hurley (✉) · B. A. Matache · M. Shah
K. A. Campbell
New York University Langone Health, Department of Orthopedic Surgery, New York, NY, USA

M. J. Alaia, K. J. Jones (eds.), *Revision Anterior Cruciate Ligament Reconstruction*,
https://doi.org/10.1007/978-3-030-96996-7_24

Several systematic reviews with mid-term follow-up have been published comparing revision to primary ACLR, and all have shown inferior outcomes after revision reconstruction [4, 8, 9]. Grassi et al. [4] compared the two procedures in a meta-analysis and found worse International Knee Documentation Committee (IKDC) and Lysholm scores and a higher failure rate and rate of arthritic development in patients who underwent a revision procedure. These results were both statistically and clinically significant. In their systematic review, the same authors found a >10% overall re-rupture rate at 5 years after revision ACLR, with one third of studies actually reporting a rate of >25%. Furthermore, arthritic changes were seen in up to 92% of patients. Additionally, they found a higher incidence of complications such as anterior knee pain, knee stiffness, and harvest-related fracture of the patella as compared to primary ACLR.

The Multi-Centre ACL Revision Study (MARS) group [10], which has 10-year follow-up data on the largest series of ACL revisions in the literature, demonstrated that 2-year patient-reported outcomes after revision ACLR were positively correlated with baseline scores, male sex, and time elapsed from previous ACLR. In contrast, predictors of poor outcome after revision surgery included prior lateral meniscectomy and the presence of grade 3/4 chondrosis in either the trochlear groove or the medial tibial plateau.

Outcomes: Return to Play

There is scant literature on the topic of return to play after revision ACLR. In a systematic review, Glogovac et al. [11] were only able to identify 13 studies totaling 1160 patients that reported on this outcome after revision ACLR. The authors found that 56–100% of patients were able to return to play, but only 13–69% were able to return to their pre-injury level of participation. A similar systematic review by Grassi et al. [12] reported an 85.3% pooled rate of return to play, defining this as return to any sporting activity at any level. However, when considering a return to pre-injury level of participation, the rate was only 53.4%. This highlights that while patients may be able to return to their sport of choice after a revision ACLR, they may be physically or psychologically limited in their ability to perform at their previous level [13].

Several studies have identified factors which may be associated with increased rates of successful return to play after revision ACLR, namely, young age and autograft use. Anand et al. [14] found that patients under 25 years old were twice as likely to be able to return to their pre-injury level of sport. Additionally, Webster et al. [15] showed that patients younger than 25 had significantly higher rates of return to play than older patients, with almost two thirds of those under 25 able to return to their pre-injury level. However, there does also appear to be an age threshold below which patients have a lower rate of return to play, as demonstrated by Christino et al. [16] who found a less than 40% rate of return to pre-injury level of play in pediatric patients. This may be as a result of a number of factors, including skeletal immaturity and psychological non-readiness [17].

The second factor that has been shown to affect the rate of return to play after revision ACLR is graft choice. Studies have demonstrated higher rates of return to play with autograft as compared to allograft use; however, this may be confounded by the fact that autograft use is more prevalent in younger patients as compared to older patients undergoing revision ACLR. Keizer et al. [18] compared autograft to allograft bone-patella-tendon-bone (BPTB) graft choice in revision ACLR and found a significantly higher rate of return to play with autograft use. Similarly, Legnani et al. [19] compared autograft to allograft hamstring tendon graft choice and showed a quicker time to return to play in the autograft group, but no significant difference in the overall rate of return to play. Glogovac et al. [11] noted in their systematic review that the four studies with the highest rate of return to play at preinjury levels (67–69%) used autograft, whereas the two studies with the lowest rates of return (17–40%)

used allograft. They concluded that autograft use may be associated with superior return to play metrics after revision ACLR.

Outcomes: Graft Choice

As with primary ACLR, the choice of graft for revision surgery can play a major role in patient outcomes. However, in contrast to primary reconstruction, autograft options may be limited depending on what grafts were previously harvested. In addition, the presence of tunnel dilation may obviate the use of an autograft and instead necessitate the use of a larger graft, such as an Achilles allograft. Considerations such as these are important and unique to patients undergoing revision ACLR.

Grassi et al. [20] evaluated the literature on graft choice in the setting of revision ACLR and found that autografts performed significantly better than allografts with improved knee laxity and lower failure rates and reoperation rates. Furthermore, they found that irradiated allografts performed worse than non-irradiated ones. These findings mirror those seen after primary ACLR. Similarly, the MARS group evaluated the effect of graft choice on outcomes and found that the use of autograft reduced the risk of recurrence by three-fold as compared to allograft. Additionally, they showed that patients treated with a hamstring tendon autograft fared better in terms of recurrence than those who received a BPTB autograft, although this may be confounded by the significant differences in patient demographics between groups.

Despite an improved understanding of how to best perform revision ACLR and treat associated pathologies, there still exists a lack of comparative and high-level studies comparing graft options in this population. Furthermore, emerging graft options such as the distal quadriceps tendon have shown promise in the revision setting but have not been extensively studied in the literature [21]. Further research is required to better guide surgical decision-making with regard to graft selection during revision ACLR.

Outcomes: Staging

The decision to stage a revision ACLR is dependent on a number of factors, including previous tunnel placement and tunnel width. LaPrade et al. [22] compared the outcomes of 88 patients who underwent revision ACLR in either single stage or two stages. Their criteria for staging were a tunnel diameter greater than 14 mm or unavoidable malpositioned tunnels (Fig. 24.1). They found no significant differences in terms of the failure rate, patient-reported outcomes, or patient satisfaction scores between groups at a mean follow-up of 3 years. Specifically, 6.1% of patients who had a staged ACLR experienced a graft re-tear during that period, as opposed to 10.3% of those who were treated in a single stage. Given these findings and the fact that patients who undergo a two-staged procedure are subjected to two separate anesthetics and lengthy rehabilitation programs, most surgeons advocate performing revision ACLR in a single stage whenever possible.

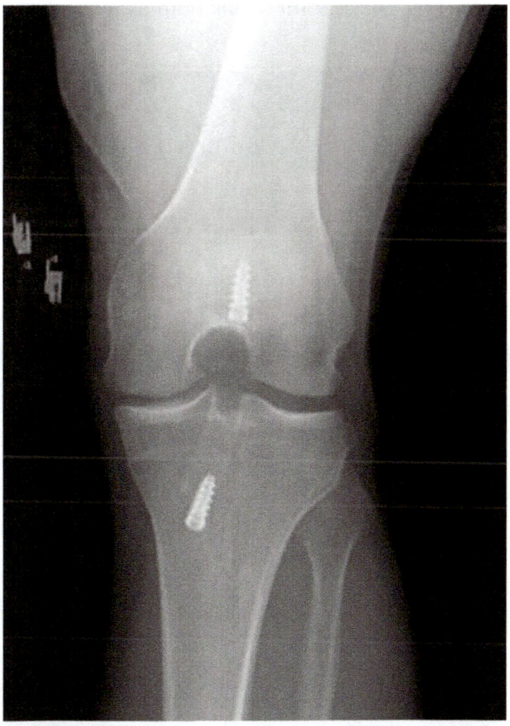

Fig. 24.1 Malpositioned tunnels

Outcomes: Concomitant Procedures

Lateral Extra-articular Augmentation

Extra-articular augmentation of the lateral side of the knee is an old concept that has been recently reintroduced as a means of reducing the recurrence rates after primary and revision ACLR. Different techniques for achieving this exist, with the two most commonly studied ones being the lateral extra-articular tenodesis (LET) or modified Lemaire procedure and the anterolateral ligament (ALL) reconstruction. Although the literature is still inconclusive as to which patients most benefit from the addition of either of these procedures to a revision ACLR, commonly reported indications include a high-grade preoperative pivot shift test, a desire to return to high-risk sports, and ligamentous laxity with associated knee recurvatum [23].

In a LET, a distally based strip of the central portion of the iliotibial band is harvested, passed deep to the lateral collateral ligament, and fixed just proximal and posterior to the lateral epicondyle (Fig. 24.2). It functions both as a checkrein to internal rotation of the tibia on the femur and in protecting the ACL. Given the relative low morbidity of performing this procedure, many surgeons are increasingly advocating for its use in the setting of revision ACLR to reduce the risk of recurrence in this high-risk population. Grassi et al. [24] performed a systematic review on this subject and identified 12 studies with 851 patients included. They found a failure rate of the combined procedure of only 3.6% at 5-year follow-up, which is significantly less than what has been reported in the literature for patients undergoing revision ACLR in isolation. Additionally, 74% of patients were able to return to play, but only 41% were able to do so at their previous level of participation. Furthermore, the complication rate was low (1.9%), and most were of the minor variety, such as hematoma. In a recent landmark clinical trial, Getgood et al. [23] evaluated the addition of a LET to primary ACLR using hamstring tendon autograft in a high-risk patient population and showed a significantly reduced re-rupture rate in the intervention group at 2 years after surgery (25% vs. 40%). However, such studies are lacking in the context of revision ACLR.

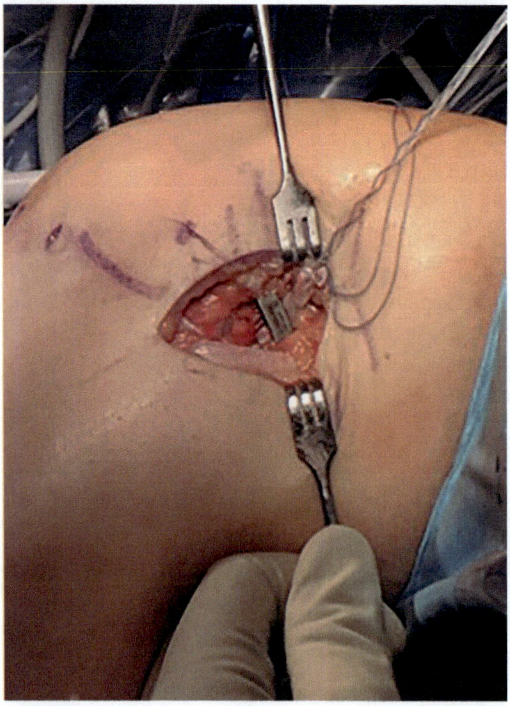

Fig. 24.2 Lateral extra-articular tenodesis

In contrast to LET, ALL reconstruction utilizes a free tendon graft to augment the lateral side of the knee and requires the creation of an additional tunnel on the tibia for distal fixation. Several authors have examined the effect of adding an ALL reconstruction in the setting of revision ACLR. Lee et al. [25] compared 45 patients who underwent combined revision ACL and ALL reconstruction to a control group of 42 patients who underwent revision ACLR alone. They found significantly reduced rotational laxity and higher rate of return to play in the intervention group at 38.2 months after surgery.

High Tibial Osteotomy

High tibial osteotomy (HTO) is indicated in the setting of revision ACLR for patients with coronal plane malalignment, excessive sagittal plane posterior tibial slope, or medial meniscal insufficiency.

Coronal plane alignment is one of the most important factors to consider in the context of revision ACL surgery. Anatomical alignment of the knee is defined as 5–7° of valgus, with the mechanical axis line of the lower extremity passing just medial to the lateral tibial spine [26]. Failure to address significant or asymmetric varus in the setting of ACLR has been shown to result in a higher incidence of graft re-rupture due to the supraphysiologic and non-anatomic stresses experienced by the graft [27]. This is commonly achieved through either a medial opening wedge (MOW) or lateral closing wedge (LCW) osteotomy of the proximal tibia (Fig. 24.3).

Excessive posterior tibial slope, defined as greater than 12° on a perfect lateral projection of the tibial plateau, has been shown to cause increased anterior tibial translation relative to the femur [27]. This, in turn, imparts excessive force on the ACL which, in the setting of revision, increases the re-rupture risk. Gupta et al. [28] performed a systematic review on combined revision ACLR and HTO, with 7 studies and 77 patients included. Overall, there were no failures reported with this approach, and 88% of patients demonstrated a negative pivot shift postoperatively. Furthermore, despite the higher incidence of arthrofibrosis known to occur with combined procedures in the knee, only one reoperation consisting of an arthroscopic lysis of adhesions for knee stiffness was reported in the included studies. Additionally, the authors found a paucity of data on the rate of return to play after combined ACLR and HTO, with only seven athletes' outcomes being reported and six having successfully returned to play.

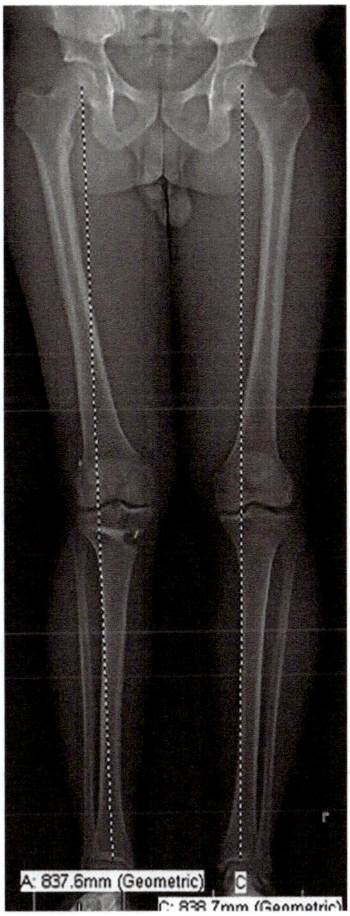

Fig. 24.3 Post-operative X-ray showing HTO alongside ACLR

The role of the posterior horn of the medial meniscus as a secondary stabilizer against internal rotation of the tibia relative to the femur has been well established [29]. In patients with combined ACL and medial meniscal insufficiency, failure to address the medial compartment has been shown to result in persistent posteromedial rotatory instability, which imparts excessive force on the reconstructed ACL and increases the risk of re-rupture [29]. Means of correcting this include performing a concomitant meniscal allograft transplantation (MAT) of the medial meniscus, which is discussed in detail below, and/or a valgus-producing HTO. A valgus-producing HTO reduces the effects of a deficient posterior horn of the medial meniscus by shifting the weight-bearing line away from the medial compartment. However, it is important to note that unless there is concomitant asymmetric varus malalignment present, the weight-bearing line should not be shifted as far as Fujisawa's point, as patients will perceive this drastic unilateral change in knee alignment.

Meniscal Allograft Transplantation

Meniscal allograft transplantation (MAT) is performed in the setting of revision ACLR in

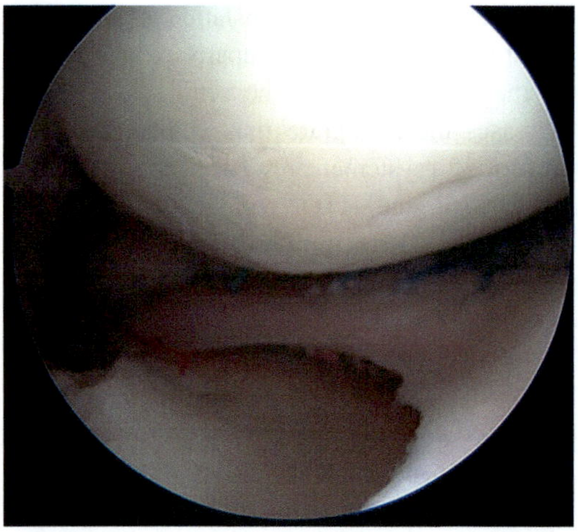

Fig. 24.4 Meniscal allograft transplantation

patients with symptomatic meniscal insufficiency (Fig. 24.4). Meniscal insufficiency can be a cause of pain and can contribute to rotational stability of the knee. There is a linear relationship between meniscus removed and the contact stresses in the knee joint, with total meniscectomy having been shown to increase peak contact stresses by 235% [30]. In those with meniscal insufficiency, they have been shown to result in poor long-term outcomes and increased risk of osteoarthritis [31]. Thus, meniscal allograft transplantation (MAT) can be utilized in those with meniscal insufficiency to restore normal tibiofemoral contact pressures [32].

Zaffagani et al. [33] evaluated 18 patients undergoing combined revision ACLR and MAT, at a mean of 4 years follow-up. They found a significant reduction in pain and improvement in functional outcome scores, with a high patient satisfaction rate, with better outcomes in those with medial MAT than lateral. Overall, 13 patients were able to return to play, and only 1 of the 5 that were unable to return was unable to do so as a result of residual symptoms. Additionally, four patients required further surgery: two for meniscal graft failure, one of which was treated with a HTO, and two for persistent pain.

Outcomes: Re-revision ACLR

There is limited literature reporting on the outcomes of re-revision ACLR. Liechti et al. [34] performed a systematic review in 2016 on the subject and identified only 6 studies with 214 patients included. Overall, they found that while the majority of patients had successful outcomes after re-revision ACLR, the patient-reported outcomes were inferior compared to primary ACLR. Specifically, the re-rupture rate after re-revision ACLR was shown to equal 15%, but the numbers were too low to identify independent risk factors for failure. However, based on the evidence gathered from revision ACL literature, anatomical factors such as notch morphology and tibial slope may play a role in recurrent ACL tears if these are not appropriately addressed at the time of surgery.

In a retrospective cohort study, Chen et al. [7] compared patients undergoing revision and re-revision ACLR and found significant differences in terms of the mechanism of injury inducing the re-tears. In the first-time revision reconstruction group, the most common mechanism of re-tear was a traumatic incident. Conversely, in the re-revision group, the most common mechanism was an atraumatic re-tear. They also showed that those undergoing re-revisions also required a higher rate of staging procedures to address excessive tunnel dilation. This may be due to the fact that patients with multiply-revised ACL tears are likely to have associated pathologies and/or anatomical risk factors that were unaddressed at the time of previous surgery that place them at high risk of re-rupture with normal activities of daily living. Overall, they found those undergoing re-revision ACLR had lower activity levels at final follow-up. Wegryzn et al. [35] found significantly higher rates of severe articular degeneration and meniscal after re-revision ACLR. They found that these factors strongly correlated with negative outcomes and may explain the worse outcomes with re-revision ACL.

Conclusion

Revision anterior cruciate ligament reconstruction is one of the most challenging entities to treat for the practicing sports medicine surgeon. While advancements in terms of graft choice, surgical technique and implants, and rehabilitation have resulted in improved outcomes in this population, re-rupture rates remain elevated as compared to primary reconstruction. A heightened level of suspicion about the presence of associated pathologies and anatomical abnormalities is important when treating these patients, as is setting appropriate patient expectations prior to surgery. Further research into this field will help refine indications and improve outcomes after revision anterior cruciate ligament reconstruction.

References

1. Sanders TL, Maradit Kremers H, Bryan AJ, Larson DR, Dahm DL, Levy BA, et al. Incidence of anterior cruciate ligament tears and reconstruction: a 21-year population-based study. Am J Sports Med. 2016;44(6):1502–7.
2. Gifstad T, Foss OA, Engebretsen L, Lind M, Forssblad M, Albrektsen G, et al. Lower risk of revision with patellar tendon autografts compared with hamstring autografts: a registry study based on 45,998 primary ACL reconstructions in Scandinavia. Am J Sports Med. 2014;42(10):2319–28.
3. Group M, Wright RW, Huston LJ, Spindler KP, Dunn WR, Haas AK, et al. Descriptive epidemiology of the Multicenter ACL Revision Study (MARS) cohort. Am J Sports Med. 2010;38(10):1979–86.
4. Grassi A, Ardern CL, Marcheggiani Muccioli GM, Neri MP, Marcacci M, Zaffagnini S. Does revision ACL reconstruction measure up to primary surgery? A meta-analysis comparing patient-reported and clinician-reported outcomes, and radiographic results. Br J Sports Med. 2016;50(12):716–24.
5. Borchers JR, Kaeding CC, Pedroza AD, Huston LJ, Spindler KP, Wright RW, et al. Intra-articular findings in primary and revision anterior cruciate ligament reconstruction surgery: a comparison of the MOON and MARS study groups. Am J Sports Med. 2011;39(9):1889–93.
6. Brophy RH, Wright RW, David TS, McCormack RG, Sekiya JK, Svoboda SJ, et al. Association between previous meniscal surgery and the incidence of chondral lesions at revision anterior cruciate ligament reconstruction. Am J Sports Med. 2012;40(4):808–14.
7. Chen JL, Allen CR, Stephens TE, Haas AK, Huston LJ, Wright RW, et al. Differences in mechanisms of failure, intraoperative findings, and surgical characteristics between single- and multiple-revision ACL reconstructions: a MARS cohort study. Am J Sports Med. 2013;41(7):1571–8.
8. Grassi A, Kim C, Marcheggiani Muccioli GM, Zaffagnini S, Amendola A. What is the mid-term failure rate of revision ACL reconstruction? A systematic review. Clin Orthop Relat Res. 2017;475(10):2484–99.
9. Wright RW, Gill CS, Chen L, Brophy RH, Matava MJ, Smith MV, et al. Outcome of revision anterior cruciate ligament reconstruction: a systematic review. J Bone Joint Surg Am. 2012;94(6):531–6.
10. Group M, Wright RW, Huston LJ, Haas AK, Allen CR, Anderson AF, et al. Predictors of patient-reported outcomes at 2 years after revision anterior cruciate ligament reconstruction. Am J Sports Med. 2019;47(10):2394–401.
11. Glogovac G, Schumaier AP, Grawe BM. Return to sport following revision anterior cruciate ligament reconstruction in athletes: a systematic review. Arthroscopy. 2019;35(7):2222–30.
12. Grassi A, Zaffagnini S, Marcheggiani Muccioli GM, Neri MP, Della Villa S, Marcacci M. After revision anterior cruciate ligament reconstruction, who returns to sport? A systematic review and meta-analysis. Br J Sports Med. 2015;49(20):1295–304.
13. Baez SE, Hoch MC, Hoch JM. Psychological factors are associated with return to pre-injury levels of sport and physical activity after ACL reconstruction. Knee Surg Sports Traumatol Arthrosc. 2020;28(2):495–501.
14. Anand BS, Feller JA, Richmond AK, Webster KE. Return-to-sport outcomes after revision anterior cruciate ligament reconstruction surgery. Am J Sports Med. 2016;44(3):580–4.
15. Webster KE, Feller JA, Kimp AJ, Whitehead TS. Revision anterior cruciate ligament reconstruction outcomes in younger patients: medial meniscal pathology and high rates of return to sport are associated with third ACL injuries. Am J Sports Med. 2018;46(5):1137–42.
16. Christino MA, Tepolt FA, Sugimoto D, Micheli LJ, Kocher MS. Revision ACL reconstruction in children and adolescents. J Pediatr Orthop. 2020;40(3):129–34.
17. McPherson AL, Feller JA, Hewett TE, Webster KE. Smaller change in psychological readiness to return to sport is associated with second anterior cruciate ligament injury among younger patients. Am J Sports Med. 2019;47(5):1209–15.
18. Keizer MNJ, Hoogeslag RAG, van Raay J, Otten E, Brouwer RW. Superior return to sports rate after patellar tendon autograft over patellar tendon allograft in revision anterior cruciate ligament reconstruction. Knee Surg Sports Traumatol Arthrosc. 2018;26(2):574–81.
19. Legnani C, Zini S, Borgo E, Ventura A. Can graft choice affect return to sport following revision anterior cruciate ligament reconstruction surgery? Arch Orthop Trauma Surg. 2016;136(4):527–31.

20. Grassi A, Nitri M, Moulton SG, Marcheggiani Muccioli GM, Bondi A, Romagnoli M, et al. Does the type of graft affect the outcome of revision anterior cruciate ligament reconstruction? A meta-analysis of 32 studies. Bone Joint J. 2017;99-B(6):714–23.
21. Haner M, Bierke S, Petersen W. Anterior cruciate ligament revision surgery: ipsilateral quadriceps versus contralateral semitendinosus-gracilis autografts. Arthroscopy. 2016;32(11):2308–17.
22. Mitchell JJ, Chahla J, Dean CS, Cinque M, Matheny LM, LaPrade RF. Outcomes after 1-stage versus 2-stage revision anterior cruciate ligament reconstruction. Am J Sports Med. 2017;45(8):1790–8.
23. Getgood AMJ, Bryant DM, Litchfield R, Heard M, McCormack RG, Rezansoff A, et al. Lateral extra-articular tenodesis reduces failure of hamstring tendon autograft anterior cruciate ligament reconstruction: 2-year outcomes from the STABILITY study randomized clinical trial. Am J Sports Med. 2020;48(2):285–97.
24. Grassi A, Zicaro JP, Costa-Paz M, Samuelsson K, Wilson A, Zaffagnini S, et al. Good mid-term outcomes and low rates of residual rotatory laxity, complications and failures after revision anterior cruciate ligament reconstruction (ACL) and lateral extra-articular tenodesis (LET). Knee Surg Sports Traumatol Arthrosc. 2020;28(2):418–31.
25. Lee DW, Kim JG, Cho SI, Kim DH. Clinical outcomes of isolated revision anterior cruciate ligament reconstruction or in combination with anatomic anterolateral ligament reconstruction. Am J Sports Med. 2019;47(2):324–33.
26. Luo CF. Reference axes for reconstruction of the knee. Knee. 2004;11(4):251–7.
27. Dejour D, Saffarini M, Demey G, Baverel L. Tibial slope correction combined with second revision ACL produces good knee stability and prevents graft rupture. Knee Surg Sports Traumatol Arthrosc. 2015;23(10):2846–52.
28. Gupta A, Tejpal T, Shanmugaraj A, Horner NS, Simunovic N, Duong A, et al. Surgical techniques, outcomes, indications, and complications of simultaneous high tibial osteotomy and anterior cruciate ligament revision surgery: a systematic review. HSS J. 2019;15(2):176–84.
29. Gupta R, Kapoor A, Mittal N, Soni A, Khatri S, Masih GD. The role of meniscal tears and meniscectomy in the mechanical stability of the anterior cruciate ligament deficient knee. Knee. 2018;25(6):1051–6.
30. Baratz ME, Fu FH, Mengato R. Meniscal tears: the effect of meniscectomy and of repair on intraarticular contact areas and stress in the human knee. A preliminary report. Am J Sports Med. 1986;14(4):270–5.
31. Ode GE, Van Thiel GS, McArthur SA, Dishkin-Paset J, Leurgans SE, Shewman EF, et al. Effects of serial sectioning and repair of radial tears in the lateral meniscus. Am J Sports Med. 2012;40(8):1863–70.
32. Verma NN, Kolb E, Cole BJ, Berkson MB, Garretson R, Farr J, et al. The effects of medial meniscal transplantation techniques on intra-articular contact pressures. J Knee Surg. 2008;21(1):20–6.
33. Zaffagnini S, Grassi A, Romandini I, Marcacci M, Filardo G. Meniscal allograft transplantation combined with anterior cruciate ligament reconstruction provides good mid-term clinical outcome. Knee Surg Sports Traumatol Arthrosc. 2019;27(6):1914–23.
34. Liechti DJ, Chahla J, Dean CS, Mitchell JJ, Slette E, Menge TJ, et al. Outcomes and risk factors of rerevision anterior cruciate ligament reconstruction: a systematic review. Arthroscopy. 2016;32(10):2151–9.
35. Wegrzyn J, Chouteau J, Philippot R, Fessy MH, Moyen B. Repeat revision of anterior cruciate ligament reconstruction: a retrospective review of management and outcome of 10 patients with an average 3-year follow-up. Am J Sports Med. 2009;37(4):776–85.

Index

M. J. Alaia, K. J. Jones (eds.), *Revision Anterior Cruciate Ligament Reconstruction*,
https://doi.org/10.1007/978-3-030-96996-7

V

W

GPSR Compliance

The European Union's (EU) General Product Safety Regulation (GPSR) is a set of rules that requires consumer products to be safe and our obligations to ensure this.

If you have any concerns about our products, you can contact us on ProductSafety@springernature.com

In case Publisher is established outside the EU, the EU authorized representative is:

Springer Nature Customer Service Center GmbH
Europaplatz 3
69115 Heidelberg, Germany

Batch number: 10732807

Printed by Printforce, the Netherlands